Classics in Mathematics

Roger C. Lyndon • Paul E. Schupp

Combinatorial Group Theory

Springer
Berlin
Heidelberg
New York
Barcelona
Hong Kong
London
Milan
Paris
Singapore
Tokyo

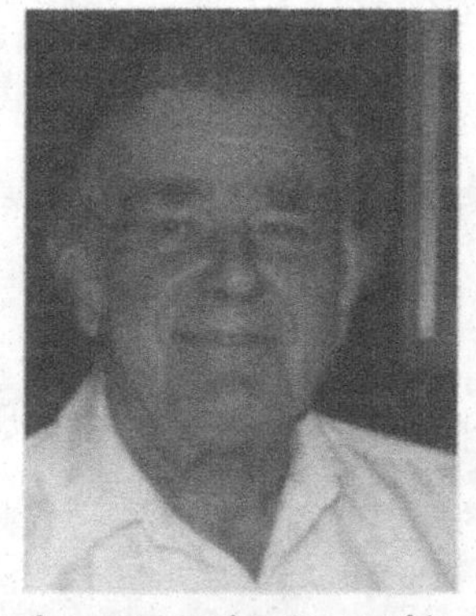

Roger Lyndon, born on Dec. 18, 1917 in Calais (Maine, USA), entered Harvard University in 1935 with the aim of studying literature and becoming a writer. However, when he discovered that, for him, mathematics required less effort than literature, he switched and graduated from Harvard in 1939. After completing his Master's Degree in 1941, he taught at Georgia Tech, then returned to Harvard in 1942 and there taught navigation to pilots while, supervised by S. MacLane, he studied for his Ph.D., awarded in 1946 for a thesis entitled *The Cohomology Theory of Group Extensions*.
Influenced by Tarski, Lyndon was later to work on model theory. Accepting a position at Princeton, Ralph Fox and Reidemeister's visit in 1948 were major influencea on him to work in combinatorial group theory. In 1953 Lyndon left Princeton for a chair at the University of Michigan where he then remained except for visiting professorships at Berkeley, London, Montpellier and Amiens.
Lyndon made numerous major contributions to combinatorial group theory. These included the development of "small cancellation theory", his introduction of "aspherical" presentations of groups and his work on length functions. He died on June 8, 1988.

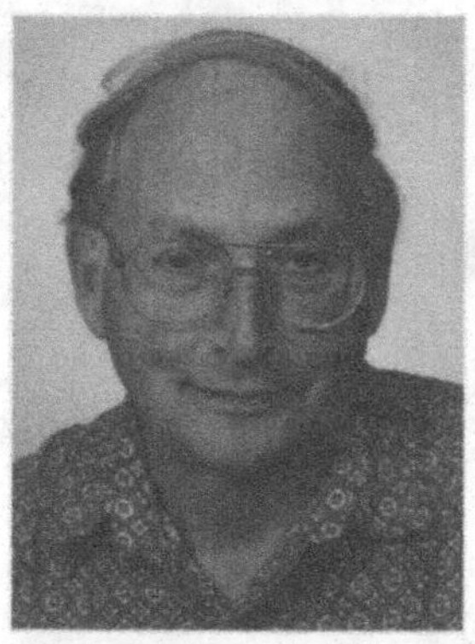

Paul Schupp, born on March 12, 1937 in Cleveland, Ohio was a student of Roger Lyndon's at the University of Michigan where he wrote a thesis of "Dehn's Algorithm and the Conjugacy Problem". After a year at the University of Wisconsin he moved to the University of Illinois where he remained. For several years he was also concurrently Visiting Professor at the University Paris VII and a member of the Laboratoire d'Informatique Théorique et Programmation (founded by M. P. Schutzenberger).
Schupp further developed the use of cancellation diagrams in combinatorial group theory, introducing conjugacy diagrams, diagrams on compact surfaces, diagrams over free products with amalgamation and HNN extensions and applications to Artin groups. He then worked with David Muller on connections between group theory and formal language theory and on the theory of finite automata on infinite inputs. His current interest is using geometric methods to investigate the computational complexity of algorithms in combinatorial group theory.

Roger C. Lyndon • Paul E. Schupp

Combinatorial Group Theory

Reprint of the 1977 Edition

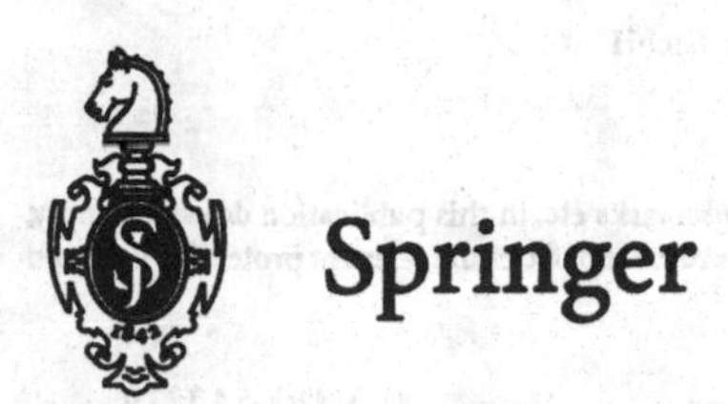

Roger C. Lyndon †

Paul E. Schupp
University of Illinois
Department of Mathematics
273 Altgeld Hall
1409 West Green Street
Urbana, IL 61801-2917
USA

Originally published as Vol. 89 of the
Ergebnisse der Mathematik und ihrer Grenzgebiete

Cataloging-in-Publication Data applied for

Die Deutsche Bibliothek - CIP-Einheitsaufnahme

Lyndon, Roger C.:
Combinatorial group theory / Roger C. Lyndon; Paul E. Schupp. - Reprint of the 1977 ed. - Berlin; Heidelberg; New York; New York; Barcelona; Hong Kong; London; Milan; Paris; Singapore; Tokyo: Springer, 2001
ISBN 3-540-41158-5

Mathematics Subject Classification (2000): 20Exx, 20Fxx, 57Mxx, 68Qxx

ISSN 1431-0821
ISBN 3-540-41158-5 Springer-Verlag Berlin Heidelberg New York

Springer-Verlag Berlin Heidelberg New York
a member of BertelsmannSpringer Science+Business Media GmbH

Printed in Germany

Printed on acid-free paper SPIN 10734588 41/3142ck-5 4 3 2 1 0

Roger C. Lyndon   Paul E. Schupp

Combinatorial Group Theory

With 18 Figures

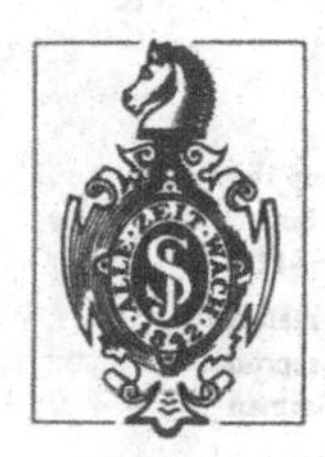

Springer-Verlag
Berlin Heidelberg New York 1977

Roger C. Lyndon
University of Michigan, Dept. of Mathematics,
Ann Arbor, MI 48104/U.S.A.

Paul E. Schupp
University of Illinois, Dept. of Mathematics,
Urbana, IL 61801/U.S.A.

AMS Subject Classification (1970)
Primary: 20Exx, 20E25, 20E30, 20E35, 20E40, 20Fxx, 20F05, 20F10, 20F15, 20F25, 20F55, 20H10, 20H15, 20J05
Secondary: 57A05, 55A05, 02F47, 02H15

ISBN 3-540-07642-5 Springer-Verlag Berlin Heidelberg New York
ISBN 0-387-07642-5 Springer-Verlag New York Heidelberg Berlin

Library of Congress Cataloging in Publication Data. Lyndon, Roger C. Combinatorial group theory. (Ergebnisse der Mathematik und ihrer Grenzgebiete; bd. 89). 1. Groups, Theory of. 2. Combinatorial analysis. I. Schupp, Paul E., 1937-. joint author. II. Title. III. Series. QA171.L94. 512'.22. 76-12537.

Printed in Germany.

Typesetting in Japan. Printing and bookbindung: Konrad Triltsch, Würzburg.
2141/3140-543210

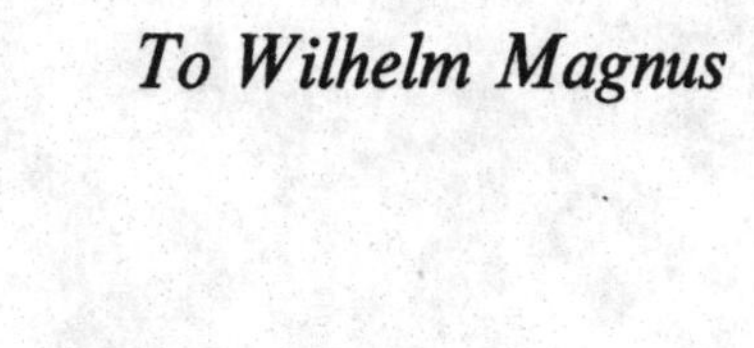

To Wilhelm Magnus

Preface

The first formal development of group theory, centering around the ideas of Galois, was limited almost entirely to finite groups. The idea of an abstract infinite group is clearly embodied in the work of Cayley on the axioms for a group, but was not immediately pursued to any depth. There developed later a school of group theory, in which Schmidt was prominent, that was concerned in part with developing for infinite groups results parallel to those known for finite groups. Another strong influence on the development of group theory was the recognition, notably by Klein, of the role of groups, many of them infinite, in geometry, as well as the development of continuous groups initiated by Lie. A major stimulus to the study of infinite discontinuous groups was the development of topology: we mention particularly the work of Poincaré, Dehn, and Nielsen. This last influence is especially important in the present context since it led naturally to the study of groups presented by generators and relations.

Recent years have seen a steady increase of interest in infinite discontinuous groups, both in the systematic development of the abstract theory and in applications to other areas. The connections with topology have continued to grow. Since Novikov and Boone exhibited groups with unsolvable word problem, results in logic and decision problems have had a great influence on the subject of infinite groups, and through this connection on topology.

Important contributions to the development of the ideas initiated by Dehn were made by Magnus, who has in turn been one of the strongest influences on contemporary research. The book *Combinatorial Group Theory*, by Magnus, Karrass, and Solitar, which appeared in 1966 and immediately became the classic in its field, was dedicated to Dehn. It is our admiration for that work which has prompted us to give this book the same title. We hope that our intention has been realized of taking a further step towards a systematic and comprehensive exposition and survey of the subject.

We view the area of combinatorial group theory as adequately delineated by the book of Magnus, Karrass, and Solitar. It is not necessary for us to list here the topics we discuss, which can be seen from the table of contents. However, we would like to note that there are two broad methods running through our treatment. The first is the 'linear' cancellation method of Nielsen, which plays an important role in Chapters I and IV; this is concerned with the formal expression of an element of a group in terms of a given set of generators for the group. The second is the more geometric method, initiated by Poincaré and Dehn, which includes many of the more recent developments in 'small cancellation theory'; this method, which plays a role in Chapters II, III, and especially V, concerns the formal expression of an element of a normal subgroup N of a group G in terms of conjugates of a given set of elements whose normal closure in G is N.

We have put considerable emphasis on connections with topology, on arguments of a primitive geometric nature, and on connections with logic. In our presentation we have tried to combine a fairly self-contained exposition at a modest level with a reasonably adequate source of reference on the topics discussed. This, together with the fact that the individual chapters were written separately by the two authors, although in close collaboration, has led to considerable variation of style, which we have nonetheless sought to adapt to the subject matter.

While we do not feel it necessary to defend our inclusions, we do feel some need to justify our omissions. There are, of course, many important branches of group theory, for example, most of the theory of finite groups, that no one would claim as part of combinatorial group theory. A borderline area, with which we have made no attempt to deal here, is that of infinite groups subject to some kind of finiteness condition. Beyond these there remain a number of important topics that we believe do belong to combinatorial group theory, but which we have mentioned only briefly if at all, on the grounds that we could not hope to improve on existing excellent treatments of these topics. We list some of these topics.

1. *Commutator calculus and Lie theory*. An excellent treatment is given in Chapter 5 of the book of Magnus, Karrass, Solitar (1966). The 'Alberta notes' of Philip Hall have been republished in 1970.

2. *Varieties of groups*. The definitive work here is the book of H. Neumann (1967).

3. *Linear groups*. Treatments germaine to our topic are given by Dixon (1973) and by Wehrfritz (1973).

4. *Groups acting on trees*. This powerful method of Bass and Serre is central to our topic. An account of this theory is contained in the widely circulated notes of Serre (1968/1969), which are intended to appear in the Springer Lecture Notes series.

5. *Ends of groups*. The development of this subject by Stallings (1968, 1968, 1970, 1971) and Swan (1969) is also central to our subject; a lucid and comprehensive account, from a somewhat different point of view, is given in the book of Cohen (1972).

6. *Cohomology theory*. Of a number of excellent sources, the book of Gruenberg (1970) seems nearest to the spirit of our discussion.

We wish also to draw attention to a few other books that are especially relevant to our topic. For a history of group theory up to the early part of this century we refer to Wussing (1960). The book of Kurosh, in its various editions and translations, remains, along with the book of Magnus, Karrass, and Solitar, the classic source for information on infinite groups. The book of Coxeter and Moser (1965) contains, among other things, presentations for a large number of groups, mainly of geometric origin. We have borrowed much from the book of Zieschang, Vogt, and Coldewey (1970). On the subject of Fuchsian groups from a combinatorial point of view we recommend, in addition to the work just cited, the Dundee notes of Macbeath (1961) and the book of Magnus (1974). For an elementary exposition of the basic connections between topology and group theory we refer to Massey (1967). For a thorough discussion of decision problems in group theory we refer to Miller (1971).

Acknowledgements

The suggestion that such a book as this be written was made in a letter from Springer Editor Peter Hilton, written from Montpellier. It is fitting that the completed manuscript should now be submitted from Montpellier.

The first author (R.C.L.) presented the first draft of some of this work in a seminar at Morehouse College, Atlanta University, in the Fall of 1969. Later versions were developed and presented in lectures at the University of Michigan and during a short visit at Queen Mary College, University of London. Much of the work was done at the Université des Sciences et Techniques du Languedoc, Montpellier, in the year 1972/73 and in the present year, and, for a shorter period, at the University of Birmingham. He is grateful for the hospitality of these universities, and also the Ruhr-Universität Bochum. He gratefully acknowledges support of the National Science Foundation (U.S.A.) and the Science Research Council (U.K.).

The second author (P.E.S.) is grateful to the University of Illinois for an appointment to the Center for Advanced Study, University of Illinois, during the academic year 1973/74. He is also grateful for the hospitality of Queen Mary College, London, and to the University of Manitoba for various periods during the preparation of this book.

We are both greatly indebted to colleagues and students, both at the universities named above and elsewhere, for discussion and criticism. For help with the manuscript we are grateful to Mme. Barrière and to Mrs. Maund. For great help and patience with editorial matters we are grateful to Dr. Alice Peters and to Roberto Minio of Springer-Verlag.

Postscript, February 1977. We have taken advantage of the time before going to press to bring the manuscript more up to date by adding a few new passages in the text and by substantial additions to the bibliography.

R.C.L., Montpellier 1974

P.E.S., Urbana 1974

Table of Contents

Notation

We have tried to use only standard notation, and list below only a few usages that might offer difficulty.

Set theory

$\varnothing$ is the empty set.
$X - Y$ is set difference, where Y is contained in X.
$X + Y$ is union, where X and Y are disjoint.
$\{x_1, \ldots, x_n\}$ is the unordered n-tuple, $(x_1, \ldots, x_n)$ the ordered n-tuple; when there is no ambiguity we write $x_1, \ldots, x_n$ for either.
$X \subset Y$ or $X \subseteq Y$ denotes inclusion, proper or not; $X \subsetneq Y$ denotes strict inclusion.
$|X|$ denotes the cardinal of the set X (except in special contexts).

General

$\mathbb{N}$, $\mathbb{Z}$, $\mathbb{Q}$, $\mathbb{R}$, $\mathbb{C}$ denote the (non negative) natural numbers, the integers, the rationals, the reals, the complex numbers.
$\mathbb{GL}(n, K)$, $\mathbb{SL}(n, K)$, $\mathbb{PL}(n, K)$, $\mathbb{PSL}(n, K)$ denote the general, special, projective, and projective special linear group of degree n over the ring K.

Group theory

1 denotes the trivial group, $\mathbb{Z}$(or C) the infinite cyclic group, $\mathbb{Z}_n$(or C_n) the cyclic group of order n.
$\langle U \rangle$ or $Gp(U)$ denotes the subgroup of G generated by the subset U, and according to context, the free group with basis U.
$\langle X; R \rangle$, $(X; R)$, $\langle x_1, \ldots, x_n; r_1, \ldots, r_n \rangle$, as well as several other variants, denote the presentation with generaters $x \in X$ and relators $r \in R$, or the group so presented.
$H < G$ or $H \leq G$ means that H is a subgroup of G.
$H \lhd G$ means that H is a normal subgroup of G.
$|G|$ is the order of G (finite or infinite), except in special contexts.
$|G\colon H|$ is the index of H in G.

$|w|$, for w an element of a free group with basis X, is the length of w as a reduced word relative to the basis X.
$[h, k] = h^{-1}k^{-1}hk$ (occasionally, where indicated, $hkh^{-1}k^{-1}$).
$[H, K]$ is the subgroup generated by all $[h, k]$ for $h \in H$, $k \in K$.
$C_G(H)$, $N_G(U)$ are the centralizer and normalizer in G of the subset U.
G_p or $\text{Stab}_G(p)$ is the stabilizer of p under action of G.
Aut G is the automorphism group of G.
$G \times H$ is the direct product.
$G * H$, $*\{G_i: i \in I\}$, or $*G_i$ denotes the free product.
$G \underset{A}{*} H$ denotes the free product of G and H with $A = G \cap H$ amalgamated; $\langle G, H; A = B, \phi \rangle$ denotes the free product of (disjoint) groups G and H with their subgroup A and B amalgamated according to the isomorphism $\phi: A \to B$.
$\langle G, t; t^{-1}at = \phi(a), a \in A \rangle$ denotes the indicated HNN extension of G.
Transformations that occur as elements of groups will ordinarily be written on the right: $x \mapsto xT$; other functions will occasionally be written on the left, e.g., $\chi(G)$ for the characteristic function of a group G.

Note on Format

The notation (I.2.3) refers to Proposition 2.3 of Chapter I (to be found in section 2). Similarly, (I.2) refers to that section, and (I) to Chapter I.

A date accompanying a name, e.g., Smith, 1970, refers to a paper or book listed in the bibliography.

A proof begins and ends with the mark □. This mark immediately following the statement of a proposition means that no (further) proof will be given.

Chapter I. Free Groups and Their Subgroups

1. Introduction

Informally, a group is free on a set of generators if no relation holds among these generators except the trivial relations that hold among any set of elements in any group. We make this precise as follows.

Definition. Let X be a subset of a group F. Then F is a *free group with basis X* provided the following holds: if ϕ is any function from the set X into a group H, then there exists a unique extension of ϕ to a homomorphism ϕ^* from F into H.

We remark that the requirement that the extension be unique is equivalent to requiring that X generate F.

Proposition 1.1. *Let F_1 and F_2 be free groups with bases X_1 and X_2. Then F_1 and F_2 are isomorphic if and only if X_1 and X_2 have the same cardinal.*

□ Suppose that f_1 is a one-to-one correspondence mapping X_1 onto X_2, and let $f_2 = f_1^{-1}$. The maps f_1 and f_2 determine maps $\phi_1: X_1 \to F_2$ and $\phi_2: X_2 \to F_1$. These have extensions to homomorphisms $\phi_1^*: F_1 \to F_2$ and $\phi_2^*: F_2 \to F_1$. Now $\phi_1^*\phi_2^*: F_1 \to F_1$ acts as the identity $f_1 f_2 = i_{X_1}$ on X_1, and hence is an extension of the inclusion map $X_1 \to F_1$. Since the identity $i_{F_1}: F_1 \to F_1$ also extends this inclusion map, by uniqueness we have $\phi_1^*\phi_2^* = i_{F_1}$. Similarly; $\phi_2^*\phi_1^* = i_{F_2}$. It follows that ϕ_1^* is an isomorphism from F_1 onto F_2.

It remains to show that F determines $|X|$. The subgroup N of F generated by all squares of elements in F is normal, and F/N is an elementary abelian 2-group of rank $|X|$. (If X is finite, $|F/N| = 2^{|X|}$, finite; if $|X|$ is infinite, $|F/N| = |X|$). □

Corollary 1.2. *All bases for a given free group F have the same cardinal, the rank of F.* □

We remark that a free group of rank 0 is trivial.

Proposition 1.3. *If a group is generated by a set of n of its elements (n finite or infinite), then it is a quotient group of a free group of rank n.*

□ We assume now the existence of a free group with an arbitrary given set as basis; this will be proved below (1.7). Let G be generated by the set $S \subseteq G$, $|S| = n$, let f be a one-to-one correspondence from a set X onto S, and let F be free with X as basis. Then f determines a map $\phi: X \to G$, which extends to a homomorphism ϕ^*: $F \to G$. Since the image S of X generates G, ϕ^* maps F onto G. □

The class of free groups can be characterized without reference to bases. This results from the circumstance that, in the category of groups, projective objects are free.

Definition. A group P is *projective* provided the following holds: if G and H are any groups and if γ is a map from G onto H and π a map from P into H, then there exists a map ϕ from P into G such that $\phi\gamma = \pi$.

Definition. A map ρ from a group G onto a subgroup S is a *retraction*, and S is a *retract* of G, provided thet $\rho^2 = \rho$, or, equivalently, that the restriction of ρ to S is the identity on S.

Proposition 1.4. *The projective groups are precisely the retracts of free groups.*

□ Let P be projective. In the definition, take $H = P$ with $\pi = i_P$, the identity on P, and, by (1.3), let G be free with γ from G onto P. By the definition of projectivity, there exists $\phi: P \to G$ with $\phi\gamma = i_P$. Let $R = P\phi \leqslant G$, and let $\rho = \gamma\phi$. Then $G\rho = G\gamma\phi = P\phi = R$, and $\rho^2 = \gamma\phi\gamma\phi = \gamma i_P \phi = \gamma\phi = \rho$. Thus ρ is a retraction and R is a retract of G. Since $P\phi = R$ and $\phi\gamma = i_P$, it follows that ϕ is an isomorphism from P onto R. Since R is a retract of a free group, so is P. □

We remark that although the subgroup of a free group generated by part of a basis is obviously a retract, not every retract of a free group is of this sort; for a counterexample see Magnus, Karrass, and Solitar, p. 140.

For the following we assume, (2.11) below, that every subgroup of a free group is free.

Corollary 1.5. *The projective groups are precisely the free groups.* □

We turn now to the existence of free groups. This follows from principles of universal algebra (see Cohn 1965), but we prefer an explicit construction. Let a set X be given; in anticipation we call the elements of X *generators*. Let Y be a set disjoint from X with a one-to-one correspondence $\eta: X \to Y$. If $x \in X$ and $x\eta = y$ we write also $y\eta = x$ (thus η becomes an involution on the set $X \cup Y$). We write $y = x^{-1}$ and $x = y^{-1}$, and we call x and y *inverse* to each other. We write $Y = X^{-1}$ and $X^{\pm 1} = X \cup X^{-1}$. The elements of $X^{\pm 1}$ are *letters*.

A *word* is a finite sequence of letters, $w = (a_1, \ldots, a_n)$, $n \geqslant 0$, all $a_i \in X^{\pm 1}$. If $n = 0$, then $w = 1$, the *empty word*. The set $W = W(X)$ of all words is a semigroup under juxtaposition (in fact, it is the free (unital) semigroup with basis $X^{\pm 1}$). With harmless ambiguity we write a_i for the one-letter word (a_i); this permits us to write $w = a_1 \ldots a_n$, a product of one-letter words. We extend the involution η to W by defining $w\eta = w^{-1} = a_n^{-1} \ldots a_1^{-1}$. Then η is an involutory antiautomorphism: $(uv)^{-1} = v^{-1}u^{-1}$, $1^{-1} = 1$.

We define the *length* $|w|$ of $w = a_1 \ldots a_n$ to be $|w| = n$. Clearly $|uv| = |u| + |v|$, $|1| = 0$.

An *elementary transformation* of a word w consists of inserting or deleting a part of the form aa^{-1}, $a \in X^{\pm 1}$. Two words w_1 and w_2 are equivalent, $w_1 \sim w_2$, if there is a chain of elementary transformations leading from w_1 to w_2. This is obviously an equivalence relation on the set W; moreover, it preserves the structure of W as unital semigroup with involutory antiautomorphism: $u_1 \sim u_2$ and $v_1 \sim v_2$ implies that $u_1v_1 \sim u_2v_2$, and $u_1 \sim u_2$ implies that $u_1^{-1} \sim u_2^{-1}$. Thus we may pass to the quotient semigroup $F = W/\sim$, which is evidently a group. We shall see that it is a free group with basis the images of the $x \in X$.

A word w is *reduced* if it contains no part aa^{-1}, $a \in X^{\pm 1}$. Let W_0 be the set of reduced words. We shall show that each equivalence class of words contains exactly one reduced word. It is clear that each equivalence class contains a reduced word, since successive deletion of parts aa^{-1} from any word w must lead to a reduced word. It will suffice then to show that distinct reduced words u and v are not equivalent. We suppose then that $u = w_1, w_2, \ldots, w_n = v$ is a chain from u to v, with each w_{i+1} an elementary transform of w_i $(1 \leqslant i < n)$, and, indeed, with $N = \sum |w_i|$ a minimum. Since $u \neq v$ and u and v are reduced, we have $n > 1$, $|w_2| > |w_1|$, and $|w_{n-1}| > |w_n|$. It follows that for some $i (1 < i < n)$, $|w_i| > |w_{i-1}|, |w_{i+1}|$. Now w_{i-1} is obtained from w_i by deletion of a part aa^{-1} and w_{i+1} by deletion of a part bb^{-1}. If these two parts coincide, then $w_{i-1} = w_{i+1}$, contrary to the minimality of N. If these two parts overlap without coinciding, then w_i has a part $aa^{-1}a$, and w_{i-1} and w_{i+1} are both obtained by replacing this part by a, hence again $w_{i-1} = w_{i+1}$. In the remaining case, where the two parts are disjoint, we may replace w_i by the result w' of deleting both parts to obtain a new chain with $N' = N - 4$, contrary to the minimality of N.

There is an alternative proof of the above, due to van der Waerden (1945; see also Artin 1947). For each $x \in X$ define a permutation $x\Delta$ of W_0 by setting $w(x\Delta) = wx$ if wx is reduced and $w(x\Delta) = u$ if $w = ux^{-1}$. Let Π be the group of permutations of W_0 generated by the $x\Delta$, $x \in X$. Let Δ^* be the multiplicative extension of Δ to a map $\Delta^*: W \to \Pi$. If $u_1 \sim u_2$, then $u_1\Delta^* = u_2\Delta^*$; moreover $1(u\Delta^*) = u_0$ is reduced with $u_0 \sim u$. It follows that if $u_1 \sim u_2$ with u_1, u_2 reduced, then $u_1 = u_2$. We note that Δ^* induces an isomorphism of $F = W/\sim$ with Π.

Proposition 1.6. *F is a free group with basis the set $[X]$ of equivalence classes of elements from X, and $\|[X]\| = |X|$.*

□ Let H be any group, and let ϕ map the set $[X]$ of equivalence classes $[x]$ of elements $x \in X$ into H. To show that $\|[X]\| = |X|$, we observe that if $x_1, x_2 \in X$ and $x_1 \neq x_2$, then $[x_1] \neq [x_2]$, since the two one-letter words x_1 and x_2 are reduced. Then ϕ determines a map $\phi_1 = X \to H$ with $[x]\phi = x\phi_1$. Define an extension ϕ_1^* of ϕ_1 from W into H by setting $w\phi_1^* = (x_1^{e_1} \ldots x_n^{e_n})\phi_1^* = (x_1\phi_1)^{e_1} \ldots (x_n\phi_1)^{e_n}$, $x_i \in X$, $e_i = \pm 1$. If w_1 and w_2 are equivalent, then $w_1\phi_1^* = w_2\phi_1^*$, whence ϕ_1^* maps equivalent words onto the same element of H, thereby inducing a map $\phi^*: F \to H$ that is clearly a homomorphism and an extension of ϕ. □

Corollary 1.7. *If X is any set, there exists a free group F with X as basis.* □

Proposition 1.8. *Let ϕ be a homomorphism from a group G onto a free group F with basis X, and let ϕ map a subset S of G one-to-one onto X. Then the subgroup* $\mathrm{Gp}(S)$ *of G generated by S is free with S as basis.*

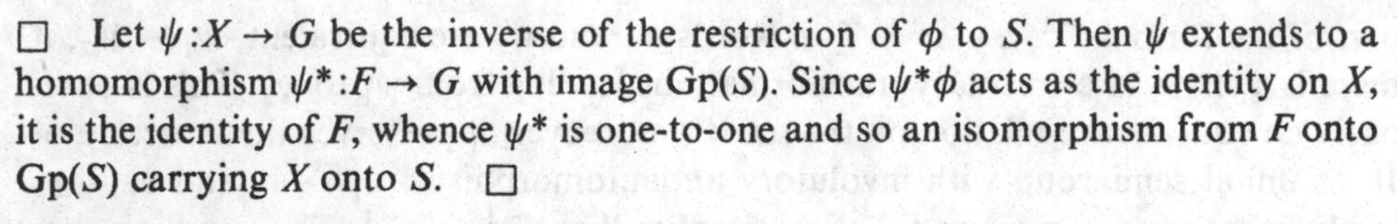
□ Let $\psi: X \to G$ be the inverse of the restriction of ϕ to S. Then ψ extends to a homomorphism $\psi^*: F \to G$ with image Gp(S). Since $\psi^*\phi$ acts as the identity on X, it is the identity of F, whence ψ^* is one-to-one and so an isomorphism from F onto Gp(S) carrying X onto S. □

Proposition 1.9. *Let X be a subset of a group G such that $X \cap X^{-1} = \varnothing$. Then X is a basis for a free subgroup of G if and only if no product $w = x_1 \ldots x_n$ is trivial, where $n \geqslant 1$, $x_i \in X^{\pm 1}$, and all $x_i x_{i+1} \neq 1$.*

□ Suppose first that some such $w = 1$. Let ϕ map X injectively into a basis Y for a free group F. Since $(x_1\phi) = \ldots (x_n\phi) \neq 1$ in F, ϕ cannot be extended to a homomorphism from Gp(X) into F. It follows that X is not a basis for Gp(X).

Suppose now that no such $w = 1$. Let F be a free group with a basis Y in one-to-one correspondence with X under $\phi: Y \to X$. Let ϕ^* be the unique extension of ϕ to a homomorphism $\phi^*: F \to G$. If u is any non-trivial reduced word in F, then, by our hypothesis, $w = u\phi^* \neq 1$; thus ϕ^* is a monomorphism. Since $Y\phi^* = X$, $F\phi^* =$ Gp(X), and ϕ^* is an isomorphism from F onto Gp(X) carrying Y onto X. Since F is free with basis Y, it follows that Gp(X) is free with basis X. □

In a free group F with given basis X, the words serve as names for the elements of F in much the same way as matrices serve as names for linear transformations. Thus, if w is a word, one often speaks of the group element w; this ambiguity must always be resolved from the context. For economy in what follows, when we speak of a free group F it will be understood that X is a basis for F, and in contrast to the usage above, the notation $|w|$ will always refer henceforth to the length of (the reduced word for) w with respect to the basis X.

If u and v are elements of F one has always $|uv| \leqslant |u| + |v|$; in fact, supposing u and v reduced one has for certain u_1, v_1, and z that $u = u_1 z$, $v = z^{-1} v_1$, and $uv = u_1 v_1$ reduced. One says the parts z and z^{-1} have *cancelled*. It is the study of the possibilities for such cancellation in forming the product of two or more words that underlies the method of Nielsen, to which we now turn.

2. *Nielsen's Method*

The main tool in the theory of free groups, and certain related groups, is *cancellation theory*. Let F be a free group with basis X. The words w over X then serve as names for the elements of F; in contrast to the usage above, the notation $|w|$ will denote henceforth the length of the reduced word equivalent to w. We say $w = u_1 \ldots u_n$ *reduced* to mean that not only does the equation $w = u_1 \ldots u_n$ hold in F, but also that $|w| = |u_1| + \cdots + |u_n|$; we say also that the equation holds *without cancellation* (*on the right side*). In general, given u_1 and u_2 in F, there exist unique a_1, a_2, and b such that $u_1 = a_1 b^{-1}$, $u_2 = b a_2$, $u_1 u_2 = a_1 a_2$, all reduced, and we say that the parts b^{-1} of u_1 and b of u_2 have *cancelled*. Note that $|u_1 u_2| = |u_1| + |u_2| - -2|b| \leqslant |u_1| + |u_2|$. For a product of more than two elements the situation can naturally be considerably more complicated. The method of Nielsen rests upon showing that certain reasonable hypotheses limit the possibilities for such cancellation; in particular, *local* hypotheses on the amount of cancellation in a product of two or three factors lead to *global* conclusions on the amount of cancellation in a product of arbitrarily many factors.

Cancellation arguments of this sort were first applied by Nielsen to prove the Subgroup Theorem; this is very roughly related to the problem, given a subset U of the free group F, of characterizing the elements w of the subgroup $\mathrm{Gp}(U)$ generated by U. An equally important problem is that of characterizing the elements of the normal closure of U in F. Nielsen's arguments could well be called *linear* in that they deal essentially with linear arrays of symbols and transformations of them. In contrast, the second problem leads naturally to the consideration of 2-dimensional configurations, and what may be called *geometric cancellation theory*. We deal here only with the *linear* theory; the *geometric* theory will be discussed in Chapters III and V.

Nielsen first proved in 1921 by the present methods that every finitely generated subgroup of a free group is itself a free group; this is the Nielsen Subgroup Theorem. Schreier (see 3.8) using somewhat different methods proved the same conclusion without the hypothesis that the subgroup be finitely generated; this is the Nielsen-Schreier Subgroup Theorem. This more general result can also be obtained by an extension of Nielsen's method (see 2.9 below). However, the conceptually simplest proofs of these results are of a primitive topological nature (see III.3.3 below). We give a version of Nielsen's proof of his Subgroup Theorem here partly because of its elementary nature, partly because of its close analogy with a familiar argument from linear algebra, but mainly to introduce the method with a view to its many further important applications.

In considering subsets of a group G it is often technically convenient to think of them as well ordered, that is to think of them as *vectors* $U = (u_1, u_2, \ldots)$, finite or infinite. However we shall not hesitate to use the same symbol U for the corresponding unordered set, and indeed in many contexts we shall find it natural to deal rather with the set $U^{\pm 1}$ consisting of all u and u^{-1} for u in U.

We define three types of transformation on a vector $U = (u_1, u_2, \ldots)$, as follows:

(T1) replace some u_i by u_i^{-1};
(T2) replace some u_i by $u_i u_j$ where $j \neq i$;
(T3) delete some u_i where $u_i = 1$.

In all three cases it is understood that the u_h for $h \neq i$ remain unchanged. These are the *elementary Nielsen transformations*; a product of such transformations is a *Nielsen transformation*, *regular* if there is no factor of type (T3), and otherwise *singular*.

It is easy to see that each transformation of type (T1) or (T2) has an inverse which is a regular Nielsen transformation, whence the regular Nielsen transformations form a group. It is easy to see that this group contains every permutation fixing all but finitely many of the u_i, and also that it contains every transformation carrying u_i into one of $u_i u_j$, $u_i u_j^{-1}$, $u_j u_i$, $u_j^{-1} u_i$, where $j \neq i$ (and fixing all u_h for

$h \neq i$). We sometimes extend the nomenclature by counting these among the regular elementary Nielsen transformations.

Proposition 2.1. *If U is carried into V by a Nielsen transformation, then* $\mathrm{Gp}(U) = \mathrm{Gp}(V)$.

□ This is obvious for an elementary Nielsen transformation, and hence follows by induction. □

We now consider $U = (u_1, u_2, \ldots)$ where each u_i is in F, a free group with basis X. As usual, $|w|$ denotes the length of the reduced word over X representing w. We consider elements v_1, v_2, v_3 of the form $u_i^{\pm 1}$, and call U *N-reduced* if for all such triples the following conditions hold:

(N0) $v_1 \neq 1$;
(N1) $v_1 v_2 \neq 1$ implies $|v_1 v_2| \geqslant |v_1|, |v_2|$;
(N2) $v_1 v_2 \neq 1$ and $v_2 v_3 \neq 1$ implies $|v_1 v_2 v_3| > |v_1| - |v_2| + |v_3|$.

Proposition 2.2. *If $U = (u_1, \ldots, u_n)$ is finite, then U can be carried by a Nielsen transformation into some V such that V is N-reduced.*

□ Suppose first that U does not satisfy (N1). Then, perhaps after a permutation of $U^{\pm 1}$, some $|u_i u_j| < |u_i|$, where $u_i u_j \neq 1$. Since it is easy to see that $|u^2| < |u|$ is impossible in a free group, we have $j \neq i$. But now a transformation (T2) replacing u_i by $u_i u_j$ diminishes the sum $\sum |u_i|$. By induction we can suppose this sum reduced to its minimum, and hence that U satisfies (N1). After transformations (T3) we may suppose that U satisfies also (N0).

We now consider a triple $v_1 = x$, $v_2 = y$, $v_3 = z$ such that $xy \neq 1$ and $yz \neq 1$. By (N1) $|xy| \geqslant |x|$ and $|yz| \geqslant z$, whence the part of y that cancels in the product xy is no more than half of y, and likewise the part that cancels in the product yz. We thus have $x = ap^{-1}$, $y = pbq^{-1}$, $z = qc$, all reduced, such that $xy = abq^{-1}$ and $yz = pbc$, both reduced. If $b \neq 1$, it follows that $xyz = abc$ reduced, whence $|xyz| = |x| - |y| + |z| + |b| > |x| - |y| + |z|$, and (N2) holds for this triple. Suppose now that $b = 1$, that is, that $x = ap^{-1}$, $y = pq^{-1}$, $z = qc$, where (N2) is indeed violated. Note that we have $|p| = |q| \leqslant \frac{1}{2}|x|, \frac{1}{2}|z|$, and $p \neq q$.

In this case we have the option, by transformations of type (T2) that do not alter $\sum |u_i|$, to replace $x^{-1} = pa^{-1}$ by $(xy)^{-1} = qa^{-1}$, or to replace $z = qc$ by $yz = pc$. To avoid the situation described above we need only exercise a preference for words whose left hand halves begin with one of p or q over those beginning with the other. Technically, we suppose the set $X \cup X^{-1}$ of letters well-ordered. This induces a lexicographical well-ordering $u < v$ on the reduced words in F. We define the *left half* of a word w to be the initial segment $L(w)$ of length $\left[\dfrac{|w| + 1}{2}\right]$. Finally we define a well-ordering of the pairs $\{w, w^{-1}\}$ as follows: $\{w_1, w_1^{-1}\} \prec \{w_2, w_2^{-1}\}$ if and only if either $\min\{L(w_1), L(w_1^{-1})\} < \min\{L(w_2), L(w_2^{-1})\}$ or else these two minima are equal and $\max\{L(w_1), L(w_1^{-1})\} < \max\{L(w_2), L(w_2^{-1})\}$. We shall write simply $w_1 \prec w_2$ if $\{w_1, w_1^{-1}\} \prec \{w_2, w_2^{-1}\}$. Now suppose that $x = ap^{-1}$, $y = pq^{-1}$, and $z = qc$ as above. If $p < q$ (lexicographically) then $yz = pc \prec z =$

qc; while if $q < p$, then $xy = aq^{-1} \prec x = ap^{-1}$. We now suppose the set of u_i transformed by (T2) to reduce the rank of the u_i, under the relation $u \prec u'$, as far as possible. The properties (N0) and (N1) remain valid, while the argument just given shows that no triple x, y, z of the sort described can occur, whence (N2) also is valid. □

We remark that, except in the case that $U^{\pm 1} = \{1\}$, the condition (N0) is a consequence of (N2); for if $1, u \in U^{\pm 1}$ where $u \neq 1$, the triple $u, 1, u^{-1}$ would violate (N2).

The next step in Nielsen's argument we give in a slightly stronger form which has been used (for free products) to good effect by Zieschang (1970).

Proposition 2.3. *Let U (finite or infinite) satisfy* (N0) *through* (N2). *Then one may associate with each u in $U^{\pm 1}$ words $a(u)$ and $m(u)$, with $m(u) \neq 1$, such that*

$$u = a(u)m(u)a(u^{-1})^{-1} \text{ reduced,}$$

and such that if

$$w = u_1 \ldots u_t, t \geqslant 0, u_i \in U^{\pm 1}, \text{ and all } u_i u_{i+1} \neq 1,$$

then $m(u_1), \ldots, m(u_t)$ remain uncancelled in the reduced form of w. [*This conclusion can be made more explicit as follows: for each i, $1 \leqslant i \leqslant t$,*

$$|w| = |u_1 \ldots u_{i-1} a(u_i)| + |m(u_i)| + |a(u_i^{-1})^{-1} u_{i+1} \ldots u_t|.]$$

□ For each $u \in U^{\pm 1}$ let $a(u)$ be the longest initial segment of u that cancels in any product $vu \neq 1$, $v \in U^{\pm 1}$. By (N2) the initial segment $a(u)$ and the terminal segment $a(u^{-1})^{-1}$ do not exhaust u, whence we have $u = a(u)m(u)a(u^{-1})^{-1}$ for some $m(u) \neq 1$. Now, for w as above, let w' be the result, in the unreduced word $u_1 \ldots u_t$, of performing all cancellation between adjacent factors u_i, u_{i+1}. Then $w' = m'_1 \ldots m'_t$ where m'_i is a *middle* segment of u_i containing $m(u_i)$. Since the $m'_i \neq 1$ and there is no cancellation between m'_i and m_{i+1}, w' is reduced, hence the reduced word for w. □

Corollary 2.4. *If U satisfies* (N0) *through* (N2) *and $w = u_1 \ldots u_t$, $t \geqslant 0$, $u_i \in U^{\pm 1}$, all $u_i u_{i+1} \neq 1$, then $|w| \geqslant t$.* □

Proposition 2.5. *If U satisfies* (N0) *through* (N2) *then* Gp(U) *is free with U as a basis.*

□ This follows directly from (1.9) and corollary (2.4). □

Proposition 2.6 (The Nielsen Subgroup Theorem). *Every finitely generated subgroup of a free group is free.*

□ Let F be free with basis X and let G be generated by a finite subset U of F. By (2.2) U can be carried by a Nielsen transformation into V such that V is N-reduced. By (2.1) $G = \text{Gp}(U) = \text{Gp}(V)$. By (2.4) G is free with V as basis. □

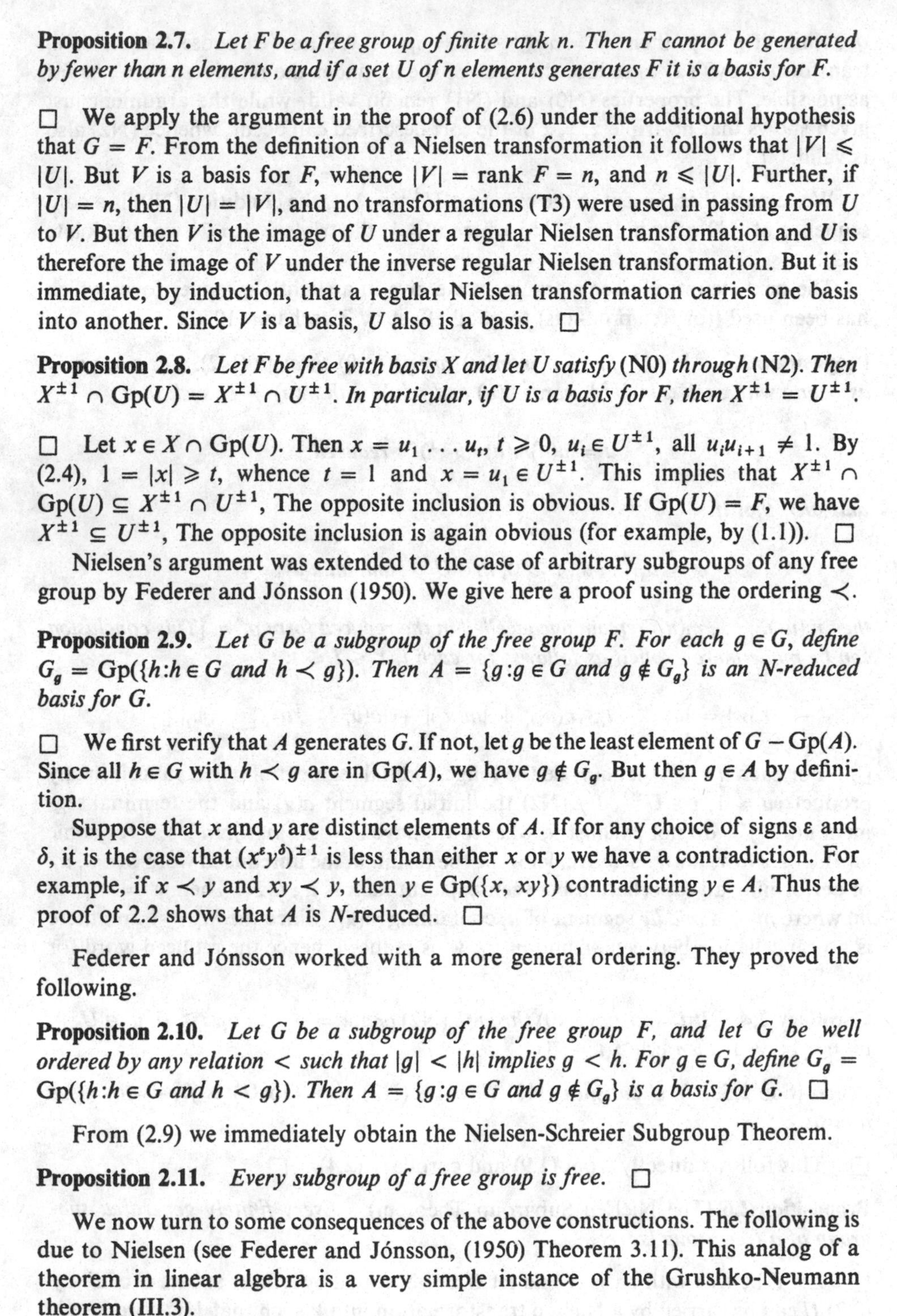

Proposition 2.7. *Let F be a free group of finite rank n. Then F cannot be generated by fewer than n elements, and if a set U of n elements generates F it is a basis for F.*

□ We apply the argument in the proof of (2.6) under the additional hypothesis that $G = F$. From the definition of a Nielsen transformation it follows that $|V| \leqslant |U|$. But V is a basis for F, whence $|V| = \text{rank } F = n$, and $n \leqslant |U|$. Further, if $|U| = n$, then $|U| = |V|$, and no transformations (T3) were used in passing from U to V. But then V is the image of U under a regular Nielsen transformation and U is therefore the image of V under the inverse regular Nielsen transformation. But it is immediate, by induction, that a regular Nielsen transformation carries one basis into another. Since V is a basis, U also is a basis. □

Proposition 2.8. *Let F be free with basis X and let U satisfy* (N0) *through* (N2). *Then $X^{\pm 1} \cap \text{Gp}(U) = X^{\pm 1} \cap U^{\pm 1}$. In particular, if U is a basis for F, then $X^{\pm 1} = U^{\pm 1}$.*

□ Let $x \in X \cap \text{Gp}(U)$. Then $x = u_1 \ldots u_t$, $t \geqslant 0$, $u_i \in U^{\pm 1}$, all $u_i u_{i+1} \neq 1$. By (2.4), $1 = |x| \geqslant t$, whence $t = 1$ and $x = u_1 \in U^{\pm 1}$. This implies that $X^{\pm 1} \cap \text{Gp}(U) \subseteq X^{\pm 1} \cap U^{\pm 1}$, The opposite inclusion is obvious. If $\text{Gp}(U) = F$, we have $X^{\pm 1} \subseteq U^{\pm 1}$, The opposite inclusion is again obvious (for example, by (1.1)). □

Nielsen's argument was extended to the case of arbitrary subgroups of any free group by Federer and Jónsson (1950). We give here a proof using the ordering $\prec$.

Proposition 2.9. *Let G be a subgroup of the free group F. For each $g \in G$, define $G_g = \text{Gp}(\{h : h \in G \text{ and } h \prec g\})$. Then $A = \{g : g \in G \text{ and } g \notin G_g\}$ is an N-reduced basis for G.*

□ We first verify that A generates G. If not, let g be the least element of $G - \text{Gp}(A)$. Since all $h \in G$ with $h \prec g$ are in $\text{Gp}(A)$, we have $g \notin G_g$. But then $g \in A$ by definition.

Suppose that x and y are distinct elements of A. If for any choice of signs ε and δ, it is the case that $(x^\varepsilon y^\delta)^{\pm 1}$ is less than either x or y we have a contradiction. For example, if $x \prec y$ and $xy \prec y$, then $y \in \text{Gp}(\{x, xy\})$ contradicting $y \in A$. Thus the proof of 2.2 shows that A is N-reduced. □

Federer and Jónsson worked with a more general ordering. They proved the following.

Proposition 2.10. *Let G be a subgroup of the free group F, and let G be well ordered by any relation $<$ such that $|g| < |h|$ implies $g < h$. For $g \in G$, define $G_g = \text{Gp}(\{h : h \in G \text{ and } h < g\})$. Then $A = \{g : g \in G \text{ and } g \notin G_g\}$ is a basis for G.* □

From (2.9) we immediately obtain the Nielsen-Schreier Subgroup Theorem.

Proposition 2.11. *Every subgroup of a free group is free.* □

We now turn to some consequences of the above constructions. The following is due to Nielsen (see Federer and Jónsson, (1950) Theorem 3.11). This analog of a theorem in linear algebra is a very simple instance of the Grushko-Neumann theorem (III.3).

Proposition 2.12. *Let ϕ be a homomorphism from a finitely generated free group F*

onto a free group G. Then F has a basis $Z = Z_1 \cup Z_2$ such that ϕ maps $Gp(Z_1)$ isomorphically onto G and maps $Gp(Z_2)$ to 1.

□ Let F have an ordered basis $X = (x_1, \ldots, x_n)$. The sequence $(x_1\phi, \ldots, x_n\phi)$ of elements of G can be carried by a series of elementary Nielsen transformations into a sequence $(u_1, \ldots, u_n)$ where for some m, $0 \leqslant m \leqslant n$, $u_1, \ldots, u_m$ is a Nielsen reduced basis for G and $u_{m+1} = \cdots = u_n = 1$. The corresponding series of elementary Nielsen transformations will then transform X into a basis $Z = (z_1, \ldots, z_n)$ for F such that $z_i\phi = u_i$, $1 \leqslant i \leqslant n$. The result follows. □

Proposition 2.13. *Let U be an N-reduced subset of a free group F and $w = u_1 \ldots u_n$ where each $u_i \in U^{\pm 1}$ and no $u_i u_{i+1} = 1$. Then $|w| \geqslant n$ and $|w| \geqslant |u_1|, \ldots, |u_n|$.*

□ We saw in the proof of (2.3) that some part of each u_i remained in w, whence $|w| \geqslant n$. The same argument reveals that in passing from $u_i \ldots u_j$ to $u_i \ldots u_j u_{j+1}$ at most half of u_{j+1} cancels, whence $|u_i \ldots u_j| \leqslant |u_i \ldots u_{j+1}|$. By iteration of this and its symmetric counterpart we have $|u_i| \leqslant |u_i u_{i+1}| \leqslant \cdots \leqslant |u_i \ldots u_n|$, and $|u_i \ldots u_n| \leqslant |u_{i-1} \ldots u_n| \leqslant \cdots \leqslant |u_1 \ldots u_n| = |w|$. □

Hoare (1970), using abstract length functions (see I.9 below), has defined a set U to be *weakly reduced* if no product $u_i^{\varepsilon_i} \ldots u_n^{\varepsilon_n}$, $n \geqslant 1$, $u_i \in U$, $\varepsilon_i = \pm 1$, $u_i^{\varepsilon_i} u_{i+1}^{\varepsilon_{i+1}} \neq 1$, is shorter than a proper subproduct. This concept is weaker than that of an N-reduced set, but permits simpler and more elegant arguments. The existence of a weakly reduced generating set for a free group is easily proved, and suffices to derive all the usual consequences.

When we speak of an element w or a set of elements w_i in a free group F with basis X as given, we understand that words representing these elements are given. It is immaterial whether we require these words to be reduced or not. Thus the *word problem* for the free group F is trivial: given a word w, it represents the element 1 of F if and only if the reduced form for w is in fact 1. The *conjugacy problem* is only slightly less trivial.

Proposition 2.14. *If F is a free group, then F has solvable conjugacy problem.*

□ A word $w = y_1 \ldots y_n$, $y_i \in X^{\pm 1}$, is *cyclically reduced* if it is reduced and $y_n y_1 \neq 1$. Clearly, every element w of F has reduced form $w = a^{-1} w_1 a$ where w_1 is cyclically reduced. Given two words to test for conjugacy, we can effectively calculate cyclically reduced conjugates. Therefore it suffices to decide if two cyclically reduced words are conjugate. We prove by induction on c that if both w and its conjugate $w' = c^{-1} w c$ are cyclically reduced, then w' is a cyclic permutation of w. For, if $c \neq 1$, $|w'| = |w|$, and w cyclically reduced, requires that there be cancellation between c^{-1} and w, or between w and c, but not both. If, say, the first case holds, then $c = yd$ and $w = yu$, reduced, for $y \in X^{\pm 1}$, and $w' = d^{-1} y^{-1} yuyd = d^{-1}(uy)d$, whence the result follows by induction. □

Proposition 2.15. *If F is free and $w \in F$, $w \neq 1$, then $|w| < |w^2| < \ldots$*

□ Write $w = a^{-1} w_1 a$, w_1 cyclically reduced. Then $w^n = a^{-1} w_1^n a$, reduced, and $|w^n| = 2|a| + n|w_1|$. □

Proposition 2.16. *A free group is torsion free: if $w^n = 1$ for $n \neq 0$, then $w = 1$.*

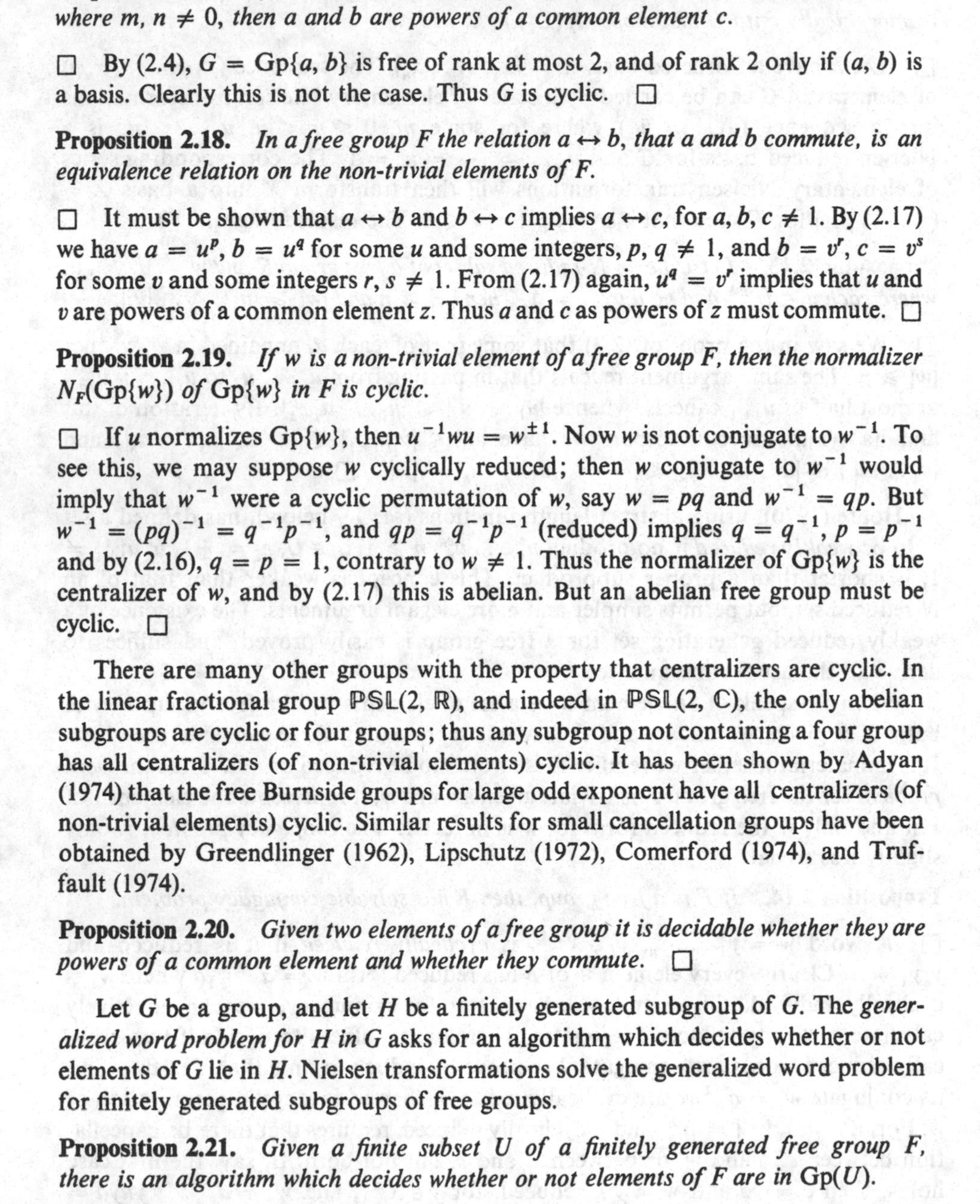

Proposition 2.17. *If a, b are elements of a free group F such that a^m and b^n commute, where $m, n \neq 0$, then a and b are powers of a common element c.*

□ By (2.4), $G = \text{Gp}\{a, b\}$ is free of rank at most 2, and of rank 2 only if (a, b) is a basis. Clearly this is not the case. Thus G is cyclic. □

Proposition 2.18. *In a free group F the relation $a \leftrightarrow b$, that a and b commute, is an equivalence relation on the non-trivial elements of F.*

□ It must be shown that $a \leftrightarrow b$ and $b \leftrightarrow c$ implies $a \leftrightarrow c$, for $a, b, c \neq 1$. By (2.17) we have $a = u^p$, $b = u^q$ for some u and some integers, $p, q \neq 1$, and $b = v^r$, $c = v^s$ for some v and some integers $r, s \neq 1$. From (2.17) again, $u^q = v^r$ implies that u and v are powers of a common element z. Thus a and c as powers of z must commute. □

Proposition 2.19. *If w is a non-trivial element of a free group F, then the normalizer $N_F(\text{Gp}\{w\})$ of $\text{Gp}\{w\}$ in F is cyclic.*

□ If u normalizes $\text{Gp}\{w\}$, then $u^{-1}wu = w^{\pm 1}$. Now w is not conjugate to w^{-1}. To see this, we may suppose w cyclically reduced; then w conjugate to w^{-1} would imply that w^{-1} were a cyclic permutation of w, say $w = pq$ and $w^{-1} = qp$. But $w^{-1} = (pq)^{-1} = q^{-1}p^{-1}$, and $qp = q^{-1}p^{-1}$ (reduced) implies $q = q^{-1}$, $p = p^{-1}$ and by (2.16), $q = p = 1$, contrary to $w \neq 1$. Thus the normalizer of $\text{Gp}\{w\}$ is the centralizer of w, and by (2.17) this is abelian. But an abelian free group must be cyclic. □

There are many other groups with the property that centralizers are cyclic. In the linear fractional group $\mathbb{PSL}(2, \mathbb{R})$, and indeed in $\mathbb{PSL}(2, \mathbb{C})$, the only abelian subgroups are cyclic or four groups; thus any subgroup not containing a four group has all centralizers (of non-trivial elements) cyclic. It has been shown by Adyan (1974) that the free Burnside groups for large odd exponent have all centralizers (of non-trivial elements) cyclic. Similar results for small cancellation groups have been obtained by Greendlinger (1962), Lipschutz (1972), Comerford (1974), and Truffault (1974).

Proposition 2.20. *Given two elements of a free group it is decidable whether they are powers of a common element and whether they commute.* □

Let G be a group, and let H be a finitely generated subgroup of G. The *generalized word problem for H in G* asks for an algorithm which decides whether or not elements of G lie in H. Nielsen transformations solve the generalized word problem for finitely generated subgroups of free groups.

Proposition 2.21. *Given a finite subset U of a finitely generated free group F, there is an algorithm which decides whether or not elements of F are in $\text{Gp}(U)$.*

□ The ordering $\prec$ on F can be effectively calculated. In the process of Nielsen reducing U, we pass successively from U through a sequence of sets $U_1, \ldots, U_m = V$ where each U_{i+1} is obtained from U_i by an elementary Nielsen transformation, each $U_{i+1} \prec U_i$, and no elementary Nielsen transformation applied to V yields a set W with $W \prec V$. The proof of (2.2) shows that V is N-reduced. Since there are only finitely many elementary Nielsen transformations, V is effectively calculable from U. By (2.13), $w \in \mathrm{Gp}(V)$ if and only if $w = v_1 \ldots v_n$ for some $v_i \in V^{\pm 1}$ and $n \leqslant |w|$. By testing all such sequences, one can decide if w is equal to such a product. □

The next proposition is due to Moldavanskii (1969).

Proposition 2.22. *Let F be a free group. Then there is an algorithm which, given two finite subsets U and V of F, decides whether $G = Gp(U)$ is conjugate to a subgroup of $H = Gp(V)$, and whether G is conjugate to H itself.*

□ Let m be the greatest length of any element of U or V. We shall prove the following.

(∗) If $w^{-1}Gw \subseteq H$ for some $w \in F$, then $w^{-1}Gw$ is conjugate in H to $w_0^{-1}Gw_0$ for some $w_0 \in F$ of length $|w_0| \leqslant m$.

We shall first prove that the assertion of the proposition follows from (∗), and then will prove (∗). Assume (∗). It is easy to see that we may suppose F finitely generated. Then the number of $w \in F$ with $|w| \leqslant m$ is finite. For each such w and each $u \in U$ we can decide whether $w^{-1}uw \in H$. Thus we can decide whether $w^{-1}Uw \subseteq H$ and so whether $w^{-1}Gw \subseteq H$. We do this for all w with $|w| \leqslant m$. By virtue of (∗) this settles the question whether any conjugate of G is contained in H. By (∗) again, G is conjugate to H just in case $w^{-1}Gw = H$ for some w of length $|w| \leqslant m$. We have already seen how to find all w with $|w| \leqslant m$ such that $w^{-1}Gw \subseteq H$. For each such w we can now decide whether $V \subseteq w^{-1}Gw$, and so whether $w^{-1}Gw = H$.

It remains to prove (∗). We put aside the trivial case that $G = 1$. Otherwise, replacing G by a conjugate, we may suppose that U contains a non-trivial cyclically reduced element. We may assume that V is a Nielsen reduced set of generators for H. Now suppose that $w^{-1}Gw \subseteq H$ for a certain $w \in F$. If $w_0 = gwh$ for some $g \in G$ and $h \in H$, then $w_0^{-1}Gw_0$ is conjugate in H to $w^{-1}Gw$. Thus the validity of (∗) for w is equivalent to its validity for w_0. We choosen such w_0 of minimal length; it will suffice to show that $|w_0| \leqslant m$. We now simplify notation by writing w instead of w_0.

From here on we argue by contradiction, assuming that $|w| > m$, that is that $|w| > |u|,|v|$ for all $u \in U$ and $v \in V$. Now some $u \in U$ is non-trivial and cyclically reduced; we fix such a u. Then one of $w^{-1}u$ and uw is reduced; by symmetry we suppose that uw is reduced. The minimality of w, that is, of its length among all elements of the double coset GwH, implies that $|w^{-1}u| \geqslant |w^{-1}|$, whence no more than half of u cancels in the product $w^{-1}u$, and hence no more than half in the product $w^{-1}uw$. Since $|w| > |u|$, this implies that more than half of the factor w^{-1} remains in the product $w^{-1}uw$, while all of the factor w remains.

Since $w^{-1}uw \in H$, we have $w^{-1}uw = v_1 \ldots v_n$ for some $n \geqslant 1$, with all $v_i \in V^{\pm 1}$ and no $v_i v_{i+1} = 1$. Maintaining our previous assumptions, we suppose w chosen to make n a minimum. We show that $v_n \neq v_1^{-1}$. For suppose that $v_n = v_1^{-1}$. Since V is Nielsen reduced and no $v_i v_{i+1} = 1$, the product $w^{-1}uw = v_1 \ldots v_{n-1}v_1^{-1}$ ends in at least half of v_1^{-1}. Since it also ends in all of w, and $|w| > |v_1|$, this implies that at least half of v_1 cancels in the product $w_0 = wv_1$, whence $|w_0| \leqslant |w|$ and, in fact, by the minimality of w, $|w_0| = |w|$. But $w_0^{-1}uw_0 = v_2 \ldots v_{n-1}$, contrary to the minimality of n. We have shown that $v_n \neq v_1^{-1}$.

Now $w^{-1}uw = v_1 \ldots v_n$ begins with at least half of v_1 and also with at least half of w^{-1}. Since $|w| > |v_1|$ this implies that w^{-1} begins with at least half of v_1.

But the minimality of w implies that $|wv_1| \geqslant |w|$, whence w^{-1} begins with no more than half of v_1. In short, $w^{-1}uw$ begins with exactly half of v_1. Similarly, it ends with exactly half of v_n. Suppose that $|v_1| \leqslant |v_n|$. Since w^{-1} begins with half of v_1 and w ends with half of v_n, it follows that half of v_1 cancels in the product $v_n v_1$ and all of it in the product $v_n v_1 v_2$. Since $v_n v_1 \neq 1$ and $v_1 v_2 \neq 1$, this contradicts the fact that V is Nielsen reduced. Similarly, if $|v_n| \leqslant |v_1|$, we obtain a contradiction from the fact that v_n cancels entirely in the product $v_{n-1} v_n v_1$. □

The next two propositions are easy consequences of the arguments just given.

Proposition 2.23. *Given finite subsets $U_1, \ldots, U_n$ and $V_1, \ldots, V_n$ of a free group F, it is decidable whether there exists $w \in F$ such that all $w^{-1}\mathrm{Gp}(U_i)w \subseteq \mathrm{Gp}(V_i)$, or such that all $w^{-1}\mathrm{Gp}(U_i)w = \mathrm{Gp}(V_i)$.* □

Proposition 2.24. *Given elements $u_1, \ldots, u_n$ and $v_1, \ldots, v_n$ of a free group F, it is decidable whether there exists $w \in F$ such that $w^{-1}u_i w = v_i$ for all i.* □

The generalized word problem has been discussed for free products by Mikhailova (1958, 1959, 1966, 1968), and for nilpotent products by Shchepin (1965); see also Shchepin (1968), Klassen (1970).

The next two propositions are due to Federer and Jónsson (1950).

Proposition 2.25. *Let F be free with finite basis X, and let A be part of some basis for F. Then F has a basis $A \cup B$ such that the longest element of B is no longer than the longest element of A.*

□ We have that $A \cup B$ is a basis for F for some B. Let m be the maximum length of a in A. Since replacing A by the standard method by N-reduced A' replaces m by $m' \leqslant m$, we may suppose A is N-reduced. We may suppose B is N-reduced. If any $b \in B$ has length $|b| \leqslant m$, we may remove it from B and adjoin it to A; thus we may suppose $|b| > m$ for all $b \in B$. It suffices now to show that $B \neq \varnothing$ leads to a contradiction. We may suppose $N = \sum |b|$, $b \in B$, is minimal. Now, since A and B are N-reduced separately, we have $|xy| \geqslant |x|, |y|$ if $x \neq y$ and both are in $A^{\pm 1}$ or in $B^{\pm 1}$. If $x \in A^{\pm 1}$ and $y \in B^{\pm 1}$, hence $|x| \leqslant m < |y|$, and N1 failed, we would have $|xy| < |y|$ and, replacing y by xy we could diminish N. Thus N1 holds. We may suppose also that if $x = ab^{-1} \in A^{\pm 1}$ with $a \prec b$ (as in the proof of 2.2), then no element of $A^{\pm 1}$ or $B^{\pm 1}$ begins with b. Then, as before, $|xyz| > |x| - |y| + |z|$ for $y \in A^{\pm 1}$. We may suppose this inequality holds also if $x, y, z \in B^{\pm 1}$. The case remains that $y \in B^{\pm 1}$ and at least one of x, z is in $A^{\pm 1}$, say $x \in A^{\pm 1}$. Then, since $|x| < |y|$ and at most half of x cancels in xy, less than half of y cancels in xy; also at most half of y cancels in yz, whence some part of y remains in xyz, and N2 holds. We have shown that $A \cup B$ is N-reduced. Since $A \cup B$ generates F, by (2.13) all elements of $A \cup B$ have length 1. But this contradicts the existence of $b \in B$ with $|b| > m \geqslant 1$. □

In anticipation of a more general definition later we define a free group to be the *free product* of subgroups F_1 and F_2, and write $F = F_1 * F_2$, provided that $F_1 = \mathrm{Gp}(X_1)$, $F_2 = \mathrm{Gp}(X_2)$ where $X_1 \cap X_2 = \varnothing$ and $X_1 \cup X_2$ is a basis for F; in this case we say that F_1 and F_2 are *free factors* of F.

Proposition 2.26. *If U is a finite subset of a finitely generated free group F, then it is decidable whether* $\mathrm{Gp}(U)$ *is a free factor of F.*

□ By (2.5) we may suppose that U is a basis for $\mathrm{Gp}(U)$. Now if one basis for $\mathrm{Gp}(U)$ is part of a basis for F then all are. Thus it suffices to decide if U is part of a basis for F. Let $n = \mathrm{rank}(F)$, $k = |U|$, and let m be the greatest length of $u \in U$. By (2.25), if $U \cup V$ is a basis for F, then this is so for some $V = \{v_1, \ldots, v_{n-k}\}$ with all $|v_i| \leqslant m$. Given a set of elements $V = \{v_1, \ldots, v_{n-k}\}$, by reducing $U \cup V$ we can decide, by (2.5), whether $U \cup V$ is a basis for F. Thus by testing all such V with all $|v_i| \leqslant m$ we can decide whether U is part of a basis for F. □

This proposition follows also from a theorem of Whitehead (4.25) below, as well as from results of Birman and of Topping (see (I.10) below).

Proposition 2.27. *Let u and w be non-trivial elements of a free group F that do not commute. Then there exists an integer n such that $|w^{-n}uw^n| < |w^{-(n+1)}uw^{n+1}| < \ldots$.*

□ It will suffice to show that in some $w^{-n}uw^n$, $n > 0$, at least half of the initial factor w^{-n} and at least half of the terminal factor w^n remain. Let $w = a_1^{-1}w_1^n a_1$, w_1 cyclically reduced, and define $u_1 = aua^{-1}$. Then the conclusion for $w_i^{-n}u_1w_1^n$ implies the same for $w^{-n}uw^n = a^{-1}(w_1^{-n}u_1w_1^n)a$. Thus we may suppose w cyclically reduced. For sufficiently large $p > 0$ by (2.15) we have $|w^p| > |u|$ and hence $uw^p = v$ with vw reduced. Thus the infinite word (sequence of letters) $\omega = vww\ldots$ is reduced. If for some $q > 0$ a part of w^{-q} remains in $w^{-q}\omega$, then a part of w^{-q} remains in $w^{-q}vw^r = w^{-q}uw^{p+r}$, and the conclusion holds for $n \geqslant q, p + r$. Otherwise ω would begin with w^q for all $q > 0$, whence $\omega = www\ldots$ This implies that $w\omega = \omega$. Since $\omega = vww\ldots$, this gives $wvww\ldots = vwww\ldots$. But then, taking initial segments of length $|w| + |v|$ we have $wv = vw$, and w commutes with $u = vw^{-p}$, contrary to hypothesis. □

We remark that infinite words were used in Lyndon (1960); the argument here is similar to one in Lyndon and Schützenberger (1962).

3. Subgroups of Free Groups

Proposition 3.1. *A free group of rank greater than 1 contains a subgroup of infinite rank.*

□ Let x, y be distinct elements of a basis for the free group F, and U the set of all $y^{-n}xy^n$, $n \in \mathbb{Z}$. The countably infinite set U is N-reduced, hence a basis for a free subgroup $\mathrm{Gp}(U)$ of countably infinite rank. As a perhaps more natural example, the commutator subgroup $[F, F]$ has infinite rank (see Levi, 1940). □

The following theorem is due to Takahasi (1951).

Proposition 3.2. *Let F_1 be free and $F_1 \supseteq F_2 \supseteq \cdots$ where each F_{i+1} is a subgroup of F_i containing no element of any basis for F_i. Then relative to any basis for F_1, every non trivial element of F_i has length $|w| \geqslant i$; in consequence, $\bigcap F_i = 1$.*

□ Induction on i. The case $i = 1$ is trivial. Let X_i be a basis for F_i and $w \in F_{i+1}$, $w \neq 1$. Since $w \in F_{i+1} \subseteq F_i$, w is contained in the group generated by some finite subset Y of X_i, and we may suppose that Y is N-reduced; thus we have $w = y_1 \ldots y_n$, $n \geqslant 1$, $y_j \in Y^{\pm 1}$, with no $y_j y_{j+1} = 1$. By hypothesis, $n \neq 1$. If $n = 2$ and $y_2 \neq y_1$, then $y_1 y_2$ is an element of a basis for F_i, and $w \neq y_1 y_2$; if $y_2 = y_1$ and $w = y_1 y_2 = y_1^2$, then $|w| = |y_1^2| > |y_1| \geqslant i$, the last by the induction hypothesis. Finally, if $n \geqslant 3$, then, as we have seen (see 2.3), w contains at least half of y_1 and of y_n, and some letter x from y_2, whence $|w| \geqslant \frac{1}{2}|y_1| + |x| + \frac{1}{2}|y_n| \geqslant \frac{1}{2}i + 1 + \frac{1}{2}i > i$. □

The next proposition is due to Levi (1930, 1933).

Proposition 3.3. *Let F_1 be free and $F_1 \supseteq F_2 \supseteq \cdots$ where each F_{i+1} is a proper characteristic subgroup of F_i. Then $\bigcap F_i = 1$.*

□ Since any one-to-one map from one basis of F_i onto another induces an automorphism of F_i, any element of one basis can be carried into any element of another by an automorphism of F_i. Thus if the characteristic subgroup F_{i+1} of F_i contained one element of a basis for F_i it would contain all and would coincide with F_i. Thus F_{i+1} contains no basis element of F_i, and (3.2) applies to give the conclusion. □

Proposition 3.4. *The derived series of a free group has trivial intersection.*

□ If the free group F has rank 0 or 1, then $[F, F] = 1$ and the assertion is trivial. If F has rank at least 2, then $[F, F]$ is a free group of rank at least 2. It follows by induction that all terms of the derived series have rank at least 2. If F has rank at least 2, then F is nonabelian while $F/[F, F]$ is abelian, whence $[F, F] < F$. It follows that the derived series is strictly decreasing, whence (3.3) applies to give the conclusion. See also Kurosh (1955, 2nd. ed., §36). □

The analogous important fact, that the descending central series of a free group has trivial intersection, is discussed in (I.10) below.

H. Hopf (1932) asked whether a finitely generated group could be isomorphic to a proper quotient group of itself. Accordingly, a group G is called *hopfian* if every homomorphism from G onto G is an isomorphism. We consider non-hopfian groups later (see IV). The fact that finitely generated free groups are hopfian follows from the consideration of Nielsen transformations. Proofs were given by Nielsen (1921), Magnus (1939), and Federer and Jónsson (1950).

Proposition 3.5. *Every finitely generated free group is hopfian.*

□ Let F be free with basis X and ϕ a homomorphism from F onto F. Since $X\phi$ generates F, by (2.4) $|X\phi| \geqslant |X|$. Since $|X\phi| \leqslant |X|$ necessarily, $|X\phi| = |X|$. By (2.7), $X\phi$ is a basis for F, whence the map ϕ, carrying one basis into another, is an automorphism of F. □

A group G is called *co-hopfian* if every one-to-one map from G into G is onto. From (3.1) it is clear that no nontrivial free group has this property.

The union of an ascending chain of free groups is *locally free* (i.e., every finite set generates a free group) but need not be free; for example, the additive group of all rationals is locally free but not free.

Proposition 3.6. *The union of an ascending chain of free groups of bounded finite rank is hopfian.*

□ Let $F_1 \subseteq F_2 \subseteq \cdots$ where each F_i is free and of rank at most r, r finite, and let $G = \bigcup F_i$. We argue by induction on r. If $r = 0$ the assertion is trivial. We assume, that $r > 0$ and that N is a non-trivial normal subgroup of G such that $G/N \simeq G$; from this we shall derive a contradiction. Each $F_iN/N \simeq F_i/(F_i \cap N)$ as a finitely generated subgroup of the locally free group $G \simeq G/N$ is free, and, as a quotient of F_i, has rank at most r. Since $N \neq 1$ and $G = \bigcup F_i$, some $F_k \cap N \neq 1$, whence $F_i \cap N \neq 1$ for all $i \geqslant k$. If $i \geqslant k$, the images of the generators of F_i satisfy a non-trivial relation in $F_i/(F_i \cap N)$, whence $F_i/(F_i \cap N)$ has rank less than r. Now G/N is the union of the ascending chain of groups F_iN/N, $i \geqslant k$, each of rank at most $r - 1$. By the induction hypothesis G/N is hopfian, whence $G \simeq G/N$ is hopfian. □

Nielsen (1948) considered a free product $G = G_1 * \cdots * G_n$ of finitely many finite cyclic groups and the kernel K (often called the *Cartesian* of $G_1, \ldots, G_n$) of the natural map from G onto the direct product $\bar{G}$ of the G_i. He showed that K is a free group (this of course follows from the theorem of Kurosh (III.3 below)), obtained a (finite) basis for K, and gave a formula for the rank of K. Król (1965) carried out the same argument in the case that all the G_i are infinite cyclic, whence G is free and $K = [G, G]$. Lyndon (1973) observed that Nielsen's argument works for arbitrary groups G, yielding a basis for K, and that, in the case all G_i are finite (but otherwise arbitrary) Nielsen's formula for the rank of K still holds and can be given the form

$$|\bar{G}| = |G_1| \cdots |G_n| = \frac{\sum\left(1 - \dfrac{1}{|G_i|}\right) - 1}{\operatorname{rank}(K) - 1}.$$

This formula can be viewed as an extension of the Schreier formula (3.9 below) and of certain cases of the Riemann-Hurwitz formula (III.7 below); a formula containing all of these has been obtained by Chiswell (1973).

We note that a formula containing the above is obtained by Kuhn (1952) as a consequence of his proof of the Kurosh theorem; he obtains also, following Levi (1940) a generating set for $G' = [G, G]$ where $G = G_1 * G_2$ in terms of the groups $[G_i, G_i]$ and $G_i/[G_i, G_i]$, and from this obtains formulas extending those of Nielsen mentioned above and of Takahasi (1944).

The next proposition is a version of a theorem of Burns (1969) incorporating several results of M. Hall (1949); the basic ideas go back to Schreier (1927).

Proposition 3.7. *Let F be a free group with basis X and T a subset of F such that every initial segment of a (reduced) word in T itself belongs to T. Suppose an action π of F on T given such that, for all t in T, $\pi(t)$ carries 1 into t. For $w \in F$ write $\bar{w} = 1.\ \pi(w)$ and $\gamma(w) = w\bar{w}^{-1}$. Then*

(1) $t_1, t_2 \in T, x_1, x_2 \in X$, *and* $\gamma(t_1x_1) = \gamma(t_2x_2) \neq 1$ *implies that* $t_1 = t_2$ *and* $x_1 = x_2$;
(2) *the set Y of all $\gamma(tx) \neq 1$, for $t \in T$ and $x \in X$, is a basis for a free group.*

□ Let G be the group generated by all $\gamma(w)$, for $w \in F$. We show first that T is a (right) transversal for G. For all $w \in F$ we have $w = \gamma(w)\bar{w}$, $\gamma(w) \in G$, $w \in T$, whence $F = GT$. If $w \in F$, then $\bar{w} \in T$, whence $\bar{w} = 1.\ \pi(\bar{w})$ and $\bar{w}.\ \pi(w)^{-1} = 1$. Since the $\gamma(w)$ generate G, it follows that $1.\ \pi(g) = 1$ for all $g \in G$, that is, that $\bar{g} = 1$. Now suppose that $Gt_1 = Gt_2$ for $t_1, t_2 \in T$. Then $t_1 t_2^{-1} \in G$ whence $1 = 1 \cdot \pi(t_1 t_2^{-1}) = 1 \cdot \pi(t_1) \cdot \pi(t_2)^{-1}$ and $t_1 = 1 \cdot \pi(t_1) = 1 \cdot \pi(t_2) = t_2$. Thus T is a transversal.

We show next that Y generates G. For this we calculate that, for $w \in F$ and $x \in X$, $\gamma(w)\gamma(\bar{w}x) = (w\bar{w}^{-1})(\bar{w}x(\overline{\bar{w}x})^{-1}) = wx\overline{wx}^{-1} = \gamma(wx)$; here we have used the fact that since T is a transversal and $\bar{w}$ is characterized by the condition that $Gw = G\bar{w}$ with $\bar{w} \in T$, one has $Gwx = G\bar{w}x$ and $\overline{wx} = \overline{\bar{w}x}$. Since $\gamma(\bar{w}x) \in \mathrm{Gp}(Y)$ this implies that $\gamma(wx) \in \mathrm{Gp}(Y)$ if $\gamma(w) \in \mathrm{Gp}(Y)$, whence, by induction, all $\gamma(w) \in \mathrm{Gp}(Y)$, and $G = \mathrm{Gp}(Y)$.

To complete the proof we shall show that if $w = \gamma(t_1 x_1)^{e_1} \cdots \gamma(t_n x_n)^{e_n}$ where $n \geqslant 1$, $t_i \in T$, $x_i \in X$, $e_i = \pm 1$, all $\gamma(t_i x_i) \neq 1$ and for no i is $t_i = t_{i+1}$, $x_i = x_{i+1}$, and $e_i = -e_{i+1}$, then $w \neq 1$. By definition $\gamma(tx) = txt'^{-1}$ where $t' = \overline{tx} \in T$. Since $t'x^{-1} = \overline{\overline{tx}\,x^{-1}} = \overline{txx^{-1}} = \bar{t} = t$, we have that $\gamma(tx)^{-1} = t'x^{-1}t^{-1} = \gamma(t'x^{-1})$. Thus we may write $w = \gamma(t_1 y_1) \ldots \gamma(t_n y_n)$ with $y_i \in X^{\pm 1}$. We consider the possible cancellation in a product $\gamma_i \gamma_{i+1} = (t_i y_i t_i'^{-1})(t_{i+1} y_{i+1} t_{i+1}'^{-1})$. If $t_i'^{-1} t_{i+1}' = u \neq 1$, we claim that $\gamma_i \gamma_{i+1} = t_i y_i u y_{i+1} t_{i+1}'^{-1}$ reduced. For if not, supposing by symmetry that $y_i u$ were not reduced we would have $t_i' y_i^{-1}$ an initial segment of t_{i+1}, hence $t_i' y_i^{-1} \in T$, and $\gamma_i^{-1} = \gamma(t_i' y_i^{-1}) = 1$, $\gamma_i = 1$. Thus the part y_i can be lost in the product only in case $t_i' = t_{i+1}$, whence $\gamma_i \gamma_{i+1} = t_i y_i y_{i+1} t_{i+1}'^{-1}$, and, in addition, $y_i = y_{i+1}$. This implies that the pair γ_i, γ_{i+1} violates the hypothesis on w (thereby establishing (1)). It now follows that in the reduced form for w all the letters y_i remain, whence $w \neq 1$. □

We postpone for the moment the uses to which Burns puts this proposition, and derive from it two of the results that Schreier first obtained by this method. The first is the Nielsen-Schreier subgroup theorem.

Proposition 3.8. *Every subgroup of a free group is free.*

□ Let F be free with basis X and let H be a subgroup of F. By a *partial Schreier transversal* for H in F we mean a set T such that the cosets Ht for $t \in T$ are distinct, and such that every initial segment of an element of T belongs to T. Since the union of an ascending chain of such partial transversals is one, there exists a maximal partial Schreier transversal T. If $t \in T$, $x \in X^{\pm 1}$ and $tx \notin HT$, then we could adjoin tx to T, contrary to the maximality of T. Thus T is a Schreier transversal.

Under right multiplication F permutes the cosets Ht; this induces an action π of F on T by the formula $Htw = H(t \cdot \pi(w))$. Thus T and π satisfy the hypotheses of (3.7). We shall verify that G of the conclusion coincides with H. First, $w \in H\bar{w}$ implies that $\gamma(w) = w\bar{w}^{-1} \in H$, whence $G \subseteq H$. Second, $w \in H$ implies that $\bar{w} = \bar{1} = 1$, whence $w = \gamma(w) \in G$, and it follows that $H \subseteq G$. □

Proposition 3.9. *If F is free of finite rank greater than* 1 *and H has finite index $|F{:}H|$, then H has finite rank and*

$$|F{:}H| = \frac{\mathrm{rank}(H) - 1}{\mathrm{rank}(F) - 1}.$$

☐ Let $f = \text{rank}(F)$, $h = \text{rank}(H)$, and $j = |F:H| = |T|$. The number d of pairs $t \in T$, $x \in X$ such that $\gamma(tx) = 1$ is the number of pairs for which $tx \in T$, and hence the number of pairs $t_1, t_2 \in T$ such that $t_1 = t_2 y$ reduced, for $y \in X^{\pm 1}$. Now every $t_1 \in T$ determines such a pair except $t_1 = 1$, whence $d = |T| - 1 = j - 1$. Thus $h = (|T| \cdot |X|) - d = jf - (j - 1)$, and $h - 1 = j(f - 1)$, as required. ☐

Remark. The preceeding proposition, and especially its proof, have a geometric interpretation, as will be made clear later. This formula is closely related to the Riemann-Hurwitz formula (III.7 below).

The following proposition of Burns is a strengthened version of a theorem of M. Hall, and provides a partial converse to the preceding proposition. See also Tretkoff (1975).

Proposition 3.10. *Let F be a free group, A a finite subset of F, and H a finitely generated subgroup of F that is disjoint from A. Then H is a free factor of a group G, of finite index in F and disjoint from A.*

☐ Let F have basis X. Let T_1 be a Schreier transversal for H in F. If $w \in F$ we write $\overline{w}$ for the representative of w in T_1, defined by the condition $Hw = H\overline{w}$, $\overline{w} \in T_1$. By (3.7), H has a basis Y_1 consisting of all non-trivial $\gamma(tx) = tx\overline{tx}^{-1}$ for $t \in T_1$, $x \in X$. Let T_2 consist of all $t \in T_1$ and $\overline{tx} \in T_1$ for such $\gamma(tx) \in Y_1$, together with $\bar{a}$ for all $a \in A$. Thus $T_2 \subseteq T_1$. Let T consist of all initial segments of elements of T_2; since $T_2 \subseteq T_1$ and T_1 is a Schreier system, $T \subseteq T_1$. Since H is finitely generated, Y_1 is finite; since also A is finite, T_2 is finite, and therefore T is finite.

For given $x \in X$ let T_x be the set of all $t \in T$ such that $\overline{tx} \in T$. Define $\rho(x): T_x \to T$ by $t \cdot \rho(x) = tx$. Then $\rho(x)$ is one-to-one, since $t_1 \cdot \rho(x) = t_2 \cdot \rho(x)$ implies $\overline{t_1 x} = \overline{t_2 x}$, $Ht_1 x = Ht_2 x$, $Ht_1 = Ht_2$, and, since $t_1, t_2 \in T_1$, $t_1 = t_2$. Thus we may extend $\rho(x)$ to a permutation $\pi(x)$ of T; this defines an action π of F on T. If $t \in T$, $x \in X$ and $tx \in T$, then $tx \in T_1$, $\overline{tx} = tx$, and $t \cdot \pi(x) = t\bar{x}$. Interchanging t and tx, this says that $t \in T$, $x \in X$ and $tx^{-1} \in T$ implies that $t \cdot \pi(x^{-1}) = tx^{-1}$. If $t = y_1 \ldots y_n$, $y_i \in X^{\pm 1}$, we have inductively that $1 \cdot \pi(t) = 1 \cdot \pi(y_1) \ldots \pi(y_n) = 1y_1 \ldots y_n = t$. Thus T and π satisfy the hypotheses of (3.7).

Let G and Y be related to T and π as in (3.7). Since T is a transversal of G and T is finite, G has finite index. Let $\gamma = \gamma(tx) \neq 1$ belong to the basis Y_1 for H; then by the definition of T is follows that t, $tx \in T$, and by the definition of π that $t \cdot \pi(x) = tx$. Consequently $\gamma = tx(t \cdot \pi(x))^{-1} \neq 1$ belongs to the basis Y for G. Now $Y_1 \subseteq Y$ implies that H is a free factor of G. Finally, to see that G is disjoint from A, let $a \in A$. Since $H \cap A = \varnothing$, $a \neq 1$, and $\bar{a} \in T$, $\bar{a} \neq 1$, whence $\bar{a} \notin G$. Since $Ha = H\bar{a}$, $a\bar{a}^{-1} \in H \subseteq G$, and thus $\bar{a} \notin G$ implies $a \notin G$. ☐

The following proposition is due to Greenberg (1960).

Proposition 3.11. *If a finitely generated subgroup H of a free group F contains a non-trivial normal subgroup of F, then it has finite index in F.*

☐ Suppose that $N \subseteq H$, where $1 \neq N \lhd F$. By (3.10), some $G = H * K$ has finite index in F. Suppose H had infinite index; then $H \neq G$ whence $K \neq 1$. Let G have basis $X = X_1 \cup X_2$ with $H = \text{Gp}(X_1)$, $K = \text{Gp}(X_2)$. Let $1 \neq u \in N \subseteq H, 1 \neq k \in K$. Since N is normal, $k^{-1}uk \in N \subseteq H$. But $k^{-1}uk$ is clearly not a word in the generators X_1 for H. Thus H cannot have infinite index. ☐

The following is an immediate corollary.

Proposition 3.12. *Every nontrivial finitely generated normal subgroup of a free group has finite index.* □

We give Burns' proof of a theorem of Howson (1954); see also Karrass and Solitar (1969).

Proposition 3.13. *The intersection of two finitely generated subgroups of a free group is itself finitely generated.*

□ Let F be free with finitely generated subgroups H and K. By (3.10) there exist $H' = H * U$ and $K' = K * V$ of finite index in F. By the Kurosh Subgroup Theorem (see III.3 below), the fact that H is a free factor of H' implies that $H \cap K'$ is a free factor of $H' \cap K'$; again, K a free factor of K' implies $H \cap K$ is a free factor of $H \cap K'$. Thus $H \cap K$ is a free factor of $H' \cap K'$. Since H' and K' have finite index, so does $H' \cap K'$. ($H' \cap K'$ is the stabilizer of (H', K') under the action by right multiplication of F on the finite set of pairs of cosets (H's, K's).) By (3.9), $H' \cap K'$ has finite rank. Therefore the free factor $H \cap K$ of $H' \cap K'$ also has finite rank. □

The *Howson property* of a group G, that two finitely generated subgroups H and K of G have finitely generated intersection $H \cap K$, was shown by B. Baumslag (1966) to be preserved under direct products, and a generalization of it, in which H, K and $H \cap K$ are required to have additional properties, was studied by Moldavanskii (1968). However, not every group G has this property. Indeed Karrass–Solitar (1969) give an example of a group G with a single defining relator that lacks the Howson property: G contains finitely generated subgroups H and K whose intersection $H \cap K$ is not finitely generated. Of necessity, at least one of H and K must have infinite index; here both do. In their example H and K are free normal subgroups of G, equivalent under an automorphism of G, and $H \cap K = [G, G]$.

H. Neumann (1956; addendum 1957) gave bounds for the rank of the intersection of two finitely generated subgroups of a free group in terms of the ranks of the two groups. Greenberg (1960) showed that Fuchsian groups have the Howson property, and Burns (1974) obtains bounds for this case. Burns (1972) studies the Howson property for free products with amalgamation.

We next give the example of Karrass and Solitar (1969) of a group for which the Howson property fails.

Proposition 3.14. *In the group $G = (x, y; x^{-1}y^2x = y^2)$, the normal closures H and K of x and of $z = xy$ are free normal subgroups of rank* 2, *while $H \cap K = [G, G]$ is a free normal subgroup of infinite rank.*

□ Let $G = (x, y; xy^2x^{-1} = y^2)$. Setting $z = xy$, Tietze transformations give $G = (z, y; zy^2z = y^2)$, whence G has an automorphism α carrying x into z and fixing y. Let H be the normal closure of x in G, and let $K = H\alpha$, the normal closure of z. Let κ be the canonical map of G onto $G_0 = G/[G, G]$, free abelian on the images x_0 and y_0 of x and y. Then $H\kappa = \langle x_0 \rangle$ and $K\kappa = \langle x_0y_0 \rangle$. If $g \in G$ and $g\kappa = x_0^a y_0^b$, then $g \in H$ iff $b = 0$ and $g \in K$ iff $a = b$, whence $g \in H \cap K$ iff $a = b = 0$, that is, $H \cap K = [G, G]$.

G has center $Z = \langle y^2 \rangle$ and $H \cap Z = 1$. Thus $H \simeq \bar{H}$, the image of H in $\bar{G} = G/Z = (\bar{x}, \bar{y}; \bar{y}^2 = 1) = \langle \bar{x} \rangle * \langle \bar{y} \rangle$ is the free product of infinite cyclic $\langle \bar{x} \rangle$ and $\langle \bar{y} \rangle$ of order 2. Since $\bar{H}$, the normal closure of $\bar{x}$ in $\bar{G}$, does not contain $\bar{y}$, it meets no conjugate of $\langle \bar{y} \rangle$ non-trivially, and, by the Kurosh Subgroup Theorem, it is a free group. Now $\bar{g} \in \bar{G}$ lies in $\bar{H}$ iff it has an even number of factors $\bar{y}$, that is, if $\bar{g}$ is of the form $\bar{g} = \Pi(\bar{x}^{a_i}\bar{y}\bar{x}^{b_i}\bar{y}) \cdot x^c$. Let $u = \bar{y}\bar{x}\bar{y}$; then $\bar{g} = \Pi(\bar{x}^{a_i}\bar{u}^{b_i}) \cdot \bar{x}^c$. Thus $\bar{x}$ and $\bar{u}$ generate $\bar{H}$, and since $\bar{x}\bar{u} \neq \bar{u}\bar{x}$, they form a basis for $\bar{H}$. It follows that the elements x and $u = y^{-1}xy$ of H, which map into $\bar{x}$ and $\bar{u}$, form a basis for H. Therefore H and $K = H\alpha$ are free groups of rank 2.

Now H has also a basis consisting of x and $v = x^{-1}u = [x, y]$. Further, $H/(H \cap K)$, where $H \cap K = [G, G]$, is infinite cyclic with generator the image of x. It follows that $H \cap K$ is the normal closure in H of the basis element v. Thus $H \cap K$ has N-reduced basis (relative to x, v) consisting of all $x^{-i}vx^i$, $i \in \mathbb{Z}$, and hence has infinite rank. □

The following is a theorem of Greenberg (1960); see also Karrass and Solitar (1969).

Proposition 3.15. *If a finitely generated subgroup H of a free group is contained in no subgroup of infinite rank, then H has finite index in F.*

□ We may suppose that F has rank greater than 1. By (3.10), some $H' = H * U$ has finite index. If $U = 1$ we are done. Suppose $U \neq 1$. Then U is infinite and is disjoint from the kernel N of the natural retraction from $H' = H * U$ onto U. It follows that N has infinite index in H' and so also in F. By (3.12.), N has infinite rank. Since $H \subseteq N$, this contradicts the hypothesis. □

The next proposition (Karrass and Solitar 1969) contains a converse to the preceding proposition.

Proposition 3.16. *If H is a finitely generated subgroup of a free group F of rank greater than 1 and H has finite index in F, then H is properly contained in no subgroup of F of rank as great as that of H.*

□ We assume that F has rank greater than 1. Let $H \subseteq G \subseteq F$. Now $|F{:}H|$ finite implies that $|F{:}G|$ and $|G{:}H|$ are finite. By (3.9) we have

$$|F{:}G| = \frac{\operatorname{rank}(G) - 1}{\operatorname{rank}(F) - 1} \geqslant 1, \text{ whence rank } (G) > 1.$$

By (3.9) again we have

$$|G{:}\,H| = \frac{\operatorname{rank}(H) - 1}{\operatorname{rank}(G) - 1} \geqslant 1, \text{ whence } \operatorname{rank}(G) \leqslant \operatorname{rank}(H) \text{ with equality}$$

only if $|G{:}H| = 1$, that is, if $G = H$. □

The next two propositions are from Karrass and Solitar (1969).

Proposition 3.17. *If H is a finitely generated subgroup of a free group F that has*

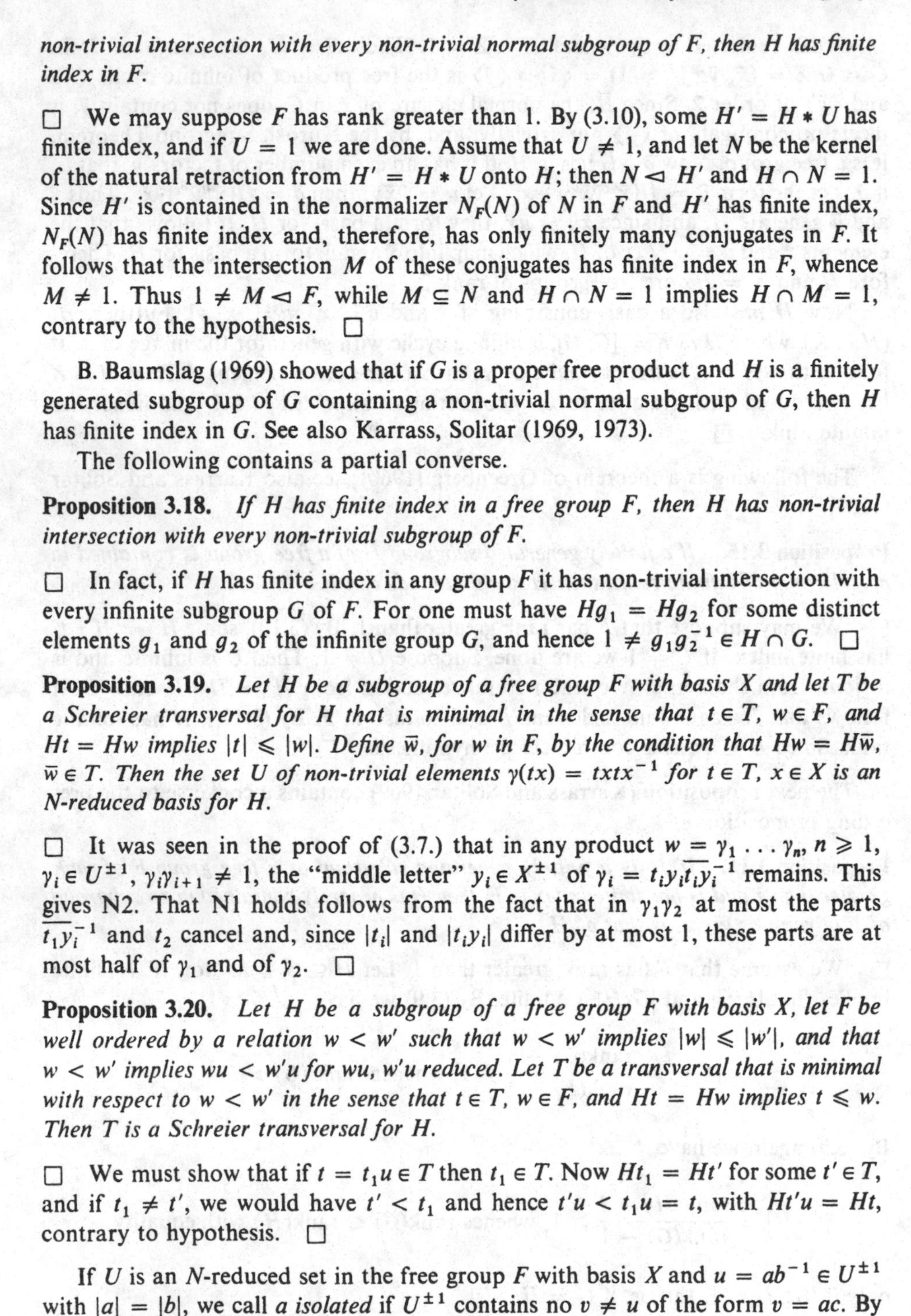

non-trivial intersection with every non-trivial normal subgroup of F, then H has finite index in F.

□ We may suppose F has rank greater than 1. By (3.10), some $H' = H * U$ has finite index, and if $U = 1$ we are done. Assume that $U \neq 1$, and let N be the kernel of the natural retraction from $H' = H * U$ onto H; then $N \lhd H'$ and $H \cap N = 1$. Since H' is contained in the normalizer $N_F(N)$ of N in F and H' has finite index, $N_F(N)$ has finite index and, therefore, has only finitely many conjugates in F. It follows that the intersection M of these conjugates has finite index in F, whence $M \neq 1$. Thus $1 \neq M \lhd F$, while $M \subseteq N$ and $H \cap N = 1$ implies $H \cap M = 1$, contrary to the hypothesis. □

B. Baumslag (1969) showed that if G is a proper free product and H is a finitely generated subgroup of G containing a non-trivial normal subgroup of G, then H has finite index in G. See also Karrass, Solitar (1969, 1973).

The following contains a partial converse.

Proposition 3.18. *If H has finite index in a free group F, then H has non-trivial intersection with every non-trivial subgroup of F.*

□ In fact, if H has finite index in any group F it has non-trivial intersection with every infinite subgroup G of F. For one must have $Hg_1 = Hg_2$ for some distinct elements g_1 and g_2 of the infinite group G, and hence $1 \neq g_1 g_2^{-1} \in H \cap G$. □

Proposition 3.19. *Let H be a subgroup of a free group F with basis X and let T be a Schreier transversal for H that is minimal in the sense that $t \in T$, $w \in F$, and $Ht = Hw$ implies $|t| \leqslant |w|$. Define $\overline{w}$, for w in F, by the condition that $Hw = H\overline{w}$, $\overline{w} \in T$. Then the set U of non-trivial elements $\gamma(tx) = tx\overline{tx}^{-1}$ for $t \in T$, $x \in X$ is an N-reduced basis for H.*

□ It was seen in the proof of (3.7.) that in any product $w = \gamma_1 \ldots \gamma_n$, $n \geqslant 1$, $\gamma_i \in U^{\pm 1}$, $\gamma_i \gamma_{i+1} \neq 1$, the "middle letter" $y_i \in X^{\pm 1}$ of $\gamma_i = t_i y_i \overline{t_i y_i}^{-1}$ remains. This gives N2. That N1 holds follows from the fact that in $\gamma_1 \gamma_2$ at most the parts $\overline{t_1 y_i}^{-1}$ and t_2 cancel and, since $|t_i|$ and $|t_i y_i|$ differ by at most 1, these parts are at most half of γ_1 and of γ_2. □

Proposition 3.20. *Let H be a subgroup of a free group F with basis X, let F be well ordered by a relation $w < w'$ such that $w < w'$ implies $|w| \leqslant |w'|$, and that $w < w'$ implies $wu < w'u$ for wu, $w'u$ reduced. Let T be a transversal that is minimal with respect to $w < w'$ in the sense that $t \in T$, $w \in F$, and $Ht = Hw$ implies $t \leqslant w$. Then T is a Schreier transversal for H.*

□ We must show that if $t = t_1 u \in T$ then $t_1 \in T$. Now $Ht_1 = Ht'$ for some $t' \in T$, and if $t_1 \neq t'$, we would have $t' < t_1$ and hence $t'u < t_1 u = t$, with $Ht'u = Ht$, contrary to hypothesis. □

If U is an N-reduced set in the free group F with basis X and $u = ab^{-1} \in U^{\pm 1}$ with $|a| = |b|$, we call a *isolated* if $U^{\pm 1}$ contains no $v \neq u$ of the form $v = ac$. By (N2), in such u at least one of a, b is isolated.

The following two propositions are from Karrass and Solitar (1969).

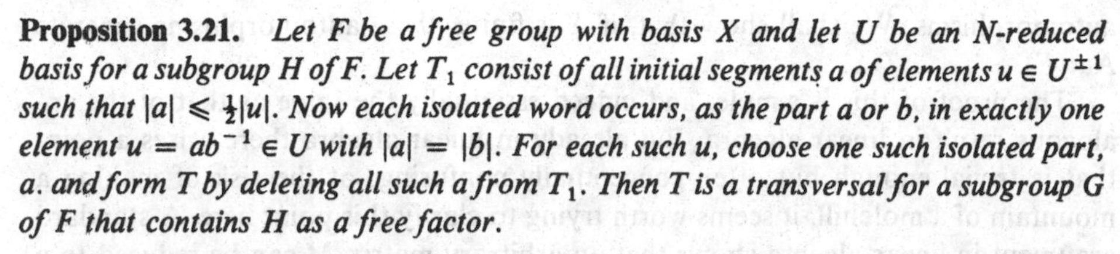

Proposition 3.21. *Let F be a free group with basis X and let U be an N-reduced basis for a subgroup H of F. Let T_1 consist of all initial segments a of elements $u \in U^{\pm 1}$ such that $|a| \leqslant \frac{1}{2}|u|$. Now each isolated word occurs, as the part a or b, in exactly one element $u = ab^{-1} \in U$ with $|a| = |b|$. For each such u, choose one such isolated part, a, and form T by deleting all such a from T_1. Then T is a transversal for a subgroup G of F that contains H as a free factor.*

□ Since T is closed under formation of initial segments we can, as in the proof of (3.8.), define an action π of F on T such that $t \in T$ implies that $1 \cdot \pi(t) = t$. By (3.7) the set Y of elements $\gamma(tx) = tx(t \cdot \pi(x))^{-1} \neq 1$ for $t \in T$, $x \in X$ are a basis for a subgroup G of F with transversal T. Now each $u \in U$ can be written $u = t_1 y t_2^{-1}$, $t_1, t_2 \in T$, and $y \in X^{\pm 1}$, where $|t_1| = |t_2|$ if $|u|$ is odd and where $|t_1|$ and $|t_2|$ differ by 1 if $|u|$ is even. In either case, $u = \gamma(t_1 y) \in Y^{\pm 1}$. Thus, after possibly replacing some $u \in U$ by u^{-1}, we have $U \subseteq Y$ and thus H is a free factor of G. □

Proposition 3.22. *Let the notation be as above, and assume that X and U are finite. Then T is finite, and H has finite index in F if and only if $(|X| - 1). |T| = |U| - 1$.*

□ Since U is finite, T is finite. We may suppose that $|X| > 1$. Assume now that H has finite index j in F. Since $G = H * K$ for some K, and $|G:H|$ is finite, $K = 1$; thus $G = H$, T is a transversal for H, and $j = |T|$. The equation now follows by (3.9.) Assume now that the equation holds. Since G has finite index $|T|$ and basis Y, we have $(|X| - 1). |T| = |Y| - 1$. This, with the equation, implies that $|U| = |Y|$. Since $U \subseteq Y$ and Y is finite, this implies that $U = Y$ and $H = G$, of finite index. □

The above enables one to decide, given a finite set U in a free group F, whether $\mathrm{Gp}(U)$ has finite index.

4. Automorphisms of Free Groups

The key to the study of automorphisms of a free group is the following simple observation. If F is a free group with basis X, then every automorphism of F carries X onto another basis, and, conversely, every one-to-one map from X onto any basis for F determines an automorphism. The situation here is entirely analogous to that in linear algebra. Using this observation, and the method introduced earlier, Nielsen (1924) obtained a finite presentation for the automorphism group $\mathrm{Aut}(F)$ of a finitely generated free group. We shall follow his ideas in obtaining generators for $\mathrm{Aut}(F)$, but we shall use more recent developments of his ideas to obtain a finite presentation.

From the definition of a free group F with basis X, any mapping ϕ of X into F defines an endomorphism of F, which we also denote by ϕ. We consider in particular the following endomorphisms. For any x in X, let α_x be the endomorphism carrying x into x^{-1} and leaving $X - x$ fixed. For any x, y in X, where $x \neq y$, let β_{xy} be the endomorphism carrying x into xy and leaving $X - x$ fixed. In both cases it is easy to see that the image of X is another basis, whence the α_x and β_{xy} are automorphisms. We shall show that, if X is finite, these automorphisms generate Aut(F).

The proof of this is simple, and indeed essentially the same as that of the analogous result in linear algebra. But already in linear algebra there arises a point that is trivial enough but often conceptually confusing; at the risk of making a mountain of a molehill, it seems worth trying to clarify this point here. A standard argument in linear algebra shows that an arbitrary matrix M can be reduced to a certain canonical form M^* by elementary row transformations, that is, $PM = M^*$ where P is a product of elementary matrices. If M is square and invertible, then $M^* = I$, an identity matrix, and from $PM = M^* = I$ one deduces that $M = P^{-1}$, and concludes that the general linear group is generated by the elementary transformations. Some confusion in this argument sometimes arises from the fact that in applying successive elementary row transformations to M we are building up the product P by multiplying successive elementary matrices in *reverse order*.

To make the parallel as clear as possible we introduce a 'matrix' notation for endomorphisms of free group F, relative to a fixed basis X. With the endomorphism ϕ we associate as matrix the ordered set $U = (u_1, u_2, \ldots)$ where $u_i = x_i\phi$, viewed as a word over X. If ψ is a second endomorphism, there are two natural ways of applying ψ to U; the first yields $U\psi = (u_1\psi, u_2\psi, \ldots)$, while the second yields $V = (v_1, v_2, \ldots)$ where each v_i is obtained from the u_j in the same way as $x_i\psi$ was obtained from the x_j, that is, if $x_i\psi = \psi_i(x_1, x_2, \ldots)$, then $v_i = \psi_i(u_1, u_2, \ldots)$. Inspection shows that $U\psi$ is in fact the matrix for the composite $\phi \circ \psi$ while V is that for $\psi \circ \phi$. If we identify endomorphisms with their matrices (of course keeping X fixed) the above discussion comes to nothing more than a rule for multiplying matrices.

We remark this "matrix" calculus for endomorphisms of a free group, although mildly suggestive (see Lyndon 1966), has hardly proved useful with the exception of H. Neumann's application of similar ideas in the study of varieties (1967). The usual computational machinery, as well as the concepts of determinants, traces, etc. is conspicuously lacking. Some of this machinery can be regained by replacing these "matrices" by matrices in the usual sense over some ring, for example, over the integral group ring of $F/[F, F]$, as in done in the Fox calculus (see I.10).

Birman (1974) has shown that if $x_1, \ldots, x_n$ is a basis for a free group F, and $u_1, \ldots, u_n$ are elements of F, then the endomorphism defined by $x_i \mapsto u_i$ is an automorphism if and only if the Fox Jacobian $\left(\frac{\partial u_i}{\partial x_j}\right)$, with entries in the group ring $\mathbb{Z}F$, is invertible. Topping (1973) had established independently certain cases of this result. It has been established that if Φ is free metabelian with basis $x_1, \ldots, x_n$ and $u_1, \ldots, u_n$ are elements of Φ, then the map defined by $x_i \mapsto u_i$ is an automorphism if and only if the Fox Jacobian, evaluated now over the integer group ring of $\Phi/[\Phi, \Phi]$, has determinant $\pm g$ for some $g \in \Phi/[\Phi, \Phi]$.

One further observation. In the notation introduced above, application of the elementary Nielsen transformations of types (T1) and (T2) to $U = (u_1, u_2, \ldots)$ amounts simply to premultiplication by certain α_x and β_{xy}, that is, passage from U to $V = \alpha_x U$ or $V = \beta_{xy} U$. For this reason we refer to the α_x and β_{xy} also as elementary (regular) Nielsen transformations.

We now prove the result stated above, but in a slightly generalized form.

Proposition 4.1. *Let F be free with basis X, and let $\mathrm{Aut}_f(F)$ be the subgroup of $\mathrm{Aut}(F)$ generated by the elementary Nielsen transformations α_x and β_{xy}. Then $\mathrm{Aut}_f(F)$ is dense in $\mathrm{Aut}(F)$ in the sense that if $u_1, \ldots, u_n$ are elements of F and $\alpha \in \mathrm{Aut}(F)$, there exists $\beta \in \mathrm{Aut}_f(F)$ such that $u_1\alpha = u_1\beta, \ldots, u_n\alpha = u_n\beta$. In particular, if F has finite rank, then $\mathrm{Aut}_f(F) = \mathrm{Aut}(F)$.*

□ For the proof we confine ourselves to the more difficult case that $X = (x_1, x_2, \ldots)$ is infinite. Now, for some finite subset $Y = (x_1, \ldots, x_p)$ of X, one has $u_1, \ldots, u_n$ in Gp Y. Clearly it suffices to find $\beta \in \mathrm{Aut}_f(F)$ such that $x_i\alpha = x_i\beta$, $1 \leqslant i \leqslant p$. Since $X\alpha^{-1}$ is a basis for F, the finite set Y is contained in $\mathrm{Gp}(Z\alpha^{-1})$ for some finite subset Z of X; clearly we may suppose that $Y \subseteq Z = (x_1, \ldots, x_q)$, $p \leqslant q$.

Let $U = Z\alpha^{-1} = (u_1, \ldots, u_q)$, $u_i = x_i\alpha^{-1}$. By (2.2) some Nielsen transformation β carries U into $\beta U = V$, reduced. Since $\mathrm{Gp}V = \mathrm{Gp}U = \mathrm{Gp}(Z\alpha^{-1}) = (\mathrm{Gp}Z)\alpha^{-1}$ has rank q, the transformation β is regular. Since $Y \subseteq \mathrm{Gp}(Z\alpha^{-1}) = \mathrm{Gp}\, V$, by (2.8) $Y \subseteq V^{\pm 1}$, and after an inessential change in β and so in $V = \beta U$, we may suppose that $V = (x_1, \ldots, x_p, v_{p+1}, \ldots, v_q)$ for some $v_{p+1}, \ldots, v_q$. We have $V = \beta U = \beta Z\alpha^{-1}$.

Now Z is an initial segment of X, whence $Z\alpha^{-1}$ is the initial segment of the same length q of $X\alpha^{-1}$. Because β consists of transformations involving only the first q components of a matrix, $\beta Z\alpha^{-1}$ is the same as the initial segment of length q of $\beta X\alpha^{-1}$. Thus V is the initial component of length q of $\beta X\alpha^{-1}$. But X is the matrix of the identity automorphism, whence $\beta X\alpha^{-1} = \beta\alpha^{-1}$. In particular, for $1 \leqslant i \leqslant p$, the i-th component x_i of V is the i-th component $x_i\beta\alpha^{-1}$ of $\beta\alpha^{-1}$; but then $x_i = x_i\beta\alpha^{-1}$ and $x_i\beta = x_i\alpha$, as was to be proved. □

One may give a characterization of $\mathrm{Aut}_f(F)$ that does not depend on reference to a fixed basis.

Proposition 4.2. *An automorphism α belongs to $\mathrm{Aut}_f(F)$ if and only if F has a basis X such that α fixes all but finitely many elements of X.*

□ If α is an elementary Nielsen transformation with respect to a given basis X it clearly fixes all but finitely many elements of X; but then the same is true of any product of such transformations. Suppose conversely that an automorphism α fixes all elements x_i for $i \geqq n$ of a basis $X = (x_1, x_2, \ldots)$. Then $X\alpha = (u_1, \ldots, u_n, x_{n+1}, x_{n+2}, \ldots)$ is a basis for F, and by a regular Nielsen transformation γ fixing all x_i for $i > n$ we can minimize $\Sigma|v_i|$, where $X\alpha\gamma = (v_1, \ldots, v_n, x_{n+1}, x_{n+2}, \ldots)$. Then $X\alpha\gamma$ will satisfy (N1), while (N0) follows from the fact that $X\alpha\gamma$ was a basis. Further regular Nielsen transformations permit us to establish also (N2). By (2.8), $x_1, \ldots, x_n \in (X\alpha\gamma)^{\pm 1}$, hence are among the $v_i^{\pm 1}$, and an inessential modification of γ permits us to suppose that $v_1 = x_1, \ldots, v_n = x_n$. But now $\alpha\gamma = 1$ and $\alpha = \gamma^{-1}$, in $\mathrm{Aut}_f(F)$. □

Remark. If F is free with a countably infinite basis X, then the symmetric group on X is isomorphically embedded in $\mathrm{Aut}(F)$ which is therefore uncountable, while $\mathrm{Aut}_f(F)$ is clearly countably generated and therefore countable.

The β_{ij} and α_i provide a reasonable set of generators for Aut(F). One could be more economical. On the other hand, we shall sometimes count as elementary N-transformations all transformations that carry some x_i into an element $x_i x_j^{\pm 1}$ or $x_j^{\pm 1} x_i$, $j \neq i$ (fixing all $x_k \neq x_i$), together with all automorphisms that permute the set $X^{\pm 1}$.

If F has infinite rank the transformations given above do not generate Aut(F), but only the subgroup of those automorphisms that fix all but finitely many of the given basis elements. Description of a set of generators for the infinite case (following the proof of (4.1.) above, or by analogy with the commutative case) presents only notational inconvenience.

Dyer and Formanek (1975) have shown the following.

Proposition 4.3. *If F is free of finite rank $r > 1$, then* Aut(F) *is complete; that is,* Aut(F) *has trivial center, and every automorphism of* Aut(F) *is inner.* □

By virtue of an observation of Burnside (1911), the proof reduces to showing that the group of inner automorphisms of F is characteristic in Aut(F). In a second paper (1976), they show that Aut(N) is complete, where N is now a free nilpotent group of class 2, and of rank $r \neq 0, 1, 3$.

Before proceeding further we clarify further the connection with the commutative theory. For this we assume F of finite rank and write $F' = [F, F]$ (the commutator subgroup of F) and $\bar{F} = F/F'$. Now $\bar{F}$ is a free abelian group, or $\mathbb{Z}$-module, with basis the image $\bar{X}$ of X in $\bar{F}$. Adopting additive notation for $\bar{F}$, we have Aut($\bar{F}$) $\simeq \mathbb{GL}(n, \mathbb{Z})$, where $n = |X|$. The Nielsen generators for Aut(F) induce the following generators for Aut($\bar{F}$):

$$\bar{\beta}_{ij}: \bar{x}_i \mapsto \bar{x}_i + \bar{x}_j \text{ where } j \neq i \text{ (transvections);}$$

$$\bar{\alpha}_i: \bar{x}_i \mapsto -\bar{x}_i \text{ (reflections).}$$

Let U be an ordered set of elements of F, with corresponding elements $\bar{u}_i \in \bar{F}$ of the form $\bar{u}_i = \Sigma c_{ij}\bar{x}_j$, $c_{ij} \in \mathbb{Z}$. Then Nielsen reduction of U (relative to the fixed basis X) induces a transformation of the matrix $C = (c_{ij})$ to 'echelon form' by elementary row transformations (without using column transformations). Replacing U by its image under an automorphism of F (a process that will be considered in connection with Whitehead's theorem, (4.19 below)) corresponds to column transformations.

Nielsen (1932) obtained not only generators, as above, for Aut(F), but also defining relations; from these B. Neumann (1932; see also B. Neumann and H. Neumann 1951) derived generators and relations for Aut($\bar{F}$).

We give below (4.17) a treatment by McCool of these matters; see also Coxeter and Moser (1965, p. 89).

It is, of course, an elementary fact that the $\bar{\beta}_{ij}$ and $\bar{\alpha}_i$ generate Aut($\bar{F}$) $\simeq \mathbb{GL}(n, \mathbb{Z})$ for n finite. From this we have the following.

Proposition 4.4. *The natural map from* Aut(F) *into* Aut($\bar{F}$) *is an epimorphism.* □

A. W. Mostowski has proved the analogous result where F is replaced by the free group of an arbitrary variety; see P. M. Neumann (1965).

The kernel of this map clearly contains the group of inner automorphisms of F, but for $n > 2$, is larger, since, for example, the automorphism $\alpha: x_2 \mapsto x_1^{-1}x_2x_1$, $x_3 \mapsto x_2^{-1}x_3x_2$ is clearly not an inner automorphism. The following proposition is due to Nielsen (1917, see also Chang, 1960).

Proposition 4.5. *Let F be free of rank 2. Then the kernel of the natural map from* $\mathrm{Aut}(F)$ *onto* $\mathrm{Aut}(\bar{F}) \simeq \mathbb{GL}(2, \mathbb{Z})$ *is the group of inner automorphisms of F.*

□ Clearly the group I of inner automorphisms is contained in the kernel K. For the converse we use the fact that $G = \mathbb{GL}(2, \mathbb{Z})$ is generated by

$$A = \begin{pmatrix} 0 & -1 \\ 1 & 1 \end{pmatrix}, \quad B = \begin{pmatrix} 0 & -1 \\ 1 & 0 \end{pmatrix}, \quad \text{and} \quad C = \begin{pmatrix} 0 & 1 \\ 1 & 0 \end{pmatrix},$$

with defining relations (see Coxeter-Moser, 1965, Chapter 7)

$$A^6 = 1, A^3B^2 = 1, (AC)^2 = 1, \quad \text{and} \quad (BC)^2 = 1.$$

(For example, the above is easily derived from the known structure of $\mathbb{PSL}(2, \mathbb{Z})$ as free product.) Now the following elements of $\mathrm{Aut}(F)$:

$$\alpha: \begin{cases} x \mapsto y^{-1} \\ y \mapsto xy \end{cases}, \quad \beta: \begin{cases} x \mapsto y^{-1} \\ y \mapsto x \end{cases}, \quad \text{and} \quad \gamma: \begin{cases} x \mapsto y \\ y \mapsto x \end{cases}$$

clearly map onto A, B, and C. To show that the natural map from $\mathrm{Aut}(F)/I$ onto G is an isomorphism, and hence $K = I$, it suffices to verify that the elements α^6, $\alpha^3\beta^2$, $(\alpha\gamma)^2$, and $(\beta\gamma)^2$ of $\mathrm{Aut}(F)$ lie in I; but this is an easy computation. □

If g is an element of finite order n in $\mathbb{GL}(2, \mathbb{Z})$, its eigenvalues must be roots of the cyclotomic polynomial $\Phi_n(x)$, which must therefore divide the characteristic polynomial of g, and hence have degree at most 2. It follows that $n = 1, 2, 3, 4$, or 6. Meskin (1974) observes that $\mathbb{GL}(2, \mathbb{Z})$ has three conjugacy classes of elements of order 2, and one each of orders 3, 4, and 6. He proves the following.

Proposition 4.6. *If F is a free group of rank 2, then* $\mathrm{Aut}(F)$ *has elements of finite order n only for $n = 1, 2, 3, 4$. There are four conjugacy classes of elements of order 2, one of order 3, and one of order 4.* □

(For torsion in $\mathbb{GL}(n, K)$, $n \geqslant 1$ and K any field see Speiser (1924, p. 210), and Volvachev (1965).)

For any group G, those automorphism of G that induce the identity on $\bar{G} = G/[G, G]$ have been called *IA automorphisms* by Bachmuth. We write $IA(G)$ for the kernel of the natural map from $\mathrm{Aut}(G)$ into $\mathrm{Aut}(\bar{G})$; we shall return to these groups later. We write $JA(G)$ for the group of inner automorphisms of G. (This unfortunately nearly reverses the notation of Baumslag and Taylor (1968).) Clearly $JA(G)$ is a normal subgroup of $IA(G)$ for any group G.

We have seen that $JA(F) = IA(F)$ for F free of rank 2, but that $JA(F)$ is a proper subgroup of $IA(F)$ if F is free of rank greater than 2. Baumslag and Taylor (1968) have shown that, for any free group F, the quotient $IA(F)/JA(F)$ is torsion free. We give a version of their proof.

Lemma 4.7. *Let F be free, let $\alpha \in IA(F)$, and suppose $\alpha^N \in JA(F)$ for some $N \geqslant 1$. Then if x is any element of a basis X for F and F_n is any term of the descending central series for F, there is an element $k \in F_n$ such that $x\alpha$ is conjugate to xk.*

□ The assertion in trivial for $n = 1$ and is contained in the hypothesis that $\alpha \in IA(F)$ for $n = 2$. We argue by induction on n, assuming for some $n \geqslant 2$ that $x\alpha$ is conjugate to xk for some $k \in F_n$. We shall use two well known facts concerning commutator structure (see Magnus-Karrass-Solitar, Chapter 5). The first is utterly elementary: $\alpha \in IA(F)$ and $k \in F_n$ implies that $k\alpha \equiv k$ (modulo F_{n+1}). It follows that $x\alpha^N \equiv xk^N$. By hypothesis, $\alpha^N \in JA(F)$ whence $x\alpha^N = u^{-1}xu = x[x, u]$ for some $u \in F$. It follows that $k^N \equiv [x, u]$ (modulo F_{n+1}). From standard knowledge of the module F_n/F_{n+1}, the fact that x is a member of a basis and $[x, u] \equiv k^N$ (modulo F_{n+1}) implies that, for some v, $[x, v] \equiv k$ (modulo F_{n+1}). If γ is conjugation by v^{-1}, then $x\alpha$ is conjugate to $x\alpha\gamma$, and, since $x\alpha$ is conjugate to xk, this is conjugate to $(xk)\gamma = x\alpha k \equiv x[x, v]^{-1}k \equiv x$ (modulo F_{n+1}). Thus $x\alpha$ is conjugate to xk' for some $k' \in F_{n+1}$. This completes the induction. □

Proposition 4.8. *If two elements u and v of a free group F are not conjugate in F, then for each prime p there is a homomorphism from F onto a finite p-group P such that the images of u and v in P are not conjugate.*

□ We follow a proof indicated by Baumslag and Taylor, who acknowledge suggestions of G. Higman.

Without loss of generality we can suppose that each generator occurs in u or in v.

Let X be a basis for F. We argue by induction on the sum $|u| + |v|$ of the lengths of u and v. If the images $\bar{u}$ and $\bar{v}$ of u and v in $\bar{F} = F/[F, F]$ are distinct, then $g = \bar{u}^{-1}\bar{v}$ is a non-trivial element of the finitely generated free abelian group $\bar{F}$, and has non trivial image in the abelian p-group $\bar{F}/\bar{F}^{p^e}$ for sufficiently large e. The images of u and v in this abelian group are then distinct and therefore not conjugate. This disposes incidentally of the case that F has rank at most 1, and thus of the initial case of the induction.

We may assume then that $\bar{u} = \bar{v}$ and that $\bar{F}$ has rank at least 2. Thus there exists a map $\bar{\phi}$ from $\bar{F}$ onto $\mathbb{Z}$ with $\bar{u} = \bar{v}$ in its kernel. This induces a map ϕ from F onto $\mathbb{Z}_p$ with u and v in the kernel N of ϕ. Since $X\phi$ generates $\mathbb{Z}_p$, $x_1\phi \neq 1$, for some x_1 in X, hence $x_1\phi$ generates $\mathbb{Z}_p$. Thus $T = \{1, x_1, \ldots, x^{p-1}\}$ is a transversal for N in F, and the method of Schreier (see 3.8 above) provides for N a basis Y consisting of all non-trivial elements of the from $\tau(t, x) = tx\overline{tx}^{-1}$ for $t \in T$, $x \in X$, and $\overline{tx}$ the representative of tx in T. As before we write $\tau(t, x^{-1}) = \tau(tx^{-1}, x)^{-1}$. Then if w in N has the form $w = s_1 \ldots s_n$, $s_i \in X \cup X^{-1}$, w is expressed relative to Y in the form $w' = \prod_{i=1}^{n} \tau(s_1 \ldots s_{i-1}, s_i)$. Thus $|w'| \leqslant |w|$. If w begins with x_1 the first factor in the product for w' is $\tau(1, x) = 1$, whence $|w'| < |w|$.

Now u and v are in N and one of them, say u, contains x_1. After possibly replacing both by their inverses and replacing u by a cyclic permutation of itself, we may suppose that u begins with x_1. Thus $|u'| < |u|$ and $|v'| \leqslant |v|$, whence the induction hypothesis applies.

We conclude that there is a normal subgroup K_1 of N such that $P_1 = N/K_1$ is a finite p-group and that the images of u and v in P_1 are not conjugate. Since N has finite index p in F and K_1 is normal in N, K_1 has only finitely many conjugates $K_1, \ldots, K_m$ (with $m = 1$ or $m = p$) in F. Let $K = \bigcap K_i$. There is a natural homomorphism from $P = N/K$ into the direct product of the $P_i = N/K_i$; since these are all isomorphic to the finite p-group P_1, P is a finite p-group. Moreover, the natural map from N onto P_1 factors through P, whence the images of u and v in P are not conjugate. Since N has index p in F and K is normal in F, $P = N/K$ has index p in $P' = F/K$. Thus P' is a finite p-group, and the image of F by a map under which the images of u and v are not conjugate. □

We mention in passing that the above proposition is very closely related to the concept of conjugacy separability; see A. W. Mostowski (1966), Stebe (1970, 1971), and especially Blackburn (1963).

Proposition 4.9. *If u and v are elements of a free group F that are not conjugate in F, then, for some n, their images in F/F_n are not conjugate.*

□ By the preceding proposition there is some finite p-group $P = F/N$ in which the images of u and v are not conjugate. Now $P_n = 1$ for some n, whence $F_n \subseteq N$ and the map from F onto P factors through F/F_n. The images of u and v in F/F_n cannot be conjugate, else the images in P would be conjugate also. □

Lemma 4.10. *If $\alpha \in IA(F)$ for F free and $\alpha^N \in JA(F)$ for some $N \geqslant 1$, then $x\alpha$ is conjugate to x for each element x of a basis for F.*

□ This follows immediately from (4.7) and (4.9). □

Proposition 4.11. (Baumslag-Taylor) *If $\alpha \in IA(F)$ for F a free group, and $\alpha^N \in JA(F)$ for some $N \geqslant 1$, then $\alpha \in JA(F)$.*

□ This is trivial if F has rank less than 2. Assume that F has rank at least 2, with distinct basis elements $x, y, \ldots$. By (4.10), after multiplying α by an inner automorphism we may suppose that $x\alpha = x$. If $y\alpha$ is not of the form $u^{-1}yu$ for some $u = x^a$, then by (4.10) it is of this form for some $u = x^h v x^k$ where v is non-trivial and begins and ends with letters other than x, x^{-1}. Now xy is also an element of a basis for F, whence $(xy)\alpha$ is conjugate to xy. But $(xy)\alpha = (x\alpha)(y\alpha) = xx^{-k}vx^{-h}yx^h vx^k$ has cyclically reduced form $xvx^{-h}yx^h v$ which is longer than xy, and hence is not conjugate to xy. We conclude that $y\alpha = x^{-a}yx^a$ for some a. If F has rank 2, then α is conjugation by x^a, and we are done. Otherwise, if z is any other element of our basis, by the same argument we have that $z\alpha = x^{-b}zx^b$ for some b. Now yz is an element of a basis for F, whence $(yz)\alpha$ is conjugate to yz. But $(yz)\alpha = x^{-a}yx^{a-b}zx^b$ has cyclically reduced form $x^{b-a}yx^{a-b}z$; which is longer than yz and hence not conjugate to yz unless $a = b$. This shows that there is a single integer a such that α carries each element of the basis into its conjugate under x^a, and hence that α is conjugation by x^a. □

Corollary 4.12. *If F is a free group, $IA(F)/JA(F)$ is torsion free.* □

Corollary 4.13. *If F is a free group, $IA(F)$ is torsion free.*

□ If F has rank less than 2 the assertion is trivial. Otherwise F has trivial center, hence is isomorphic to JA, and F is torsion free. The result now follows immediately from (4.12). □

Corollary 4.14. *If G is any finite subgroup of* Aut(F) *for F free of rank n, then the natural homomorphism from* Aut(G) *onto* Aut($F/[F, F]$) $\simeq$ $\mathbb{GL}(n, \mathbb{Z})$ *maps G isomorphically onto a subgroup of* $\mathbb{GL}(n, \mathbb{Z})$. □

Corollary 4.15. *If the free group F of rank n has an automorphism of order N for some integer N, then* $\mathbb{GL}(n, \mathbb{Z})$ *has an element of order N.* □

Let $SA(F)$, for F free, be the preimage of $\mathbb{SL}(n, \mathbb{Z})$ under the natural map from Aut(F) onto $\mathbb{GL}(n, \mathbb{Z})$; then, for $n \geqslant 1$, $SA(F)$ has index 2 in Aut(F). The elements of $SA(F)$ are the *proper automorphisms* of F.

We remark that the study of the automorphism group of a free group can be generalized to the study of the automorphism group of a free product; for this see Fouxe-Rabinovitch (1940, 1941), also Kurosh (1955).

Nielsen (1924) showed for $n \leqslant 3$ and Magnus (1935) for all n that, if F is free of rank n, then $IA(F)$ is generated by the automorphisms $\alpha_{ijk}: x_i \mapsto x_i[x_j, x_k]$ (and $x_h \mapsto x_h$ for $h \neq i$) for all i, j, k with $j \neq k$. Nielsen showed that $IA(F)$ is the normal closure in Aut(F) of $\alpha_{112}: x_1 \mapsto x_2^{-1}x_1x_2$.

The study of the kernel $IA(F)$ and image $\mathbb{GL}(n, \mathbb{Z})$ of the natural map from Aut(F) into Aut($F/[F, F]$) can be generalized. Indeed, if ϕ is any homomorphism from a group G onto a group H, one can ask what elements of Aut(H) are induced under ϕ by elements of Aut(G), what elements of Aut(G) leave invariant the kernel of ϕ and so induce automorphisms of H, and which among these induce the identity automorphism of H.

Andreadakis (1965) showed that if F is free of rank $q > 2$ then the natural map μ_n from Aut(F) into Aut(F/F_n), where $n \geq 2$ and F_n is the n-th term of the descending central series for F, is not an epimorphism; and he showed that the kernels of the μ_n are a central series for Aut(F) and have trivial intersection. He showed that on the other hand, if $n \geqslant m$, then the natural map from Aut(F/F_n) into Aut(F/F_m) is indeed an epimorphism. Andreadakis obtained many more results too technical to cite here. Some of Andreadakis' results were obtained independently by Bachmuth (1965).

Bachmuth (1965) studied similar problems for the free metabelian groups $\Phi = F/F''$, where F'' is the second derived group of the free group F. He showed that if F has rank $q = 2$ then, in analogy with Nielsen's result, $IA(\Phi) = JA(\Phi)$, but that, for $q > 2$, although $JA(\Phi)$ as a quotient group of Φ is metabelian, $IA(\Phi)$ is not even solvable.

Bachmuth (1965) introduced a matrix representation of $IA(\Phi)$, based on a matrix representation for Φ discovered by Magnus (1935). Let R be a commutative ring over $\mathbb{Z}$ containing independent invertible elements $s_1, \ldots, s_q$ and $t_1, \ldots, t_q$. Magnus showed that the map μ from Φ into $\mathbb{GL}(n, R)$ defined by

$$x_i\mu = \begin{pmatrix} s_i & t_i \\ 0 & 1 \end{pmatrix}$$

is a monomorphism. For w in F we shall write $\bar{w}$ for its image in Φ and w° for its image in $F^\circ = F/[F, F]$. It will be convenient to identify the s_i with x_i°, and hence F°

with the subgroup of the multiplicative group of R generated by the s_i. Bachmuth observed that for any w in F,

$$\bar{w}\mu = \begin{pmatrix} w^\circ & b(w) \\ 0 & 1 \end{pmatrix},$$

where $b(w) = \sum u_i t_i$ and in fact $u_i = (\partial w/\partial x_i)^\circ$ where $\partial w/\partial x_i$ is the Fox derivative (see 10 below) and the operator $^\circ$ has been extended from the natural map from F into F° to the induced map from the group ring $\mathbb{Z}F$ of F to the group ring $\mathbb{Z}F^\circ$ of F°. Consequently, if we write $t_i = dx_i$, we have

$$\bar{w}\mu = \begin{pmatrix} w & dw \\ 0 & 1 \end{pmatrix}^\circ$$

where $dw = \sum(\partial w/\partial x_i)dx_i$. Now Bachmuth shows that, under the map μ, every automorphism $\alpha \in IA(\Phi)$ induces an automorphism $\bar{\alpha}$ of $\Phi\mu$ given by

$$\begin{pmatrix} s_i & dx_i \\ 0 & 1 \end{pmatrix}^\circ \bar{\alpha} = \begin{pmatrix} x_i & d(x_i\alpha) \\ 0 & 1 \end{pmatrix}^\circ,$$

whence the map B carrying each α in $\mathrm{Aut}(\Phi)$ into its Jacobian $(\partial(x_i\alpha)/\partial x_j)^\circ$ is a faithful representation of $IA(\Phi)$ by matrices of degree q over the commutative ring $\mathbb{Z}F^\circ$. This representation, which underlies many of Bachmuth's further results, Chein (1968) has called the *Bachmuth representation.*

We digress to note that $\mathrm{Aut}(F)$ has a similar faithful matrix representation B' over the non-commutative ring $\mathbb{Z}F$, carrying each $\alpha \in \mathrm{Aut}(F)$ into its Jacobian

$$\alpha B' = \left(\frac{\partial(x_i\alpha)}{\partial x_j}\right).$$

Indeed the same is true for the multiplicative semigroup of endomorphisms α of F, for given $\alpha B' = (b_{ij})$ one can (see 10 below) recover α by virtue of the formula $x_i\alpha - 1 = \sum b_{ij}(x_j - 1)$. Birman (1973) has shown that an endomorphism α is invertible, that is, is an automorphism, just in case the matrix $\alpha B'$ is invertible. Topping (1974) has shown, among other things, that if F is free with basis $\{x, y\}$, then $w \in F$ is an element of some basis just in case there exist elements p, q in $\mathbb{Z}F$ such that $p(\partial w/\partial x) + q(\partial w/\partial y) = 1$.

Bachmuth (1966) shows that in $\mathrm{Aut}(\Phi/\Phi_n)$ the intersection of the natural image of $\mathrm{Aut}(\Phi)$ with the kernel of the natural map into $\mathrm{Aut}(\Phi/\Phi_{n-1})$ is a free abelian group and determines its rank. He shows also that the natural images in $\mathrm{Aut}(\Phi/\Phi_q)$ of $\mathrm{Aut}(F)$ and $\mathrm{Aut}(\Phi)$ coincide and, for $q \geqslant 2$, are a proper subgroup of $\mathrm{Aut}(\Phi/\Phi_q)$. He raises the question whether the natural map from $\mathrm{Aut}(F)$ into $\mathrm{Aut}(\Phi)$ is in fact an epimorphism. Chein (1972) shows that for $q = 3$ the natural map from $IA(F)$ into $IA(\Phi)$ is not an epimorphism, and indeed that the natural image in $\mathrm{Aut}(\Phi/\Phi_q)$ of $IA(F)$ has index 2 in the image of $IA(\Phi)$.

All the papers mentioned contain results beyond those cited above. In particular

Chein (1968) contains further results on Aut(Φ) and the groups Aut(Φ/Φ_n), and a paper of Bachmuth (1967) with a sequel by Bachmuth and Mochizuki (1967) considers similar problems for the groups $F/F''(F')^m$ where $(F')^m$ is the group generated by all m-th powers of elements from $F' = [F, F]$, and $F'' = [F', F']$.

We conclude with mention of a classical result of Nielsen (1967; see also Zieschang, 1964, and Rosenberger, 1972), that if $G = (X; r)$ is the canonical presentation of the fundamental group of a closed 2-manifold, with a single defining relator, and F is free with basis X (see II.1 below), then every automorphism of G is induced by an automorphism of F. This is not true for all one-relator presentations. See McCool-Pietrowski (1973) and Zieschang (1969).

Let G be the fundamental group of a surface, or more generally a Fuchsian group, and let $G = F/N$, F free. Then relations between Aut(F) and Aut(G) have been obtained by Peczynski, Rosenberger, Nielsen, and Zieschang. See I.5 below.

We turn now to two central problems in the theory of the automorphism groups of free groups, which were posed by Whitehead (1936). The first is, given two finite ordered sets $U = (u_1, \ldots, u_n)$ and $V = (v_1, \ldots, v_n)$ in a free group F to decide if there is an automorphism α of F carrying U into V, that is, such that $u_i\alpha = v_i$ for $1 \leqslant i \leqslant n$; the second is to decide if there is an automorphism α carrying Gp(U) *into* Gp(V). The first problem was solved by Whitehead himself by topological methods involving dimensions as high as 4. A proof in the spirit of combinatorial group theory was given by Rapaport (1958); the proof we shall give below is a revision by Higgins and Lyndon (1974) of her proof. More recently Waldhausen (unpublished), using essentially the theory of 3-manifolds, has given short solutions of both problems. We shall give also a refinement of the argument of Higgins and Lyndon by McCool (1973), from which he obtains a presentation for the automorphism group of a finitely generated free group and for certain stabilizers in a free group.

We remark that, in the language of "matrices" introduced earlier, if we view U and V as matrices, the problem whether Gp(U) = Gp(V) is that of left equivalence: whether $V = PU$ for nonsingular P; the first Whitehead problem is that of whether $V = UQ$ for some nonsingular Q; the second Whitehead problem is that of whether $V = PUQ$ for nonsingular P and Q.

We remark also that, as we have seen already (2.14, 2.21), the analogs of Whitehead's problems for inner automorphisms have rather easy solutions.

We begin by introducing some ideas that play an essential role in the proof of Whitehead's theorem, and which have also some intrinsic interest. First, we define a *cyclic word* of length n to be a cyclically ordered set of n letters a_i indexed by elements i from $\mathbb{Z}_n$; we shall usually understand a cyclic word to be reduced in the sense that $a_i a_{i+1} \neq 1$ for all i (indices taken modulo n). A cyclic word may also be thought of as the set of all cyclic permutations of a given cyclically reduced word; accordingly, the cyclic words are in one-to-one correspondence with the conjugacy classes in the free group F.

With each cyclic word w we associate a function $\phi_w: X^{\pm 1} \times X^{\pm 1} \to \mathbb{Z}$ by defining $\phi_w(x, y)$, for x and y in $X^{\pm 1}$, to be the number of segments of one of the forms xy^{-1} or yx^{-1} in w. Note that $\phi_w^{-1} = \phi_w$. We shall often suppress reference to the word w and write $\phi_w(x, y) = x.\, y$; if $A, B \subseteq X^{\pm 1}$, we define $A.\, B$ to be the sum of $a.\, b$ for all $a \in A$, $b \in B$. This function clearly has the following properties:

$$A.B \geqslant 0, \quad A.B = B.A, \quad (A + B).C = A.C + B.C$$

(we write $A + B$ instead of $A \cup B$ to carry the implication that $A \cap B = \emptyset$),

$$a.a = 0, \quad a.X^{\pm 1} = \text{the number of letters } a \text{ or } a^{-1} \text{ in } w.$$

This function $\phi_w(x, y)$ is closely related to the *star graph* (or *coinitial graph*) discussed below (I.7); apart from a minor change of notation, the star graph has vertex set $X^{\pm 1}$ and $\phi_w(x, y)$ undirected edges connecting x and y for each pair $x, y \in X^{\pm 1}$.

We now define a *Whitehead automorphism* of F to be an automorphism τ of one of the following two kinds:

1) τ permutes the elements of $X^{\pm 1}$;
2) for some fixed 'multiplier' $a \in X^{\pm 1}$, τ carries each of the elements $x \in X^{\pm 1}$ into one of x, xa, $a^{-1}x$, or $a^{-1}xa$.

Let Ω be the set of all Whitehead transformations. If τ is of the second type we write $\tau = (A, a)$, where A consists of all $x \in X^{\pm 1}$ such that $x\tau = xa$ or $x\tau = a^{-1}xa$, including a but excluding a^{-1}. It is clear that

$$(A, a)^{-1} = (A - a + a^{-1}, a^{-1});$$

moreover, if $A' = X^{\pm 1} - A$, the complement of A, it is easily checked that

$$(*) \qquad (A', a^{-1})(A, a)^{-1} = (X^{\pm 1} - a, a^{-1}) = \kappa,$$

the inner automorphism carrying each x into axa^{-1}, and hence, for any cyclic word w, that

$$(**) \qquad w(A, a) = w(A', a^{-1}).$$

If w is a cyclic word and $\tau = (A, a)$ a Whitehead transformation of the second type, we define $D(\tau, w) = |w\tau| - |w|$; we shall often write $D(\tau)$ instead of $D(\tau, w)$.

Proposition 4.16. *Let w be a cyclic word and $\tau = (A, a)$; then $D(\tau, w) = A.A' - a.X^{\pm 1}$.*

□ Let w' be the unreduced cyclic word obtained from w by replacing each letter x in w by $x\tau$ without cancellation. Let w'' be the result of deleting all parts aa^{-1} and $a^{-1}a$ from w'. We show first that w'' is reduced. A letter a^{-1} can be introduced in the passage from w to w' only preceding a letter x from w, where $x \neq a^{\pm 1}$; similarly, a letter a can be introduced only following a letter y from w where $y \neq a^{\pm 1}$. Thus w' can contain no part $a^{-1}a$. Suppose next that a part aa^{-1} arises from a part yx of w, yielding $yaa^{-1}x$ in w'; then in w'' we have again yx, reduced. Suppose now that one of the letters in a part aa^{-1}, say the letter a, was already present in w, while the letter a^{-1} was not. We have then yax in w going into either $yaa^{-1}x$ or $yaaa^{-1}x$ in w' and thence into yx or yax in w''; in the first case $y \neq x^{-1}$, and in the second $y \neq a^{-1}$, whence the resulting part of w'' is reduced.

Now $D(\tau, w)$ is evidently equal to $D_1 - D_2$ where D_1 is the number of letters $a^{\pm 1}$ introduced in passing from w to w' that remain in $w\tau = w''$ and D_2 is the number of $a^{\pm 1}$ in w that are lost in passing from w' to w''. If a letter a in w' arises from a letter $x\tau$ in w, then x is xa or $a^{-1}xa$ (and $x \neq a^{\pm 1}$), whence $x \in A - a$; if x occurs in a part xy^{-1} of w, then the newly introduced letter a fails to cancel iff $y \in A'$. Similarly, a letter a^{-1} in w' arising from a letter x^{-1} in w fails to cancel iff x^{-1} occurs in a part yx^{-1} with $y \in A'$ and $x \in A - a$. Thus $D_1 = (A - a)\cdot A'$. A letter a present in w cancels in w'' iff it occurs in a part ax^{-1} with $x \in A - a$; similarly a letter a^{-1} from w can cancel if and only if it occurs in a part xa^{-1} with $x \in A - a$. Thus $D_2 = (A - a)\cdot a$. We have now that $D(\tau, w) = D_1 - D_2 = (A - a)\cdot A' - (A - a)\cdot a = A\cdot A' - (A' + A)\cdot a + a\cdot a = A\cdot A' - a\cdot X^{\pm 1} + 0$. □

We first prove Whitehead's theorem in the following rather restricted form.

Proposition 4.17. *Let w and w' be cyclic words, let $w' = w\alpha$ for some $\alpha \in \mathrm{Aut}(F)$, and suppose $|w'| \leqslant |w|$. Then $\alpha = \tau_1 \ldots, \tau_n$, $n \geqslant 0$, where $\tau_1, \ldots, \tau_n \in \Omega$, and where, for $0 < i < n$, one has $|w\tau_1 \ldots, \tau_i| \leqslant |w|$ with strict inequality unless $|w'| = |w|$.*

Lemma 4.18. *Let w be a cyclic word and $u = w\sigma$, $v = w\tau$ where $\sigma, \tau \in \Omega$. Assume that $|u| \leqslant |w|$ and $|v| \leqslant |w|$ with at least one inequality strict. Then $\sigma^{-1}\tau = \rho_1 \ldots \rho_n$, $n \geqslant 0$, where $\rho_1, \ldots, \rho_n \in \Omega$ and where, for $0 < i < n$, $|u\rho_1 \ldots \rho_i| < |w|$.*

□ We derive the proposition from the lemma. Let w and $w' = w\alpha$ be given, satisfying the hypothesis of the proposition. Since the Nielsen transformations are among the Whitehead transformations, and generate $\mathrm{Aut}(F)$, we can write $\alpha = \tau_1 \ldots, \tau_n$, $n \geqslant 0$, where $\tau_1, \ldots, \tau_n \in \Omega$. Let $m = \max\{|w\tau_1 \ldots, \tau_i| : 0 < i < n\}$. If the conclusion of the proposition does not hold for this representation of α as a product of Whitehead transformations, then $n \geqslant 2$ and either $m \geqslant |w| > |w'|$ or $m > |w| = |w'|$. It will suffice to show that, in this case, we can obtain a new representation for α as a product of Whitehead transformations with $m' \leqslant m$ and such that the value $|w\tau_1 \ldots \tau_i| = m$ is attained for fewer indices i.

Suppose then that $n \geqslant 2$ and $m \geqslant |w| > |w'|$ or $m > |w| = |w'|$. Let i be the largest index such that $|w_i| = m$, where $w_i = w\tau_1 \ldots \tau_i$. Then $|w_{i-1}| \leqslant |w_i| > |w_{i+1}|$. Apply the lemma, with $w = w_i$, $\sigma = \tau_i^{-1}$, $\tau = \tau_{i+1}$; then $\tau_i\tau_{i+1} = \rho_1 \ldots \rho_k$, $k \geqslant 0$, all $\rho_i \in \Omega$, and with all $|w_{i-1}\rho_1 \ldots \rho_j| < |w_i| = m$ for $0 < j < k$. Replacing the pair τ_i, τ_{i+1} in the sequence $\tau_1, \ldots, \tau_n$ by the sequence $\rho_1, \ldots, \rho_k$ now gives a new representation for α with the required properties. □

We turn now to the proof of the lemma. We suppose then that w is a cyclic word, that $u = w\sigma$, $v = w\tau$, with $\sigma, \tau \in \Omega$, and that $|u| \leqslant |w|$, $|v| \leqslant |w|$ with either $|u| < |w|$ or $|v| < |w|$. Note that

$$(***) \qquad |w| > \tfrac{1}{2}(|u| + |v|).$$

Let w, $u = w\sigma$, and $v = w\tau$ be as above, with $\sigma = (A, a)$, $\tau = (B, b)$, and let $\bar{\sigma} = (A', a^{-1})$, $\bar{\tau} = (B, b^{-1})$. Then the hypothesis remains valid with σ replaced by $\bar{\sigma}$ or τ by $\bar{\tau}$, since, by (**), $u = w\bar{\sigma}$ and $v = w\bar{\tau}$. We observe that if the conclusion holds with σ replaced by $\bar{\sigma}$, then it holds as originally stated. Suppose then that $\rho_1, \ldots, \rho_n$ are elements of Ω such that $\sigma^{-1}\tau = \rho_1 \ldots, \rho_n$ and that $|u\rho_1 \ldots, \rho_i| < |w|$ for $1 < i < n$. By (*), $\bar{\sigma} = \sigma\kappa$, where κ is conjugation by $\bar{a}$. Thus $\sigma^{-1} = \kappa^{-1}\bar{\sigma}^{-1}$ and $\sigma^{-1}\tau = \kappa^{-1}\rho_1 \ldots \rho_n$. Now $\kappa \in \Omega$ and $|u\kappa| = |u|$, whence the conclusion holds for the sequence $\kappa, \rho_1, \ldots, \rho_n$ provided $|u\kappa| = |u| < |w|$. If this is not the case, then $|v| < |w|$. Then $\sigma^{-1}\tau = \rho_1 \ldots, \rho_n\lambda$ where λ is a conjugate of κ, hence also an inner automorphism, and so a product of inner automorphisms $\lambda_1, \ldots, \lambda_m \in \Omega$. Now $\sigma^{-1}\tau = \rho_1 \ldots \rho_n\lambda_1 \ldots \lambda_m$, and $|u\rho_1 \ldots \rho_n\lambda_1 \ldots \lambda_i| = |v\lambda_1 \ldots \lambda_i| = |v| < |w|$, and the conclusion holds for the sequence $\rho_1, \ldots, \rho_n, \lambda_1, \ldots, \lambda_m$.

In view of this, in proving the lemma not only may we freely interchange σ and τ, by symmetry, but we may replace σ by $\bar{\sigma}$ or τ by $\bar{\tau}$.

Case 1: τ permutes the letters. Here $|v| = |w|$, whence $|u| < |w|$. We take $n = 2$ with $\rho_1 = \tau$ and $\rho_2 = \tau^{-1}\sigma^{-1}\tau$.

In view of this case we may suppose, by symmetry, that neither σ nor τ is a permutation of the letters; thus we may write $\sigma = (A, a)$ and $\tau = (B, b)$.

Case 2: $A \cap B = \varnothing$ and $b = a^{-1}$. Here we may take $n = 1$ with $\rho_1 = \sigma^{-1}\tau = (A + B - a, a^{-1})$.

Case 3: $A \cap B = \varnothing$ and $a^{-1} \in B'$. Here we take $n = 2$ with $\rho_1 = \tau$ and $\rho_2 = \tau^{-1}\sigma^{-1}\tau$. To verify that $\rho_2 \in \Omega$ we check that $\tau^{-1}\sigma\tau$ is σ if $b^{-1} \in A'$ and is $(A + B - b, a)$ if $b^{-1} \in A$. It remains to show that $|u\tau| < |w|$. For this, let w' and u' be the unreduced cyclic words obtained by applying τ to w and u. The occurrences of letters $x \in B - b$ in w correspond one-to-one with those in $u = w\sigma$. It follows that $|w'| - |w| = |u'| - |u|$. Now w and u are obtained from w' and u' by deleting all parts bb^{-1}; we show that u' contains as many parts bb^{-1} as w' (in fact, the same number).

A part bb^{-1} in w' must occur in a context $p' = xbb^{-1}$, $bb^{-1}y^{-1}$ or $xbb^{-1}y^{-1}$ arising from a part p of w of one of the forms $p = xb^{-1}$, by^{-1}, or xy^{-1}, where $x, y \in B - b$. Since $x, y, b \in A$, such a part p of w occurs intact in $u = w$, and thus gives rise to an occurrence of bb^{-1} in u'. This establishes that $|u\tau| - |u| \leqslant |w\tau| - |w|$; using (*) and the fact that $w\tau = v$, we obtain $|u\tau| \leqslant |u| + |v| - |w| < 2|w| - |w| = |w|$.

Case 4: $A \cap B = \varnothing$, general case. Note that $A \cap B = \varnothing$ implies that $a \neq b$. By Case 2, we may suppose that $a \neq b^{-1}$. By Case 3, we may suppose that $a^{-1} \in B$ and $b^{-1} \in A$. Define $\sigma' = (A, b^{-1})$ and $\tau' = (B, a^{-1})$. Now, from (4.5) and the definitions of σ' and τ' we have that $D(\sigma') + D(\tau') = D(\sigma) + D(\tau)$; from (*) we have $D(\sigma) + D(\tau) = |u| + |v| - 2|w| < 0$. It follows that $D(\sigma') + D(\tau') < 0$ and one term is negative, say $D(\tau') < 0$. We take $n = 3$ with $\rho_1 = \sigma^{-1}\tau' = (A + a + a^{-1}, a^{-1})(B, a^{-1}) = (A + B - a, a^{-1})$, with ρ_2 the automorphism carrying a into b^{-1} and b into a^{-1} and fixing all other letters, and with $\rho_3 = (B - a^{-1} + a - b + b^{-1}, a)$. Computation shows that $\tau'^{-1}\tau = \rho_2\rho_3$ whence $\sigma^{-1}\tau = \rho_1\rho_2\rho_3$. Now $D(\tau') = |w\tau'| - |w| < 0$, and $u\rho_1 = (w\sigma)(\sigma^{-1}\tau') = w\tau'$, whence $|u\rho_1| < |w|$. Since ρ_2 is a permutation, $|u\rho_1\rho_2| = |u\rho_1| < |w|$.

Case 5: $A \cap B \neq \varnothing$. We shall reduce this case to Case 4. Observe that by (***)

$D(\sigma) + D(\tau) < 0$ and hence, by (4.5), that

$$(\dagger) \qquad A.A' + B.B' - a.X^{\pm 1} - b.X^{\pm 1} < 0.$$

We write

$$A_1 = A, \quad A_2 = A', B_1 = B, \quad B_2 = B', \quad \text{and} \quad P_{ij} = A_i \cap B_j.$$

Now

$$A.A' + B.B' = A_1.A_2 + B_1.B_2 = P_{11}.P'_{11} + P_{22}.P'_{22} + 2P_{12}.P'_{21}$$
$$\geqslant P_{11}.P'_{11} + P_{22}.P'_{22};$$

similarly, interchanging B_1 and B_2 gives

$$A.A' + B.B' \geqslant P_{12}.P'_{12} + P_{21}.P'_{21}.$$

Thus ($\dagger$) gives

$$(\dagger\dagger) \qquad \begin{cases} P_{11}.P'_{11} + P_{22}.P'_{22} - a.X^{\pm 1} - b.X^{\pm 1} < 0, \\ P_{12}.P'_{12} + P_{21}.P'_{21} - a.X^{\pm 1} - b.X^{\pm 1} < 0. \end{cases}$$

Let x stand for any one of a, a^{-1}, b, b^{-1}, and let $P(x)$ be that P_{ij} which contains x; note that $x^{-1} \notin P(x)$. We shall show that, for at least one choice of x, the transformation $(P(x), x)$ decreases $|w|$. If the $P(x)$ are distinct for the four choices of x, from (4.16) and ($\dagger\dagger$) we have

$$\Sigma D(P(x), x) = \Sigma P(x).P(x)' - \Sigma x.X^{\pm 1}$$
$$= \Sigma P_{ij}.P'_{ij} - 2(a.X^{\pm 1} + b.X^{\pm 1}) < 0$$

whence some $D(P(x), x) < 0$. In the remaining case some P_{ij} contains none of $a_1 = a$, $a_2 = a^{-1}$, $b_1 = b$, and $b_2 = b^{-1}$. Since $a_i \in A_i = P_{i1} + P_{i2}$, we have $a_i \in P_{ik}$ for $k \neq j$; similarly, $b_j \in P_{hj}$ for $h \neq i$. Either $i = k$ and $h = j$ or else $i \neq k$ and $h \neq j$; in either case, by ($\dagger\dagger$) we have

$$D(P(a_i), a_i) + D(P(b_j), b_j) = P_{ik}.P'_{ik} + P_{hj}.P'_{hj} - a.X^{\pm 1} - b.X^{\pm 1} < 0$$

and again some $D(P(x), x) < 0$.

Interchanging σ and τ if necessary we can suppose that x is a or a^{-1}, and, by (**), that $x = a$. Then $P(x)$ is P_{11} or P_{12}, and by (**) applied to τ we can suppose that $P(x) = P_{12}$. We now have $a \in B'$ and $D(A \cap B', a) < 0$. Let $\theta = (A \cap B', a)$ and $w_1 = w\theta$; then $|w_1| < |w|$. Let $\rho_1 = \sigma^{-1}\theta = (A' \cup B' - a^{-1}, a)$; then $w_1 = u\rho_1$. We now have $|w_1| < |w|$, $|v| \leqslant |w|$ where $w_1 = w(A \cap B', a)$ and $v = w(B, b)$. Since $A \cap B'$ and B are disjoint, by Case 4 we can find $\rho_2, \ldots, \rho_n \in \Omega$ such that $\theta^{-1}\tau = \rho_2 \ldots \rho_n$ with $|w_1\rho_1 \ldots \rho_i| < |w|$ for $0 < i < n$. The sequence $\rho_1, \rho_2, \ldots, \rho_n$ therefore satisfies the conclusions of the lemma. $\square$

Proposition 4.19. *Let w_1 and w_2 be elements of a free group F. Then it is decidable whether there is an automorphism of F carrying w_1 into w_2.*

□ We may suppose F finitely generated. Let (w_1) and (w_2) be the cyclic words associated with w_1 and w_2. Since there are only finitely many Whitehead transformations we may determine by trial and error whether any of them diminishes the length of (w_1), and, if so, we can replace (w_1) by a shorter image; thus we can replace (w_1) by a cyclic word that cannot be shortened further by any Whitehead transformation. By (4.17), (w_1) now has minimal length among all of its images under $\mathrm{Aut}(F)$. We can suppose (w_2) minimal in the same sense. Now there cannot exist an automorphism carrying (w_1) into (w_2) unless they have the same length; suppose they both have length n. The set V of cyclic words in F of length n is finite. Take these as vertices of a graph and introduce an edge from $(w) \in V$ to $(w') \in V$ just in case some Whitehead transformation carries (w) into (w'). By (4.17) there exists an automorphism carrying (w_1) into (w_2) if there is a connected path leading from (w_1) to (w_2).

The above argument enables us to determine if there exists an automorphism $\alpha \in \mathrm{Aut}(F)$ such that $(w_1)\alpha = (w_2)$, and to find such α if one exists. But now $(w_1)\alpha = (w_2)$ is equivalent to $w_1\alpha$ being conjugate to w_2, and hence to the existence of $\alpha' \in \mathrm{Aut}(F)$ such that $w_1\alpha' = w_2$. □

We now modify (4.17) by considering not a single cyclic word w but a finite set of cyclic words $w_1, \ldots, w_t$, and we replace consideration of the length $|w|$ of w by the sum of the lengths $\Sigma|w_h|$ of $w_1, \ldots, w_t$. Then the proof of (4.17) goes through without further change, yielding the following.

Proposition 4.20. *Let $w_1, \ldots, w_t$ and $w'_1, \ldots, w'_t$ be cyclic words such that $w_1\alpha = w'_1, \ldots, w_t\alpha = w'_t$ for some $\alpha \in \mathrm{Aut}(F)$, and assume that $\sum|w'_h|$ is minimal among all $\sum|w_h\alpha'|$ for $\alpha' \in \mathrm{Aut}(F)$. Then $\alpha = \tau_1 \ldots \tau_n$, $n \geqq 0$, where $\tau_1, \ldots, \tau_n \in \Omega$ and where, for $0 < i < n$, one has $\sum|w_h\tau_1 \ldots \tau_i| \leqslant \sum|w_h|$ with strict inequality unless $\sum|w_h| = \sum|w'_h|$.* □

By the same argument as in the first part of the proof of (4.9.) we establish the following.

Proposition 4.21. *Let $w_1, \ldots, w_t$ and $w'_1, \ldots, w'_t$ be cyclic words in a free group F. Then it is decidable whether there is an automorphism $\alpha \in \mathrm{Aut}(F)$ such that $w_1\alpha = w'_1, \ldots, w_t\alpha = w'_t$.* □

We turn now to arguments of McCool (1974) obtaining a refinement of (4.18) and deriving from it the analog (4.23 below) of (4.17) for ordinary, non-cyclic words, and also a presentation for the automorphism group of a finitely generated free group.

Let F be free of finite rank n, with basis $X = \{x_1, \ldots, x_n\}$. Let Ω be the set of Whitehead transformations relative to X, and let $A = \mathrm{Aut}(F)$. Since Ω contains the Nielsen transformations, Ω generates A. We consider presentations with generators mapping onto the set Ω. More explicitly, let $\tilde{\Omega}$ be a set in one-to-one correspondence with Ω, let Φ be free with basis $\tilde{\Omega}$, and let ϕ be the map from Φ onto A carrying each $\tilde{\sigma} \in \tilde{\Omega}$ into corresponding $\sigma \in \Omega$. Let $N \lhd \Phi$ be the kernel of ϕ. We shall describe a finite set $R \subseteq N$ for which it will be shown that the normal closure of R in Φ is N, hence that A has a presentation (see II.1 below) $A = (\tilde{\Omega}; R)$.

If $r = \tilde{u}\tilde{v}^{-1} \in N$, with $\tilde{u}\phi = u$, $\tilde{v}\phi = v$, then in A a relation $u = v$ holds. We shall follow common practice in describing R not by listing the elements $r \in R$ directly, but rather by listing corresponding relations $u = v$. Here u and v are written as products $u = \sigma_1^{e_1} \ldots \sigma_h^{e_h}$, $v = \tau_1^{f_1} \ldots \tau_k^{f_k}$, $e_i, f_i = \pm 1$, of elements of Ω and their inverses, and it is understood that corresponding r is the product

$$r = \tilde{\sigma}_1^{e_1} \ldots \tilde{\sigma}_n^{e_n}(\tilde{\tau}_1^{f_1} \ldots \tilde{\tau}_k^{f_k})^{-1}.$$

By definition, Ω is the union of two sets Ω_1 and Ω_2 with only 1 in common: here Ω_1 consists of all $\sigma \in \Omega$ that permute the elements of $L = X \cup X^{-1}$, and Ω_2 of all elements $\sigma \in \Omega$ of the form $\sigma = (A, a)$. The set Ω_1 evidently generates the subgroup A_1 of A, of order $2^n.n!$, consisting of all $\alpha \in A$ that effect a permutation of L. If Φ_1 is the subgroup of Φ generated by $\tilde{\Omega}_1$, then the restriction ϕ_1 of ϕ to Φ_1 maps Φ_1 onto A_1. Clearly the kernel N_1 of ϕ_1 is the normal closure in Φ_1 of some finite set R_1. We suppose such R_1 chosen, and will obtain R in the form $R = R_1 \cup R_2$.

We now describe R_2 as consisting of all $r \in \Phi$ defined by relations of the forms (R1) through (R6) below. Here we write $\bar{a}$ and $\bar{b}$ for a^{-1} and b^{-1}.

(R1) $$(A, a)^{-1} = (A - a + \bar{a}, \bar{a}).$$

(R2) $$(A, a)(B, a) = (A \cup B, a)$$
$$\text{where } A \cap B = \{a\}.$$

(R3) $$(B, b)^{-1}(A, a)(B, b) = (A, a)$$
$$\text{where } A \cap B = \varnothing, \bar{a} \notin B, \bar{b} \notin A.$$

(R4) $$(B, b)^{-1}(A, a)(B, b) = (A + B - b, a)$$
$$\text{where } A \cap B = \varnothing, \bar{a} \notin B, \bar{b} \in A.$$

(R5) $$(A, a)(A - a + \bar{a}, b) = (a, \bar{b}, \bar{a}, b)(A - b + \bar{b}, a)$$
$$\text{where } b \in A, \bar{b} \notin A, a \neq b$$

and $(a, \bar{b}, \bar{a}, b)$ denotes the automorphism induced by the indicated cyclic permutation of L.

(R6) $$\sigma^{-1}(A, a)\sigma = (A\sigma, a\sigma)$$
$$\text{where } \sigma \in \Omega_1.$$

It is immediate that $R \subseteq N$. We denote by N_2 the normal closure of R_2 in Φ. It is convenient to observe that N_2 contains all relations of the following three forms.

(R7) $$(A, a) = (L - \bar{a}, a)(A', \bar{a}) = (A', \bar{a})(L - \bar{a}, a)$$

(R8)
$$(L - b, \bar{b})(A, a)(L - \bar{b}, b) = (A, a)$$
where $b \neq \bar{a}$ and $b, \bar{b} \in A'$.

(R9)
$$(L - b, \bar{b})(A, a)(L - \bar{b}, b) = (A', \bar{a})$$
where $b \neq a$, $b \in A$, and $\bar{b} \in A'$.

These follow from the following calculation, where only relations of the forms (R1) through (R6) are used. For (R7), we have by (R2) and (R1), that

$$(L - \bar{a}, a) = (A, a)(L - A - \bar{a} + a, a) = (L - A - \bar{a} + a, a)(A, a)$$
$$= (A, a)(A', \bar{a})^{-1} = (A', \bar{a})^{-1}(A, a).$$

For (R8), we have by (R4) that

$$(A' - b, \bar{b})(A, a) = (A, a)(L - b - a, \bar{b})$$

whence, using (R2)

$$\begin{aligned}(L - b, \bar{b})(A, a)(L - \bar{b}, b) &= (A + \bar{b}, \bar{b})(A' - b, \bar{b})(A, a)(L - \bar{b}, b)\\ &= (A + \bar{b}, \bar{b})(A, a)(L - b - a, \bar{b})(L - \bar{b} - a, b)(a + b, b)\\ &= (A + \bar{b}, \bar{b})(A, a)(a + b, b);\end{aligned}$$

by (R4) and (R1)

$$\begin{aligned}(A + \bar{b}, \bar{b}) &= (A - a + \bar{a}, \bar{a})^{-1}(a + \bar{b}, b)(A - a + \bar{a}, \bar{a})\\ &= (A, a)(a + b, b)^{-1}(A, a)^{-1},\end{aligned}$$

whence

$$(L - b, \bar{b})(A, a)(L - \bar{b}, b) = (A, a).$$

For (R9) observe first that, by (R2) and (R6)

$$\begin{aligned}(L - b, \bar{b})(A, a) &= (L - b, \bar{b})(A - b, a)(a + b, a)\\ &= (A - b, a)(L - b, \bar{b})(a + b, a)\end{aligned}$$

while by (R1)

$$(A', \bar{a})^{-1} = (A' - \bar{a} + a, a).$$

Combining and using (R2) gives

$$\begin{aligned}&(A', \bar{a})^{-1}(L - b, \bar{b})(A, a) =\\ &\quad = (L - \bar{a} - b, a)(L - b - a, \bar{b})(a + \bar{b}, \bar{b})(a + b, a).\end{aligned}$$

Now (R5) gives

$$(L - \bar{a} - \bar{b}, b)(L - \bar{a} - b, a) = \sigma(L - a - \bar{b}, b)$$

where $\sigma = (a, b, \bar{a}, \bar{b})$. By (R1) we have

$$(L - \bar{a} - b, \bar{b})^{-1}(L - \bar{a} - b, a) = \sigma(L - a - b, \bar{b})^{-1}$$

and

$$(L - \bar{a} - b, a)(L - b - a, \bar{b}) = (L - \bar{a} - b, \bar{b})\sigma,$$

thus

$$(A', \bar{a})^{-1}(L - b, \bar{b})(A, a) = (L - \bar{a} - b, \bar{b})\sigma(a + \bar{b}, \bar{b})(a + b, a).$$

By (R5) again,

$$\sigma(\bar{a} + \bar{b}, \bar{b})(\bar{a} + b, \bar{a}) = \sigma(a + \bar{b}, \bar{b}),$$

whence, using (R2) and (R1),

$$\begin{aligned}(A', \bar{a})^{-1}(L - b, \bar{b})(A, a) &= \\ &= (L - \bar{a} - b, \bar{b})(\bar{a} + \bar{b}, \bar{b})(\bar{a} + b, \bar{a})(a + b, a) \\ &= (\bar{L} - b, \bar{b}).\end{aligned}$$

This completes the proof of R9.

If $\sigma_1, \ldots, \sigma_h \in \Omega$, we say a relation $\sigma_1 \ldots \sigma_h = 1$ *holds modulo* N_2 provided $\tilde{\sigma}_1 \ldots \tilde{\sigma}_n \in N_2$; in other words, the relation is a consequence of (R1) through (R6). Since the free group F' with basis $X' = \{x_1, \ldots, x_{n-1}\}$ is a subgroup of F, it is natural to view $A' = \mathrm{Aut}(F')$ as a subgroup of A, and the set Ω' of Whitehead transformations of F' as a subset of Ω. It is clear what it means, for $\sigma_1, \ldots, \sigma_h \in \Omega'$, to say that $\sigma_1 \ldots \sigma_h = 1$ holds modulo N_2'. With this terminology, we may state McCool's refinement of (4.18).

Proposition 4.22. *Let u, v, w be cyclic words over F, with $u = w\sigma$, $v = w\tau$ for $\sigma, \tau \in \Omega$, with $|u|, |v| \leqslant |w|$ and either $|u| < |w|$ or $|v| < |w|$. Then there exist $\rho_1, \ldots, \rho_r \in \Omega$ such that*

(A) $\sigma^{-1}\tau = \rho_1 \ldots \rho_r$ *and that*
(B) $|u\rho_1 \ldots \rho_i| < |w|$ *for* $0 < i < r$. *Moreover,*
(C) *the relation* $\sigma^{-1}\tau = \rho_1 \ldots \rho_r$ *holds modulo* N_2;
(D) *if* $\sigma, \tau \in \Omega'$, *then* $\rho_1, \ldots, \rho \in \Omega'$, *and* $\sigma^{-1}\tau = \rho_1 \ldots \rho_r$ *modulo* N_2'.

□ The proof of (4.18) yields in each case a sequence $\rho_1, \ldots, \rho_r$ such that $\sigma^{-1}\tau = \rho_1 \ldots \rho_r$ and $|u\rho_1 \ldots \rho_i| < |w|$ for $0 < i < r$. We call such a sequence a *direct path*. In certain cases this path satisfies (A) and (B). However, certain of these paths are obtained by replacing some $\sigma = (A, a)$ by $\bar{\sigma} = (A', \bar{a})$, or $\tau = (B, b)$ by $\bar{\tau} = (B', \bar{b})$; if, say, $\sigma \in \Omega'$ then $x_n \notin A$ whence $x_n \in A'$ and $\bar{\sigma} \in \Omega'$, and the path obtained need not lie in Ω'. In each such case we obtain a second path that does lie in Ω'.

Note that, by symmetry, we may interchange σ and τ. This leaves us with three special cases to which the general case will be reduced. These are as follows: Case I; $\tau \in \Omega_1$; Case II; $\sigma, \tau \in \Omega_2$ and $A \cap B = \emptyset$; Case III; $\sigma, \tau \in \Omega_2$ and $A \subseteq B$. In Case I the lemma clearly holds with $\rho_1 = \tau$, $\rho_2 = \tau_1^{-1}\sigma\tau$. We enumerate subcases of II and III in such a way that if (A, a) and (B, b) lie in Subcase III.i, then (A, a) and $(B', \bar{b})$ lie in Subcase II.i.

Subcase	1	2	3	4	5
Case II. $A \cap B = \emptyset$	$b = \bar{a}$	$\bar{a} \in B'$, $\bar{b} \in A'$	$\bar{a} \in B'$, $\bar{b} \in A$	$a \in B$, $\bar{b} \in A'$	$b \neq \bar{a}, \bar{a} \in B$ $\bar{b} \in A$
Case III. $A \subseteq B$	$b = a$	$\bar{a} \in B$, $b \in A'$	$\bar{a} \in B$, $b \in A$	$\bar{a} \in B$, $b \in A'$	$b \neq a, \bar{a} \in B$, $b \in A$

For each case II.i, a path $\rho_1, \ldots, \rho_r$ satisfying (A) and (B) is given in the proof of (4.18). Inspection shows that each $\rho_i = (C, c)$ for some $C \subseteq A \cup B$, $c = a^{\pm 1}$, $b^{\pm 1}$; it follows that if $\rho, \tau \in \Omega'$, then each $\rho_i \in \Omega'$, whence $\rho_1, \ldots, \rho_r \in \Omega'$. To establish that $\sigma^{-1}\tau = \rho_1 \cdots \rho_r$ holds modulo N_2', we modify the chain that will be given below by replacing L by $L' = X' \cup X'^{-1}$ and taking all complements within L'. To establish (C), in each case a chain of equations establishing that $\sigma^{-1}\tau = \rho_1 \cdots \rho_r$ is exhibited such that it can be seen by inspection that each step is effected by a relation of one of the types (R1) through (R9).

For each case III.i, the pair σ, $\bar{\tau}$ falls under II.i, yielding a path $\rho_1' \cdots \rho_n'$ as above, with $\sigma^{-1}\bar{\tau} = \rho_1' \cdots \rho_n'$. From this equation, which holds modulo N_2, we obtain suitable $\rho_1, \ldots, \rho_n$ and a proof again that (A) through (D) hold. For convenience, we treat the cases in the order II.1, III.1, ..., II.5, III.5.

Case II.1. Here $r = 1$, $\rho_1 = (A + B - a, \bar{a})$.

The chain of equations is the following:

$$(A, a)^{-1}(B, \bar{a}) = (A - a + \bar{a}, \bar{a})(B, \bar{a}) = (A + B - a, \bar{a}).$$

Case III.1. Again $r = 1$, $\rho_1' = (A + B' - a, \bar{a})$.

By II.1 we have that $\sigma^{-1}\tau = \rho_1'$ modulo N_2. We take $\rho_1 = (A' \cap B + a, a)$, and, using the above equation, obtain the following chain:

$$\begin{aligned}(A, a)^{-1}(B, a) &= (A, a)^{-1}(B', \bar{a})(L - \bar{a}, a)\\ &= (A + B' - a, \bar{a})(L - \bar{a}, a)\\ &= (A' \cap B + a, a).\end{aligned}$$

Case II.2. $\rho_1 = (B, b), \rho_2 = (A, a)^{-1}$.

Chain: $(A, a)^{-1}(B, b) = (B, b)(A, a)^{-1}$.

Case III.2. $\rho'_1 = (B, \bar{b}), \rho'_2 = (A, a)^{-1}$,

$\rho_1 = (B, b), \rho_2 = (A, a)^{-1}$.

Chain:
$$\begin{aligned}(A, a)^{-1}(B, b) &= (A, a)^{-1}(B', \bar{b})(L - \bar{b}, b)\\ &= (B', \bar{b})(A, a)^{-1}(L - \bar{b}, b)\\ &= (B, b)(L - b, \bar{b})(A, a)^{-1}(L - \bar{b}, b)\\ &= (B, b)(A, a)^{-1}.\end{aligned}$$

Case II.3. $\rho_1 = (B, b), \rho_2 = (A + B - b, a)^{-1}$.

Chain:
$$\begin{aligned}(A, a)^{-1}(B, b) &= (B, b)(B, b)^{-1}(A, a)^{-1}(B, b)\\ &= (B, b)(A + B - b, a)^{-1}.\end{aligned}$$

Case III.3. $\rho'_1 = (B', \bar{b}), \rho'_2 = (A + B' - \bar{b}, a)^{-1}$;

$\rho_1 = (B, b), \rho_2 = (A' \cap B + \bar{b}, \bar{a})^{-1}$.

Chain:
$$\begin{aligned}(A, a)^{-1}(B, b) &= (A, a)^{-1}(B', \bar{b})(L - \bar{b}, b)\\ &= (B', \bar{b})(A + B' - \bar{b}, a)^{-1}(L - \bar{b}, b)\\ &= (B, b)(L - b, \bar{b})(A + B' - \bar{b}, a)^{-1}(L - \bar{b}, b)\\ &= (B, b)(A' \cap B + \bar{b}, \bar{a})^{-1}.\end{aligned}$$

Case II.4. $\rho_1 = (A + B - a, b), \rho_2 = (A, a)^{-1}$;

this is obtained from II.3 by interchanging σ and τ.

Case III.4. $\rho'_1 = (A + B' - a, \bar{b}), \rho'_2 = (A, a)^{-1}$.

$\rho_1 = (A' \cap B + a, b), \rho_2 = (A, a)^{-1}$.

Chain:
$$\begin{aligned}(A, a)^{-1}(B, b) &= (A, a)^{-1}(B', \bar{b})(L - \bar{b}, b)\\ &= (A + B' - a, \bar{b})(A, a)^{-1}(L - \bar{b}, b)\\ &= (A' \cap B + a, b)(L - b, \bar{b})(A, a)^{-1}(L - \bar{b}, b)\\ &= (A' \cap B + a, b)(A, a)^{-1}.\end{aligned}$$

Case II.5. There are two cases (see Case 4 in the proof of (4.18)).

Case II.5a $|w(B, \bar{a})| < |w|$.

Here $\rho_1 = (A + B - a, \bar{a})$, $\rho_2 = (a, \bar{b}, \bar{a}, b)$, $\rho_3 = (B - \bar{a} + a - b + \bar{b}, a)$.

$$\begin{aligned}\text{Chain: } (A, a)^{-1}(B, b) &= (A - a + a, a)(B, \bar{a})(B - \bar{a} + a, a)(B, b)\\ &= (A + B - a, \bar{a})(B - \bar{a} + a, a)(B, b)\\ &= (A + B - a, \bar{a})(a, \bar{b}, \bar{a}, b)(B - \bar{a} + a - b + \bar{b}, a).\end{aligned}$$

Case II.5b $|w(A, \bar{b})| < |w|$. By symmetry we have $\rho_1 = (A - a + \bar{a}, \bar{b})$, $\rho_2 = (a, \bar{b}, \bar{a}, b)$, $\rho_3 = (A + B - \bar{b}, \bar{b})$.

Case III.5a $|w(B', \bar{a})| < |w|$.

$$\rho_1' = (A + B' - a, \bar{a}),\ \rho_2' = (a, b, \bar{a}, \bar{b}),\ \rho_3' = (\bar{a} + a - \bar{b} + b, a)$$
$$\rho_1 = (A' \cap B + a, a),\ \rho_2 = (a, b, \bar{a}, \bar{b}),\ \rho_3 = (B + \bar{b} - b + \bar{a} - a, a).$$

$$\begin{aligned}\text{Chain: } (A, a)^{-1}(B, b) &= (A, a)^{-1}(B', \bar{b})(L - \bar{b}, b)\\ &= (A + B' - a, \bar{a})(a, b, \bar{a}, \bar{b})(B' - \bar{a} + a - \bar{b} + b, a)\\ &\quad (L - \bar{b}, b)\\ &= (A' \cap B + a, a)(L - a, \bar{a})(a, b, \bar{a}, \bar{b})(B' - \bar{a} + a - \bar{b}\\ &\quad + b, a)(L - \bar{b}, b)\\ &= (A' \cap B + a, a)(a, b, \bar{a}, \bar{b})(L - b, \bar{b})(B' - a + a -\\ &\quad \bar{b} + b, a)(L - \bar{b}, b)\\ &= (A' \cap B + a, a)(a, b, \bar{a}, \bar{b})(B + \bar{a} - a + \bar{b} - b, \bar{a})\end{aligned}$$

Case III.5b $|w(A, b)| < |w|$.

$$\rho_1' = (A - a + \bar{a}, b),\ \rho_2' = (a, b, \bar{a}, \bar{b}),\ \rho_3' = (A + B' - b, \bar{b}).$$
$$\rho_1 = (A - a + \bar{a}, b),\ \rho_2 = (a, b, \bar{a}, \bar{b}),\ \rho_3 = (A' \cap B + b, b).$$

$$\begin{aligned}\text{Chain: } (A, a)^{-1}(B, b) &= (A, a)^{-1}(B', \bar{b})(L - \bar{b}, \bar{b})\\ &= (A - a + \bar{a}, b)(a, b, \bar{a}, \bar{b})(A + B' - b, \bar{b})(L - \bar{b}, b)\\ &= (A - a + \bar{a}, b)(a, b, \bar{a}, \bar{b})(A' \cap B + b, b).\end{aligned}$$

The treatment of special cases is now complete. For the general case, if none of $A \cap B = \emptyset$, $A \subseteq B$, $B \subseteq A$ holds, we have as in the proof of (4.18) that some $|w(P(x), x)| < |w|$, and, interchanging σ and τ if necessary, we can assume that $x = a$ or $x = \bar{a}$, hence that $|w\pi| < |w|$ for π one of $(A \cap B, a)$, $(A \cap B', a)$, $(A' \cap B, \bar{a})$, or $(A' \cap B', \bar{a})$. It follows that $|w\pi| < |w|$ for π one of $(A \cap B, a)$, $(A \cap B', a)$, $(A' \cap B, \bar{a})$, or $(A \cup B, a)$. For π of the latter form, let $u_1 = w\pi$, hence $u_1 = u\sigma^{-1}\pi$. By II.1 or III.1 we have that $\sigma^{-1}\pi = \rho_1$ holds modulo N_2 for some $\rho_1 \in \Omega$, and indeed $\rho_1 \in \Omega'$ if $\sigma, \tau \in \Omega'$. Now II or III gives $\pi^{-1}\tau = \rho_2 \cdots \rho_r$ in accordance with the lemma, whence $\sigma^{-1}\tau = \rho_1 \cdots \rho_r$ as required. □

An immediate consequence of (4.12) is the following.

Proposition 4.23. *Let $U = (u_1, \ldots, u_m)$, $V = (v_1, \ldots, v_m)$, and $W = (w_1, \ldots, w_m)$, all u_i, v_i, w_i elements of F, and let $\sigma, \tau \in \Omega$ be such that $u_i = w_i\sigma$, $v_i = w_i\tau$ for $1 \leqslant i \leqslant m$. Defining $|W| = \Sigma|w_i|$, suppose that $|U|, |V| \leqslant |W|$ and either $|U| < |W|$ or $|V| < |W|$. Then there exist $\rho_1, \ldots, \rho_r \in \Omega$ such that the relation $\sigma^{-1}\tau = \rho_1 \cdots \rho_r$ holds modulo N_2 and that $|U\rho_1 \cdots \rho_i| < |W|$ for $0 < i < r$.*

□ Let F^* have basis $X^* = \{x_1, \ldots, x_{n+1}\}$; then all $u_i, v_i, w_i \in F \subseteq F^*$. Define cyclic words

$$u = (u_1 x_{n+1} \cdots u_m x_{n+1}),\ v = (v_1 x_{n+1} \cdots v_m x_{n+1}),\ w = (w_1 x_{n+1} \cdots w_m x_{n+1})$$

in F. Then $u = w\sigma$, $v = w\tau$, $|u|, |v| \leqslant |w|$, and either $|u| < |w|$ or $|v| < |w|$. By (4.22) there exist $\rho_1, \ldots, \rho_r \in \Omega'$ such that the relation $\sigma^{-1}\tau = \rho_1 \cdots \rho_r$ holds modulo N_2, and that $|u\rho_1 \cdots \rho_i| < |w|$ for $0 < i < r$. But $|u\rho_1 \cdots \rho_i| < |w|$ implies $|U\rho_1 \cdots \rho_i| < |W|$. □

Proposition 4.24. *Let $U = (u_1, \ldots, u_m)$, all $u_i \in F$, let $\alpha \in \mathrm{Aut}(F)$, and $|U\alpha| \leqslant |U|$. Then $\alpha = \rho_1 \cdots \rho_r$, $\rho_i \in \Omega$, such that $|U\rho_1 \cdots \rho_i| \leqslant |U|$ for $1 \leqslant i \leqslant r$, with strict inequality unless $|U\alpha| = |U|$.*

□ This follows from (4.23) exactly as (4.17) followed from (4.18). □

Proposition 4.25. *Let $U = (u_1, \ldots, u_m)$, $V = (v_1, \ldots, v_m)$, all $u_i, v_i \in F$. Then it is decidable whether there exists $\alpha \in \mathrm{Aut}(F)$ such that $U\alpha = V$.*

□ This follows from (4.15) exactly as (4.19) followed from (4.18). □

The following is McCool's primary result on presentations for the automorphism groups of free groups.

Proposition 4.26. *For F free of finite rank, $A = \mathrm{Aut}(F)$ has a finite presentation*

$$A = (\Omega; R).$$

More informally, A is generated by the set Ω of Whitehead transformations and every relation among the elements of Ω follows from relations among the elements of Ω_1 together with relations of the forms (R1) *through* (R6).

□ It suffices to show that if $\sigma_1, \ldots, \sigma_n \in \Omega$ and $\sigma_1 \cdots \sigma_n = 1$, then this relation is a consequence of the relations R. Let $U = (x_1, \ldots, x_n)$ and $U_i = U\sigma_1 \cdots \sigma_i$; thus $U_0 = U_k = U$. Let $m = \max\{|U_i|\} \geqslant n$; we argue by induction on m and on the number of U_i with $|U_i| = m$. If $m = n$, then each $\sigma_i \in \Omega_1$, and $\sigma_1 \cdots \sigma_n = 1$ is a relation among elements of Ω_1. If $m > n$ and i is the last index with $|U_i| = m$, then $1 < i < m$ and $|U_{i-1}| \leqslant |U_i|$, $|U_{i+1}| < |U_i|$. By (4.22), $\sigma_i\sigma_{i+1} = \rho_1 \cdots \rho_k$ modulo N_2 for some $\rho_j \in \Omega$, and such that $|U_{i-1}\rho_1 \cdots \rho_j| < |U_i| = m$ for $0 < j \leqslant k$. Thus the given relation follows modulo N_2 from the relation $\sigma_1 \cdots \sigma_{i-1}\rho_1 \cdots \rho_k\sigma_{i+2} \cdots \sigma_h$. Now this relation has either $m' < m$ or else $m' = m$ with fewer occurrences of the value m, whence, by the inductive hypothesis, it is a consequence of the relations R. It follows that $\sigma_1 \cdots \sigma_h = 1$ is a consequence of R. □

McCool (1973) derives from (4.17) the presentation for $A = \mathrm{Aut}(F)$ given by Nielsen (1924). As generators Nielsen takes a subset $\Omega^0 = \Omega_1^0 \cup \Omega_2^0$ of Ω, comprising certain Nielsen transformations. Specifically, Ω_1^0 consists of the permutations (x_i, x_j) for all $i \neq j$ and (x_i, x_i^{-1}) for all i. The set Ω_2^0 consists of all

$$(x_i + x_j, x_j): x_i \mapsto x_i x_j, \text{ for } i \neq j, \text{ and all}$$

$$(x^{-1} + x_j^{-1}, x_j^{-1}): x_i \mapsto x_j x_i, \text{ for } i \neq j.$$

It is clear that Ω_1^0 generates A_1 and that Ω^0 generates A. Nielsen takes for defining relations a set $R^0 = R_1^0 \cup R_2^0$ where R_1^0 defines A_1 and where R_2^0 consists essentially of all relations in McCool's set R_2 that involve only the generators in Ω^0.

To prove that Nielsen's R^0 is a full set of defining relations McCool modifies Nielsen's presentation by Tietze transformations. First he adjoins as new generators the inverses of the elements in Ω_2^0, adjoining the obvious defining relations. Second, he adjoins all (A, a) not already present (that is, with $|A| > 2$) introducing for each a defining relation of the form $(A, a) = (a_1 + a, a) \cdots (a_r + a, a)$ where $a_1, \ldots, a_r$ and a are the distinct elements of A. He then uses these last relations, and induction on $|A|$ for the (A, a) involved, to show that all relations in R_2 follow.

Nielsen observed also that $\mathrm{Aut}(F)$ is in fact generated by any set of generators for A_1 together with a single element from Ω_2. Thus A is generated by the permutations (x_1, x_2), (x_1, x_1^{-1}), $(x_1, x_2, \ldots, x_n)$ together with the transformation $x_1 \mapsto x_1 x_2$; Nielsen gave a set of defining relations in terms of these generators. B. H. Neumann (1932) reduced the number of generators to three. (For these last matters, see Coxeter-Moser 1965, p. 85; Magnus-Karrass-Solitar 1966, p. 162.)

From a result of Nielsen (1924) and Magnus (1934), $IA(F)$ is the normal closure in $\mathrm{Aut}(F)$ of the single element $\alpha = (x_1 + x_1^{-1} + x_2, x_2): x_1 \mapsto x_2^{-1} x_1 x_2$. Thus from either of the above presentations for $\mathrm{Aut}(F)$ a presentation for $\mathrm{Aut}(F)/IA(F) \simeq \mathbb{GL}(n, \mathbb{Z})$ can be obtained by adding the further defining relation $\alpha = 1$.

We remark that the special question of deciding whether some $\alpha \in \mathrm{Aut}(F)$ carries given $W = (w_1, \ldots, w_n)$ into a sequence W' of basis elements was already resolved by an earlier theorem of Federer and Jónsson (2.26 above). Even so, the present method is usually easier to apply; for example, a very brief calculation shows that no Whitehead transformation diminishes the length of the word $xyx^{-1}y^{-1}$, or the word x^2 (viewed as cyclic words in the basis elements x, y), whence it follows that neither element of F is a member of any basis.

Hoare (preprint) has obtained a substantial simplification of the proof of Whitehead's Theorem, and also of McCool's finite presentation of $\mathrm{Aut}(F)$ for F a finitely generated free group, by analyzing the geometry of the star graph (coinitial graph).

5. *Stabilizers in* Aut(*F*)

We next examine the stabilizer in $\mathrm{Aut}(F)$ of a given set of words or cyclic words. Before turning to a far reaching result of McCool we mention some more special results.

One might expect that if w were a sufficiently irregular word containing all the generators, then its stabilizer A_w would be small, or even trivial; as an extreme example, in the free group of rank 1 the stabilizer of any non-trivial element is trivial. On the other hand results of Nielsen and Zieschang, which we cite below, show that in certain important special cases A_w can be very large. The first of these results is the following, due to Nielsen (1918); see also Stebe (1972, p. 117).

Proposition 5.1. *Let F be a free group of rank 2 with a basis $\{x, y\}$, and let w be the cyclic word determined by the commutator $[x, y]$. Then every automorphism of F carries w into w or into w^{-1}, whence A_w is the group $SA(F)$ of proper automorphisms of F, of index 2 in* Aut(F).

□ It is routine to verify that every elementary Nielsen automorphism carries w into w or w^{-1}, with the proper automorphisms fixing w and the improper ones carrying w into w^{-1}. □ See also Malcev (1962).

It is well known that no analogous result holds for free groups of rank greater than 2 (see Magnus-Karrass-Solitar, p. 165). This is contained in the following.

Proposition 5.2. *Let F be a free group of rank at least 2 and w a non-trivial element of F, with (w) the associated cyclic word. Then the image $\bar{A}_{(w)}$ of $A_{(w)}$ has infinite index in $\bar{A} =$ Aut$(F)/JA(F)$ except in the case that w has the form $w = [x, y]^k$, $k \neq 0$, where $\{x, y\}$ is a basis for F.*

□ Suppose $\bar{A}_{(w)}$ has finite index. Then the orbit $\{(w)\alpha\colon \alpha \in \text{Aut}(F)\}$ is finite, and the lengths of the $(w)\alpha$ are bounded, say $|(w)\alpha| < B$ for all $\alpha \in \text{Aut}(F)$. Clearly w must involve all generators in any basis for F. Suppose that a, a^{-1}, b, c are distinct elements of $X^{\pm 1}$, and that (w) has a part bc^{-1}. If α is the automorphism $\alpha\colon b \to ba$, then α^N inserts N letters a between b and c^{-1}, none of which can cancel. Thus $|(w)\alpha^N| \geqslant N$, unbounded for increasing N, contrary to $|(w)\alpha^N| < B$. Fixing a, we conclude that if $b \neq a, a^{-1}$, then (w) has no part bc^{-1} for $c \neq a, a^{-1}, b$. But (w) reduced has no part bb^{-1}. We conclude that some $a^i \neq 1$ lies between each pair of successive occurrences of letters b, c^{-1} other than a, a^{-1}. The same with a and b exchanged shows that all $i = \pm 1$. Now every alternate letter is a or a^{-1}; similarly, every alternate letter is b or b^{-1}. Moreover, if (w) contained a part aba, then, for $\alpha\colon a \to ab$, the transformation α^N would yield $|(w)\alpha^N| \geqslant N$, as before. Thus, after a permutation of a, a^{-1}, b, b^{-1}, $w = [a, b]^k$, $k \neq 0$. Finally, $\{a, b\}$ is a basis, for if X contained a further element c, then as before $\alpha^N\colon a \to ac^N$ would yield $(w)\alpha^N$ of unbounded length. □

In certain cases, $A_{(w)}$ can be very small, and in a sense this is a typical situation.

Suppose that, for w in F, free of rank n, every Whitehead transformation α that is neither a permutation of $X^{\pm 1}$ nor an inner automorphism increases the length of (w). Then it follows from (4.17) that $\bar{A}_{(w)}$ is contained in the image in $\bar{A}$ of the subgroup of Aut(F) consisting of automorphisms that permute $X^{\pm 1}$, whence $|\bar{A}_{(w)}| \leqslant n!2^n$. The two smallest examples are (1) $w = x^3y^3$ with $\{x, y\}$ a basis, where $|\bar{A}_{(w)}| = 2$; and (2) $w = x^2y^2x^{-1}y^{-1}$ with $\{x, y\}$ a basis, where $|\bar{A}_{(w)}| = 1$.

As a different sort of converse to (5.1), it was shown by Dehn, Magnus, and Nielsen (see Magnus, 1930) that if F is free of rank 2 with basis $\{x, y\}$ and an endomorphism α of F fixes $w = [x, y]$, then α is an automorphism. Zieschang (1968) showed that if F has a basis $\{x_1, \ldots, x_{2g}\}$ and $w = [x_1, x_2] \cdots [x_{2g-1}, x_{2g}]$, then every endomorphism that fixes w is an automorphism. The determination of $\bar{A}_{(w)}$ for w of the latter form, or for $w = x_1^2 \cdots x_n^2$, corresponds to a classical problem arising in topology and analysis upon which little progress had been made until the result (5.5) of McCool.

Zieschang (1962) studies A_w for $w = x_1^{a_1} \cdots x_n^{a_n}$, all $a_i \geq 1$, in the free group F with basis $\{x_1, \ldots, x_n\}$. As noted, the case that all $a_i = 2$ (and $n \geq 3$) is difficult. If all $a_i = 1$, hence $w = x_1 \cdots x_n$, it was shown by Artin (1947) that A_w is a braid group B. If all $a_i > 2$, it was shown by Zieschang (1962) that A_w consists of all automorphisms that have the form $x_i \mapsto u_i x_{i\pi} u_i^{-1}$, for π a permutation, that belong to the braid group B.

Zieschang (1962) also shows that two elements $w = x_1^{a_1} \cdots x_n^{a_m}$ and $z = x_1^{b_1} \cdots x_n^{b_n}$ of a free group with basis $\{x_1, x_2, \ldots\}$, where all $a_i, b_i \geq 2$, are equivalent under an automorphism of F if and only if $m = n$ and the b_i are a permutation of the a_i.

□ We sketch a proof of this. Clearly if the latter condition is fulfilled, w and z are equivalent. Suppose now that w and z are equivalent. By inspection, the length of neither can be diminished by a Whitehead transformation. By (4.17), $|w| = |z|$ and there is a sequence of words $w_0 = w, w_1, \ldots, w_t = z$ such that all $|w_i| = |w|$ and that each $(w_{i+1}) = (w_i)\alpha_i$ for some Whitehead transformation α_i. For each x_j, let c_{ij} be the number of occurrences of letters x_j and x_j^{-1} in w_i, and let C_i be the ordered set $(c_{i1}, c_{i2}, \ldots)$. Now if α_i permutes $X^{\pm 1}$, clearly C_{i+1} is a permutation of C_i. If $\alpha_i = (A, a)$ where $a = x_k^{\pm 1}$, then clearly all the c_{ij} are unchanged for $j \neq k$. Since also $|w| = \sum_j c_{ij}$ is unchanged, it follows that c_{ik} also is unchanged, and $C_{i+1} = C_i$. We conclude that $C_0 = (a_1, \ldots, a_n, 0, 0, \ldots)$ is a permutation of $C_t = (b_1, \ldots, b_n, 0, 0, \ldots)$. □

Zieschang (1962) computes the group A_w for all words $w = x^a y^b$ in the free group F of rank 2 with basis $\{x, y\}$.

□ We give a version of his argument. Without loss of generality, we may suppose, $a, b \geq 0$. We may put aside the case $w = 1$, and if either $a = 1$ or $b = 1$, then w is a basis element and we may suppose $w = x$. Thus we may suppose that either $w = x^a$, $a \geq 1$, or $w = x^a y^b$, $a, b \geq 2$. We treat separately five cases.

Case 1: $w = x^a$, $a \geq 1$. If θ fixes w it must fix its unique a-th root x. Since $x\theta = x$ and $y\theta$ must generate F, $y\theta$ must have the normal form $y\theta = x^h y^{\pm 1} x^k$. Thus $\alpha: y \mapsto xy$ and $\beta: y \mapsto yx^{-1}$ are a basis for a free abelian subgroup A' of A_w, of rank 2, and A_w is the split extension of A' by the involution $\varepsilon: y \mapsto y^{-1}$ where conjugation by ε exchanges α and β.

Case 2: $w = x^a y^b$, $a, b > 2$, $a \neq b$. No Whitehead transformation except permutations fixes the length of the cyclic word (w), and only the trivial permutation fixes (w). Thus A_w consists entirely of inner automorphisms, and is an infinite cyclic group generated by $\omega = \kappa_w$, carrying each element u of F into wuw^{-1}.

Case 3: $w = x^a y^a$, $a > 2$. Here there is a single non-trivial permutation $\pi: x \leftrightarrow y$ preserving (w), yielding an outer automorphism $\alpha = \pi\kappa_{x^a}$; $x \mapsto x^a y x^{-a}$,

$y \mapsto x$ carrying w into itself. Now $\alpha^2 = \omega$, whence A_w is infinite cyclic with generator α.

Case 4: $w = x^2y^b$, $b > 2$. Here there are essentially two sequences of Whitehead transformations preserving the length of (w) and with non-trivial product. The first is $\sigma_1, \ldots, \sigma_b, \pi$ where $\sigma_1 = \cdots = \sigma_b = \sigma: x \mapsto xy^{-1}$ and $\pi: y \mapsto y^{-1}$. Now $\sigma^b\pi: x \mapsto xy^b$, $y \mapsto y^{-1}$ carries w into xy^bx; thus $\alpha = \sigma^b\pi\kappa_x: x \mapsto x^2y^bx^{-1}$, $y \mapsto xy^{-1}x^{-1}$ is in A_w. The other sequence is $\tau_1 = \cdots = \tau_n = \tau: x \mapsto y^{-1}x$ followed by π, with $\tau^b\pi: x \mapsto y^bx$, $y \mapsto y^{-1}$ carrying w into $y^bxy^bxy^{-b}$. However, the element $\tau^b\pi\kappa_{xy^b}$ of A_w is again α. Now $\alpha^2 = \omega$, whence again A_w is infinite cyclic with generator α.

Case 5: $w = x^2y^2$. The image $\bar{A}_w$ of A_w under the natural map from Aut(F) onto $\mathbb{GL}(2, \mathbb{Z})$ stabilizes the vector $\bar{w} = (2, 2)$. By Nielsen's result (4.5) the kernel of this map is the group of inner automorphisms of F, whence it follows that if B is any subgroup of A_w mapping onto $\bar{A}_w$, then $A_w = JB$ where J is the set of inner automorphisms in A_w. In fact, J is infinite cyclic with generator ω and is central in A_w.

In $\mathbb{GL}(2, \mathbb{Z})$, the transformation $\bar{\alpha} = \begin{pmatrix} 0 & 1 \\ 1 & 0 \end{pmatrix}$, with determinant -1, stabilizes (2,2). Calculation shows that if any transformation $T = \begin{pmatrix} p & q \\ r & s \end{pmatrix}$ with determinant $+1$ stabilizes (2,2), then $T = \bar{\beta}^q = \begin{pmatrix} q+1 & q \\ -q & -(q-1) \end{pmatrix}$ where $\bar{\beta} = \begin{pmatrix} 2 & 0 \\ -1 & 1 \end{pmatrix}$. Thus $\bar{\alpha}$ and $\bar{\beta}$ generate $\bar{A}_w$. Calculation shows that the elements $\alpha: x \mapsto x^2y^2x^{-1}$, $y \mapsto xy^{-1}x^{-1}$ and $\beta: x \mapsto x^2y$, $y \mapsto y^{-1}x^{-1}y$ of Aut(F) belong to A_w. Since α and β map onto $\bar{\alpha}$ and $\bar{\beta}$, the group B generated by α and β maps onto $\bar{A}_w$. It follows that α, β, and γ generate A_w.

Let $\gamma: x \mapsto x^2yx^{-2}$, $y \mapsto x$. Then calculation shows that $\alpha^2 = \gamma^2 = \omega$ and that $\alpha\gamma = \beta\omega$, whence A_w is generated by α and γ. Now $\bar{A}_w = A_w/J$ has generators $\bar{\alpha}$ and $\bar{\gamma}$ satisfying relations $\bar{\alpha}^2 = \bar{\gamma}^2 = 1$, and since $\bar{\beta} = \bar{\alpha}\bar{\gamma}$, has infinite order, $A_w = (\bar{\alpha}, \bar{\gamma}; \bar{\alpha}^2 = \bar{\gamma}^2 = 1)$. Now each element of A_w has uniquely the form $\omega^m\delta$ for δ a product of alternate factors α and γ. From this it follows that A_w has a presentation $(\alpha, \gamma, \omega: \alpha^2 = \gamma^2 = \omega)$, and hence that $A_w = (\alpha, \gamma; \alpha^2 = \gamma^2)$. □

The following result was established by Dyer and Scott (1975).

Proposition 5.3. *If F is a finitely generated free group and α an automorphism of F of finite order, then the set of elements of F fixed by α is a free factor of F.* □

The following observation was made by Shenitzer (1955).

Proposition 5.4. *Let F be a free group with basis X and w an ordinary or cyclic word of minimal length under the action of* Aut(F). *If exactly n elements of X occur in w, then at least n elements of X occur in every $w\alpha$ for α in* Aut(F).

□ By (4.17) there is a chain $w\alpha = u_0, u_1, \ldots, u_t = w$ where each $u_{i+1} = u_i\alpha_i$ for some Whitehead transformation σ_i and where each $|u_{i+1}| \leqslant |u_i|$. If $w\alpha$ contained fewer elements of X than w, some u_{i+1} would have to contain more elements of X than u_i. This would require that $\sigma_i = (A, x^{\pm 1})$ for some x from X that does not occur in u_i but does occur in u_{i+1}. But then u_{i+1} would be the result of inserting one or more occurrences of $x^{\pm 1}$ in u_i, contrary to the fact that $|u_{i+1}| \leqslant |u_i|$. □

The two preceding results imply the following.

Proposition 5.5. *Let F be free with basis X and w an ordinary word of minimal length under the action of* Aut(F) *and which contains every element of X. Then the stabilizer of w in* Aut(F) *is torsion-free.*

☐ The hypothesis implies that X is finite. Let α be an element of finite order in the stabilizer of w. By (5.3.) the fixed point set H of α is a free factor of F. Now w is in H, while by (5.4.) w is not contained in any proper free factor of F. It follows that $H = F$ and hence $\alpha = 1$. ☐

Note that if F has basis $\{x, y\}$ and w is the cyclic word $w = (xyx^{-1}y^{-1})$, then w is fixed by the automorphism $\alpha: x \mapsto y^{-1}, y \mapsto x$, of order 4. However, one can assert the following.

Proposition 5.6. *If w is a cyclic word of minimal length containing all the elements of a basis for F, and α an automorphism of finite order n that fixes w, then n divides $|w|$.*

☐ Let $W = \{w_1, \ldots, w_m\}$ be the ordinary words that correspond to w; then m divides $|w|$. Let G be the group generated by α. Since no non trivial element of G fixes any of the w_i, each orbit under the action of G on W has length n. Thus n divides m and therefore $|w|$. ☐

We now give a very important theorem of McCool (1975) concening stabilizers in Aut(F) of a finite sequence of cyclic words.

Proposition 5.7. *Let F be free with finite basis X and let $U = (u_1, \ldots, u_m)$ be a finite sequence of cyclic words over X. Let A_U be the subgroup of $A =$ Aut(F) stabilizing each of the cyclic words $u_1, \ldots, u_m$. There exists an effective procedure associating with each such U a finite presentation for A_U.*

☐ We shall construct effectively a finite 2-complex K whose fundamental group is isomorphic to A_U. To begin we may suppose that U is minimal in the sense that $|U| = |u_1| + \cdots + |u_m|$ cannot be diminished by any automorphism of F. As vertex set K^0 for K we take the set of all $V = U\alpha$, α in A, such that $|V| = |U|$. This set is obviously finite, and by Whitehead's theorem it can be determined effectively. We now form the 1-skeleton K^1 of K by introducing a directed edge $e = e(V, \tau)$ from V to $V\tau$ whenever V and $V\tau$ are in K^0 and τ is in Ω; we take $e^{-1} = (V\tau, \tau^{-1})$. Again it is clear that K^1 is finite and that its construction is effective.

We next define a morphism φ from the groupoid of paths in K^1 into a free group Φ with basis Ω by assigning to each edge $e = e(V, \tau)$ the label $e\phi = \tau$. We complete the construction of K as follows: if p is a (reduced) loop in K^1 whose label $p\phi$ is one of the relators in the set R of (4.26), we attach a 2-cell with boundary p.

The identity on Ω induces a homomorphism θ from Φ onto A. If p is a loop at U in K, then $p\phi\theta$ is evidently an element of A_U. Moreover, in view of (4.26), if p and p' are homotopic loops at U in K, then $p\phi\theta = p'\phi\theta$. Thus $\phi\theta$ induces a homomorphism $\bar{\phi}$ from $\pi(K; U)$ into A_U.

Since U is minimal, it follows from (4.17) that if $|U\alpha| = |U|$ for some α in A, then $\alpha = \tau_1 \cdots \tau_g$ where the τ_i are in Ω and each $U\tau_1 \cdots \tau_i$ is in K^0. Thus there is a loop p at U in K with $p\phi\theta = \alpha$. This shows that $\bar{\phi}$ is an epimorphism.

It remains to show that $\bar{\phi}$ is a monomorphism, that is, that if p is a loop at U in

K with $p\phi\theta = 1$, then p is homotopic to 1 in K. Let such p be a product $p = e_1 \cdots e_k$ of edges e_i with labels $e_i\phi = \tau_i$ in Ω. Let Z be the set of all cyclic words of length 2, that is, $Z = (x_i x_j; i \leqslant j)$, and let $z(p) = \max\{|Z\tau_1 \cdots \tau_i| : 0 \leqslant i \leqslant k\}$. We argue by induction on $z(p)$.

Inspection shows that Z is minimal, whence the initial case of the induction is that where $z(p) = Z$. It is easily seen that $|Z\alpha| = |Z|$ for α in A in fact implies that α is in Ω_1. Thus $z(p) = Z$ implies that all $|Z\tau_1 \cdots \tau_i| = |Z|$ whence all $\tau_1 \cdots \tau_i$ are in Ω_1 and therefore all τ_i are in Ω_1. It follows that the relation $\tau_1 \cdots \tau_k = 1$ in A is a consequence of the relators r from R_1 of (4.26). Since all $|U\tau_1 \cdots \tau_i| = |U|$, it follows from the construction of K that p is homotopic to 1 in K.

For the inductive step we suppose that $z(p) > |Z|$ and that the conclusion holds for all p' such that $z(p') < z(p)$. Let $W = (U^z, Z) = (U, \ldots, U, Z)$, where the part U is repeated $z = z(p)$ times. We write $U_i = U\tau_1 \cdots \tau_i$, $Z_i = Z\tau_1 \cdots \tau_i$ and $W_i = W\tau_1 \cdots \tau_i$; evidently $W_i = (U_i^z, Z_i)$ and $|W_i| = z|U_i| + |Z_i| = z|U| + |Z_i|$.

Let h be the largest index such that $|Z_h| = z$; since $Z_0 = Z_h = Z$, $0 < h < k$. It will suffice to show that p is homotopic to p' such that the value z is assumed by $|Z_i'| = |Z\tau_1' \cdots \tau_i'|$ only for those indices $i < h$ for which $|Z_i| = z$. From the choice of h we have that $|W_{h-1}| \leqslant |W_h|$ and $|W_{h+1}| < |W_h|$. From (4.18, 4.26) it follows that R contains a relator of the form $r = \tau_h\tau_{h+1}(\sigma_1 \cdots \sigma_t)^{-1}$ such that all $|W_{h-1}\sigma_1 \cdots \sigma_j| < |W_h|$ for $1 \leqslant j \leqslant t$. We propose to obtain p' from p by replacing the two edges $e_h e_{h+1}$ of p by a path with label $\sigma_1 \cdots \sigma_t$; to show that there is such a loop p' in K, homotopic to p, it remains to show that all $|U_{h-1}\sigma_1 \cdots \sigma_j| = |U|$ for $1 < j < t$.

For this, we have that $|W_{h-1}\sigma_1 \cdots \sigma_j| < |W_h|$, that is, $z|U_{h-1}\sigma_1 \cdots \sigma_j| + |Z_{h-1}\sigma_1 \cdots \sigma_j| \leqslant z|U| + z$; it follows that $z|U_{h-1}\sigma_1 \cdots \sigma_j| < z|U| + z(p)$. Suppose that $|U_{h-1}\sigma_1 \cdots \sigma_j| \geqslant |U| + 1$; then we should have $z(|U| + 1) < z|U| + z$, a contradiction. This completes the proof. □

McCool obtains in a similar way an analogous result for the subgroup of A effecting a permutation of the u_i and u_i^{-1} lying within a prescribed group; and he obtains analogous results for ordinary words instead of cyclic words.

In the case that U consists of a single cyclic quadratic word, McCool (unpublished) has shown that $\text{Aut}(F) \simeq \pi_1(K_0)$ where K_0 is a finite 2-complex constructed as in the proof of (5.7), but now with an edge from a vertex V to $V\tau$ only in case τ is an elementary Nielsen transformation.

An important consequence of McCool's results concerns mapping class groups (for a discussion of these see Magnus-Karrass-Solitar, pp. 172–179). Let M be a closed 2-manifold; then the mapping class group $\mathcal{M}(M)$ is defined to be the group of all autohomomorphisms of M modulo the subgroup of those deformable to the identity. By a theorem of Nielsen (1927), (see also Harvey and Maclachlan (to appear)) $\mathcal{M}(M)$ is isomorphic to $\text{Out}(\pi(M))$, the group of all automorphisms of $\pi(M)$ modulo inner automorphisms. Now the fundamental group $\pi(M)$ has a presentation with a single relator, $\pi(M) = (X; r)$; by another theorem of Nielsen (1927) every automorphism of $\pi(M)$ is induced by an automorphism of the free group F with basis X, which must necessarily leave the normal closure N of r invariant. (A proof of this result of Nielsen has been given by Zieschang (1966), and a proof by small cancellation theory has been given by Schupp (unpublished).)

By a theorem of Magnus (II.5.8 below), such an automorphism of F must carry r into a conjugate of r or r^{-1}. Let A_U be the stabilizer of the unordered couple $U = \{(r), (r)^{-1}\}$ where (r) and $(r)^{-1}$ are the cyclic words determined by r and r^{-1}, and let Out_U be A_U modulo the group of inner automorphisms of F. Then we have a map f from Out_U onto $\text{Out}(\pi(M))$ and so onto $\mathcal{M}(M)$. The kernel K of this map has been determined by Birman (1969): apart from trivial cases it is the image of $\pi(M)$ under a natural and explicit injection g. Thus, in all interesting cases, we have an exact sequence

$$1 \to \pi(M) \to \text{Out}_U \to \mathcal{M}(M) \to 1.$$

It follows that $\mathcal{M}(M)$ is finitely presented, and that such a presentation can be obtained effectively. Analogous results hold in the more general case that M is the quotient space of the hyperbolic plane under action of a Fuchsian group.

Hatcher and Thurston (unpublished), using Morse theory, have obtained a general formula yielding uniformly a finite presentation for each of these groups.

6. *Equations over Groups*

The problem of adjunction of elements to groups was introduced by B. H. Neumann (1943), in analogy with the corresponding problem in the theory of fields. For example, given a group G and an element g of G, one may ask if G can be embedded in a group H such that g is the square of some element x of H, $g = x^2$. More generally, let W be a set of elements $w_j = w_j(\gamma_1, \ldots, \gamma_m; \xi_1, \ldots, \xi_n)$ in the free group Φ with basis the set of distinct elements $\gamma_1, \ldots, \gamma_m, \xi_1, \ldots, \xi_n$, let G be a given group and $g_1, \ldots, g_m$ given elements of G. Then one asks for all homomorphisms ϕ from Φ into a group H containing G such that all $\gamma_i\phi = g_i$ and all $w_j\phi = 1$. It is natural to refer to the *system W of equations* $w_j(g_1, \ldots, g_m; \xi_1, \ldots, \xi_n) = 1$ with *coefficients* g_i in G and *unknowns* ξ_k and to speak of the set of $x_k = \xi_k\phi$ as a 'solution'.

A variant of this problem is that of the solution of *equations in a group G*, that is, with the further restriction that $H = G$ and so that the elements $x_k = \xi_k\phi$ are to be found in G itself, and a further specialization concerns systems of equations $w_j = w_j(\xi_1, \ldots, \xi_n)$ *without coefficients*. These latter problems, to which we shall return, have been studied almost exclusively in the case that W consists of a single equation $w = 1$, and that the group G is free.

The first important result on the adjunction problem is a theorem of B. H. Neumann (1943) concerning the adjunction of roots.

Proposition 6.1. *Let G be any group and, for an index set I, let g_i, for all i in I, be elements of G and m_i be positive integers. Then G can be embedded in a group H containing elements x_i such that, for all i in I, $x^{m_i} = g_i$.*

□ Obvious arguments reduce the problem to the solution of a single equation $\xi^m = g$. Let C be a cyclic group with generator x and of order mn if g has finite order n, otherwise of infinite order. Then the subgroups $A = \mathrm{Gp}(x^m)$ of C and $A' = \mathrm{Gp}(g)$ of G are isomorphic. By a theorem of Schreier (1927), the free product H of C and G with A and A' amalgamated according to the isomorphism carrying x^m into g contains C and G isomorphically; moreover, in H, one has $x^m = g$. □

A second important result in this area is a theorem of Higman, Neumann, and Neumann (1949).

□ **Proposition 6.2.** *Let G be any group and, for an index set I, let g_i and g'_i be elements of G. Then G can be embedded in a group H containing an element x such that, for each i in I, $x^{-1}g_ix = g'_i$, if and only if there exists an isomorphism from $\mathrm{Gp}\{g_i\}$ onto $\mathrm{Gp}\{g'_i\}$ carrying each g_i onto g'_i.* □

The necessity of the condition is obvious, and shows that equations over groups do not always have solutions. The sufficiency again involves, classically, free products with amalgamation, and is indeed the prototype for the extensive and important theory of what are called HNN-extensions, which will be treated later (see IV. 2 below). We accordingly defer the proof of (6.1) and (6.2), and of further results in this direction, which for the most part depend on special but very basic techniques to be treated later.

A very comprehensive result of Gerstenhaber and Rothaus (1962) shows, by topological means, that if a group G can be embedded in a compact connected Lie group then a system $w_1 = 1, \ldots, w_n = 1$ of n equations over G in n unknowns $\xi_1, \ldots, \xi_n$ has a solution provided the determinant of the exponent sums e_{ij} of the ξ_j in the w_i does not vanish. Application of this result yields a partial solution to a problem attributed to Kervaire by Magnus-Karrass-Solitar (p. 403) and to Laudenbach by Serre (Problems, Conference Canberra, 1973). Let $G = (X; R)$ and $G^* = (X^*; R^*)$ where X^* contains one additional generator not in X and R^* contains one additional relator; the problem asks whether $G \neq 1$ implies that $G^* \neq 1$. The observation that this problem, in the case that G is finite, could be solved by such methods was brought to our attention (indirectly) by A. Casson (unpublished); the details of the argument below are due to P. Neumann.

Proposition 6.3. *Let G be a finite group, X an infinite cyclic group, and N the normal closure of a single element in the free product $G * X$. If $G \neq 1$, then $(G * X)/N \neq 1$.*

□ Let X have generator x and let N be the normal closure of an element $w = g_1x^{e_1} \cdots g_nx^{e_n}$, where each g_i is in G and each e_i is in $\mathbb{Z}$. If the exponent sum $e = e_1 + \cdots + e_n$ is not ± 1, the image of x in $G^* = (G * X)/N$ is evidently not trivial. We may suppose then that $e = 1$.

Let G be embedded in a unitary group U. Since U is arcwise connected we can, for each $i = 1, \ldots, n$, define a path $\gamma_i \colon [0, 1] \to U$ such that $\gamma_i(0) = 1$ and $\gamma_i(1) = g_i$. We now define a map $\gamma \colon U \times [0, 1] \to U$ by setting $\gamma(h, t) = \gamma_1(t)h^{e_1} \cdots \gamma_n(t)h^{e_n}$ for all $h \in U$, $t \in [0, 1]$. Since $e = 1$, $\gamma(\cdot, 0)$ is the identity map on U, and it follows from easy topological considerations that $\gamma(\cdot, 1)$ maps U onto all of U. Therefore there exists h in U such that $\gamma(h, 1) = g_1h^{e_1} \cdots g_nh^{e_n} = 1$. It follows that there exists a map ϕ from G^* into U that is the identity on G and carries x into h. Since $G^*\phi$ contains G, if $G \neq 1$ then $G^* \neq 1$. □

We turn now to the problem of the solution of equations in groups. This problem had an independent origin, in mathematical logic, and, specifically, in the theory of models. The *elementary language* of group theory may be taken to consist of first order logic in which the sole non-logical constant is a binary function symbol, to be interpreted as denoting group multiplication; this elementary language, in particular, does not permit one to speak directly of set theoretical concepts such as the order of an element, or of subgroups or chains of subgroups. The *elementary theory* of a set of groups then consists of all sentences in the elementary language of groups that are valid in all groups of the set. There are two natural and long unsolved problems in this context: first, do free groups of distinct ranks have distinct elementary theories, and, second, is the elementary theory of the class of all free groups decidable?

We digress to discuss briefly the first question. It is a trivial observation that among free groups those of rank 0 (that is, that are trivial) are distinguished by the elementary sentence $\forall x.(xx = x)$, and that those of rank at most 1 (that is, that are cyclic) are distinguished by the sentence $\forall x \forall y.(xy = yx)$. But it is not known if, for example, exactly the same elementary sentences are true in free groups of rank 2 and in free groups of rank 3. By way of comparison, we cite a sentence which, as observed by Tarski (unpublished), singles out among free abelian groups precisely those of rank at most 2; this is the following sentence:

$$\exists x\, \exists y\, \forall z\, \exists u.\ (u^2 = z \text{ or } u^2 = zx \text{ or } u^2 = zy \text{ or } u^2 = zxy).$$

Partial results on the problem under discussion have been obtained by Sacerdote (1972, 1973).

We turn now to the question of the decidability of the theory of a set of free groups: given a sentence in the elementary language of group theory, can we decide if it holds in all groups in the set? If the set is empty or contains only trivial groups an affirmative answer is immediate. For the set of free groups of rank 1 (that is, of infinite cyclic groups), the positive solution of this problem is a classical result of Pressburger (1929). By way of comparison, we remark that the elementary theory of free abelian groups, and indeed of all abelian groups, is decidable, while that of free non-abelian semigroups is known to be undecidable.

It is in this contex that R. L. Vaught (unpublished) posed the following test problem: does the sentence

$$\forall x\, \forall y\, \forall z.\ (x^2 y^2 z^2 = 1 \Rightarrow xy = yx)$$

hold in all free groups? A positive solution was obtained by Lyndon (1959) and further results were obtained by G. Baumslag (1959), Schenkman (1959), Stallings (1959), Schützenberger (1959), and by Lyndon and Schützenberger (1962) who showed that any elements x, y, z of a free group that satisfy a relation $x^m y^n z^p = 1$ for $m, n, p \geqslant 2$ are all contained in a cyclic subgroup. Schützenberger (1959) showed also that the equation $[x, y] = z^k$, for $k > 1$, in a free group implies that x, y, and z lie in a cyclic subgroup, whence in fact $z = 1$; otherwise put, no non-trivial commutator in a free group is a proper power. This result follows also from later more general results of Karrass, Magnus, and Solitar (1960) and G. Baumslag and Steinberg (1961).

The analogous problem for free metabelian groups (that is, groups F/F'' where F'' is the second derived group of the free group F) was studied by Baumslag and Mahler (1965) and by Lyndon (1966). The solution of Vaught's problem was extended by Wicks (1974) to free products. He showed that if G is a free product of two groups, each without elements of order 2 and satisfying the condition that $x^2y^2z^2 = 1$ implies $xy = yx$, then G also satisfies this condition.

Similar problems for semigroups have been studied by Lentin (1965, 1972); see also Nivat (1970). A formula for semigroups, established by Lentin, has been proved for groups by Piollet (1974); this is closely related to the Hoare-Karrass-Solitar version of the Riemann-Hurwitz formula (III.7.8 below).

The solution of the problem of Vaught can be restated as follows: if x, y, z are elements of a free group F such that $x^2y^2z^2 = 1$, then the free subgroup U of F generated by x, y, and z has rank at most 1. This can be generalized as follows. Let W be any system of equations $w_j(\xi_1, \ldots, \xi_n) = 1$, and define the *inner rank* $\mathrm{Ir}(W)$ of the system to be the maximum rank of subgroups U of free groups F generated by solutions $x_k = \xi_k\phi$ of the system W. If Φ is the free group with basis $\xi_1, \ldots, \xi_n$ and G the quotient group obtained from Φ by setting all $w_j = 1$, then $\mathrm{Ir}(W)$ is evidently the maximal rank of free homomorphic images of G. One is led thus to define the inner rank $\mathrm{Ir}(G)$ of an arbitrary group G to be the maximal rank of free homomorphic images of G; this is in a sense dual to the concept of 'outer rank', that is, the minimal rank of free groups F such that G is a homomorphic image of F, or, more simply, the least cardinal of a set of generators for G. This concept has arisen independently in the study of fundamental groups of 3-manifolds, and has led Jaco (1972) to the following theorem, for which he gives a geometric proof.

Proposition 6.4. *Let $G = G_1 * G_2$, free product. Then* $\mathrm{Ir}(G) = \mathrm{Ir}(G_1) + \mathrm{Ir}(G_2)$.

□ First, let ϕ_i $(i = 1, 2)$ map G_i onto F_i free, of maximal rank $\mathrm{Ir}(G_i)$. Then ϕ_1 and ϕ_2 have a common extension to a map ϕ from G onto $F = F_1 * F_2$, free, of rank $\mathrm{Ir}(G_1) + \mathrm{Ir}(G_2)$. This shows that $\mathrm{Ir}(G) \geqslant \mathrm{Ir}(G_1) + \mathrm{Ir}(G_2)$. For the opposite inequality, suppose that ϕ is a map of G onto F free of maximal rank $\mathrm{Ir}(G)$. If $F_1 = G_1\phi$ and $F_2 = G_2\phi$, we have an induced map of $F_1 * F_2$ onto F, whence it follows that the rank of F is no greater than that of $F_1 * F_2$, that is, that $\mathrm{Ir}(G) \leqslant \mathrm{Ir}(G_1) + \mathrm{Ir}(G_2)$. □

It is known (see Zieschang (1962)) that if w is strictly quadratic in $x_1, \ldots, x_n$, then $\mathrm{Ir}(w) = [n/2]$, the greatest integer in $n/2$. This follows from (7.13) below, but in the case that $w = x_1^2 \cdots x_n^2$ it is contained in a more general result of Lyndon, Morris Newman, and McDonough (1973). We give a slightly stronger version (Lyndon 1973) of their result, which depends on a lemma from linear algebra.

Lemma 6.5. *Let q be an integer, $q > 1$, and $A = (\alpha_{ij})$ an n-by-m matrix with entries in a field K. We assume that K contains an element ω such that $\omega^q = -1$.*

Suppose that for all $i_1, \ldots, i_q$, where $1 \leqslant i_h \leqslant m$, one has

$$\textstyle\sum_{j=1}^{m} \alpha_{i_1 j} \cdots \alpha_{i_q j} = 0$$

Then rank$(A) \leqslant m/2$.

□ We may assume that V is a vector space over K with basis $e_1, \ldots, e_m$. If, for $1 \leqslant i \leqslant q$, $a_i = \sum_j \alpha_{ij} e_j$, we define

$$P(a_1, \ldots, a_q) = \textstyle\sum_{j=1}^{m} \alpha_{i_1 j} \cdots \alpha_{i_q j}.$$

A subset S of V will be called *null* if $P(a_1, \ldots, a_q) = 0$ for all $a_1, \ldots, a_q \in S$; since P is clearly multilinear, in this case the subspace N generated by S is null. We shall prove that if N is a null subspace of dimension n, then $n \leqslant m/2$.

The case $m = 1$ is trivial, and we argue by induction on m. We assume that $m \geqslant 2$, that $n > m/2$, and derive a contradiction; note that the hypotheses imply that $n \geqslant 2$. Let $a_1, \ldots, a_n$, as above, be a basis for N, and let $A = (\alpha_{ij})$. Clearly transformation of A by elementary row transformations or by permutation of columns does not alter the situation. Thus we may arrange that the upper lefthand corner of A has the form $\begin{pmatrix} 1 & 0 \\ 0 & 1 \end{pmatrix}$, and then that it has the form $\begin{pmatrix} 1 & \omega \\ 0 & 1 \end{pmatrix}$, hence that

$$A = \left(\begin{array}{cc|c} 1 & \omega & a_1' \\ 0 & 1 & a_2' \\ \hline \multicolumn{2}{c|}{0} & A' \end{array}\right)$$

Let V' be the subspace, of dimension $m - 2$, generated by $e_3, \ldots, e_m$. Then a_1', a_2' and $a_3, \ldots, a_n$ lie in V'. We show that $a_1', a_3, \ldots, a_n$ form a null set. First, if $b_1, \ldots, b_q$ come from this set and not all are a_1', then the first two components contribute nothing to $P(b_1, \ldots, b_q)$, whence its value is unaltered by replacing a_1' by a_1, and hence, by hypothesis, is 0. The case remains that all $b_j = a_1'$, but here, by hypothesis, $P(a_1, \ldots, a_1) = 0$, while $P(a_1, \ldots, a_1) = 1^q + \omega^q + P(a_1', \ldots, a_1')$, and, since $\omega^q = -1$, $P(a_1', \ldots a_1') = 0$.

Now the hypothesis that $n > m/2$ implies that $n - 1 > (m - 2)/2$, and by the induction hypothesis, the $n - 1$ elements of the null set $a_1', a_3, \ldots, a_n$ cannot be independent. Since the set $a_3, \ldots, a_n$ is by hypothesis independent, it follows that a_1' is a linear combination of these elements. Thus, by a further row transformation, we can arrange that $a_1' = 0$. But now $P(a_1, a_2, \ldots, a_2) = 0 + \omega.1^{q-1} = \omega \neq 0$, a contradiction. □

We venture the conjecture that if r is the least positive number such that K contains elements $\omega_1, \ldots, \omega_r \neq 0$ with $\omega_1^q + \cdots + \omega_r^q = 0$, then, for A as above, rank $(A) \leqslant m/r$.

For the application below we note that if K has finite characteristic p and if $q \equiv p$ (modulo 2), we may always take $\omega = -1$.

Proposition 6.6. *Let $N > 1$ be an integer and $u_1, \ldots, u_m$ elements of a free group such that $u_1^N \cdots u_m^N = 1$. Then the group generated by $u_1, \ldots, u_m$ has rank $n \leqslant m/2$.*

□ Let the free group F generated by $u_1, \ldots, u_m$ have a basis $x_1, \ldots, x_n$. Let $\bar{F} = F/F'$, where $F' = [F, F]$; then $\bar{F}$ is free abelian with basis the images $\bar{x}_i$ of the x_i. Let $\bar{\bar{F}} = \bar{F}/\bar{F}^p$, p a prime; then $\bar{\bar{F}}$, written additively, is a vector space over $\mathbb{Z}_p$ with basis the images $\bar{\bar{x}}_i$ of the x_i. Let $u_j \equiv \prod_{i=1}^n x_i^{a_{ij}}$ (modulo F'); then in $\bar{\bar{F}}$ the images $\bar{\bar{u}}_j = \sum_{i=1}^n \alpha_{ij}\bar{\bar{x}}_i$, where the α_{ij} are the images in $\mathbb{Z}_p$ of the integers a_{ij} from $\mathbb{Z}$. Let $A = (\alpha_{ij})$. If the m-by-n matrix A had rank less than n, then the elements $\bar{\bar{u}}_j$ would generate a proper subspace of $\bar{\bar{F}}$, contrary to the fact that the u_j generate F. Thus $\operatorname{rank}(A) = n$, and it remains to show that $\operatorname{rank}(A) \leqslant m/2$.

We choose a prime p dividing N and write $N = qM$ where $q = p^e$ for some $e > 1$ and p does not divide M. Let $\tilde{R}$ be the associative ring of polynomials over $\mathbb{Z}_p$ in non-commuting indeterminates $\tilde{X}_1, \ldots, \tilde{X}_n$, and let $\tilde{J}$ be the ideal in $\tilde{R}$ generated by the $\tilde{X}_i$. Let $R = \tilde{R}/\tilde{J}^{qp}$, and let X_i be the image of $\tilde{X}_i$ in R and J the image of $\tilde{J}$. (We note in passing that R is finite, with additive basis over $\mathbb{Z}_p$ consisting of all the monomials in the X_i of degree less than qp.)

The elements $1 + X_i$ of R have multiplicative inverses

$$(1 + X_i)^{-1} = 1 - X_i + \cdots + (-X_i)^{qp-1},$$

and hence generate a subgroup G of the multiplicative group of R. (Hence G is finite, and in fact a p-group of exponent p^{e+1}.)

Let μ be the homomorphism from F onto G defined by $x_i\mu = 1 + X_i$. It is easy to see that if $u_j \equiv \prod x_i^{a_{ij}}$ (modulo F'), then

$$x_i^a\mu = 1 + aX_i + C_i, \quad C_i \in J^2,$$
$$u_j\mu = 1 + \textstyle\sum a_{ij}X_i + C_j, \; C_j \in J^2.$$

Then

$$\begin{aligned} u_j^q\mu &= (1 + \textstyle\sum \alpha_{ij}X_i + C_j)^q \\ &= 1 + (\textstyle\sum \alpha_{ij}X_i + C_j)^q \\ &= 1 + (\textstyle\sum \alpha_{ij}X_i)^q, \end{aligned}$$

and

$$(u_j^N)\mu = 1 + M(\textstyle\sum \alpha_{ij}X_i)^q.$$

Thus

$$(u_1^N \cdots u_m^N)\mu = 1 + M \textstyle\sum_{j=1}^m (\sum_{i=1}^n \alpha_{ij}X_i)^q.$$

Since $u_1^N \cdots u_m^N = 1$, and p does not divide M, one has

$$\textstyle\sum_{j=1}^m (\sum_{i=1}^n \alpha_{ij}X_i)^q = 0.$$

The coefficient of $X_{i_1} \cdots X_{i_q}$ in $(\sum \alpha_{ij}X_i)^q$ is $\alpha_{i_1 j} \cdots \alpha_{i_q j}$, and thus in $\sum(\sum \alpha_{ij}X_i)^q$

is $P(a_{i_1}, \ldots, a_{i_q}) = \sum_j \alpha_{i_1 j} \cdots \alpha_{i_q j}$. Thus all $P(a_{i_1}, \ldots, a_{i_q}) = 0$, and, by the lemma, $\text{rank}(A) \leqslant m/2$. □

The result just obtained asserts that, if $N > 1$, then $\text{Ir}(x_1^N \cdots x_m^N) \leqslant m/2$; it is easy to see, setting $x_2 = x_1^{-1}$, $x_4 = x_3^{-1}$, and so forth, that this inequality is sharp.

The following corollary was raised as a problem; for $N = 2$, by Newman (see Lyndon and Newman, 1973), and proved by Lyndon, McDonough, and Newman (1973).

Corollary 6.7. *For every $n \geqslant 0$ and $N > 1$ there is a product of n N-th powers in a group G that is not expressible as a product of fewer than n N-th powers.*

□ By (6.6), if G is free with basis $x_1, \ldots, x_n$ and $x_1^N \cdots x_m^N = u_1^N \cdots u_m^N$, then, after transposing, we have that $n = \text{rank}(G) \leqslant (n + m)/2$, whence $n \leqslant m$. The proof of (6.6) shows in fact that, in the corollary, G may be taken to be a finite p group for any p dividing N. □

We have mentioned that every word strictly quadratic in $x_1, \ldots, x_n$ is equivalent, under an automorphism of F, to a word of one of the two forms $w = x_1^2 \cdots x_g^2$ $(g \leqslant n)$ or $w = [x_1, x_2] \cdots [x_{2g-1}, x_{2g}]$ $(2g \leqslant n)$. This is proved below (7.6) and also (7.14). We state a partial analog of (6.7).

Proposition 6.8. *If F is free with a basis of distinct elements $x_1, \ldots, x_{2g}$ and there are elements $u_1, \ldots, u_{2m}$ of F such that*

$$[x_1, x_2] \cdots [x_{2g-1}, x_{2g}] = [u_1, u_2] \cdots [u_{2m-1}, u_{2m}],$$

then $m \geqslant g$.

□ The proof is analogous to that of (6.6). □

In the same vein, we note that it was proved by Newman and Lyndon (1973) that, although $[x, y] = (x^{-1}y^{-1})^2(yxy^{-1})^2y^2$, the equation $[x, y] = u_1^2u_2^2$ does not admit any solution in general, and in particular for x and y distinct elements of a basis for a free group. We give two theorems that contain this result. To state the first we use the notation $F_1 = F$, $F_{n+1} = [F_n, F]$ for the descending central series of a group F.

Proposition 6.9. *If w is a product of two squares in a free group F and w is in F_n for some n, then the image of w in F_n/F_{n+1} is a square.*

□ Let $w = u^2v^2$ and $w \in F_n$. If $n = 1$ we have $w \equiv (uv)^2$ modulo F_2. Assume now that $n > 1$, whence $w \in F_2$, $(uv)^2 \equiv 1$ modulo F_2, and, since F/F_2 is torsion free, $uv = k \in F_2$. Now $v = u^{-1}k$ and $w = u^2(u^{-1}k)^2 = [u, k]k^2 \equiv k^2$ modulo F_3. Here, exceptionally, we have written $uku^{-1}k^{-1} = [u, k]$. We show by induction on $n \geqslant 2$ that $w \in F_n$ implies $k \in F_n$. This has been established for $n = 2$; assume it now for some $n \geqslant 2$. If $w \in F_{n+1}$ then $w \in F_n$ and, by the induction hypothesis, $k \in F_n$. But then $[u, k] \in F_{n+1}$, and from the equation $w = [u, k]k^2$ it follows that $k^2 \in F_{n+1}$. Since F_n/F_{n+1} is torsion free, $k \in F_{n+1}$. This completes the induction. Suppose now that $w \in F_n$, $n \geqslant 2$. We have shown that this implies that $k \in F_n$, whence $[u, k] \in F_{n+1}$ and $w = [u, k]k^2 \equiv k^2$ modulo F_{n+1}. □

We remark that it follows from this that, if $x_1, \ldots, x_n$ are elements of a basis for F, and $x_1 \neq x_2$, then $w = [[\cdots[[x_1, x_2], x_3]\cdots], x_n]$ is not a product of two squares.

The leading idea in the proof of the following theorem is due to McDonough (see Lyndon-McDonough-Newman, 1973).

Proposition 6.10. *Let F be a free group with a basis of distinct elements $x_1, \ldots, x_{2n}$. Then there exist elements $u_1, \ldots, u_m$ in F such that*

$$[x_1, x_2] \cdots [x_{2n-1}, x_{2n}] = u_1^2 \cdots u_m^2$$

if and only if $m \geqslant 2n + 1$.

□ We show first that this equation has a solution for $m = 2n + 1$ hence trivially for $m \geqslant 2n + 1$. We use the fact, already mentioned, that there is a representation $[x_1, x_2] = u_1^2 u_2^2 v^2$. We use also the easy fact (see, for example, Massey, Ch. I) that for any elements a, b, c of any group there are elements u, v, w such that $a^2[b, c] = u^2 v^2 w^2$. Suppose inductively that $[x_1, x_2] \cdots [x_{2n-3}, x_{2n-2}] = u_1^2 \cdots u_{2n-2}^2 v^2$. Then we may write

$$v^2[x_{2n-1}, x_{2n}] = u_{2n-1}^2 u_{2n}^2 v'^2.$$

For the converse, we suppose that the equation holds. Let $G = F/F''(F')^2$ (we may even set each $x^2 = 1$, to make G a finite 2-group). We write x_i and u_i also for the images of these elements in G. Let $c_{ij} = [x_i, x_j]$. Then each element u of G has a unique expression

$$u = \prod_{i=1}^n x_i^{a_i} \cdot \prod_{i<j} c_{ij}^{d_{ij}} \quad \text{for } a_i \in \mathbb{Z}, \quad d_{ij} \in \mathbb{Z}_2.$$

Then

$$u^2 = \prod x_i^{2a_i} \prod_{i<j} c_{ij}^{a_i a_j}.$$

Since all x_i^2 and all c_{ij} are in the center of G, we have

$$u_1^2 \cdots u_m^2 = \prod_{i=1}^n x_i^{2\Sigma_k a_{ik}} \prod_{i<j} c_{ij}^{\Sigma_k a_{ik} a_{jk}}.$$

If α_{ik} is the image of a_{ik} under the canonical map from $\mathbb{Z}$ onto $\mathbb{Z}_2$, if A is the matrix $A = (\alpha_{ij})$ over $\mathbb{Z}_2$, and $a_i = (\alpha_{i1}, \ldots, \alpha_{im})$ the i-th row of A, then from the relation $u_1^2 \cdots u_m^2 = [x_1, x_2] \cdots [x_{2n-1}, x_{2n}]$ we conclude that, taking inner products

$$a_i \cdot a_j = \begin{cases} 1 \text{ if } \{i, j\} = \{2h - 1, 2h\} \text{ for } 1 < h < n \\ 0 \text{ otherwise.} \end{cases}$$

We conclude $A.A^{\mathrm{Tr}} = B$, where A^{Tr} is the transpose of A, and B is the direct sum of n matrices of the form $\begin{pmatrix} 0 & 1 \\ 1 & 0 \end{pmatrix}$, and hence has rank $2n$. It follows that $\operatorname{rank}(A) \geqslant 2n$. But the equation $a_i.a_i = \sum_{j=1}^m a_{ij} = 0$.

for each i implies that the sum of the m columns of A is 0, whence rank$(A) \leqslant m - 1$. Therefore $m - 1 \geqslant 2n$. □

It is clear that every group G admits a homomorphism onto the trivial group, whence $\operatorname{Ir}(G) \geqslant 0$; alternatively, every system W of equations without coefficients admits a trivial solution. It is also easily decidable for G finitely generated whether G has $\operatorname{Ir}(G) \geqslant 1$, that is, whether G admits a homomorphism onto an infinite cyclic group; for this is the case if and only if $G/[G, G]$ has an element of infinite order. For W a system of equations in the finite set $\xi_1, \ldots, \xi_n$ and a_{ji} the coefficient sum of ξ_i in w_j, this is equivalent to the condition that the matrix (a_{ji}) have rank less than n. At the other extreme, if W is a finite set of equations in the finite set $\xi_1, \ldots, \xi_n$, and W is not trivial, it follows from (1.7) that $\operatorname{Ir}(W) < n$. If η is an element of some basis for Φ and all w_j are contained in the normal closure of η in Φ, then evidently the projection ϕ from Φ into Φ by setting $\eta \to 1$ defines a solution of rank $n - 1$, whence $\operatorname{Ir}(W) \geqslant n - 1$. Steinberg (1965) has proved the following partial converse.

Proposition 4.11. *If $W = \{w\}$ for w a non-trivial element of a free group Φ of rank n, then $\operatorname{Ir}(W) = n - 1$ if and only if w lies in the normal closure of an element in a basis for Φ.* □

Another result in this direction was obtained by Baumslag and Steinberg independently. See Baumslag and Steinberg (1965), Baumslag (1965), and Steinberg (1965).

Proposition 4.12. *Let $W = w$ where $w = w_1(\xi_1, \ldots, \xi_{n-1})\xi_n^k$ and w_1 is not a member of any basis for Φ, free on $\xi_1, \ldots, \xi_n$, where w_1 is not a proper power, and $k > 1$. Then $\operatorname{Ir}(W) < n - 1$.* □

The case $w = [\xi_1, \xi_2]\xi_3^k$ is contained in a result of Schützenberger cited above.

Stallings (1976) cites an example due to Lyndon of a 1-relator group $G = (x_1, \ldots, x_n; r)$, for r a product of $n(n-1)/2$ factors $[x_i^{a_{ij}}, x_j^{a_{ij}}]^{b_{ij}}$, $i < j$, where all a_{ij} are distinct and all $a_{ij}b_{ij} = 2^N$ for some fixed N. That has no non-abelian free quotient group.

We turn now to some generalities about solutions of systems of equations in a free group. First, we make two obvious observations.

Proposition 6.13. *If W is a set of words in the free group Φ, and $W' = W\alpha$ is the image of W under some automorphism α of Φ, then $\operatorname{Ir}(W') = \operatorname{Ir}(W)$.* □

Proposition 6.14. *If W is a set of words in the free group Φ, and W° is obtained from W by setting some generator ξ_i equal to 1, then $\operatorname{Ir}(W) \geqslant \operatorname{Ir}(W^\circ)$.* □

In connection with (6.13 and 6.14) we note that if ϕ is any solution for the system W, in that $W\phi = 1$, and $W' = W\alpha$, then $\phi' = \alpha^{-1}\phi$ is a solution for the system W'. Let ϕ be any solution, and define $|\phi| = \sum|\xi_i\phi|$, where length is taken relative to any fixed basis for the free group $U = \Phi\phi$. An elementary Nielsen transformation of Φ, of the form $\xi \mapsto \xi\eta$, where ξ and η are among the $\xi^{\pm 1}$, will be called a *regular* transformation *attached* to W if some cyclic conjugate of an element of W contains a part $(\xi\eta^{-1})^{\pm 1}$. A transformation of the form $\xi_i \mapsto 1$ will be called a *singular* transformation *attached* to W if ξ_i occurs in some (cyclically reduced conjugate of an) element w of W. Now, if W is not trivial and no $\xi_i\phi = 1$, then a sequence of regular elementary transformations attached to W carries W and ϕ into W' and ϕ' such that $|\phi'| \leqslant |\phi|$ and that some $\xi_i\phi' = 1$. Now ϕ' induces a solution ϕ'' of W'' obtained from W' by the singular transformation $\xi_i \mapsto 1$. Iteration of this process, which either decreases the number of ξ_i occurring in W or, leaving this number fixed, decreases $|\phi|$, must ultimately lead to W^* and ϕ^* where W^* is trivial. It is evident that $U = \Phi\phi = \Phi\phi^*$ and that $U = \Phi\phi^*$ has rank at most $n - s$, for s the number of singular transformations employed. Moreover, the value of ϕ^* can be chosen arbitrarily on the $n - s$ elements ξ_i in the new basis for Φ that have not been annihilated by singular transformations. We speak of a sequence of transformations $\tau_1, \ldots, \tau_t$ as being attached to W if, for $0 \leqslant i < t$, τ_i is a regular or singular transformation attached to $W\tau_1 \cdots \tau_{i-1}$. We have established the following.

Proposition 6.15. $\operatorname{Ir}(W) = n - s$, *where s is the minimum number of singular transformations in a sequence attached to W and reducing W to triviality.* □

The application of this proposition appears to be feasible only in the case that W is essentially quadratic; that is, that W consists of a set of powers $w = s^{m(s)}$ of elements from a set S such that each generator ξ_i occurs (as ξ_i^{+1} or ξ_i^{-1}) at most twice in the elements of S. For, in this case, the number of W' obtainable from W by sequences attached to W is finite. For this reason, and even more because of their importance in connection with the study of groups with planar Cayley diagrams and with Fuchsian groups, we turn special attention to quadratic sets.

7. Quadratic Sets of Word

Most of what follows is to be found in Hoare, Karrass, Solitar (1971, 1972), although, as they acknowledge, the ideas go back to Nielsen (1918) and are implicit in the standard procedure for classifying compact 2-manifolds (see for example Massey 1967). They had been used in a context similar to the present one by Lyndon (1959) and Zieschang (1964).

Let F be free with basis X and S a set of cyclic words over F. We call S *quadratic* over a subset X_0 of X if no element s of S contains any x from X (as x^{+1} or x^{-1}) except x in X_0, and if S contains such x at most twice. We call S *strictly quadratic* over X_0 if, moreover, each x in X_0 occurs in S exactly twice. For any subset S of a free group F with basis X, we define the *incidence graph* $J(S)$ to be the undirected graph with S as vertex set and an edge from s_1 to s_2 (with label x) whenever some element x in X occurs in both elements s_1 and s_2 of S. We call S *connected* just in case $J(S)$ is connected.

The following is obvious.

Proposition 7.1. *For some index set I, with $0 \notin I$, it is possible to partition X into sets X_0 together with X_i, for all i in I, and S into connected sets S_i, for all i in I, such that X_0 is the set of x in X that occur in no s in S, and that, for each i in I, X_i is precisely the set of x in X that occur in S_i.* □

For our purposes, this reduces the study of subsets S of F to the case that S is connected and contains all x in X.

We use the following lemmas.

Lemma 7.2. *Let T be an undirected tree containing some infinite path. Then it is possible to assign an orientation to the edges of T in such a way that T contains no infinite descending path and that T contains no maximal element.*

□ Let v_0 be any vertex of T; then there is an infinite path out of v_0. Let T_0 consist of the union of all infinite paths out of v_0. We orient T_0 upward out of v_0; by definition T_0, thus oriented, contains no maximal element, while every descending path in T_0 ends at v_0. Each component K of the complement of T_0 in T is attached to T_0 at a unique point v and, by the definition of T_0, contains no infinite path. We orient each such K upward toward v. It is now immediate that T, with the given orientation, contains no infinite descending chain and no maximal element. □

Lemma 7.3. *Let X_0 be a partially ordered subset of X satisfying the descending chain condition. For each x in X_0 let p_x and q_x be elements of F containing x' in X_0 only for $x' < x$. Then there is an automorphism of F carrying each x in X_0 into $p_x x q_x$.*

□ Let α be the endomorphism of F defined by setting $x\alpha = p_x x q_x$ for each x in X_0, and $x\alpha = x$ for each x in $X - X_0$. It suffices to construct an endomorphism β inverse to α. Clearly it is necessary and sufficient that $x\beta = (p_x\beta)^{-1}x(q_x\beta)^{-1}$ for each x in X_0, with $x\beta = x$ for all x in $X - X_0$. Because the order on X_0 satisfies the descending chain condition, it is possible to use the conditions above to give a recursive definition of β. □

The next three propositions deal with the three possibilities for S a connected quadratic set over X.

Proposition 7.4. *Let S be quadratic over X, connected, and infinite. Then some automorphism of F carries S into a subset of X.*

□ Let J be the incidence graph of S. By hypothesis, J is connected. Therefore there exists a maximal tree T in S containing all the vertices of J. Because T is infinite but locally finite, by König's Lemma, T contains an infinite path. We orient T in accordance with (7.2). Because T, oriented thus, contains no maximal element, each vertex s is joined to some higher vertex s' by an edge with label $x = x(s)$. We choose such an $x = x(s)$ for each s in S, and denote by X_0 the set of all such $x = x(s)$. Since S is quadratic, and x occurs both in s and s', it occurs exactly once in s whence (replacing s by s^{-1} if necessary) we can suppose that $s = p_x x q_x$ for some words p_x and q_x not containing x. The orientation on T induces an order on the set S of vertices, satisfying the descending chain condition, and hence on the set X_0 of elements $x(s)$ for s in S. From the definitions it follows that p_x and q_x contain x' in X_0 at most for $x' = x(s')$ where s' is immediately below s. Thus the conditions of (7.3) are satisfied, and the inverse of the automorphism given there carries each s into $x(s)$, and thus S into the subset X_0 of X. □

Proposition 7.5. *Let S be quadratic over X, but not strictly quadratic, finite, and connected. Then there is an automorphism of F carrying S into a subset of X.*

□ Let J and T be as before. Because S is not strictly quadratic, there exists s_0 in S containing a generator x_0 in X that occurs in no other s' in S. We orient T upward toward s_0. We choose $x_0 = x(s_0)$ in X_0, and the remaining $x = x(s)$ in X_0 as before. Since T is finite the induced order on X_0 again satisfies the descending chain condition, and the conclusion follows as before from (7.3). □

If S is any set of cyclic words in a free group F, we say that a Nielsen transformation α is *attached* to S if α is singular and deletes a letter that occurs in S or if α is regular and some occurrence of a letter introduced into S by α cancels in passing to the reduced from of of $S\alpha$; in the latter case, for certain letters x and y, $x\alpha = xy$ while some element of S has a part $(xy^{-1})^{\pm 1}$. If S is finite and quadratic, evidently α is attached to S if and only if $|S\alpha| \leqslant |S|$. We say that a sequence of Nielsen transformations $\alpha_1, \ldots, \alpha_n$ is attached to S if, for $1 \leqslant i \leqslant n$, α_i is attached to $S\alpha_1 \cdots \alpha_{i-1}$.

Proposition 7.6. *Let S be strictly quadratic over X, finite, and connected. Then some automorphism α of F carries S into $S' = S\alpha$ of the following sort: $S' = \{s_1, \ldots, s_n\}$ where $s_1 = x_1, \ldots, s_{n-1} = x_{n-1}$ and $s_n = x_1 \cdots x_{n-1}q$, where $x_1, \ldots, x_{n-1}$ are in X and q has either the form $q = [y_1, y_2] \cdots [y_{2g-1}, y_{2g}]$ or $q = y_1^2 \cdots y_g^2$, where the y_i are distinct elements of $X - \{x_1, \ldots, x_{n-1}\}$. Moreover, this can be accomplished by a sequence of transformations attached to S.*

□ We prove first only that S' can be obtained as described with q required only to be strictly quadratic in a subset X_0 of X not containing any of $x_1, \ldots, x_{n-1}$. If $n \leqslant 1$ there is nothing to prove. We argue by induction, supposing that $k < n$ and that $s_1 = x_1, \ldots, s_k = x_k$, with S' still strictly quadratic over some subset X_0 of X, and connected. If $k = n - 1$, the hypotheses imply that s_n contains each of $x_1, \ldots, x_k$ exactly once, and each other x_i that occurs at all exactly twice. A sequence of elementary transformations (attached to S') replacing x_1 by some conjugate of $x_1^{\pm 1}$ reduces s_n to the form $x_1 r$; and iteration of this process reduces s_n to the form $x_1 \cdots x_{n-1}q$, where q is strictly quadratic in X_0 as required. If $k < n - 1$, the connectedness of S' implies that s_{k+1} contains some x_{k+1} distinct from $x_1, \ldots$, x_k. We may suppose that $s_{k+1} = x_{k+1}u$, where u does not contain x_{k+1}. Now a sequence of transformations attached to S' carries s_{k+1} into x_{k+1} leaving $s_1, \ldots$, s_k unchanged. Moreover, the resulting system S'' is evidently strictly quadratic in some subset X_0 of X, finite, and connected. This completes the inductive proof of the assertion under consideration.

It remains to prove that if $w = pq$, where q is strictly quadratic in a set X_0 of generators that do not occur in p, then a sequence of transformations attached to w carries w into an element $w' = pq'$ where q' is of one of the two forms described above. We observe first that a sequence of transformations of the required sort carries $px^2[y, z]r$ into $px^2y^2z^2r$. Therefore, for an argument by induction on the length of q, it suffices to show that pq can be carried into one of the forms px^2q' or $p[x, y]q'$. If q contains some x in X_0 twice with the same exponent, we may suppose that $q = uxvxz$. We can carry xv into x, hence q into $q' = ux^2v^{-1}z$. Now carrying x into $u^{-1}xu$ transforms q' into $q'' = x^2uv^{-1}z$. In the remaining case each x in q occurs once as x^{+1} and once as x^{-1}. If we pick a pair $x^{\pm 1}$ and $x^{\mp 1}$ as close together as possible, some $y^{\pm 1}$ will occur between, with $y^{\mp 1}$ not between. After permuting x, x^{-1}, y, y^{-1} if necessary, we have that $q = uxvyzx^{-1}ty^{-1}s$. A transformation replacing vyz by y carries q into the form $q' = uxyx^{-1}t'y^{-1}s'$. A transformation replacing $x^{-1}t'$ by x^{-1} carries q into the form $q'' = u'xyx^{-1}y^{-1}s'$. Finally, conjugating x and y by u' yields $q''' = [x, y]\, u's'$. □

With any set S of cyclic words over the free group F with basis X we associate the *star graph* $\Sigma(S)$. (This graph is called the *coinitial graph* by Hoare-Karrass-Solitar. It appears implicitly in Neuwirth (1968) where L denotes the number of components of $\Sigma(S)$, and also in Santani (1967).) The vertex set of Σ is the set $L = X \cup X^{-1}$ of letters. An undirected edge is introduced, connecting vertices y_1 and y_2, for each occurrence in S of a part $y_1^{-1}y_2$ or $y_2^{-1}y_1$. (We count a cyclic word y of length 1 as containing an occurrence of a part yy, and hence giving rise to one edge joining y^{-1} to y.) We observe that $\Sigma(S)$ is the graph of the function $\phi_S(y_1, y_2) = y_1 \cdot y_2$ introduced in connection with Whitehead transformations (except that the x and x^{-1} have been exchanged) in that $y_1 \cdot y_2$ is exactly the number of edges joining y_1 and y_2 (or, properly, y_1^{-1} and y_2^{-1}).

A finite set S will be called *minimal* if no automorphism of F diminishes $|S| = \Sigma|s|$, $s \in S$. Note that if S is not connected, then $\Sigma(S)$ splits into components $\Sigma(S_i)$ where the S_i are the connected components of S; moreover, each x that does not occur in S gives rise to a pair of isolated point x and x^{-1} in $\Sigma(S)$. Even if S is connected and contains all the generators, $\Sigma(S)$ need not be connected. However, we have the following.

Proposition 7.7. *If S is connected, minimal, and contains all x in X, then $\Sigma(S)$ is connected.*

□ Suppose that $\Sigma(S)$ is not connected. Then the set L of vertices can be partitioned into two non-empty sets A and A' such that no edge joins a vertex of A to one of A', that is, with $A.A' = \varnothing$. If we had $A = A^{-1}$ and so also $A' = A'^{-1}$, then S could be partitioned into sets S_1 containing only generators that occur in A and S_2 containing only generators from A'; since S is connected, this is impossible. Therefore some a occurs in A with a^{-1} in A'. If σ is the Whitehead transformation $\sigma = (A, a)$, then by (4.16) $|S\sigma| - |S| = A.A' - a.L = -a.L < 0$, whence $|S\sigma| < |S|$, contrary to the minimality of S. We conclude that $\Sigma(S)$ is connected. □

Note that if S is quadratic there are at most two edges at each vertex and that if S is strictly quadratic, and contains all the generators, there are exactly two edges at each vertex, whence, if S also is finite, $\Sigma(S)$ is a union of cycles. We now establish a partial converse to (7.7).

Proposition 7.8. *Let S be finite and strictly quadratic and $\Sigma(S)$ connected. Then S is connected, minimal, and contains all the generators.*

□ It is immediate that S is connected and contains all the generators. Note that since Σ is a union of disjoint cycles, it is impossible to partition the vertex set L into two parts A and A' such that $A.A' = 1$. Suppose now that S were not minimal, hence by (4.17), that $|S\sigma| < |S|$ for some Whitehead transformation $\sigma = (A, a)$. By (4.16) we have $|S\sigma| - |S| = A.A' - a.L < 0$ and hence $A.A' < a.L = 2$.

Since $A.A' \neq 1$, this implies that $A.A' = 0$, contrary to the hypothesis that Σ is connected. We conclude that S is minimal. □

Recall that if S is finite and strictly quadratic then $|S\sigma| \leqslant |S|$ for σ an elementary Nielsen transformation just in case σ is attached to S. We write $k(S)$ for the number of components of $\Sigma(S)$, excluding isolated points.

Proposition 7.9. *If σ is an elementary Nielsen transformation attached to the finite strictly quadratic set S, then either $|S\sigma| = |S|$ and $k(S\sigma) = k(S)$ or $|S\sigma| = |S| - 2$ and $k(S\sigma) = k(S) - 1$.*

□ We may suppose that σ is given by $x \mapsto xy$ where S contains a part xy^{-1}; now S will contain a second part $(xz)^{\pm 1}$ for some z in L. If $z \neq y^{-1}$ then $|S\sigma| = |S|$, and parts $xy^{-1}t$ and $(xz)^{\pm 1}$ of S are replaced by parts xt and $(xyz)^{\pm 1}$ in S. Thus $\Sigma(S\sigma)$ is obtained from $\Sigma(S)$ by replacing arcs $z—x^{-1}—y^{-1}$ and $y—t$ by arcs $z—y^{-1}$ and $y—x^{-1}—t$. This clearly leaves $k(S)$ unchanged. If $z = y^{-1}$ then $|S\sigma| = |S| - 2$, and parts $xy^{-1}t$ and $(xy^{-1}s)^{\pm 1}$ of S are replaced by parts xt and $(xs)^{\pm 1}$ in S. Thus $\Sigma(S\sigma)$ is obtained by replacing the cycle $x^{-1}y^{-1}$, with two vertices x^{-1} and y^{-1}, and arc $t—y—s$ of $\Sigma(S)$ by the single arc $t—x^{-1}—s$. This clearly diminishes $k(S)$ by 1. □

For the sake of a later result we insert here a proposition dealing with a set S that is not reduced.

Proposition 7.10. *Let S be a finite and strictly quadratic set of cyclic words, but not reduced. Let S' be obtained by deleting a part xx^{-1} from S. Then $k(S') = k(S) - 1$, except in the case that xx^{-1} is an element of S.*

□ If xx^{-1} is not an element of S, then a part $yxx^{-1}z$ of S is replaced by a part yz in S'. Thus an arc $y^{-1}—x—z$ together with a cycle with a single vertex x^{-1} are replaced by a single arc $y^{-1}—z$. If xx^{-1} belongs to S, then two cycles, each with a single vertex x or x^{-1}, are lost. □

Proposition 7.11. *Let S be strictly quadratic and minimal, and let S' be the result of setting $x \mapsto 1$ for some x that occurs in S. Then either $|S'| = |S| - 2$ and $|k(S') - k(S)| \leqslant 1$ or else $|S'| = |S| - 4$ and $k(S') = k(S)$.*

□ Let S_1 be the possibly unreduced set obtained from S by setting $x \mapsto 1$. If S_1 is in fact reduced, then $S' = S_1$ and $|S'| = |S| - 2$. If S contains either two elements x and x^{-1}, or a single element x^2, then $\Sigma(S)$ contains a cycle xx^{-1} and $\Sigma(S')$ is obtained by deleting this cycle, whence $k(S') = k(S) - 1$. Otherwise, since S_1 is reduced, S contains parts $(uxv)^{\pm 1}$ and $(wxv)^{\pm 1}$ (where we do not exclude coincidences among $u^{\pm 1}, \ldots, z^{\pm 1}$) which are replaced in S' by parts $(uv)^{\pm 1}$ and $(wz)^{\pm 1}$. Thus arcs $u^{-1}—x—w^{-1}$ and $v—x^{-1}—z$ in $\Sigma(S)$ are replaced by arcs $u^{-1}—v$ and $w^{-1}—z$ in $\Sigma(S')$. If the two mentioned arcs occur on the same cycle and in the same sense in $\Sigma(S)$, then this is replaced by a different cycle in $\Sigma(S')$, and $k(S)$ is unchanged. If the two arcs appear on the same cycle but in opposite senses, then this cycle is replaced by two in $\Sigma(S')$, and $k(S') = k(S) + 1$. If the two arcs occur on different cycles of $\Sigma(S)$, these are replaced by a single cycle in $\Sigma(S')$, and $k(S') = k(S) - 1$.

We suppose now that S_1 is not reduced. Inspection shows that since S is minimal it cannot contain a part $(u^{-1}x^2u)^{\pm 1}$, a part $(u^{-1}v^{-1}xvu)^{\pm 1}$, or a pair of parts $(u^{-1}xu)^{\pm 1}$ and $(v^{-1}xv)^{\pm 1}$. It follows that S must contain parts $(uv^{-1}xvw)^{\pm 1}$ and $(zxt)^{\pm 1}$ going into reduced parts $(uw)^{\pm 1}$ and $(zt)^{\pm 1}$ in S'. Now arcs u^{-1}—v^{-1}—w and z^{-1}—x—v—x^{-1}—t of $\Sigma(S)$ are replaced by arcs u^{-1}—w and z^{-1}—t in $\Sigma(S')$, whence $k(S)$ is unchanged. □

Proposition 7.12. *Let q and q' be minimal strictly quadratic cyclic words, and suppose that q' is obtained from q by a sequence of transformations attached to q that contains exactly one singular transformation. Then $|q'| = |q| - 2$ or $|q'| = |q| - 4$.*

□ Since the hypothesis is not affected by applying to q any sequence of regular transformations attached to q, we may suppose that the sequence begins with a singular transformation $\alpha: x \mapsto 1$. If $q = x^2$ then $q' = 1$ and we are done. If $k(q\alpha) = k(q) = 1$, then $q\alpha$ is minimal and so $|q'| = |q\alpha|$; by (7.11), $|q'| = |q| - 2$ or $|q'| = |q| - 4$. The case remains that $k(q\alpha) \neq 1$; then, by (7.11), $k(q\alpha) = 2$ and $|q\alpha| = |q| - 2$. By (7.9) the sequence has the form $\alpha, \beta_1, \ldots, \beta_n$ where the β_i are regular and for some k, $|q\alpha\beta_1 \cdots \beta_{k-1}| = |q\alpha| = |q| - 2$ and $k(q\alpha\beta_1 \cdots \beta_{k-1}) = k(q\alpha) = 2$, while $|q\alpha\beta_1 \cdots \beta_k| = |q\alpha| - 2 = |q| - 4$ and $k(\alpha\beta_1 \cdots \beta_k) = k(q\alpha) - 1 = 1$. By (7.8) $q'' = q\alpha\beta_1 \cdots \beta_k$ is minimal, and the sequence $\beta_{k+1}, \ldots, \beta_n$ does not alter either q'' or $k(q'')$. Thus $|q'| = |q''| = |q| - 4$. □

Proposition 7.13. *If q is a minimal strictly quadratic cyclic word, then* $\mathrm{Ir}(q) = [|q|/4]$, *the greatest integer in* $|q|/4$.

□ It is easy to see, taking $x_2 \mapsto x_1^{-1}, x_4 \mapsto x_3^{-1}, \ldots$, and the last $x_n \mapsto 1$ if the number n of generators is odd, that $\mathrm{Ir}(q) \geqslant n/2$. For the converse, if $\mathrm{Ir}(q) = n - s$, then by (6.15) there is a chain of transformations attached to q, carrying q into 1, and containing s singular transformations. Thus we have a sequence $q_0 = q$, $q_1, \ldots, q_s = 1$ where each q_i is strictly quadratic and is obtainable from q_{i-1} by a sequence attached to q_{i-1} and containing exactly one singular transformation. Now additional regular transformations will carry q_i into some minimal q_i'. Clearly $|q_i'| \leqslant |q_i|$, while by (7.11) $|q_i'| \geqslant |q_{i-1}| - 4$, whence $|q_i| \geqslant |q_{i-1}| - 4$. It follows that $0 = |q_s| \geqslant |q_0| - 4s = |q| - 4s$, hence that $\mathrm{Ir}(q) = n - s \leqslant n - |q|/4 = n - n/2 = n/2$. □

Proposition 7.14. *Let S be a finite minimal strictly quadratic set of cyclic words. Then* $\mathrm{Ir}(S) = [|S|/4]$.

□ By a sequence of regular transformations attached to S we can suppose by (7.6) that S, still minimal, has the form $S = \{x_1, \ldots, x_p, x_1 \cdots x_p q\}$ for q minimal and strictly quadratic in the remaining basis elements $x_{p+1}, \ldots, x_n$. It is evident that $\mathrm{Ir}(S) = \mathrm{Ir}(q)$, whence the conclusion follows by (7.13). □

This proposition is stated in Zieschang (1965); see also Jaco (1972). An analogous but somewhat more delicate result has been obtained by Lentin (see 1969) in his study of equations in free semigroups; Piollet (1974) has obtained Lentin's formula for free groups, thereby giving a slightly sharper form of (7.14). See also Shapiro and Sonn (1974).

8. Equations in Free Groups

We turn now to equations in free groups that contain constants; examples show that the description of all solutions requires parameters that run over elements of a free group F and also parameters running through the set $\mathbb{Z}$ of integers. To attack this problem, Lyndon (1960) introduced the concept of an *R-group*, where R is any unital ring. Specifically, an R-group is to be a group G equipped with an operation of R on G, that is, a map $G \times R \mapsto G$, written $(g, r) \mapsto g^r$, and subject to the following axioms: $g^1 = g$, $g^{(r+s)} = g^r g^s$, $g^{(rs)} = (g^r)^s$, $(g^{-1}hg)^r = g^{-1}h^r g$. The category of R-groups can be viewed as the noncommutative analog of that of R-modules. The concept of $\mathbb{Z}$-group reduces simply to that of group. The possibility of raising a group element to a power that is a real number, not necessarily an integer, is familiar from the theory of Lie groups. Philip Hall (1957) has suggested, in connection with the multiplication formula for elements expressed as power products according to the *collection process*, the possibility of taking exponents from a ring R more general than $\mathbb{Z}$ that contains, along with each r, appropriate analogs of the binomial coefficients $\binom{r}{k}$ for all $k \in \mathbb{Z}$. Groups of this sort have been studied by Kargapolov, Remeslennikov, Romanovskii, Romankov, Curkin (1969), who have solved the word problem and a number of other algorithmic problems for certain such groups.

Lyndon considered only the case that R is the ring of all polynomials with integer coefficients in a finite set of indeterminates $v_1, \ldots, v_n$. It follows from general principles of universal algebra that there exists a free R-group (in the usual sense of universal algebra) F^* with given basis $x_1, \ldots, x_m$, and it is easy to see that F^* contains the ordinary free group F with the same basis. Now every assignment $v_1\phi = k_1, \ldots, v_n\phi = k_n$ of values $k_1, \ldots, k_n \in \mathbb{Z}$ to the indeterminates $v_1, \ldots, v_n$ determines a retraction ϕ from R onto $\mathbb{Z}$, and likewise a retraction ϕ' from F^* onto F. Lyndon proved the following.

Proposition 8.1. *Let R, F^*, and F be as above. Suppose that w is an element of F^* such that for each retraction ϕ: R onto $\mathbb{Z}$, with induced ϕ': F^* onto F, one has $w\phi' = 1$. Then $w = 1$.* □

Proposition 8.2. *For R and F^* as above, the word problem for F^* is solvable.* □

Lyndon (1970) applied these ideas to the solution of equations over free groups containing arbitrary constants but only a single unknown. Let Φ be free with basis $\xi_1, \ldots, \xi_n$ and let $w(\xi_1, \ldots, \xi_n) \in \Phi$. Let F be a free group with basis $X_1, \ldots, X_m$ and let $u_2, \ldots, u_n$ be given elements of F. The problem then is to determine all $x \in F$ such that setting $\xi_1\phi = x$, $\xi_2\phi = u_2, \ldots, \xi_n\phi = u_n$ determines $\phi: \Phi \to F$ such that $w\phi = 1$. More informally, given $u_2, \ldots, u_n \in F$ one asks for all $x \in F$ such that $w(x, u_2, \ldots, u_n) = 1$. A *parametric word* w is in this context an element of the free R-group F^* with basis $x_1, \ldots, x_m$, where R contains some sufficiently large number of indeterminates v_i. The *set of values* of a parametric word w is the set of elements $w\phi' \in F$ for all retractions ϕ': F^* onto F determined by retractions ϕ: R onto $\mathbb{Z}$. Lyndon obtained the following theorem.

Proposition 8.3. *Let R, F^*, F, w, and $u_2, \ldots, u_n$ be as above. Then there exists a finite set $W \subseteq F^*$ of parametric words such that the set of all values of elements $w \in W$ comprises exactly those $x \in F$ such that $w(x, u_2, \ldots, u_n) = 1$.* □

Lorents (1963) extended this result to finite systems of equations in one unknown, showing that the set of solutions is given by a finite set of parametric words of the forn $ab^\mu cd^\nu e$ in two parameters μ and ν. He showed also (1963) that it is decidable if solutions exist, and showed (1965) the same for systems in two unknowns. Appel (1968) showed that the set of solutions for a single equation in one unknown is given by a finite set of words of the form $ab^\mu c$ in a single parameter μ, and Lorents (1968) established the same for finite systems of equations in one unknown. Appel (1968) showed that for three or more unknowns the set of all solutions is not given by any finite set of parametric words. See also Hmelevskii (1966, 1967) and Aselderov (1969).

A somewhat related problem is the *substitution problem.* Again let $w(\xi_1, \ldots, \xi_n)$ be an element of a free group Φ with basis $\xi_1, \ldots, \xi_n$. Let g be any element of a group G. Then one asks whether there exists a homomorphism ϕ: Φ into G such that $w\phi = g$. In other words, does g have the form $g = w(u_1, \ldots, u_n)$ for some elements $u_1, \ldots, u_n$ of G? We shall consider here only the case that G is free. If $n = 1$ the problem is trivial, since $w = \xi^m$ for some $m \in \mathbb{Z}$, and it is routine to decide if a given element g of the free group G is an m-th power. The first significant result was that of Wicks (1962) who treated the case that $w = [\xi_1, \xi_2] = \xi_1^{-1}\xi_2^{-1}\xi_1\xi_2$, and obtained the following solution.

Proposition 8.4. *An element g of a free group G is a commutator iff, for some u, v, w in G, g has the reduced form $g = uvwu^{-1}v^{-1}w^{-1}$.* □

Wicks (1971, 1972) has recently obtained further results in this direction. Schupp (1969) proved the following.

Proposition 8.5. *Let $w(\xi_1, \xi_2)$ be any element of Φ free with basis ξ_1, ξ_2. Let G be a free group and g any element of G. Then it is decidable whether there exists a homomorphism ϕ from Φ into G such that $w\phi = g$.* □

The special case of (6.8) asserting that the product of two commutators is not in general itself a commutator (observed by Brenner, unpublished) can be derived more easily from (8.4). See also Malcev (1962) and Edmonds (1975).

9. Abstract Length Functions

All that has gone so far is based on the ideas of Nielsen, and in particular the simple but extremely important idea of calculating the amount of cancellation in passing to the reduced form of a product of reduced words in a free group. As will be seen later, quite analogous ideas enter in other contexts, expecially in the study of free products, of free products with amalgamation, and of Higman-Neumann-Neumann extensions. Anyone who has drawn pictures to clarify these arguments will recognize that they have an essentially geometric character, albeit concerned only with the rather simple geometry of segments of a line. There can be no doubt that this form of argument has further applications, where the fact that the lengths of words are integers (essential for proofs by induction) does not enter; indeed the approach we are about to sketch arose from observation of the close analogy between cancellation arguments in the theory of free R-groups F^* (as discussed above) and that of ordinary free groups, and the few results stated below concerning groups with real valued length functions gives some promise of further applications. In the discussion that follows we anticipate by discussing together both length functions in free groups and in free products.

In an attempt to axiomatize Nielsen's arguments, Lyndon (1963) put forth the following axioms. First, we have an arbitrary group G, and a function from G into $\mathbb{N}$, the natural numbers, which we write as $g \mapsto |g|$. For convenience we define $d(g, h) = \frac{1}{2}\{|g| + |h| - |gh^{-1}|\}$; this quantity is either an integer or a half integer, and in the case of the usual length function in a free group evidently denotes the length of the longest terminal segment common to g and h. We now state the axioms:

(A1) $$|x| \geqslant 0 \text{ and } |x| = 0 \text{ iff } x = 1;$$

(A2) $$|x^{-1}| = |x|;$$

(A3) $$d(x, y) \geqslant 0;$$

(A4) $$d(x, y) \geqslant d(x, z) \text{ implies } d(y, z) = d(x, z);$$

(A5) $$d(x, y) + d(x^{-1}, y^{-1}) \geqslant |x| = |y| \text{ implies } x = y.$$

These are evidently true for the usual length function in a free group F relative to a given basis X, and are also true for the usual length function in a free product $F = F_1 * \cdots * F_n$ relative to the given decomposition. In a free product one has non-trivial 'nonarchimedean' elements x, that is such that $|x^2| \leqslant |x|$ (these are the elements of the free factors and their conjugates). On the other hand, in a free group the following axiom is satisfied (see 2.15):

(A0) $$x \neq 1 \text{ implies } |x| < |x^2|.$$

In the presence of A0 the axiom A5 becomes redundant. In stating the next two results we pass over the matter of a rather inconsequential technical adjustment of the length function.

Proposition 9.1. *Let G be any group equipped with a length function satisfying axioms A0, . . . , A4. Then G is a free group and, moreover, G can be embedded in a free group F with basis X such that the given length function on G is the restriction to G of the length function on F relative to the basis X.* □

Proposition 9.2. *Let G be a group equipped with a length function satisfying* *axioms* A1, . . . , A5. *Then G can be embedded in a free product F such that the given length function on G is the restriction to G of the length function of F relative to the given decomposition.* □

The first theorem of course contains the subgroup theorem of Nielsen; the second, stated in fuller detail, contains the theorems of Kurosh and of Grushko-Neumann (III.5 below 7).

The question naturally arises of what groups have length functions satisfying the above axioms, but with values in some ordered abelian group other than $\mathbb{Z}$. The case of groups with length functions satisfying A0, . . . , A5 and with values in the additive group of reals has been studied by Harrison (1962), but appears to be very difficult. It is a reasonable conjecture that such a group is a subgroup of a free product F of replicas F_i of the additive group $\mathbb{R}$ of reals, with length function defined as follows: if $w = w_1 \cdots w_k$ with consecutive w_i nontrivial elements of distinct F_j, then $|w| = \Sigma|w_i|$, where length $|w_i|$ in F_j corresponds to ordinary absolute value in $\mathbb{R}$. In this direction she has proved the following.

Proposition 9.3. *Every maximal abelian subgroup of G is isomorphic to a subgroup of* $\mathbb{R}$. □

Proposition 9.4. *Every subgroup of G generated by two elements is either free or abelian.* □

She has partial results concerning subgroups generated by three elements.

Abstract length functions have been used by Nivat (1970).

Chiswell (1970) has shown that if a group G is equipped with an integer valued length function satisfying A1, A2, and A4, and such that $d(x, y)$ is always an integer, then G acts on a tree T, with a vertex P_0, in such a way that, for all x in G, $|x|$ is the length of the reduced path in T from P_0 to xP_0. He then shows that A5 holds if and only if the stabilizer of each (directed) edge is trivial, and that A0 holds if and only if the stabilizer of each vertex is trivial and no element of G inverts an edge. From the theory of Serre and Bass (Serre 1968/69) it follows from A5 that G is a free product, and from A0 that G is a free group. Chiswell establishes also a connection between such length functions and Stallings' bipolar structures (see IV. 6 below). For real valued length functions satisfying A1, A2, and A4, the analogous construction yields a representation of G as a group of isometries of T, equipped now with the structure of a pathwise connected and contractible metric space.

10. Representations of Free Groups; the Fox Calculus

Representations of free groups in the classical sense abound; that is, linear groups over the reals, complexes, or even over the integers, have in general an abundance of free subgroups. These have received considerable attention: see III.12, 13. We remark here that if one is concerned only with countable free groups, it is enough, by (3.1), to find linear free groups of rank 2, and, in most cases it suffices to find such free groups as subgroups of linear groups of dimension 2. (However, Bachmuth and Mochizuki (1976) raise the question of finding free subgroups of $\mathbb{GL}(2, \mathbb{C})$ of rank 3 or higher that are contained in no free subgroup of rank 2.) We shall return to such matters in (III.12) below.

We discuss here two representations of a somewhat different nature, both due to Magnus (1955; 1959). The first is a representation by non-commutative power series.

Let P be the free unital associative (but not commutative) ring with basis $\xi_1, \ldots, \xi_n$; its elements then are polynomials with integer coefficients in the non-commuting indeterminates $\xi_1, \ldots, \xi_n$. Let Π be the associated power series ring; one can view Π as the completion of P under the topology defined by powers of the *fundamental ideal* $\Delta = (\xi_1, \ldots, \xi_n)$; its elements are all formal sums $\pi = \sum_{\nu=0}^{\infty} \pi_\nu$ where each π_ν is a homogeneous polynomial of degree ν. The ideal Δ is the kernel of the map ρ from P onto $\mathbb{Z}$ defined by setting all $\xi_i \rho = 0$.

Proposition 10.1. *Let F be free with basis $x_1, \ldots, x_n$ and Π the power series ring in indeterminates $\xi_1, \ldots, \xi_n$, as above. Then the map $\mu: x_i \mapsto 1 + \xi_i$ defines an isomorphism from F into the multiplicative group $\Pi^\times$ of units in Π.*

□ In fact, the same assertion holds if we modify Π by setting all $\xi_i^2 = 0$. Suppose this done. Then, $x_i\mu = 1 + \xi_i$, $x_i^{-1}\mu = 1 - \xi_i$, whence, for all $a \in \mathbb{Z}$, $x_i^a \mu = 1 + a\xi_i$. Now if $w \in F$ with $w \neq 1$, we can write $w = x_{i_1}^{a_1} \cdots x_{i_k}^{a_k}$ with all $i_j \neq i_{j+1}$ and all $a_j \neq 0$. Then $w\mu = (1 + a_1\xi_{i_1}) \cdots (1 + a_k\xi_{i_k})$ and the total coefficient of the monomial $\xi_{i_1} \cdots \xi_{i_k}$ is $a_1 \cdots a_k \neq 0$, whence $w\mu \neq 1$. □

The coefficients of the higher terms in $w\mu$ are given by an analog of Taylor's formula, using iterated Fox differentiation (see Chen-Fox-Lyndon 1958).

Andreadakis (1965) gives an analogous representation for a free product of arbitrary cyclic groups.

A different but related representation of free groups by power series was given by Fouxe-Rabinovitch (1940, 1940; see also Lyndon, 1953).

Magnus' primary use of this representation was to establish the following result.

Proposition 10.2. *If F is a free group, and we define the descending central series by $F_1 = F$, $F_{n+1} = [F_n, F]$, then the intersection of the groups F_n is trivial.*

□ From the formula

$$(*) \quad [x, y] - 1 = x^{-1}y^{-1}(xy - yx) = x^{-1}y^{-1}((x - 1)(y - 1) - (y - 1)(x - 1)),$$

where $[x, y] = x^{-1}y^{-1}xy$, we see that if $x - 1 \in \Delta^m$ and $y - 1 \in \Delta^n$, then $[x, y] - 1 \in \Delta^{m+n}$. It follows by induction that if $w \in F_n$ then $w\mu - 1 \in \Delta^n$. Now if $w \in F_n$ for all n, then $w\mu - 1 \in \Delta^n$ for all n; since clearly the intersection of the Δ^n is 0, $w\mu = 1$, and, by (10.1), $w = 1$. □

The groups $D_n(F)$ of all w such that $w \equiv 1$ (modulo Δ^n) are commonly called the *dimension subgroups*. We give an alternative definition that applies to all groups and yields the same result for free groups. Instead of the ring Π we use the integral group ring $\mathbb{Z}G$ of the group, and define Δ to be the ideal generated by all $g - 1$ for $g \in G$; then $D_n(G)$ is defined to be the group of all g such that $g \equiv 1$ (modulo Δ^n). As we shall see below, Magnus showed that $F_n = D_n(F)$ for all n in the case that F is free; it became what Sandling (1972) rightly calls a notorious problem to settle the *dimension subgroup conjecture*, that $G_n = D_n(G)$ for all n and all groups G. This conjecture had been established in a great number of cases before Rips published a counter example in 1972. We summarize a few of these results, following Sandling 1972.

The formula (*) establishes that $G_n \subseteq D_n(G)$ for all n and all G. Suppose that, for some G and n, $G_n < D_n(G)$. Let $\bar{G} = G/G_n$; then it is easy to see that $\bar{G}_n = 1$ while $D_n(\bar{G}) \neq 1$. Thus to establish the conjecture for any n and any class of groups closed under homomorphisms, it suffices to establish for this class that $G_n = 1$ implies $D_n(G) = 1$. In particular, it suffices to consider nilpotent groups, and since we can clearly confine attention to finitely generated groups, it suffices to consider finite p-groups. Clearly $G_1 = D_1(G) = G$ for all groups G. We use the method above to give Sandling's proof of the result of Higman (see Sandling) that $G_2 = D_2(G)$ for all G. It suffices to show that $G_2 = 1$ implies $D_2(G) = 1$. Assume that $G_2 = 1$, that is, that G is abelian. Now the additive group $\mathbb{Z}G^+$ of $\mathbb{Z}G$ is free abelian with the monomials g, for $g \in G$, as basis. Define a map $\phi\colon \mathbb{Z}G^+ \mapsto G$ by setting $g\phi = g$. Since ϕ carries $(x-1)(y-1) = xy - x - y + 1$ into $xy \cdot x^{-1} \cdot y^{-1} \cdot 1 = 1$, $\Delta^2 \subseteq \operatorname{Ker}\phi$. Now, if $g \neq 1$, then $(g-1)\phi = g \cdot 1^{-1} = g \neq 1$, whence $g - 1 \notin \operatorname{Ker}\phi$ and $g - 1 \notin \Delta^2$, $g \notin D_2(G)$. This shows that $D_2(G) = 1$. See also Gruenberg (1970; Sec. 4.1).

Passi (1969) showed that if G is a p-group for $p > 2$, then $G_3 = D_3(G)$, and Moran (1972) showed that for any p-group G, $G_{p-1} = D_{p-1}(G)$. However Rips (1972) refuted the dimension subgroup conjecture by exhibiting a 2-group G with $G_4 = 1$ such that $D_4 \neq 1$.

Sandling (1972) proposed a modified definition of the dimension subgroups, which in some ways seems closer to Magnus' definition in the case of free groups. In any case, in view of Rips' counter example, it seems reasonable to turn to the correspondingly modified dimension subgroup conjecture. Let B be the set of all $g - 1$ for $g \in G$. Let L be the Lie ring in $\mathbb{Z}G$ generated by B under the Lie multiplication $u * v = uv - vu$; as usual, we define $L^1 = L$ and $L^{n+1} = L^n * L$. We now define the n-th *Lie dimension subgroup* $L_n(G)$ of G to consist of all g such that $g \equiv 1$ (modulo (L^n)) where (L^n) is the ideal in $\mathbb{Z}G$ generated by L^n.

Proposition 10.3. *For all groups G and all n, $G_n \subseteq L_n(G) \subseteq D_n(G)$.*

□ This follows immediately from the formula (*). □

Magnus (1937) established that $G_n = L_n(G) = D_n(G)$ for all n if G is a free group. In fact he established more. Let X be a basis for F and let B_0 consist of $x - 1$ for all $x \in X$; then Magnus showed that L is a free Lie ring (over the coefficient ring $\mathbb{Z}$) with B_0 as basis. He showed that if $g \in G_n$ then, in $\mathbb{Z}G$, $g = 1 + \lambda_g + \delta_g$ where λ_g is an element of L^n homogeneous of degree n and $\delta_g \in \Delta^{n+1}$. If we write the abelian groups G_n/G_{n+1} and L^n/L^{n+1} additively, then for each n the map $\lambda\colon g \mapsto \lambda_g$ is an additive map from G_n/G_{n+1} onto L^n/L^{n+1}; together these induce an additive map λ from $\bar{G} = \sum G_n/G_{n+1}$ into L. Moreover, for each m and n a pairing from G_n/G_{n+1} and G_m/G_{m+1} to G_{n+m}/G_{n+m+1} carries the images of $u \in G_n$ and $v \in G_m$ to the image of $[u, v] \in G_{n+m}$. Under this multiplication, $\bar{G}$ becomes a Lie ring and λ an isomorphism from $\bar{G}$ onto the Lie ring L.

Sandling (1972) shows that $G_n = L_n(G)$ for arbitrary G and $n \leqslant 6$, and that if G is a p-group with $(G_2)_p = 1$, then $G_n = L_n(G)$ for all n. It follows that if there is any counterexample to the conjecture that $G_n = L_n(G)$ for all n and G, it must be considerably more complicated that Rips' group.

Returning to the original dimension subgroups, we note that Zassenhaus (1940) proved results analogous of those of Magnus with $\mathbb{Z}G$ now replaced by $\mathbb{Z}_m G$ where $\mathbb{Z}_m = \mathbb{Z}/m\mathbb{Z}$, $m > 0$. In particular he introduced the *modular dimension subgroups* $D_n(p^e, G)$ for the case that $m = p^e$. Zassenhaus characterized these groups for $e = 1$ and G free, and Lazard (1954) extended this case to arbitrary G. This situation was studied further by Jennings (1941, 1955) and by Lazard (1954) who studied in great generality the connections between a discrete group and various associated Lie rings. A survey of the theory of dimension subgroups over arbitrary coefficient rings is given by Sandling (1972). We note also that Passi (see 1968) had introduced ideals in $\mathbb{Z}G$ associated with various polynomials that generalize at once the definitions of the dimension subgroups and the Lie dimension subgroups.

Before turning to Magnus' second representation we discuss briefly the Fox derivatives (Fox, 1953, 1954; Crowell and Fox, 1963).

Let F be a free group with basis X and $\mathbb{Z}F$ the group ring of F over the integers. Let $\varepsilon\colon \mathbb{Z}F \to \mathbb{Z}$ be the augmentation map, induced by the trivial map $\varepsilon_0\colon F \to 1$. In the present context we define a *derivation* $D\colon \mathbb{Z}F \to \mathbb{Z}F$ to be a linear map satisfying the rules $D1 = 0$ and

$$D(uv) = Du \cdot v\varepsilon + u \cdot Dv. \tag{1}$$

It is easy to see that D is fully determined by the Dx_i for x_i in X, and that every choice of the Dx_i defines a derivation. In fact, for certain elements $\partial u/\partial x_i$ of $\mathbb{Z}F$ one has

$$Du = \sum \frac{\partial u}{\partial x_i} Dx_i;$$

the *Fox derivatives* $\partial u/\partial x_i$ are easily calculated. If $u = y_1 \cdots y_n \in F$, with the $y_j \in X \cup X^{-1}$, then $\partial u/\partial x_i = \sum y_1 \cdots y_{j-1}(\partial y_j/\partial x_i)$ where $\partial y/\partial x_i = 0$ if $y \neq x_i^{\pm 1}$, where $\partial x_i/\partial x_i = 1$, and $\partial x_i^{-1}/\partial x_i = -x_i^{-1}$.

We remark that the map $1 - \varepsilon\colon u \mapsto u - u\varepsilon$ is a derivation, whence (1) gives

$$u - u\varepsilon = \sum \frac{\partial u}{\partial x_i}(x_i - 1). \tag{2}$$

It follows, in passing, from the fact that ε and $1 - \varepsilon$ are orthogonal retractions on $\mathbb{Z}F$ (projections), that $\mathbb{Z}F$ decomposes as $\mathbb{Z}$-module into the direct sum of $\mathbb{Z}$ and the kernel $\Delta = \mathbb{Z}F(1 - \varepsilon)$ of ε. In fact, viewed as a left ideal Δ is a free $\mathbb{Z}F$ module with basis the $x_i - 1$ for x_i in X. For supposing a relation $\sum v_i(x_i - 1) = 0$, applying each operator $\partial/\partial x_i$ shows that each $v_i = 0$. (For more on the ideal Δ and related ideals, see Cohen 1972).

Finally, we describe the second Magnus representation (see also I.4 above). Let $d\mathbb{Z}F$ be the free left $\mathbb{Z}F$ module with a basis of elements dx_i corresponding to the x_i

in X. For u in $\mathbb{Z}F$ define

$$du = \sum \frac{\partial u}{\partial x_i} dx_i,$$

in $d\mathbb{Z}F$. Then, for w in F, multiplication of matrices

$$w\mu = \begin{pmatrix} w\varepsilon & dw \\ 0 & 1 \end{pmatrix}$$

is well defined, and in fact gives a faithful representation μ of F.

We shall return to the topics discussed in this section more fully below (II.3).

11. Free Products with Amalgamation

Nielsen's method can be extended to free products, and to free products with amalgamation. In (I.9) we have indicated that this method, indeed in axiomatic form, can be applied to free products to yield the theorems of Kurosh and of Grushko and Neumann. An extension of Nielsen's method was undertaken by Zieschang (1970), who obtained a result he put to good use in the study of the ranks of Fuchsian groups (see Zieschang, 1970 and Peczynski, Rosenberger, and Zieschang, 1970). By similar methods one can obtain an analog for amalgamated products of the Kurosh Theorem. This is the result of Karrass and Solitar (1970) in a somewhat modified form. Let G be the free product of groups H_ν, $\nu \in I$, with amalgamated subgroup A, and let G^* be a subgroup of G; then the intersections $G^* \cap H_\nu^g$, $\nu \in I$, $g \in G$, generate a normal subgroup N of G^*, which is a tree product of certain of these intersections, and G^* is a (split) extension of N by a free group. One can obtain also a partial analog of the Grushko-Neumann Theorem due to Smythe (1976). As noted below, various of these results extend also to HNN-extensions, to tree products, and to more general graph products.

We present proofs only of results concerning amalgamated products; in particular, the Karrass-Solitar theorem is proved in a way that yields as a special case the theorem of H. Neumann (see IV.6.6 below) and the Kurosh Theorem (see III.5.1). The theorems of Zieschang and of Smythe follow easily by the same argument. Following an observation of Rosenberger (1974), the restrictions in Zieschang's theorem are unavoidable, and Smythe's analog of the Grushko-Neumann Theorem must remain only partial, for the examples of Burns, Karrass, Pietrowski, Purzitsky show that the natural strict analog of the Grushko-Neumann Theorem fails for amalgamated products.

Although we have followed the ideas of (I.9) especially as extended by Zieschang, our treatment is not axiomatic. Indeed any axiomatization in the spirit of (I.9), using only universally quantified axioms, would have to deal with a larger class of groups. For, as the example we give next shows, a subgroup G^* of an amalgamated product $G = \underset{A}{*} H_\nu$ need not be the amalgamated product of intersections $G^* \cap H^g$ together with any other proper subgroups of G^*.

Example. Let $A = (a; a^3)$, $H = (a, b; a^3, b^2, a^b = a)$, $K = (a, c; a^3, c^2, a^c = a^{-1})$, and let $G = H \underset{A}{*} K$.

Let $d = bc$ and $G^* = Gp(a, d)$. Then $G^* = (a, d; a^3, a^d = a^{-1})$. Note that G^* has infinite cyclic center Z with generator d^2.

Suppose now that $G^* = U \underset{B}{*} V$ with U, V, and B all distinct. Then Z must be contained in B, and $\bar{G} = G^*/Z = \bar{U} \underset{\bar{B}}{*} \bar{V}$ for $\bar{U} = U/Z$, $\bar{V} = V/Z$, $\bar{B} = B/Z$, and $\bar{U}$, $\bar{V}$, $\bar{B}$ all distinct. This implies that $\bar{G}$ have infinite order. But clearly $\bar{G} = (\bar{a}, \bar{d}; \bar{a}^3, \bar{d}^2, \bar{a}^{\bar{d}} = \bar{a}^{-1})$, the dihedral group of order 6.

We now proceed to give a proof of the theorems of Karrass-Solitar, Zieschang, and Smythe mentioned above, which we follow with some more fragmentary comments. We assume the definition and the most elementary properties of amalgamated products (see IV.2 below).

Let G be the amalgamated product of groups H_ν, for ν in an index set I, with amalgamated subgroup A. We establish some terminology and notation. If $u \in G$, then either $u \in A$ or else $u = h_1 \ldots h_m$ for some $m \geqslant 1$, where each $h_i \in H_{\nu_i} - A$ for some ν_i, and no $\nu_i = \nu_{i+1}$. In the latter case m, and the sequence $(\nu_1, \ldots, \nu_m)$, are uniquely determined by u, but not (unless $m = 1$ or $A = 1$) the factors h_i; we nonetheless call the product $h_1 \ldots h_m$ a *normal form* for u. [We are here employing a familiar abuse of language: the normal form is not the product $h_1 \ldots h_m$, which is simply the element u, but rather the sequence $(h_1, \ldots, h_m)$.] For u as above we define the *length* $|u|$ of u to be $|u| = 0$ if $u \in A$ and otherwise $|u| = m$.

We write $x \equiv u_1 \ldots u_n$, and say that the product $u_1 \ldots u_n$ is *reduced*, if $x = u_1 \ldots u_n$ and $x = |u_1| + \cdots + |u_n|$. Similarly, the notation $x \equiv p^{-1}(hk)r$ means $x = p^{-1}hkr$ and $x = |p^{-1}| + |hk| + |r|$. If $x \equiv u_1u_2 \equiv v_1v_2$ with $|u_2| = |v_2|$, then $v_2 = au_2$ for some $a \in A$, that is, $Au_2 = Av_2$.

If $x,y \in G$, then there exist p, q, r, h, and k, where either $h = k = 1$ or $|h| = |k| = |hk| = 1$, such that

$$x \equiv p^{-1}hq, \; y \equiv q^{-1}kr, \text{ and } xy \equiv p^{-1}(hk)r.$$

We say that q, or any segment of q, has *cancelled* in the product xy; in the case $|h| = |k| = |hk| = 1$, we say that the part h of x has *consolidated* with the part k of y to yield the part hk. If $x \equiv u_1u_2$ we say that x *ends* in u_2.

Following Zieschang (1970), we shall make essential use of the fact that every element $u \in G$ can be written in the form

$$u \equiv p^{-1}hq \text{ with } |p| = |q| \text{ and } |h| \leqslant 1;$$

here Ap, Aq, and AhA are uniquely determined by u. If $|h| = 1$, then $|u|$ is odd. If $|u|$ is even, either $u \in A$ and $|u| = 0$, or else we may suppose that $h = 1$ and $u \equiv p^{-1}q$. If $Ap = Aq$, we may suppose that $u \equiv p^{-1}hp$, where necessarily $|h| = 1$.

We shall use a well ordering of the cosets Ap with the following properties:

$$\text{if } |p| < |q| \text{ then } Ap < Aq;$$

$$\text{if } |p| = |q| \text{ and } p \equiv p_1 p_2,\ q \equiv q_1 q_2,\ |p_2| = |q_2|, \text{ then}$$

$$Ap_2 < Aq_2 \text{ implies } Ap < Aq.$$

It is easy to construct such an ordering, by induction on $|p|$, using the axiom of choice. In many contexts the axiom of choice is not needed: for example, if G is finitely generated, or if we are concerned only to order a family of cosets Ap that contains only finitely many Ap for each given value of $|p|$.

All the cancellation arguments we shall need below follow the same pattern, and we now prove a somewhat technically involved lemma that contains them all as special cases.

Lemma 11.1. *Let* $\sigma = (u_1, a_1, u_2, a_2, \ldots, u_t, a_t)$, $t \geqslant 1$, *where each*

$$u_i \equiv p_i^{-1} h_i q_i, \quad |p_i| = |q_i|, \quad |h_i| \leqslant 1,$$

and for each i, $1 \leqslant i < t$,

$$a_i = g_{i1} \ldots g_{in_i}, \quad g_{ij} \equiv h_{ij}^{p_{ij}}, \quad |h_{ij}| = 1, \quad \text{or} \quad g_{ij} \in A,$$

where, for each j, $1 \leqslant j \leqslant n_i$,

$$|g_{ij}| \leqslant |u_{i+1}|, \quad |g_{ij} \ldots g_{in_i} u_{i+1}| = |u_{i+1}|,$$

while $a_t \in A$. *Let*

$$w = u_1 a_1 \ldots u_t a_t.$$

Assume for each i, $1 \leqslant i \leqslant t - 1$, *the following.*

(1) $|u_i|, |u_{i+1}| \leqslant |u_i a_i u_{i+1}|$.

(2) *If* $Ap_i \leqslant Aq_i$ *then* $|u_{i+1}| < |u_i a_i u_{i+1}|$.

(3) *If* $Aq_{i+1} < Ap_{i+1}$ *then* $|u_i| < |u_i a_i u_{i+1}|$.

The following conclusions now hold.

(4) *If* $Ap_t < Aq_t$ *and* $|h_t| = 0$, *then* $w \equiv z q_t a_t$ *for some* z.

(5) *Unless* $Ap_t < Aq_t$ *and* $|h_t| = 0$, *one has* $u_t \equiv z x q_t$, $w \equiv z_1 x_1 q_t a_t$, *for some* z, z_1 *and for* $x, x_1 \in H_\nu - A$ *for some* $\nu \in I$.

(6) *If* $Aq_t < Ap_t$ *and* $|h_t| = 1$, *then* $w \equiv z_1 h_t q_t a_t$ *for some* z_1.

(7) $|u_1|, \ldots, |u_t| \leqslant |w|$.

□ It suffices to treat the case that $a_t = 1$. Let $\sigma_i = (u_1, a_1, \dots, u_i)$ and $w_i = u_1 a_1 \dots u_t a_t$. Then σ_i satisfies the same hypotheses (1, 2, 3) as $\sigma_t = \sigma$. We argue by induction. The case $i = 1$ is trivial. For the inductive step, we let $1 < i \leqslant t$, and assume (1, 2, 3) and the conclusions for w_{i-1} and deduce the conclusions for w_i.

We introduce the following simplifying notation:

$$u_i = u \equiv p^{-1}hq, |p| = |q|, |h| \leqslant 1;$$

$$u_{i+1} = v = r^{-1}ks, |r| = |s|, |k| \leqslant 1,$$

$$a_i = g = g_1 \dots g_n, \text{ where, for all } i, |g_i| \leqslant |v|, |g_i \dots g_n v| = |v|.$$

$$w_{i-1} = w'$$

If $Ap = Aq$ after refactoring u we may suppose that $p = q$ and $|h| = 1$. If $|h| = 0$, after refactoring u we can suppose $h = 1$ and $u = p^{-1}q$. We assume similarly that $Ar = As$ implies $r = s$ and $|k| = 1$, and that $|k| = 0$ implies $k = 1$. We shall use the following lemma.

Lemma 11.2. *$gv \equiv r'^{-1}k's$, where either $r' = r$ or $r' = rg^{-1}$ and $|r'| = |r|$, and where either $k, k' \in H_\nu - A$ for some $\nu \in I$, or else $k = k' = 1$.*

Proof of Lemma (11.2) reduces by induction on n to the case that $n = 1$ and $g \equiv h_*^{p_*}$, $|h_*| = 1$, or $g \in A^*$. The case $g \in A^*$ is immediate. In the remaining case we have the hypotheses that $|g| \leqslant |v|$ and $|gv| = |v|$. Now $|g| \leqslant |v|$ implies that $|p_*| \leqslant |r|$ and, if $|p_*| = |r|$, then $|k| = 1$. If $|p_*| = |r|$, then, refactoring, we may suppose $p_* = r$. We now have $g \equiv h_*^r$, $v \equiv r^{-1}ks$, with $|r| = |s|$ and $|k| = 1$. Then $|gv| = |v|$ implies that in the product $gv = r^{-1}h_*ks$ the factors h_* and k consolidate to give $h_*k = k'$, with k, k' in the same $H_\nu - A$. Thus $gv = r^{-1}k's$, as required. If $|p_*| < |r|$, then we may suppose $r \equiv r_1 h_1 p_*$ with $|h_1| = 1$, and that in $gr^{-1} = p_*^{-1}h_*h_1^{-1}r^{-1}$ the part h_*h^{-1} consolidates. Then, for $r' = rg^{-1}$, we have $|r'| = |r|$, and $gv \equiv r'^{-1}ks$, as required. This completes the proof of lemma (11.2).

We now consider the case $i = 2$, which contains the burden of the inductive argument. Here we have $\sigma_2 = (u, a, v)$. We shall use the hypotheses (1, 2, 3) to draw the conclusions, which now take the following form.

(4′) $Ar < As$ and $k = 1$ imply $w \equiv zs$ for some z.

(5′) Unless $Ar < As$ and $k = 1$, one has $v \equiv zxs$, $uav \equiv z_1x_1s$ for some z, z_1 and for $x, x_1 \in H_\nu - A$, some $\nu \in I$.

(6′) If $As < Ar$ and $|k| = 1$, then $uav \equiv z_1ks$ for some z_1.

(7′) $|u|, |v| \leqslant |uav|$.

We observe first of all that (7′) is contained in (1). To prove (4′), let $Ar < As$ and $k = 1$, hence $v \equiv r^{-1}s$ and $av \equiv r'^{-1}s$ for r' as above. By (1), $|u| \leqslant |uav|$, whence at most the part r'^{-1} of av cancels in the product, and if it does cancel there is no amalgamation. It follows that uav ends in s.

We next prove (6′). Let $As < Ar$ and $|k| = 1$. By (3), $|u| < |uav|$, whence again at most r'^{-1} cancels, and if it does cancel k does not amalgamate. Thus uav ends in ks.

We now prove (5′). By (1), $|u| \leqslant |uav|$, whence once more at most r'^{-1} cancels. If r'^{-1} cancels and $|k| = 1$, then k at most consolidates to yield some k_1 with k, k_1 in the same $H_\nu - A$, and uav ends in $k_1 s$. If r'^{-1} cancels and $k = 1$, then $|u| = |uav|$, and by (3) $Ar < As$. Since $k = 1$, $Ar \neq As$. But then $Ar < As$ and $k = 1$, contrary to the hypothesis of (5′). The case remains that less than r'^{-1} cancels. But then uav ends in s, and the preceding letter x is either left unchanged or consolidated to give a letter x_1, with x, x_1 in the same $H_\nu - A$.

This completes the proof of the case $i = 2$. It remains to treat the case $2 < i \leqslant t$. We first establish the conclusions (4′, 5′, 6′). In view of the case $i = 2$, it will suffice to show that no more of v cancels in the product $w'av$ than in uav, and that if the same amount cancels, then there is consolidation in $w'av$ only if there is consolidation in uav.

By the induction hypothesis, w' ends in q. If q does not cancel in uav, then both uav and $w'av$ end with qav, and we are done. Thus we may suppose that q cancels in uav, and so also in $w'av$. By (1), $|v| \leqslant |uav|$, whence no more of the factor u than q can cancel in the product uav.

Let $Ap \leqslant Aq$. Then by (2), $|v| < |uav|$. Since q cancels in uav, this implies that $|q| < \frac{1}{2}|u|$, whence $|h| = 1$. It also implies that h does not consolidate. Now $|h| = 1$ implies we are not in the case (4), and therefore by (5), $u \equiv zxq$, $w' \equiv z_1 x_1 q$ for some z, z_1 and for x, x_1 in the same $H_\nu - A$. Since x does not consolidate in uav, it follows that x_1 can neither consolidate nor cancel in $w'av$. This establishes the desired result for the case $Ap \leqslant Aq$.

Let $Aq < Ap$. By (1), $|v| \leqslant |uav|$, so at most q cancels in uav. If $|h| = 1$, then (5) gives $w' \equiv z_1 hq$, whence it follows that h does not cancel in $w'av$, and, further, that it consolidates in $w'av$ only if it consolidates in uav. We are done if $|h| = 1$. Let $h = 1$. By (5), $u \equiv zxq$, $w' \equiv z_1 x_1 q$ for some z, z_1 and for x, x_1 in the same $H_\nu - A$. Now $|v| \leqslant |uav|$ implies there is no consolidation or cancellation of x in uav; but this implies there is no consolidation or cancellation of x_1 in $w'av$. This completes the proof of (4′, 5′, 6′).

To prove (7′), we note that since v cancels and consolidates no more in $w'av$ than in uav, and since $|u| \leqslant |uav|$, it follows that $|w'| \leqslant |w'av|$. Now $w' = w_{i-1}$ and $w'av = w_i$, whence we have $|w_{i-1}| \leqslant |w_i|$. Since we have by induction that $|u_1|, \ldots, |u_{i-1}| \leqslant |w_{i-1}|$, we have $|u_1|, \ldots, |u_{i-1}| \leqslant |w_i|$.

It remains to show that $|u_i| \leqslant |w_i|$, that is, that $|v| \leqslant |w'av|$. This follows from the following two facts. First, $u = u_{i-1}$, $w' = w_{i-1}$, and we have thus inductively that $|u| \leqslant |w'|$. Second, we have shown that w' cancels or consolidates no more in $w'av$ than u cancels or consolidates in uav. This completes the proof of (7′), and, with it, the inductive proof of Lemma (11.1). □

We now examine the family $\mathscr{C}$ of all subgroups H_μ^p, $\mu \in I$, $p \in G$. Let $U = \bigcup \mathscr{C}$, the set of all $u = h^p$, $|h| \leqslant 1$, that is, of all $a \in A$ together with all $u \equiv h^p$, $|h| = 1$. We shall show that U is the 'tree union' of a tree with vertex groups $C \in \mathscr{C}$ together with the group A, in a sense to be made precise, and that G is obtainable from the corresponding tree product by imposing conjugating relations of the form $u^v = w$ for $u, v, w \in U$.

If $C \in \mathscr{C}$, we can write

$$C = H_{\mu_0}^p, p \equiv h_1 \ldots h_m, \ m \geqslant 0, h_i \in H_{\mu_i} - A, \text{ and } \mu_i \neq \mu_{i+1} \text{ for } 0 \leqslant i \leqslant m-1.$$

Define $C^o = A^p$. If $p \neq 1$, then $A^{h_1} \subseteq H_{\mu_1}$, whence $C^o \subseteq C' = H_{\mu_1}^{h_2 \ldots h_m}$. If $p = 1$, hence $C = H_{\mu_0}$, then $C^o = A$, and we define $C' = A$. Examination of length shows that $C \cap C' = C^o$.

We now define a graph Γ with vertex set $\mathscr{C} \cup \{A\}$. If $C = H_{\mu_0}^p$ with $p \neq 1$, we introduce an edge between C and C' and assign to it the group $C^o = C \cap C'$. To each $C = H_{\mu_0}$ we introduce an edge between C and A and assign to it the group $A = C \cap C^o = C \cap A$. Evidently Γ is a tree, which we orient upward from A as root.

We assert that U is the set theoretic tree union of the $C \in \mathscr{C}$ and A as sets: that is, U results from the disjoint union of replicas of the C and of A by identifying, for each pair C and C', the subgroups corresponding to the inclusions of the edge group C^o into C and C'. This is expressed more explicitly in the following proposition.

Proposition 11.3. *Let $C_1, C_2 \in \mathscr{C} \cup \{A\}$, and let $D = C_1 \wedge C_2$, the greatest lower bound of C_1 and C_2 in the sense of the directed tree Γ. Then $C_1 \cap C_2 \subseteq D$.*

□ If C_1 or C_2 is A, the assertion is trivial. We may suppose that $C_1 = H_{\mu_0}^p$, $C_2 = H_{\nu_0}^q$ for $p = h_1 \ldots h_m$, $q = k_1 \ldots k_n$, with the conventions established earlier. We suppose $m \geqslant n$, and argue by induction on m. The initial case, $m = n = 0$, is trivial. The case $C_1 = C_2$ also is trivial, and we assume $C_1 \neq C_2$. Let $g \in C_1 \cap C_2$. Then $g = h^p$ for some $h \in H_{\mu_0}$, and similarly $g = k^q$, $k \in H_{\nu_0}$. If $h \notin A$, then $g \equiv h^p$, normal form; but the sequence of H_μ containing the successive factors in this normal form is impossible for an element $g = k^q \in C_2$. Thus $h \in A$ and $g \in C_1^o \subseteq C_1'$. We have shown that $C_1 \cap C_2 \subseteq C_1' \cap C_2$. Evidently $C_1' \cap C_2 = D$. Now the inductive hypothesis gives $C_1' \cap C_2 \subseteq D$, whence we conclude that $C_1 \cap C_2 \subseteq D$. □

We now show that G is obtained from the tree product $\tilde{G}$ of Γ by introducing all valid relations $u^v = w$ for $u, v, w \in U$. First, the tree product $\tilde{G}$ is generated by the tree union U of Γ, and is obtained by imposing on U all the relations defining the group structure of the component groups in U, that is, all valid relations $uv = w$ for u, v, w all in some $C \in \mathscr{C}$. Let R_1 be the set of such relations; then $\tilde{G}$ has a presentation $\tilde{G} = (U; R_1)$. Let R_2 be the set of all valid relations $u^v = w$ for $u, v, w \in U$. Then our assertion takes the following form.

Proposition 11.4. $G = (U; R_1, R_2)$.

□ The assertion will follow from the following. Let $\sigma = (u_1, u_2, \ldots, u_t)$, $t \geqslant 1$, each $u_i \in U$. Then $w = u_1 \ldots u_t$ is equal to 1 only if the sequence σ can be reduced to the trivial sequence $\sigma_0 = (1)$ by a succession of steps that replace some part u_i, u_{i+1} by one of the following:

$$\alpha\colon u_i u_{i+1} \text{ provided } u_i u_{i+1} \in U;$$

$$\beta\colon u_{i+1}, u_i^{u_{i+1}}, \text{ where } |u_i^{u_{i+1}}| < |u_i|;$$

$$\gamma: u_{i+1}^{u_i^{-1}}, u_i, \text{ where } |u_{i+1}^{u_i^{-1}}| < |u_{i+1}|.$$

We may suppose that t cannot be decreased by such steps, nor $\sum |u_i|$. We may suppose also that the lexicographical rank of the sequence $|\sigma| = (|u_1|, \ldots, |u_t|)$ cannot be increased. If $u_i \in A$, $i < t$, then the transformation (γ) does not alter t or $\sum |u_i|$ and does not decrease $|\sigma|$. Thus we may suppose that all $u_i \in A$ come at the end of the sequence σ, and, in view of (α), and the minimality of t, that there is at most one such factor, that is, $u_i \notin A$ for $i < t$. After adjoining a trivial factor at the end if necessary, and reindexing, we may restore a uniform notation, assuming that $\sigma = (u_1, \ldots, u_t)$ satisfies all the previous hypotheses, and, in addition, that no $u_i \in A$, for $1 \leqslant i < t$, while $u_t \in A$. We verify that σ satisfies the hypotheses of (11.1), where we take all the $a_i = 1$ for $i < t$. Since all the $u_i \in U$, condition (2) is vacuous, while condition (1) takes the form $|u_i|, |u_{i+1}| \leqslant |u_i u_{i+1}|$. Let $u_i = u \equiv p^{-1}hp$, $u_{i+1} = v \equiv q^{-1}kq$, with $|h| = |k| = 1$, and suppose first that $|u| \leqslant |v|$. We draw a contradiction from the assumption that $|uv| < |v|$. This assumption implies that the part hp of u cancels in the product uv. Now $|u| \leqslant |v|$ implies that $|p| \leqslant |q|$. If $|p| = |q|$, cancellation of p implies that $pq^{-1} \in A$, and we may suppose that $p = q$. Now cancellation of h implies that h and k are in the same H^q. But then u, v, and uv and all in $C = H_\nu^p$, contrary to the assumption that t cannot be decreased by a step (α). If $|p| < |q|$ then hp must cancel in the product uq^{-1}, whence $|qu^{-1}| < |q|$. But this implies that $|v^{u^{-1}}| < |v|$, contrary to the minimality of $\sum |u_i|$ under steps (γ). The case $|v| \leqslant |u|$ is symmetric.

We may therefore apply (11.1) to conclude by (4) that $|u_1| \leqslant |w|$, whence $w \neq 1$. $\square$

A special case of (11.8) below says that G is in fact the tree product of a subgraph Γ_0 of Γ; but this is trivial, the subgraph Γ_0 is that with vertices A and all the H_ν, $\nu \in I$.

We now examine a subgroup G^* of G. Let $\mathscr{C}^*$ be the set of all $C^* = C \cap G^*$ for $C \in \mathscr{C}$, and let $A^* = A \cap G^*$. Let $U^* = \bigcup \mathscr{C}^*$, and let N be the subgroup of G generated by U^*. Evidently N is a normal subgroup of G^*.

We now construct a graph Γ^* analogous to Γ, with vertices labelled by $\mathscr{C}^* \cup \{A^*\}$. We do this by replacing each vertex C or A of Γ by C^* or A^*, and replacing the label C^o on an edge by $C^{o*} = C^{*o} = C^o \cap G^*$. The graph Γ^* may contain redundancies in the following sense. It may be that $C^* = C \cap G^*$, for $C = H_\mu^p$, is in fact contained in A^p, whence $C^* \subseteq C^{o*} \subseteq C'^*$; it may even be that $C^* = C'^*$. To remedy this, we form a new graph Γ^{**} as follows. If e is the edge joining C and C' in Γ, and e^* the corresponding edge in Γ^*, whose ends now bear labels C^* and C'^*, and if $C^* \subseteq C'^*$, we contract the edge e^* to a point. A vertex in Γ^{**} will then result from contracting a subtree of Γ^*. If C_0 is the label in Γ on the vertex corresponding to the root of this subtree, then all the labels on vertices of this subtree are elements C^* such that $C^* \subseteq C_0^*$. We label the vertex in Γ^{**} with the group C_0^*.

Let $\mathscr{C}^{**}$ be the set of labels on vertices of Γ^{**}. It is immediate that $\bigcup \mathscr{C}^{**} = \bigcup \mathscr{C}^* = U^*$ and that U^* is the tree union of Γ^{**}. Moreover distinct vertices of Γ^{**} bear distinct labels, so we may again identify the vertices with the labels they bear. Finally, if $C^* \in \mathscr{C}^{**}$, then there is a unique shortest p such that $C^* = H_{\mu_0}^p \cap G^*$; henceforth when we write $C^* = H_{\mu_0}^p \cap G^*$ it is always with this convention.

The proofs of (11.2) and (11.3) now yield the analogous results for Γ^{**}. The set U^* is the tree union of Γ^{**} where the vertex labels C^* and A^* are regarded only as sets. The group N results from the tree product $\tilde{N}$ of Γ^{**} by imposing the set R_2^* of all valid relations $u^v = w$ for $u, v, w \in U^*$. If we let R_1^* be the set of all valid relations $uv = w$ for u, v, w in some $C^* \in \mathscr{C}^{**}$, then N has presentation $N = (U^*; R_1^*, R_2^*)$.

We now propose to show that N is the tree product of a subtree Δ of Γ^{**}, without imposing any further relations. For this we define $\mathscr{D}$ to be the set of $C^* = C \cap G^*$, $C = H_\mu^p$, $C^* \in \mathscr{C}^{**}$, for which Ap is minimal among the conjugates of C^* in N. Let $V = \bigcup \mathscr{D}$. We must show four things:

I. The set $\mathscr{D} \cup \{A^*\}$ is the vertex set of a subtree Δ of Γ^{**}.

II. V is the tree union of Δ, regarding the vertex groups only as sets.

III. V generates N.

IV. N is the tree product of Δ.

To prove I it suffices to show that if a vertex C^* of Γ^{**} belongs to $\mathscr{D}$, then the vertex immediately below it does also, or else is A^*. Let $C^* = H_{\mu_0}^p \cap G^*$ be in $\mathscr{D}$, where $p = h_1 \ldots h_m$, normal form. Then the vertex immediately below C^* in Γ^{**} is that $C_1^* = H_{\mu_i}^{h_{i+1} \ldots h_m} \cap G^*$ with least i that lies in $\mathscr{C}^{**}$, or, if there is no such i, is A^*. Now $C_1^* = H_{\mu_i}^q \cap G^*$ where $p \equiv p_1 q$. If C_1^* were not in $\mathscr{D}$, then, for some $w \in N$, one would have $C_1^{*N} = H_{\mu_1}^{qw} \cap G^*$ where $Aqw < Aq$. But this would imply $Apw < Ap$, contrary to the assumption that $C^* \in \mathscr{D}$.

Assertion II follows immediately from (11.2).

To prove III, for each $n \geqslant 0$ let N_n be the subgroup of N generated by all $C^* = H_{\mu_0}^p \cap G^*$ in $\mathscr{C}^*$ with $|p| \leqslant n$, together with A^*, and let M_n be the subgroup generated by all such C^* that are in $\mathscr{D}$, together with A^*. We show inductively that $N_n = M_n$. If $n = 0$, since $H_{\mu_0} \cap G^*$ is in $\mathscr{D}$ unless it is contained in A^*, we have $M_0 = N_0$. For the inductive step it will suffice to show that if C^* as above is in $\mathscr{C}^*$ with C^{*w} in $\mathscr{D}$, then w is a product of elements $u \equiv k^q$ with $|q| < |p|$.

For this it will suffice to show that if $|pw| \leqslant |p|$, then w is such a product. Assume $|pw| \leqslant |p|$ where $w = u_1 \ldots u_t$, $u_i \in U$. The proof of (11.3), applied with left and right exchanged, shows that the sequence $(u_1, \ldots, u_t)$ can be transformed, without changing w, to a sequence $(a, v_1, \ldots, v_s)$ for $a \in A$ and the sequence $(v_1, \ldots, v_s)$ satisfying the symmetric counterpart of the hypothesis of (11.1). Let $p' = pa$ and $w' = v_1 \ldots v_s$. Then $|p'w'| \leqslant |p'| = |p|$. If we can show that $v_1 \equiv h^q$ with $|q| < |p|$, we will be done by induction on s. Let $v_1 \equiv k^q$. Then the conclusion (5) of (11.1), in symmetric form, gives $w' \equiv q^{-1}k'z$ with $k, k' \in H_\nu - A$ for some $\nu \in I$. Also (4) of (11.1) gives $|v_1| \leqslant |w'|$, whence q^{-1} is less than half of w'. Now $p'w' = pq^{-1}k'z$, and $|p'w'| \leqslant |p'|$ requires that q^{-1} cancel and k' consolidate. But this implies that $|p'| \leqslant |q^{-1}k'| > |q|$.

Finally, we prove IV. We have shown that N has a presentation $N = (U^*; R_1^*, R_2^*)$ where R_1^* consists of all relations of the form $uv = w$ that are valid in N, for u, v, w all in some $C^* \in \mathscr{C}^{**}$, and where R_2^* consists of all valid relations

$u^v = w$ for $u, v, w \in U^*$. We must show that N has a presentation $N = (V; T_1)$ where T_1 consists of all relations $uv = w$ for u, v, w all in some $C^* \in \mathscr{D}$.

Now $V \subseteq U^*$, and for each $u \in U^* - V$ we choose an expression $\bar{u}$ for u in terms of the set V of generators. Each $C^* \in \mathscr{C}^{**}$ is conjugate to some $C^{*z^{-1}} \in \mathscr{D}$; we choose such a z for each C^*, taking z as a particular word over V. Then each $u \in C^*$ in $\mathscr{C}^{**} - \mathscr{D}$ has the form u_0^z for some $u_0 \in C^{*z^{-1}} \in \mathscr{D}$. We choose such an expression $\bar{u} = u_0^z$ for u in terms of the set V of generators. For u in V we write $\bar{u} = u$, $z = 1$.

If $\rho: uv = w$ is a relation in R_1^*, then $\bar{u} = u_0^z$, $\bar{v} = v_0^z$, and $\bar{w} = w_0^z$, all with the same z, whence ρ expressed in terms of the set V of generators becomes $\bar{\rho}: u_0^z v_0^z = w_0^z$. But this is a consequence of the relation $u_0 v_0 = w_0$ from T_1.

Let $\rho: u^w = v$ be a relation in R_2^*. In terms of the set V of generators this takes the form $\bar{\rho}: u_0^{z_1 w_0^{z_2}} = v_0^{z_3}$; here we note that since u and v are conjugate, u_0 and v_0 lie in the same $C^* \in \mathscr{D}$. Thus ρ is equivalent to an equation of the form $\bar{\rho}: u_0^w = v_0$ where u_0 and v_0 lie in some $C^* = H_\mu^p \cap G^* \in \mathscr{D}$. Let $u_0 \equiv p^{-1}hp$ and $v_0 \equiv p^{-1}kp$, $h,k \in H_\mu - A$.

Now $w \in N$ implies by III that $w = v_1 \ldots v_s$ for some $v_i \in V$. Thus the product of the terms in the sequence $\sigma = (v_t^{-1}, \ldots, v_1^{-1}, u_0, v_1, \ldots, v_t, v_0)$ is 1, and, as we have seen in the proof of (11.1), reduces to 1 by a succession of steps (α, β, γ). We will be done if we can show that these steps are justified by T_1, that is, in each case u_i, u_{i+1} lie in the same $C^* \in \mathscr{D}$.

We pause now to prove four lemmas about amalgamated products G.

Lemma 11.5. *Let $u \equiv h^p$, $v \equiv k^q$, $h \in H_\mu - A$, $k \in H_\nu - A$, and $uv \in U$. Then, if $|p| = |q|$, one has $v \equiv k_1^p$, $\mu = \nu$, and $k_1 \in H_\mu - A$. If $|p| < |q|$, then $q \equiv q_1 p$, $|q_1| \geqslant 1$, $h = b^{q_1}$, $b \in A$, and $u = b^q$.*

$\square$ Let $|p| = |q|$. If $Ap \neq Aq$, then $uv \equiv p^{-1}h(pq^{-1})kq$, and $uv \in U$ would imply $Ap = Aq$. Thus $Ap = Aq$, $q = ap$, $a \in A$, and $v \equiv k_1^p$ for $k_1 = k^a$. Now $uv = p^{-1}(hk_1)p$, and since an element of U cannot have positive even length, the part hk must cancel or consolidate, whence $\mu = \nu$.

Let $|p| < |q|$. If $q \equiv q_1 p$ does not hold, as before uv would be reduced with the parts p^{-1} and q untouched, and $uv \in U$ would imply $q \equiv q_1 p$. Thus $q \equiv q_1 p$, $|q_1| \geqslant 1$, and $uv = p^{-1}hq_1^{-1}kq_1 p$, whence $hq_1^{-1}kq_1 \in U$. Since an element of U cannot have positive even length, h can neither remain intact nor cancel; thus h consolidates. Now $w \equiv (hq_1^{-1})kq_1 \in U$ implies $Aq_1 h^{-1} = Aq$, $q_1 h^{-1} = h^{-1}q_1$ for some $b \in A$, whence $h = b^{q_1}$, and $u = h^p = b^{q_1 p} = b^q$. $\square$

Lemma 11.6. *If $u \equiv h^p$, $|h| = 1$, $a \in A$, and $ua \in U$, then $a = b^p$, $b \in A$.*

$\square$ Here ua has reduced form $ua = p^{-1}h(pa)$, and $ua \in U$ implies that $Ap = Apa$, hence $pa = bp$ for some $b \in A$, and $a = b^p$. $\square$

Lemma 11.7. *For u, w as above, let $|u^v| \leqslant |u|$. Then either $uv \in U$, or $|q| < |p|$ and $u^v \equiv h^{p'}$ for $p' = pv$, $|p'| \leqslant |p|$.*

$\square$ If $|p| = |q|$ it follows as before that we may suppose $p = q$, and $|u^v| \leqslant |u|$ implies $|h^k| \leqslant |h|$, whence $\mu = \nu$. Let $|p| < |q|$; as before we must have $q \equiv q_1 p$ and $u^v = p^{-1}q_1^{-1}k^{-1}q_1 hq_1^{-1}kq_1 p$. Now $|u^v| \leqslant |u|$ implies that $q_1^{-1}k^{-1}q_1 hq_1^{-1}kq_1 \leqslant 1$;

now $q_1^{-1}hq_1 \in U$, and the preceding inequality implies that $q_1^{-1}hq_1 = b \in A$, $h = b^{q_1}$, $u = b^q$. We are now in the second case of (11.4), with $uv \in U$.

Let $|q| < |p|$. If q^{-1} did not cancel in pq^{-1}, we would have $|pv| > |p|$ and $u^v \equiv h^{(pv)}$. Thus $p \equiv p_1 q$, $|p_1| \geqslant 1$, and $p' = pv = p_1 hq$. The inequality now implies that h cancel or consolidate, with $|p'| < |p|$. □

Lemma 11.8. *If $u \equiv h^p$, $|h| = 1$, $a \in A$, and $|u^a| < |u|$, then $u = h_1$, $|h_1| = 1$, and $u^a = h_1^a \in A$.*

□ If $|p| > 1$, then $u^a \equiv h^{pa}$, reduced with $|u^a| = |u|$. If $|p| = 0$, that is, $p \in A$, then $u \equiv h^p$ implies $u = h_1$ with $|h_1| = 1$. Now $|u^a| < |u|$ implies $|u^a| = 0$, that is, $u^a \in A$. □

We return to the proof of IV. For a step (α), we have a pair (u, v) with $u, v \in V$, and $uv \in U$. Let $u \in C_1^* \in \mathscr{D}$, $v \in C_2^* \in \mathscr{D}$; then (11.4, 11.5) implies that u, v, and so uv are all in C_1^* or all in C_2^*, whence the relation is a consequence of T_1.

For a step (β, γ) we can suppose by symmetry, for $u \in C_1^* \in \mathscr{D}$ and $v \in C_2^* \in \mathscr{D}$, that $|u^v| < |u|$. If $u, v \in A$ the conclusion is immediate, and follows from (11.5) if exactly one is in A. By (11.4) we are done unless $|q| < |p|$ and $u^v \equiv h^{p'}$, $p' = pv$, and $|p'| < |p|$. But now $Apv < Ap$ contradicts the minimality of Ap.

This completes the proof of the following.

Proposition 11.9. *N is the tree product of Δ.* □

We show next that N has as complement in G^* a free group F.

Let the elements of G be well ordered in such a way that, if $p \equiv p^{-1}hq$, $|p| = |q|$, $|h| \leqslant 1$, and $v \equiv r^{-1}ks$, $|r| = |s|$, $|k| \leqslant 1$, then $u < v$ if $|u| < |v|$; if $|u| = |v|$ and $Ap < Ar$; or if $|u| = |v|$, $Ap = Ar$, and $Aq < As$. Let S be the set obtained from the well ordered set G^* by deleting every u that is contained in the subgroup generated by N together with all $v < u$. Let $W = S \cup S^{-1}$. For $u \in W$, we write u^* for that one of u, u^{-1} that lies in S, that is, such that $u^* \leqslant u^{*-1}$. After some preliminaries we propose to show that S is a basis for a free group F, and that $N \cap F = 1$.

We now fix some notation. We write $u \equiv p^{-1}hq$, $|p| = |q|$, $|h| \leqslant 1$; if $Ap = Aq$ we may assume $p = q$, and if $|h| = 0$, we may assume $h = 1$ and $u \equiv p^{-1}q$. We write $v = r^{-1}ks$, $|r| = |s|$, $|k| \leqslant 1$; if $Ar = As$, then $r = s$, and if $|h| = 0$, then $k = 1$ and $v \equiv r^{-1}s$. We also denote by g an element of the form $g = g_1 \ldots g_n$ where for all i, $1 \leqslant i \leqslant n$, $g_i \in U^*$, $|g_i| \leqslant |v|$, and $|g_i \ldots g_n v| = |v|$.

Lemma 11.10. *If $u \in U$, $|u| \leqslant |v|$, and $|uv| = |v|$, then $uv \equiv r'^{-1}k's$, with $r' = r$ or $r' = ru^{-1}$, $|r'| = |r|$, and with $k, k' \in H_\nu - A$ for some $\nu \in I$, or else $k = k' = 1$.*

□ Since $|uv| = |v|$ the part p of $u = h^p$ cancels in the product uv, and h consolidates. Since $|u| \leqslant |v|$, $|p| \leqslant |r|$. If $|p| = |r|$ then $Ap = Ar$ and, refactoring v, we may suppose $p = r$. Now $|u| \leqslant |v|$ implies $|k| = 1$ and that h and k consolidate to give $k' = hk$, $|k'| = 1$. Then $uv \equiv r^{-1}k's$. If $|p| < |r|$, then $r \equiv r_1 h_1 p$, $|h_1| = 1$, and $r'^{-1} = ur^{-1} \equiv p^{-1}h'r_1^{-1}$ for $h' = hh_1^{-1}$, $|h'| = 1$. □

Lemma 11.11. *For g, v as above, $gv \equiv r'^{-1}k's$ with $r' = r$ or $r' = rg^{-1}$, $|r'| = |r|$, and with $k, k' \in H_\nu - A$ for some $\nu \in I$, or else $k = k' = 1$.*

□ This follows from (11.10) by induction. □

Lemma 11.12. *If $u \in U$, $|v| < |u|$, and $|uv| \leqslant |v|$, then $|u^v| < |u|$.*

□ Again, in uv, p cancels and h consolidates or cancels against a letter h_1 of v. Thus $v \equiv p^{-1}h_1z$, $|h_1| = 1$, and $|hh_1| \leqslant 1$. Now $|v| < |u|$ implies $|z| < |p|$. Since $u^v = (h^{h_1})^z$ with $|h^{h_1}| \leqslant 1$, one has $|u^v| < |u|$. □

Lemma 11.13. *If $u \in U$ and $|v|$, $|uv| < |u|$, then $|u^v| < |u|$.*

□ From $|v| < |u|$ we have $|r| < |p|$. From $|uv| < |u|$ we conclude that at least one letter more than the part r^{-1} of v cancels in uv, and, since $|r| + 1 \leqslant |p|$, in $p' = pv$, whence $|p'| < |p|$. But $u^v = h^{p'}$ whence $|u^v| < |u|$. □

Lemma 11.14. *If $v \in W$, then $|v| < |vgv|$.*

□ Suppose that $|vgv| \leqslant |v|$. Since $v = r^{-1}ks$, $gv = r'^{-1}k's$, with $|s| = |r| = |r'|$, and the part s of the first factor v must cancel in the product, we have $As = Ar'$, and we may suppose $s = r'$, and $gv \equiv s^{-1}k''s$ for $k'' = 1$. But now $gv \in U^*$, and $g, gv \in N$ contradicts $v \in W$. □

Lemma 11.15. *If $v \in W$, then either $|v| < |v^{-1}gv|$ or $v^{-1}gv \in U^*$.*

□ Suppose that $|v^{-1}gv| \leqslant |v|$. Then $v^{-1}gv = s^{-1}k^{-1}rr'^{-1}k's$ with $|r| = |r'|$ whence $r' = ar$, $a \in A$, and $v^{-1}gv = s^{-1}(k^{-1}a^{-1}k')s$ with $|k^{-1}a^{-1}k'| \leqslant 1$. □

Lemma 11.16. *If $u, v \in W$ and $uv \neq 1$, then $|u|, |v| \leqslant |ugv|$.*

□ By hypothesis, $u \neq v^{-1}$, while by (11.13) we may assume that $u \neq v$. Thus $u^* \neq v^*$; suppose $u^* < v^*$. Then $|u| < |v|$, and if $|ugv| < |v|$, we have $(ugv)^* < v^*$, contrary to $v \in W$. The symmetric analog of this argument applies if $v^* < u^*$. □

Lemma 11.17. *If $u, v \in W$, $uv \neq 1$, and $Ap < Aq$, then $|v| < |ugv|$.*

□ We suppose $|ugv| \leqslant |v|$. By (11.15), $|u| \leqslant |v| = |ugv|$. Now in $ugv = p^{-1}hqr'^{-1}k's$ the factor q must cancel and the letter h consolidate. But $|u| \leqslant |v|$ implies $|q| \leqslant |n'|$; thus, regardless of whether $|q| = |r'|$ or $|q| < |r'|$, we have $ugv \equiv r''^{-1}k''s$, $|k''| = 1$, where r ends in q and r'' in p. Now $Ap < Aq$ implies $Ar'' < Ar$, and $(ugv)^* < v^*$, contrary to $u, v \in W$. □

We now turn to showing that S is a basis for a free group F and that $N \cap F = 1$. We consider a sequence $\sigma = (v_1, \ldots, v_s)$, $s \geqslant 1$, where each v_i is either in U^* or W, and suppose that $v_1 \ldots v_s = 1$. It will suffice to show that the product $w = v_1 \ldots v_s$ reduces to 1 by virtue of the relations holding in N, the trivial relations of the form $v_iv_{i+1} = 1$ among the elements of W, and the set R_3 of relations ρ: $u^g = v$, for $u, v \in U^*$ and $g \in N$, that define the action of W (and so F) on N. More explicitly, it will suffice to show that σ can be reduced to the trivial sequence $\sigma_0 = (1)$ by a succession of steps (α, β, γ) justified by the relations mentioned above, that is, of passages from (v_i, v_{i+1}) to (u', v') or to (z) where the equation $v_iv_{i+1} = u'v'$ or $u_iv_{i+1} = z$ is justified by these relations. We call such steps permissible.

We shall successively modify the sequence $\sigma = (v_1, \ldots, v_s)$ by permissible steps until we obtain a new sequence σ^* that satisfies the hypotheses of (11.1).

By (7) of the conclusion of (11.1) it will then follow that $v_1 \dots v_s = 1$ is possible only if σ^* is the trivial sequence $\sigma_0 = (1)$.

As in the proof of (11.3), by replacing (v_i, v_{i+1}) by $(v_i v_{i+1})$ in case $v_i, v_{i+1} \in A^*$, by inserting trivial terms $a_i = 1$, and by cyclically permuting the v_i, we can replace σ by a sequence $\tau = (u_1, a_1, u_2, a_2, \dots, u_t, a_t)$ where all the u_i are in either W or $U^* - A^*$, and all the a_i are in A^*. (We have here excluded the trivial case of our problem where all the $v_i \in A^*$.)

For the sake of our inductive argument it is necessary to consider a somewhat enlarged class of sequences τ. We shall permit the a_i to be as in the statement of (11.1) in the case that $i < t$ and u_{i+1} is in W; for $u_{i+1} \in U^* - A^*$, and for $i = t$, we continue to require that $a_i \in A^*$.

We now establish a special case of our result.

Proposition 11.18. *If all $u_i \in W$ and no $u_i u_{i+1} = 1$, then $w \neq 1$.*

□ Under our assumption that all $u_i \in W$, Proposition (11.15) provides the hypothes of (11.1). Now it follows from (7) of the conclusion of (11.1) that $w \neq 1$. □

Corollary 11.19. *S is a basis for a free group F.*

□ This follows from (11.7) by considering $\tau = (u_1, a_1, u_2, a_2, \dots, u_t, a_t)$, $t \geqslant 1$, where all the $u_t \in W$, no $u_i u_{i+1} = 1$, and all the $a_i = 1$. □

We are now prepared to embark on the details of the proof of the following.

Proposition 11.20. *G^* is the split product of N by F.*

□ Resuming the notation above, we want to transform τ by permissible steps until all triples (u_i, a_i, u_{i+1}) satisfy the hypotheses of (11.1). To simplify notation we write (u, a, v) for (u_i, a_i, u_{i+1}).

Consider first the case that $u, v \in W$. By (11.14, 11.15), the triple (u, a, v) satisfies the hypotheses of (11.1) except in the case that $uv = 1$ and $uav \in U^* - A^*$. In this case we can replace (u, a, v) by (uav), using a permissible step justified by a relation given by the action of F on N. By hypothesis a_{i-1} is a product, $a_{i-1} = g_1 \dots g_n$, of factors $g_j \in U^*$. We replace the part (a_{i-1}, u, a, v) of τ by a part $(g_1, \dots, g_n, uav)$; after possibly inserting some terms 1, this gives a new sequence τ' with the required properties. This may well increase t, but it decreases the number t_0 of $u_i \in W$.

As the first stage in our reduction of τ, we suppose t_0 reduced in this way as far as possible. Then we may assume that every triple (u, a, v) with $u,v \in W$ satisfies the hypotheses of (11.1).

Consider next the case that $u,v \in U^* - A^*$. By our general conditions on τ, this implies that $a \in A^*$. Now, exactly as in the proof of (11.3), if the triple does not satisfy the hypotheses of (11.1), we can apply a step (α, β, γ), permissible by a relation among elements of N, to decrease t, to leave t fixed while decreasing $\sum |u_i|$, or to leave both t and $\sum |u_i|$ fixed while increasing the lexicographical rank of $|\tau| = (|u_{i_1}|, \dots, |u_{i_n}|)$ where the u_{i_k} are in order those $u_i \in U^* - A^*$. By induction on these quantities, in the order mentioned, we may suppose that every triple (u, a, v) with $u, v \in U^* - A^*$ satisfies the hypotheses of (11.1).

It remains to consider triples (u, a, v) such that one of u and v is in W and the other is in $U^* - A^*$. We first establish (1) of (11.1). Suppose $u \in U^* - A^*$ and $v \in W$, and $|v| \leqslant |u|$. If (1) fails, that is, if $|uav| < |u|$, then by (11.12) with v replaced by av, we have $|u^{av}| < |u|$. But now $\sum |u_i|$ could be decreased by replacing (u, a, v) by (a, v, u^{av}), a step permissible by the action of F on N. But this contradicts our assumption that $\sum |u_i|$ cannot be decreased by any permissible step. Suppose now that $|u| < |v|$ but (1) fails, so that $|uav| < |v|$. Then $(uav)^* < v^*$ which, since $ua \in N$, contradicts the fact that v is in W. This proves (1) for $u \in U^* - A^*$ and $v \in W$. But the symmetric counterpart of this argument proves (1) for $u \in W$ and $v \in U^* - A^*$.

We next establish (3) of (11.1). Let $As < Ar$. Then $v \notin U$, whence $v \in W$ and $u \in U^* - A^*$. Suppose the conclusion of (3) fails, and $|uav| \leqslant |u|$. By (1) this implies $|uav| = |u|$ and $|v| \leqslant |u|$. Thus the part r'^{-1} of $av \equiv r'^{-1}k's$ must cancel in the product uav, and, since $|v| \leqslant |u|$ and so $|r'| \leqslant |p|$, into the part p of $u \equiv p^{-1}hp$. Then $p \equiv p_1 r'$ for some p_1. From $|uav| = |u|$ we conclude that $p' = pav = p_1 ks$ has the same length as p. Since $a \in N$ and $v \equiv r^{-1}ks \in W$, $Ar' = Ara^{-1} \geqslant Ar$, and $As < Ar \leqslant Ar'$. Since p ends in r' and p' ends in s, $Ap' < Ap$. If we replace (u, a, v) by (a, v, u') where $u' = u^{av} = p'^{-1}hp'$, we have decreased Ap_i for one of the $u_i \equiv h^{p_i}$ in τ without disturbing any of our other hypotheses. By induction we may suppose the set of ranks of these Ap_i is minimal. Then the situation described above is no longer possible, and (3) holds.

The argument just given, in symmetric form, shows that $Ap < Aq$ implies $|v| < |uav|$. To prove (2) it remains only to show that $Ap = Aq$ implies $|v| < |uav|$. Now $Ap = Aq$ implies that $u \in U^* - A^*$ and so $v \in W$. Suppose $|uav| \leqslant |v|$; then by (1) $|u| \leqslant |v| = |uav|$. Moreover $a_{i-1} \in A^*$, so $|a_{i-1}| = 0 < |v|$ and $|a_{i-1}uav| = |uav| = |av| = |v|$. Thus we can use a relation within N to replace $(u_{i-1}, a_{i-1}, u, a, v)$ by $(u_{i-1}, a_{i-1}ua, v)$, thereby decreasing t, contrary to our hypothesis on τ. This completes the proof of (2).

We have now all the hypotheses of (11.1), and by (11.1) the proof of (11.19) follows by the arguments already given. □

We assemble various of the results established above to give a version of the Karrass-Solitar Theorem.

Proposition 11.21. *Let G be the free product of subgroups H_v for v in an index set I, with a subgroup A amalgamated. Let G^* be a subgroup of G, and let N be the normal subgroup of G^* generated by the groups $C^* = p^{-1}H_v p \cap G^*$ for all p in G and all v in I. Then N is a tree product of a certain family of these groups C^*, and G^*/N is a free group.*

In order to obtain the theorem of H. Neumann (see also IV.6.6 below), we recall that all the amalgamated subgroups in the tree product N were contained in conjugates of A. Thus, if G^* has trivial intersection with all conjugates of A, then N is the free product of a certain family of the groups C^*.

The action of F on N need not be free, but it is free in the case that G^* has trivial intersection with all conjugates of A. Now F permutes the C^* in $\mathscr{C}^*$, and no non-trivial element of F fixes any C^*. Let $\mathscr{E}$ be the set of $C^* = H_\mu^p \cap G^*$ for which Ap is minimal among all conjugates of C^* by elements of G^*. Then we see, as earlier in the consideration of $\mathscr{D}$, that the subgroup E generated by the C^* in $\mathscr{E}$ is the free product of those C^*, that N is the normal closure of E in G^*, and that G^* is the free product of E and F.

We have thus the theorem of H. Neumann (1948; see IV.6.6 below).

Proposition 11.22. *Let $G = \underset{A}{*} H_\nu$, $\nu \in I$, and let G^* be a subgroup of G having trivial intersection with all conjugates of A. Then G^* is the free product of certain subgroups $H_\mu^g \cap G^*$, $\mu \in I$, $g \in G$, together with a free group.* □

The case $A = 1$ gives the theorem of Kurosh (1934; see III.5.1 below).

Zieschang was interested in finite subsets of G, and, in particular, in finite generating subsets of G. Let a finite subset $X \subseteq G$ be given. Using the same order relation as before we can apply a finite sequence of elementary Nielsen transformations to obtain a finite set Y such that $\mathrm{Gp}(X) = \mathrm{Gp}(Y)$ and that $x, y \in Y^{\pm 1}$ and $xy \neq 1$ implies that $x^*, y^* < (xy)^*$. Consider now a sequence $\sigma = (u_1, \ldots, u_t)$, $t \geqslant 1$, with all $u_i \in Y^{\pm 1}$ and $u_i u_{i+1} \neq 1$. In applying permissible transformations, as in the proof of (11.19), no reduction is obtained by conjugating transformations carrying (u, a, v) to (a, v, u^{av}) for $u \in U$, $v \in W$, or to $(v^{a^{-1}u^{-1}}, u, a)$ for $v \in U$, $u \in W$. Thus only transformations justified by the relations of N are applicable, and, in the earlier notation, $G^* = \mathrm{Gp}(Y)$ is the free product of N and F. In particular, in view of (11.11), the condition $|u_1|, \ldots, |u_t| \leqslant |w| = |u_1 \ldots u_t|$ can fail only if the analogous condition fails for some subsequence for which all the u_i lie in U. We have thus a somewhat less detailed version of the theorem of Zieschang (1970); the full detail may be recovered from the indicated proof.

Proposition 11.23. *If X is a finite subset of $G = \underset{A}{*} H_\nu$, $\nu \in I$, then X can be carried by a Nielsen transformation into a set Y with the following property. Let $u_1, \ldots, u_t \in Y^{\pm 1}$, $t \geqslant 1$, with no $u_i u_{i+1} = 1$. Then either*

$$|u_1|, \ldots, |u_t| \leqslant |u_1 \ldots u_t|$$

or else, for some h and k, $1 \leqslant h \leqslant k \leqslant t$, $u_h, \ldots, u_k$ are conjugates of elements from the H_ν and for some i, $h \leqslant i \leqslant k$,

$$|u_h \ldots u_k| < |u_i|. \quad \square$$

An immediate consequence of the construction above is the result of Smythe (1976). If ϕ is a map from a finitely generated free group F into G, then F is the free product of groups $F_0, F_1, \ldots, F_n$, where ϕ maps F_0 injectively into G and, for $1 \leqslant i \leqslant n$, $F_i\phi$ lies in some H_μ^p, $\nu \in I$, $p \in G$.

Rosenberger (1974) analyzes Zieschang's result, showing by examples that none of the alternative conclusions spelled out in the detailed statement of Zieschang's theorem can be dropped. He also illustrates with examples the failure of the analog of the Grushko-Neumann Theorem (see III.3.7) for amalgamated products. Specifically, he shows that the following two assertions may fail for an amalgamated product $G = H_1 \underset{A}{*} H_2$.

(I) *If a finite set X generates G, then it can be carried by a Nielsen transformation into a set $Y \subseteq H_1 \cup H_2$.*
(II) Rank $G \geqslant$ Rank H_1 + Rank H_2 − Rank A.
As he notes, McCool and Pietrowski (1971) have established I for the case that A is normal in G.

As counterexamples to I and II^p Rosenberger cites two out of the infinite family of Fuchsian groups exhibited by Burns, Karrass, Pietrowski, and Purzitsky (unpublished) as counterexamples (and, in fact, the only counterexamples) to an assertion of Zieschang concerning the rank of Fuchsian groups (see III.7 below). These groups have the form

$$G = (x_1, \ldots, x_n; x_1^2 = \cdots = x_{n-1}^2 = x_n^m = 1, x_1 \ldots x_n = 1),$$

for even $n \geqslant 4$ and odd $m \geqslant 3$.
Such G is generated by $X = \{x_1x_2, \ldots, x_1x_{n-1}\}$. To see this, note that

$$\text{(i)} \quad (x_1x_2)(x_3x_1)(x_1x_4) \ldots (x_1x_{n-2})(x_{n-1}x_1) = x_1 \ldots x_{n-1}x_1$$

and

$$\text{(ii)} \quad (x_2x_1)(x_1x_3)(x_4x_1) \ldots (x_{n-2}x_1)(x_1x_{n-1}) = x_2 \ldots x_{n-1}$$

lie in Gp (X), whence multiplying,

$$(x_1 \ldots x_{n-1})^2 = x_n^{-2} \in \mathrm{Gp}(X).$$

Since x_n has odd order, this implies that $x_n \in \mathrm{Gp}(X)$. Now $x_n^{-1} = x_1 \ldots x_{n-1}$, whence, by (i), $x_1 \in \mathrm{Gp}(X)$. The conclusion is now immediate.

For a counterexample to both I and II, Rosenberger takes G as above with $n = 4$. Let $H_1 = (x_1, x_2; x_1^2 = x_2^2 = 1)$, $H_2 = (x_3, x_4; x_3^2 = x_4^m = 1)$; then $A = H_1 \cap H_2 = \mathrm{Gp}(a)$ where $a = x_1x_2 = (x_3x_4)^{-1}$, and $G = H_1 \mathop{*}_A H_2$. Now G is generated by the set $X = \{x_1x_2, x_1x_3\}$, while G clearly cannot be generated by any two-element set $Y \subseteq H_1 \cup H_2$. Thus I fails. Moreover, Rank G = Rank H_1 = Rank $H_2 = 2$ and Rank $A = 1$, whence II also fails.

As an example where I holds but II fails, Rosenberger takes the group G for $n = 6$. He takes $H_1 = (x_1, x_2, x_3; x_1^2 = x_2^2 = x_3^2 = 1)$, $H_2 = (x_4, x_5, x_6; x_4^2 = x_5^2 = x_6^m = 1)$, and hence $G = H_1 \mathop{*}_A H_2$ for $A = \mathrm{Gp}(a)$ for $a = x_1x_2x_3 = (x_4x_5x_6)^{-1}$. Now G is generated by $Y = \{x_1x_2, x_1x_3, x_4x_5, x_4x_6\}$. To see this, note that $(x_5x_4)(x_4x_6)(x_1x_2) = (x_5x_6)(x_1x_2) = (x_4x_3x_2x_1)(x_1x_2) = x_4x_3 \in \mathrm{Gp}(Y)$, when $(x_1x_3)(x_3x_4) = x_1x_4$ and $(x_1x_3)(x_3x_5) = x_1x_5$ are in Gp (Y). But then $X = \{x_1x_2, \ldots, x_1x_5\} \subseteq \mathrm{Gp}(Y)$ and $G = \mathrm{Gp}(X) = \mathrm{Gp}(Y)$. Here $Y \subseteq H_1 \cup H_2$, whence I holds, while II again is violated.

Kuhn (1952) gave a subgroup theorem for $G = \mathop{*}_A H_\nu$, $\nu \in I$, in the case that A is normal, and noted the special case that A is normal and $G^* \cap A = 1$. We have noted the theorem (11.21) of H. Neumann; a different proof was given by Imrich (1975). The proof by Karrass and Solitar of their subgroup theorem for amalgamated products used the Schreier rewriting process. This method has been used by Fischer (1975) to extend their result to a subgroup theorem for tree products. Chipman (1973) establishes by a covering space argument a very general theorem concerning subgroups of a graph product of groups, where the graph is not required to be a tree. Higgins (1966) used groupoids to prove a generalization, for free products without amalgamation, of Wagner's (1965) strong form of the Grushko-Neumann Theorem. Ordman (1971), again using groupoids, gives an extension of this result to mappings of amalgamated products onto free products. Chiswell (1970) gives a proof of the Grushko-Neumann Theorem by Serre's (1968/69) method of groups acting on trees. Karrass and Solitar (1971) give a subgroup theorem for HNN groups, and Cohen (1972), again using Serre's method, proves a sharpened form of their result.

Chapter II. Generators and Relations

1. Introduction

Groups are very often described as quotient groups of free groups: $G = F/N$. If F is free with basis X and N is the normal closure in F of a set R, we say that the pair $(X; R)$ is a *presentation* for G, and, by a mild abuse of language, we write $G = (X; R)$.

If $\bar{X}$ is the set of images $\bar{x}$ in G of the elements x of X, then $\bar{X}$ generates G. If $r = r(x_1, \ldots, x_n)$ is in R, then the equation $r(\bar{x}_1, \ldots, \bar{x}_n) = 1$ holds in G. By abuse of language it is customary to speak as X as a set of *defining generators* for G and of the equations $r = 1$, for r in R, as a set of *defining relations*. The elements r themselves will be called *relators*. The elements w of N are *consequences* of the set R of defining relators.

We often simplify the set theoretic notation; instead of

$$G = (\{a, b\}; \{a^2, b^3, (ab)^2\})$$

we write

$$G = (a, b; a^2, b^3, (ab)^2).$$

It is often suggestive to list the relations $r = 1$, or equivalent equations, rather than the relators; thus, for the above presentation we write also

$$G = (a, b; a^2 = 1, b^3 = 1, a^{-1}ba = b^{-1}).$$

Finally, we may omit to list the generators if they all appear in the defining relators (or relations); thus we write

$$G = (a^2, b^3, (ab)^2).$$

Magnus-Karrass-Solitar define a presentation to be a triple (X, R, ϕ), where X and R are as above and ϕ is a homomorphism from F onto G with kernel N. This is more precise, but is a refinement that we shall not require.

A presentation $(X; R)$ is *finitely generated* if X is finite, and is *finitely related* if R is finite; one says then also that $G = (X; R)$ is finitely generated or finitely related. A presentation $(X; R)$ is *finite* if both X and R are finite; in this case $G = (X; R)$ is *finitely presented*. For a finite group G, the multiplication table provides a finite presentation: for generators we take all the elements g_i of G and for defining relations all the equations $g_i g_j = g_k$ that are valid in G. A presentation can then be thought of as a possibly abbreviated generalization of a multiplication table. Many important infinite groups have finite presentations. On the other hand, B. H. Neumann (1937) has shown that there are uncountably many non-isomorphic groups generated by two elements; from this it follows that there are many finitely generated groups that admit no finite presentation.

Clearly a group G is determined up to isomorphism by a presentation. However, we shall see that even a finite presentation may not provide much knowledge about G. If X or R is not finite, they are often described by means of parameters. Such presentations arise naturally for groups of matrices over a given ring or field; see Zassenhaus (1969), Behr and Mennicke (1968), Beetham (1971), Swan (1971).

An important case is that where X is indexed by a set I consisting of all the natural numbers or a finite set of natural numbers. It is then not difficult to define a simple code (or Gödel numbering), f, establishing a one-to-one correspondence between F and the natural numbers. In logic one defines precisely what it means for a set U of natural numbers to be *recursive* or *recursively enumerable*; intuitively, U is recursive if there is an algorithm for determining whether or not a given number belongs to U, and U is recursively enumerable if there exists an algorithm which enumerates the elements of U in some order. We carry this language over to F by saying that a subset R of F is recursive or recursively enumerable if and only if $f(R)$ is; within reason this definition is independent of the chosen code.

We say that a presentation $(X; R)$ is *recursive* if X is indexed by I, as above, and R is recursively enumerable. This usage may seem a bit strange, but we shall see that if G has a presentation with R recursively enumerable, then it has another presentation with R recursive. A remarkable theorem of G. Higman (1961) states that a finitely generated group G has a recursive presentation if and only if G can be embedded in a finitely presented group. It follows from Neumann's result cited above together with cardinality considerations that there are many finitely generated groups that admit no recursive presentation.

The *word problem* is the first of the three fundamental decision problems posed by Dehn in 1912. Given a presentation $G = (X; R)$, this asks for an algorithm for deciding, given two elements w_1 and w_2 of F, whether they represent the same element of G. Clearly this is equivalent to deciding whether an arbitrary element $w = w_1^{-1} w_2$ lies in N. If such an algorithm exists, that is, if N is recursive, one says that the presentation has *solvable word problem*. For finitely generated presentations, this property is independent of the particular presentation of G that is chosen, and one therefore usually speaks of G as having solvable word problem. A fundamental result of P. S. Novikov (1955) and, independently, Boone (1959), exhibits a finite presentation with unsolvable word problem. (See also Britton (1963), G. Higman (1961), Rotman (1973), and Section IV.7 below.)

The second of Dehn's problems is the *conjugacy problem*, to decide if arbitrary

w_1 and w_2 in F represent conjugate elements of G. The third problem is the *isomorphism problem*, to decide whether two given finite presentations define isomorphic groups. Dehn (1912) solved all three of these problems as restricted to the canonical presentations of fundamental groups of closed 2-manifolds; we shall discuss extensions of his results in Chapter V below. We note (see 5.4 below) that Magnus (1932) showed the word problem solvable for groups with a *single defining relation*, that is, with a presentation $(X; R)$ in which R consists of a single element. It is not known whether every presentation in which R has only two elements has solvable word problem. Nor is it known whether every presentation with a single defining relation has solvable conjugacy problem.

It is clear that a solution of the conjugacy problem contains a solution of the word problem. It is also intuitively plausible that the conjugacy problem is intrinsically harder than the word problem, since it contains an extra 'existential variable' in that it asks about the existence of an element u in F such that $w_1^{-1}u^{-1}w_2u$ is in N. This intuition is correct, for there exist finitely presented groups with solvable word problem but unsolvable conjugacy problem; see Fridman (1960), Collins (1969), Miller (1971).

The isomorphism problem is even more difficult. Perhaps the most striking among a multitude of results in this area is that of Adyan (1957) and Rabin (1958), showing a very special case of the isomorphism problem already unsolvable: there is no algorithm which decides, given a finite presentation, whether the group it defines is trivial. For further discussion of decision problems in group theory see Miller (1971). We shall say no more in this chapter about unsolvability results; a few solvability results will be given.

2. Finite Presentations

A basic theorem of Tietze (1908) relates different finite presentations of the same group.

Let $(X; R)$ be any presentation. Let r be any element of N and let $R' = R \cup \{r\}$. It is clear that $(X; R)$ and $(X; R')$ define isomorphic groups.

Again, let $(X; R)$ be given, let $X' = X \cup \{x\}$ where $x \notin X$, let w be any element of F, and let $R' = R \cup \{r\}$ where $r = x^{-1}w$. It is easy to see that $(X; R)$ and $(X'; R')$ define isomorphic groups.

We refer to the passage from a given presentation to a second in either of these two ways, or in the opposite direction, as a *Tietze transformation.*

Proposition 2.1. *Two finite presentations define isomorphic groups if and only if it is possible to pass from one to the other by a finite sequence of Tietze transformations.*

□ It is clear that if two presentations, finite or not, are related by a finite sequence of Tietze transformations, then they define isomorphic groups. For the converse we suppose that two finite presentations $(X_1; R_1)$ and $(X_2; R_2)$ define isomorphic groups. For $i = 1, 2$, let F_i be the free group with basis X_i and let N_i be the normal closure in F_i of the subset R_i of F_i. We may suppose we are given a group G and two maps ϕ_i from F_i onto G with kernels N_i. We may suppose that $X_1 \cap X_2 = \varnothing$. Let $X = X_1 \cup X_2$, and let F be free with basis X. Then ϕ_1 and ϕ_2 together determine a map from X into G, which extends to a homomorphism ϕ from F onto G. Indeed, if we view F_1 and F_2 as subgroups of F, ϕ is the unique common extension of ϕ_1 and ϕ_2.

For each $x \in X_1$ choose $w_x \in F_2$ such that $x\phi = w_x\phi$, and let S_1 be the finite set of words $s_x = x^{-1}w_x$. Let S_2 be defined analogously. Now we can pass from $(X_1; R_1)$ to $(X; R_1 \cup S_2)$ by a finite sequence of Tietze transformations, each introducing a new generator $x \in X_2$ and a relator $x^{-1}w_x \in S_2$ serving to *define* x in terms of X_1. Clearly the kernel N of the map ϕ from F onto G is the normal closure in F of $R_1 \cup S_2$. It is also clear that $(R_2 \cup S_1)\phi = 1$, whence $R_2 \cup S_1 \subseteq N$. By a finite sequence of Tietze transformations we can adjoin the elements of $R_2 \cup S_1$ one at a time to $R_1 \cup S_2$ to obtain a presentation $(X; R) = (X; R_1 \cup R_2 \cup S_1 \cup S_2)$ for G.

We have shown that we can pass from $(X_1; R_1)$ to $(X; R)$ by a finite sequence of Tietze transformations. By symmetry, we can pass similarly from $(X_2; R_2)$ to $(X; R)$. It follows that we can pass from $(X_1; R_1)$ to $(X_2; R_2)$. □

It should be emphasized that (2.1) does not provide an answer to the isomorphism problem even assuming the given presentations have solvable word problem. For no effective procedure is provided for choosing S_1 or S_2. Although Tietze transformations have been used to show that solvability of the word or conjugacy problem is an invariant for finite presentations of the same group, more can be proved by an even simpler argument.

Proposition 2.2. *If a given finitely generated presentation of a group has solvable word or conjugacy problem, then the same is true of every finitely generated presentation of the group.*

□ Let $(X_1; R_1)$ and $(X_2; R_2)$ be two presentations of the same group G; we assume that $(X_1; R_1)$ has solvable word (or conjugacy) problem, and that X_2 is finite. We choose a function ϕ from X_2 into F_1 such that, for each $x \in X_2$, x and $x\phi$ represent the same element of G; then ϕ extends to a homomorphism from F_2 into F_1 with the same property. This homomorphism ϕ is certainly effectively calculable: given the finite table of values $x\phi$ for $x \in X_2$, to obtain $w\phi$ for any w in F_2 one need only substitute. Now, to decide if two given elements w_1 and w_2 of F_2 represent the same (or conjugate) elements of G, one need only calculate $w_1\phi$ and $w_2\phi$ and apply the algorithm for the presentation $(X_1; R_1)$. □

Tietze transformations are useful in special cases for showing that two given presentations define isomorphic groups, and, in particular, for simplifying a given presentation. They are also useful for showing that certain invariants of finite presentations are in fact invariants of the groups presented.

We state now a result of Magnus (1934) about presentations of finitely generated groups. Let A be a finitely generated abelian group generated by a set $x_1, \ldots, x_n$ and defined by a set of relators $s_i = \prod x_j^{c_{ij}}$ qua abelian group, that is, in the sense that all relations among the x_j follow from the equations $s_i = 1$ together with commutativity. We call the matrix $M = (c_{ij})$, which may have infinitely many rows, a *relation matrix* for A. The fundamental theorem on finitely generated abelian groups and its variants give us various *canonical forms* for M, from which one can extract invariants of A.

Proposition 2.3. *Let G be a finitely generated group, let $A = G/[G, G]$ be the abelianized group, and let $M = (c_{ij})$ be a finite m-by-n relation matrix for A. Then G has a presentation $G = (x_1, \ldots, x_n; r_1, r_2, \ldots)$ such that*

$$r_i \equiv \prod x_j^{c_{ij}} \ (\textit{modulo } [F, F]) \quad \textit{for } 1 \leqslant i \leqslant m$$

and

$$r_i \equiv 1 \ (\textit{modulo } [F, F]) \quad \textit{for } i > m.$$

□ Let $G = (X; R)$ with X finite and R possibly infinite. This determines a relation matrix M for A with $n = |X|$ columns and a possibly infinite number of rows. We can choose a finite number of these rows, say the first m, such that they span the row space of M; after adding suitable integral linear combinations of these rows to the rest, we may suppose that all the remaining rows are 0. We parallel this for the presentation, multiplying all r_i after the first m by suitable products of powers of $r_1, \ldots, r_m$; then all $r_i \equiv 1$ (modulo $[F, F]$) for $i > m$. We have thus a matrix M and presentation $(X; R)$ related in the described manner.

Any other finite relation matrix M' for A can be obtained from M by a succession of (i) elementary row transformations, (ii) elementary column transformations, and (iii) transformations carrying M into $M' = \begin{pmatrix} M & 0 \\ * & 1 \end{pmatrix}$ or conversely. Now an elementary row transformation of M can be induced by replacing the corresponding r_i by r_i^{-1} or by $r_i r_j$, $j \neq i$. An elementary column transformation can be induced by replacing some x_j by x_j^{-1} or by $x_j x_k$, $k \neq j$. The third type of transformation can be induced by a Tietze transformation introducing a new generator x_{n+1} together with a new relator $r'_{m+1} = (\prod_{j=1}^{n} x_j^{c_{m+1,j}}) x_{n+1}$, or the converse. Thus we can pass by a sequence of Tietze transformations to a new presentation $(X'; R')$ inducing the relation matrix M'. □

There are several problems concerning the possible pairs of cardinals $|X| = n$ and $|R| = m$ for a presentation $(X; R)$ of a given group. The minimum value of n is evidently the *rank* $r(G)$ of G, the smallest cardinal of a set of generators for G.

By (I.2.7), this agrees with the earlier definition of the rank of a free group. Obviously $r(G) = 0$ only if $G = 1$, and $r(G) = 1$ just in case G is cyclic but not trivial. By the Grushko-Neumann Theorem (III.5), if G is a free product, $G = G_1 * G_2$, then $r(G) = r(G_1) + r(G_2)$. No satisfactory general result is known concerning the rank of an amalgamated product, but Zieschang (1970) obtained such a formula under rather restrictive conditions on the amalgamated subgroup and its position in the two components, which has proved useful in determining the ranks of Fuchsian groups; see also Rapaport, 1964, and Peczynski, Rosenberger and Zieschang, 1970. It has been shown that many of the finite simple groups have rank 2; see Coxeter (1936, 1937); Coxeter-Moser (1965); Douglas (1951); G. A. Miller

(1900, 1901, 1902, 1908, 1920); Sinkov (1936, 1937, 1938); and Macbeath (1967). Indeed, G. A. Miller (1900) showed that, with a few small exceptions, every symmetric or alternating group can be generated by an element of order 2 together with an element of order 3. In fact, G. Higman (unpublished; see Dey and Wiegold (1971)) showed that, with a few small exceptions, every alternating group can be generated by an element of order 2 together with an element of order 3, and such that their product has order 7; these groups are thus quotients of the famous *triangle group* (2, 3, 7) with presentation $G = (x^2 = y^3 = (xy)^7 = 1)$. (We return to these triangle groups in III. 7 below.) Related groups $(l, m, n; p)$ with presentations $(x^l = y^m = (xy)^n = [x, y]^p = 1)$ have been discussed by Brahana (1931), Coxeter (1940), and Sinkov (1937); see also Macbeath (1961) and Leech (1965).

The ranks of the groups of Fuchsian type, the non-cyclic groups $G = (a_1, \ldots, a_g, b_1, \ldots, b_g, x_1, \ldots, x_p; x_1^{m_1}, \ldots, x_p^{m_p}, x_1 \cdots x_p Q)$ where $Q = [a_1, b_1] \cdots [a_g, b_g]$ have also been determined. If $p = 0$ it is evident from inspection of the abelianized group that $r(G) = 2g$. If $p > 0$, it is evident that one generator can be eliminated by a Tietze transformation, whence $r(G) \leqslant 2g + p - 1$; Zieschang (1970) showed that equality holds if $g > 0$, and indeed in the majority of cases where $g = 0$. It was noted by Burns, Karrass, Pietrowski, and Purzitsky (unpublished) that if $g = 0$ and p is even, and if $m_1 = \cdots = m_{p-1} = 2$, while m_p is odd, then $r(G) = p - 2$. It has been shown by Peczynski, Rosenberger, and Zieschang (1975) that these are the only exceptions: otherwise if $g = 0$ then $r(G) = p - 1$.

Considerable attention has been given to finding economical presentations for the classical linear groups over finite fields and special rings; see Behr and Mennicke (1968); Kneser (1964); Mennicke (1967); Zassenhaus (1969); Sunday (1972).

Given a finite set S of generators for a group G, one may consider all possible presentations $G = (X; R)$ in which X maps one-to-one onto S; it is natural to ask for the smallest value of $m = |R|$. Even the case that G is trivial presents difficult problems. If $(X; R) = 1$, by abelianizing F one can see that one must have $m \geqslant n$, and, trivially, taking $R = X$, the value $m = n$ can be attained. It was conjectured by Andrews and Curtis (1965, 1966) that if the trivial group has a balanced finite presentation, $(X; R) = 1$, $m = n$ finite, then R can be transformed into X by a sequence of transformations each of which is either an elementary Nielsen transformation or else consists of replacing some element by a conjugate. This problem has been investigated extensively by Rapaport (1964, 1968, 1968, 1973). Rapaport (1973) mentions a related problem of Waldhausen: if $G = (X; R)$ is a finite presentation with $n > r(G)$ does the normal closure of R in F necessarily contain some element of a basis for F?

A problem suggested by analogy with the commutative case is the following. Let G have a finite presentation $G = (X; R)$ with $m = |R| \leqslant n = |X|$, and let $d = n - m$, the *deficiency*. Does some subset X_0 of X, of cardinal d, have as image in G a basis for a free subgroup of G? If $d = 0$ the assertion is trivial. If $d = 1$, then $G/[G, G]$ is a finitely generated infinite abelian group, whence the image of some x in X must have infinite order, that is, must be a basis for a free group of rank 1. At the other extreme, if $d = n$, that is, if R is empty, the assertion is trivial. If $d = n - 1$, that is, if R consists of a single defining relator, the conclusion follows from the Freiheitssatz (see (5.1) below). The first case remaining open is that

$G = (x_1, x_2, x_3, x_4; r_1, r_2)$; do the images of some x_i and x_j generate a free subgroup of G of rank 2? A result of Stammbach (1968) gives a sufficient condition for a positive answer to the general conjecture.

The question of the relation between $n = |X|$ and $m = |R|$ in the case that $G = (X; R)$ is a finite group has received much attention. Clearly one must have $m \geqslant n$, and every cyclic group has a presentation with $m = n = 1$. A presentation is *minimal* if n is as small as possible, that is, if $n = \operatorname{rank} G$. Frucht (1955) has shown that the cyclic groups are the only abelian groups having minimal presentations with $m = n$. Neumann (1956, see also Coxeter-Moser, 1965, p. 11), has given minimal presentations for the dihedral groups of order $2k$ in the case that k is odd; the solution of a problem of Jones (1969) shows that three relators are necessary in in the case that k is even. Neumann (1956) constructed a family of finite groups having minimal presentations with $m = n = 2$. Schur (1904) had shown that for a finite group if $m = n$ then the multiplicator is trivial, and Neumann (1965) conjectured that the converse was true; this was disproved by Swan (1965); see also Tehara (1974). Mennicke (1959) exhibited a family of finite groups having minimal presentations with $m = n = 2$. Let $G = (x_1, x_2, x_3; r_1, r_2, r_3)$ where $r_i = x_{i+1}x_ix_{i+1}x_i^{-(t+1)}$, indices modulo 3. G is trivial if $t = -1, +1$ and is infinite if $t = -2, 0$; otherwise G is finite and of rank 3. Macdonald (1962) exhibited a class of finite groups of the form $G = (a, b; c^{-1}ac = a, c^{-1}bc = b)$ where $c = [a, b]$, thus with $m = n = 2$; Wamsley (1974) showed that for such G and p an odd prime, the maximal p-quotient of G is a finite p-group with $m = n \leqslant 2$. Further groups with $m = n = 2$ were constructed by Schenkmann (1967). Mennicke (1959) conjectured that $m = n = 3$ is impossible for a minimal presentation of a finite group, and indeed that one must have $m \geqslant n(n - 1)/2$. But Kostrikin (1964; see Huppert 1967, p. 402) constructed, for n an arbitrary power of 2, a p-group admitting a minimal presentation with n generators and $m = (3n^2 + 6n)/8$ relators; later (1969) he refined this to $m = (n^2 + 3n - 1)/3$. He observes (unpublished) that if we define γ to be the infimum of m/n^2 for minimal presentations of finite groups, then, by the above result $\gamma \leqslant 1/3$, while a result of Golod and Shafarevitch (1964) shows that $\gamma \geqslant 1/4$. (But note that Golod-Shafarevitch define m as the number of defining relators of G as pro-p-group, that is, as the dimension of $H^2(G, Z/pZ)$). In fact, Golod-Shafarevitch showed that for finite groups $m \geqslant (n - 1)^2/4$; Akagawa (1968) improves this, for finite p-groups, to $m \geqslant \sqrt{p/(p + 1)}.n(n - 1)/2$.

The *deficiency* of a finite presentation $G = (X; R)$ is defined as $d = n - m = |X| - |R|$. Assume that the normal closure of R is not the normal closure of fewer than m elements. According to Baumslag and Solitar (1962) it was at one time conjectured that, for a given group G, the deficiency was the same for all presentations satisfying this assumption, or at least all minimal presentations satisfying this assumption, and a proof was attempted by Petresco (1955). However, G. Higman observed that *the Baumslag-Solitar non-hopfian group* $G = (x, y; x^{-1}y^2x = y^3)$, *which clearly has rank* 2, *is also generated by* x *together with* $z = y^4$, *but has no presentation with these two generators and only a single defining relation.*

□ We give a proof of this. Let F be free of rank 2 with generators x and y. let $r = y^3x^{-1}y^{-2}x$, let N be the normal closure of r in F, and let ϕ be the canonical map from F onto $F/N = G$. Now, in G,

$$[y^4, x] = y^{-4}x^{-1}y^4x = y^{-4}y^6 = y^2$$

(that is, the elements of F listed have the same image in G), and

$$[[y^4, x], x] = y^{-2}x^{-1}y^2x = y^{-2}y^3 = y,$$

whence G is generated by (the images of) x and $z = y^4$. Let $F_1 = \mathrm{Gp}\{x, z\}$; then the restriction ϕ_1 of ϕ to F_1 maps F_1 onto G. We assume that the kernel N_1 of ϕ_1 is the normal closure of a single element $s = s(x, z)$ of F_1, and derive a contradiction.

Let $\bar{F}$ be the normal closure of y in F; then $\bar{F}$ has a basis of elements $y_i = x^{-i}yx^i$, $i \in \mathbb{Z}$. Evidently N is contained in $\bar{F}$ and is the normal closure in $\bar{F}$ of the elements $r_i = y_i^3 y_{i+1}^{-2}$, $i \in \mathbb{Z}$. Moreover, $\bar{F}_1 = F_1 \cap \bar{F}$ has a basis of elements $z_i = y_i^4$, while N_1 is contained in $\bar{F}_1$ and is the normal closure of the elements $s_i = x^{-i}sx^i$. Replacing s by a conjugate we may suppose that $s = s(z_0, \ldots, z_k)$ for some $k \geqslant 0$; then the s_i are obtained by substitution, $s_i = s(z_i, \ldots, z_{i+k})$.

Since the relation $y^{12} = x^{-1}y^8x$ holds in G, the element $u = z_0^3 z_1^{-2}$ of $\bar{F}_1$ lies in N_1. We now invoke the Freiheitssatz (II.5.1), in *staggered form*. Since u lies in the normal closure N_1 in $\bar{F}_1$ of the s_i, and u contains only z_0 and z_1, it follows that u is a consequence of s_0 alone, and that s_0 involves at most z_0 and z_1, that is, that $k = 1$ and $s_0 = s(z_0, z_1)$. We apply the Freiheitssatz once more. In $\bar{F}$, with a basis of the y_i, the element $s_0 = s(y_0^4, y_1^4)$ is a consequence of the $r_i = y_i^3 y_{i+1}^{-2}$, whence it follows that s_0 is a consequence of r_0 alone. In other words, the relation $s(z_0, z_1)$ holds in the group $H = (y_0, y_1; y_0^3 = y_1^2)$; inspection shows that every relation between $z_0 = y_0^4$ and $z_1 = y_1^4$ in this group is a consequence of the relation $z_0^3 = z_1^2$. Thus, in $\bar{F}_1$, $s(z_0, z_1)$ is a consequence of $u = z_0^3 z_1^{-2}$. We have shown that, in $\bar{F}_1$, u is a consequence of s_0 and s_0 is a consequence of u. We invoke another theorem of Magnus (II.5.8) to conclude that $s = s_0$ is conjugate in $\bar{F}_1$, and so in F_1, to u or to u^{-1}. We conclude that N_1 is also the normal closure of the element u.

It remains, to obtain a contradiction, to show that not every relation between x and z that holds in G is a consequence of the relation $u = z^3x^{-1}z^{-2}x$. We have seen that the relation $y = [z, x, x]$ holds in G, and hence the relation $z = [z, x, x]^4$; we shall show that this relation is not a consequence of u. In terms of the z_i, we must show that the element $v = z_0^{-1}(z_1^{-1}z_0z_1^{-1}z_2)^4$ is not a consequence of the $s_i = z_i^3 z_{i+1}^{-2}$. By the Freiheitssatz once more, if v were a consequence of the s_i it would be a consequence of s_0 and s_1 alone, and thus would represent the trivial element of the group $K = (z_0, z_1, z_2; z_0^3 = z_1^2, z_1^3 = z_2^2)$. But K is the amalgamated product (see IV.2 below) of the cyclic group $K_1 = (z_0; \varnothing)$ and $K_2 = (z_1, z_2; z_1^3 = z_2^2)$ with the two infinite cyclic subgroups L_1 and L_2 generated by z_0^3 and z_1^2 amalgamated by identifying the given generators. But v can be written as $v = z_0^{-1} \cdot z_1 \cdot (z_0 \cdot (z_1^{-1}z_2z^{-1}))^3 \cdot z_0 \cdot (z_1^{-1}z_2)$ with the indicated factors alternately from K_1 and K_2, and none of them from L_1 or L_2. From the Normal Form Theorem for Amalgamated Products (III.2.5) it follows that $v \neq 1$ in K. $\square$

Rapaport (1964) obtains as a consequence of a more complicated result that if a free group F of rank r has a finite presentation $F = (X; R)$, then $d = |X| - |R| =$

r; this can be seen also by abelianizing. She concludes also that if a group G has a finite presentation $G = (X; r)$ with a single defining relator, then in any finite presentation $G = (X'; R')$ for the same group one has that $d' = |X'| - |R'| = d = |X| - 1$. In particular, invoking symmetry, two presentations for the same group, each with a single (non-trivial) defining relator, must contain the same number of generators. She gives the following example. Let $G_1 = (X_1; R_1)$, $G_2 = (X_2; R_2)$, finite presentations; then supposing as we may that $X_1 \cap X_2 = \emptyset$, their free product G has a presentation $G = (X_1 \cup X_2; R_1 \cup R_2)$. In her example, neither normal closure N_i of R_i in F_i is the normal closure of fewer than $m_i = |R_i|$ elements, but the normal closure N of $R_1 \cup R_2$ in F, free with basis $X_1 \cup X_2$, is the normal closure of fewer than $m_1 + m_2 = |R_1 \cup R_2|$ elements. She gives also an example of a finite presentation $G = (X; R)$, where the normal closure of R is not the normal closure of fewer than $m = |R|$ elements, such that there exists a presentation $G = (X \cup \{x\}; R')$, where $x \notin X$ and where the elements of X represent the same elements of G under the two presentations, and in which $|R'| = m$.

Magnus (1959) proved that if a group G has a finite presentation $G = (X; R)$ such that $d = |X| - |R| = r(G)$, then G is a free group; Stammbach (1967) has given a new proof.

Further discussion of deficiency is given in Gruenberg (1970) and in Wamsley (1970, 1973).

Higman, Neumann, and Neumann (1940) showed that every group G with a finite presentation $G = (X; R)$ can be embedded in a group $G' = (X'; R')$ such that $|X| = 2$ and $|R'| = |R|$.

If $G = F/N$, F free, in general not every automorphism of F will leave N invariant. Those that do, induce automorphisms of G, but, in general, not every automorphism of G is induced by an automorphism of F. Rosenberger (1972) calls a presentation $G = (X; R)$ *quasifree* if $\mathrm{Aut}(F)$ maps naturally onto $\mathrm{Aut}(G)$; that is, every automorphism of F leaves N invariant, and every automorphism of G is induced by one of F. He shows that if G is not free, a presentation $G = (X; r)$ for G with a single defining relator is quasifree only in case it is of the form $G = (x; x^n)$ for $n = 2, 3, 4$, or 6, or else of the form $G = (x, y; [x, y]^n)$ for some $n \neq 0$. He observes that the usual presentation for the four group, $G = (x^2, y^2, (xy)^2)$ is quasifree. He notes also that, from results of Andreadakis, Bachmuth, and Chein (see I.4), the natural presentations for F/F_2 and F/F_3, as well as $F/F''(F')^p$, p a prime, are quasifree, while for F free of rank at least 2, the natural presentations for F/F'' and for F/F_n, $n = 3$, are not quasifree.

Rosenberger (1972) calls a presentation *almost quasifree* if every automorphism of G is induced by an automorphism of F. Nielsen (1917) showed that for the fundamental group G of a closed 2-manifold, that is, for $G = ([a_1, b_1] \cdots [a_g, b_g])$ or $G = (c_1^2 \cdots c_g^2)$, the indicated presentation is almost quasifree. Rosenberger (1972) has shown that if the relator Q in the first (orientable) case is replaced by a power Q^k, the same conclusion holds; see also Purzitsky (1972). Zieschang (1970) shows that in this case any presentation $G = (X; r)$ of G with a single defining relator can be brought into the given canonical form by an automorphism induced by one of F; here $|X| = 2g$, we set $X' = (a_1, \ldots, a_g, b_1, \ldots, b_g)$; then some automorphism of F carries X into X' and r into Q. Peczynski (1973) establishes the same result in the second (non-orientable) case. Zieschang also establishes the analogous result for the groups of Fuchsian type $G = (x_1^{a_1}, \ldots, x_p^{a_p}, x_1 \cdots x_p Q)$, with the assumption that $|X| \leqslant 2g + p$. Rosenberger (1974) establishes an analogous result, in the case that $p > 0$, for presentations with $2g + p - 1$ generators. It follows that all the presentations involved are quasifree.

Despite the theorem of Magnus (II.5.8) that if r_1 and r_2 have the same normal closure in the free group F with basis X, then r_1 is conjugate to r_2 or r_2^{-1} it is not the case that if two presentations $G_1 = (X; r_1)$ and $G_2 = (X; r_2)$ define isomorphic groups there must exist an automorphism of F, free on X, carrying r_1 into r_2 or r_2^{-1}. Counterexamples were found independently by McCool and Pietrowski (1971) and Zieschang (1970). McCool and Pietrowski examine a family of groups first studied by Schreier (1924), of the form $G_{k,l} = (x, t; x^k = y^l)$, $k, l > 0$. By an ingenious but short computation using Tietze transformations, they show that if $l = pt + 2$ for some $p > 0$ and $t > 1$, then $G_{k,l}$ has also a presentation $G_{k,l} = (x, y; y = (x^k y^{-t})^p)$. Now every Whitehead transformation (see I.4) other than a permutation increases the length of both $r_1 = x^k y^{-l}$ and $r_2 = y(x^k y^{-t})^{-p}$; by (I.4.1) it follows that no automorphism of F, free with basis x, y, can carry r_1 into r_2 or r_2^{-1}.

In connection with these matters see Metzler (1973); also contrast with (5.8) below.

Pride (1974) has shown that a presentation $G = (a, b, t; u^n = 1, t^{-1}at = b^e)$ where $n \geqslant 2$, $e = \pm 1$, and u is a word containing both a and b but only with positive exponent, is almost quasifree. This includes the groups $G = ([a, t]^n)$, $q \geqslant 2$, studied by Purzitsky and by Rosenberger, and also the groups $G = ((t^{-1}a^2ta^{-3})^n)$ for $n \geqslant 2$. For $n = 1$, G is the Baumslag-Solitar non-hopfian group. Brunner (1974) has studied these groups for $n = 1$. He observes that for all $m \geqslant 0$ the pair a^{2m}, b generates G, thus determining a map ϕ_m from F free on x, y onto G that carries x to a^{2m} and y to b, with kernel N_m. He shows that if $m \neq m'$ there is no automorphism α of F such that $\phi_m = \alpha\phi_{m'}$. For each m, N_m is the normal closure of the two elements $x^{-1}[x, y^2]$ and $[x, y^{-m}xy^m]$; for $m = 1$ the second element is superfluous, while, for $m = 2$, Higman has shown (see above) that N_2 is not the normal closure of a single element. Dunwoody and Pietrowski (1973) have shown, analogously, that the trefoil group $G = (a^2 = b^3)$ has infinitely many pairs of generators that are inequivalent in the above sense, and that, relative to at least one of these pairs, G cannot be defined by a single relator. For some of the basic ideas here, see B. H. Neumann and H. Neumann, 1951.

Serre (1974) calls a group *coherent* if every finitely generated subgroup is finitely presented. G. P. Scott (1973) has shown that the fundamental group of any closed 3-manifold is coherent. Serre asks if the groups $\mathbb{SL}(3, \mathbb{Z})$, $\mathbb{GL}(n, \mathbb{Q})$, $\mathbb{SL}(n, F[t])$, $\mathbb{SL}(n, F[t, t^{-1}])$ are coherent; here F is a finite field, $F[t]$ the ring of polynomials over F in an indeterminate t, and $F[t, t^{-1}]$ that of 'L-polynomials' (Laurent polynomials) of the form $t^{-k}p(t)$, $p(t)$ an ordinary polynomial. Note that $\mathbb{GL}(n, \mathbb{Q})$ and $\mathbb{SL}(n, \mathbb{Z})$ are known not to be coherent.

Certain groups have presentations $G = (X; R)$ such that the group of automorphisms of F induced by a certain subgroup P of the symmetric group on X leaves N invariant; we may then suppose that P leaves R invariant. We shall consider below (in (II.6)) the case that $X = (x_i \colon i \in \mathbb{Z})$ and that P is the group of translations $x_i \mapsto x_{i+p}$. Clearly the symmetric groups, the alternating groups, and some other groups with a geometric definition, naturally admit presentations that are symmetric in this sense. The case that R consists of a single orbit has been examined by Emerson (1967). Given such a symmetric presentation, it is clear that P acts as a group of automorphism on G. If P has a presentation $P = (Y; Q)$, then evidently the split extension H of G by P has a presentation $H = (Y \cup X_1; Q \cup R_1)$ where X_1 is a set of representatives of the orbits of X under the action of P, and R_1 results from expressing a set of representatives of the orbits of R under P in terms of the elements of X_1 together with their conjugates under elements of P. Thus, if $G = (x_1, \ldots, x_n; r_1, \ldots, r_n)$ and the permutation $b: x_i \mapsto x_{i+1}$ (indices modulo n) carries r_j into r_{j+1}, then H has a presentation $H = (x_1, b; b^n = 1, w(x_1, b) = 1)$, where w is a word with exponent sum 0 in b.

Conway (1965, 1967) introduced a family of groups F_n with balanced presentations, as follows:

$$F_n = (x_1, \ldots, x_n; x_1x_2 = x_3, \ldots, x_{n-1}x_n = x_1, x_nx_1 = x_2);$$

we call these *Fibonacci groups*. It is not difficult to show that $F_1, \ldots, F_5$ have orders 1, 1, 8, 5, 11. Coxeter and Mendelsohn (see Conway (1967)) showed that F_6 is infinite, and Mendelsohn that F_7 is infinite. Conway (1967) stated that F_n is infinite for all sufficiently large n, and Lyndon (unpublished) showed by small cancellation theory that F_n is infinite for all $n \geqslant 11$. Johnson (1974) introduced the more general class of groups

$$F_{r,n} = (x_1, \ldots, x_n; x_ix_{i+1} \cdots x_{i+r-1} = x_{i+r}, i \text{ modulo } n).$$

Thus $F_{2,n} = F_n$. He showed that $F_{3,4}$ is infinite, that $F_{5,5}$ has order 22, while C. M. Campbell (see Johnson 1974) showed that $F_{3,6}$ has order $2^3 3^3 7$, and determined its Sylow subgroups. For further discussion of these groups see Johnson (1976).

The minimal cardinality of R with normal closure N for a group $G = (X; R)$, given X, is perhaps a rather crude way of measuring the departure of G from the free group F with basis X. For there are various measures of the *dependence* or partial redundancy of the set R of relators. A discussion of one aspect of this question, in the context of the Freiheitssatz and related matters, in given in Lyndon, 1962. A different and very fruitful measure of this independence of relators is provided by *small cancellation theory*; see Chapter V. A third way of judging the dependence of relators lies in considering the number of essentially different ways in which a given consequence of the relators can be derived; a precise form of this problem, discussed in (II.3 below), leads to cohomological considerations. We turn to one aspect of this approach in the following paragraph, and, in a succeeding paragraph, to yet another way of approaching this problem. The interrelations among these approaches are at present far from clear.

Swan (1965) considered a generalization of the concept of the deficiency of a presentation. Suppose that a group G has a free resolution (see II.3):

$$\to M_n \to \cdots \to M_1 \to M_0 \to \mathbb{Z} \to 0$$

where the M_i are free $\mathbb{Z}\mathbb{G}$ modules of finite ranks f_i. He considers the alternating sums $\mu_n = f_0 - f_1 + \cdots + (-1)^n f_n$. In particular, if G has a finite presentation $G = (X;\ R)$ one may take $f_0 = 1$, $f_1 = |X|$, $f_2 = |R|$, whence $\mu_0 = 1$, $\mu_1 = 1 - |X|$, and $\mu_2 = 1 - |X| + |R| = 1 - d$, for d the deficiency of the presentation. Now f_3 is a measure of the *sphericity* of the presentation (see III.11), that is, of the dependence among the relators, and in this sense $\mu_3 = 1 - d + f_3$ provides, in $d' = d - f_3$, a first order correction to the previous definition of the deficiency. Swan obtains extensive results relating to the possible values of these invariants of a resolution, but, unfortunately, they come near to being definitive only under the assumption that the group G is finite. We note that in the same paper he provides the counterexample mentioned earlier to a conjecture of Neumann, exhibiting a group $G = (X;\ R)$, $|R| \leqslant |X|$, such that the multiplicator $H_2(G, \mathbb{Z}) = 0$.

Wall (1961) considers the case that G has a finite resolution, that is with $M_i = 0$ for all i greater than some n. Then the *Euler-Poincaré characteristic* $\chi(G) = f_0 - f_1 + \cdots + (-1)^n f_n$ is in fact an invariant of G. Serre (1969/70, 1971) extends this definition to groups H that contain a subgroup G, of finite cohomological dimension in the above sense, by setting $\chi(H) = |H\colon G|^{-1}\chi(G)$, observing that this too is an invariant of such H; he calculates $\chi(H)$ for certain such H. Karrass-Pietrowski-Solitar (1974) axiomatize a characteristic function on a class C of groups, invariant under isomorphism, by the condition that if G and H are in C and G has finite index in H, then $\chi(G) = |H\colon G| \cdot \chi(H)$. In particular, if C contains all finite groups, then $\chi(G) = 1/|G|$ for G finite; moreover, if H and two subgroups G_1 and G_2, both of finite index, are in C, and G_1 and G_2 are isomorphic, then they must have the same index. Wall's characteristic function satisfies the further axiom that if G_1 and G_2 are in C, here the class of all groups of finite cohomological dimension, then the free product $G = G_1 * G_2$ also is in C, and $\chi(G) = \chi(G_1) + \chi(G_2) - 1$. For the class C of finite extensions of finitely generated free groups, Stallings (to appear) improves this formula to $\mu(G_1 *_A G_2) = \mu(G_1) + \mu(G_2) - \mu(A)$ in the case of an amalgamated product with the amalgamated subgroup A finite. Karrass, Pietrowski, and Solitar extend Stallings' result to one covering the case of combined finite amalgamation and finite HNN-extension. These results are related to those of Brown (1974), Chiswell (1976), Verdier (1973), and also to the Riemann-Hurwitz formula (III.7 below) and its extension by Hoare-Karrass-Solitar (to appear) to non-Euclidean crystallographic groups.

Milnor (1963) introduced the concept of the *rate of growth* of a finitely generated group. This concept had already been studied in special contexts by Krause (1953) and Svarc (1955). Let X be a finite set of generators for a group G, thus $G = F/N$ for F free with basis X. For each natural number n, let $\gamma(n)$ be the number of elements of G that are represented by elements w of F of length $|w| \leqslant n$. If a second finite set X' of generators is chosen, then the functions γ and γ' are *equivalent* in the following sense: there exist natural numbers k and k' such that for all n, one has $\gamma(n) \leqslant \gamma'(kn)$ and $\gamma'(n) \leqslant \gamma(k'n)$. Milnor asked if the function γ is always equivalent in this sense either to a polynomial in n or to an exponential function in n. He conjectured that γ is of polynomial growth if and only if G contains a nilpotent subgroup of finite index. In a second paper (1968) he observes that $\gamma(n)^{1/n}$ always converges to a value a in the interval $1 \leqslant a < \infty$, and that γ is exponential if

$a > 1$. He states there also the connection, from which these ideas arose, between the curvature of a Riemannian manifold and the rate of growth of its fundamental group. He gives some examples, and relates the general concept to the results of Kesten (1959) on the eigenvalues of random walks on groups. Wolf (1968), in addition to continuing the study of the connection with curvature, shows that if a group G has a finitely generated nilpotent subgroup of finite index, then its growth is polynomial, and that if G is polycyclic and has no finitely generated nilpotent subgroup of finite index, then its growth is exponential. Milnor (1968) shows that a solvable group that is not polycyclic has exponential growth, thereby establishing his conjecture for all finitely generated solvable groups.

Justin (1971) showed that if a finitely generated group or semigroup has a growth function satisfying $\gamma(n) < n(n + 3)/2$, then it satisfies $\gamma(n) \leqslant kn$ for some k. Adyan (1974) showed that the free Burnside group $B(m, n)$, with m generators and with exponent n, in case that it is infinite, has exponential growth. A further discussion of growth functions is given by Bass (1973).

3. *Fox Calculus, Relation Matrices, Connections with Cohomology*

We have noted already that, by virtue of the fundamental theorem on finitely generated abelian groups, if an abelian group is defined, qua abelian group, by a finite number of generators and relations, then the structure of the group can be read off from the associated relation matrix. Analogous methods are not so easily applicable to non-abelian groups, and the results they yield are not so complete. However, a method of this sort introduced by Fox has met with considerable success in the study of the groups of knots and links. For details see the books of Crowell and Fox (1963) and of Birman (1974). We sketch a few central ideas.

Let F be a free group with basis X and let $\mathbb{Z}F$ be the group ring of F over the ring $\mathbb{Z}$ of integers. For each x in X the free derivation $\partial/\partial x$: $\mathbb{Z}F \to \mathbb{Z}F$ has been described (I.10); these are characterized by the condition that $\partial/\partial x$ be a derivation and that $\partial y/\partial x = \delta_{xy}$ (Kronecker delta) for $y \in X$, or alternatively by the formula

$$(*) \qquad w - 1 = \textstyle\sum_{x \in X} \dfrac{\partial w}{\partial x}(x - 1), \qquad w \in F.$$

Let $G = (X; R)$; we denote by ϕ both the canonical map from F onto $G = F/N$ and the induced map from $\mathbb{Z}F$ onto $\mathbb{Z}G$. We write $\bar{G} = G/[G, G]$ and $\bar{\phi}$ for the map from $\mathbb{Z}F$ onto $\mathbb{Z}\bar{G}$ induced by ϕ. We shall not hesitate to use the same symbol w for an element of F and for its images in G and in $\bar{G}$ whenever the meaning is clear from the context. The *Jacobian matrix* of the presentation is the matrix

$$J = \left(\frac{\partial r_i}{\partial x_j}\right)\phi$$

over $\mathbb{Z}G$; for most purposes it is preferable to pass to the abelianized Jacobian $\bar{J} = (\partial r_i/\partial x_j)\bar{\phi}$ over the commutative ring $\mathbb{Z}\bar{G}$.

As usual, we define the *determinantal ideal* D_i, of order i, of $\bar{J}$ to be the ideal in $\mathbb{Z}\bar{G}$ generated by all i-by-i minors of $\bar{J}$. It is easy to verify that the finite sequence $D_1, D_2, \ldots$ of fundamental ideals is unaltered by Tietze transformation apart from the possible deletion or insertion of the unit ideal as D_1. Thus by (2.1) the non trivial part of the sequence $D_1, D_2, \ldots$ is an invariant of the group G. This theory arose in the case that G is the fundamental group of the complement of a knot in 3-space; here $\bar{G}$ is an infinite cyclic group, say with generator t, and the highest non-vanishing determinantal ideal is a principal ideal with generator a (monic) polynomial in t, the *Alexander polynomial* of the knot.

We sketch the connection of these ideas with cohomology theory; for more details see Gruenberg (1970).

We continue the notation above. The trivial map $\varepsilon: G \to 1$ induces the *augmentation map* $\varepsilon: \mathbb{Z}\bar{G} \to \mathbb{Z}$, with kernel K_0 the *augmentation ideal* (or *fundamental ideal*) of $\mathbb{Z}G$. It is easy to see that for $u = \sum c_g g \in \mathbb{Z}G$ ($c_g \in \mathbb{Z}$, $g \in G$), $u\varepsilon = \sum c_g$, the coefficient sum of u, and that K_0 is generated by the $x - 1$ for $x \in X$. Indeed, by virtue of the formula (*), K_0 is generated by the $x - 1$ as left ideal in $\mathbb{Z}G$. If we view $\mathbb{Z}G$ as a (free) left $\mathbb{Z}G$-module M_0, then K_0 is a submodule. Let M_1 be the free left $\mathbb{Z}G$-module with basis a set of elements δx in one-to-one correspondence with the elements x of X, and define a map $d_1: M_1 \to M_0$ by setting $d_1: \delta x \mapsto x - 1$. By construction, d_1 maps M_1 onto K_0. It is not too difficult to show that the kernel K_1 of d_1 is the submodule of M_1 consisting of all elements $\delta r = \sum(\partial r/\partial x)\delta x$ for r in N and that K_1 is generated by the elements δr for r in R. Let M_2 be the free left $\mathbb{Z}G$-module with basis a set of elements $\tilde{r}$ in one-to-one correspondence with the elements r of R, and define a map $d_2: M_2 \to M_1$ by setting $d_2: \tilde{r} \mapsto \delta r$. By construction, d_2 maps M_2 onto K_1. We shall discuss the interpretation of the kernel K_2 of d_2 below.

We have now a sequence of left $\mathbb{Z}G$-modules which can obviously be extended indefinitely to obtain a *free resolution*

$$\cdots \xrightarrow{d_3} M_2 \xrightarrow{d_2} M_1 \xrightarrow{d_1} M_0 \xrightarrow{d_0} \mathbb{Z}$$

in the following sense: the M_i are free $\mathbb{Z}G$-modules and the sequence is exact at each M_i in the sense that the image under d_{i+1} is the kernel of d_i (here we take $d_0 = \varepsilon$).

From the definitions, $K_0 \simeq M_1/K_1$, where M_1 has a basis of the δx_j and where K_1 is generated by the elements $\delta r_i = \sum(\partial r_i/\partial x_j)\delta x_j$ for $r_i \in R$. Thus the Jacobian matrix J can be viewed as a relation matrix for the left $\mathbb{Z}G$-module K_0, and $\bar{J}$ as a relation matrix for the left $\mathbb{Z}G$-module $\mathbb{Z}\bar{G} \otimes K_0$.

It can also be shown that $K_1 \simeq M_2/K_2 \simeq N/[N, N]$ where the latter has the natural structure of $\mathbb{Z}G$-module. We call $\bar{N} = N/[N, N]$ the *relation module* of the given presentation; if $G = F/N$, it clearly depends upon F and N, but not upon the choice of R. This too is to a large extent an invariant of G (see Lyndon, 1962). More precisely, if $\bar{N}_1$ and $\bar{N}_2$ are two relation modules obtained from finite presentations of the same group G, then there exist two free $\mathbb{Z}G$-modules P_1 and P_2

such that $\bar{N}_1 \oplus P_1 \simeq \bar{N}_2 \oplus P_2$. Evidently $\bar{N}$ is generated by the images of the elements r of R. Gruenberg (1970) has shown that if G is a finite group and if $\bar{N}_1$ and $\bar{N}_2$ are relation modules derived from two finite presentations such that $|X_1| = |X_2|$, then the minimum number of generators for $\bar{N}_1$ is the same as that for $\bar{N}_2$. Dunwoody (1973) showed that this need not be true if G is infinite. If G is the trefoil group $G = (a^2 = b^3)$ then the relation module $\bar{N}_1$ associated with this presentation is clearly generated by a single element; he exhibits a second presentation $G = (X_2; R_2)$ with $|X_2| = |R_2| = 2$ such that the associated relation module $\bar{N}_2$ cannot be generated by a single element. (From this it follows that N_2 is not the closure of a single element; compare Dunwoody and Pietrowski, 1973.) In this case, by a result of Lyndon (1950; see II.5 below) $\bar{N}_1 \simeq \mathbb{Z}G$, the free $\mathbb{Z}G$-module of rank 1; Dunwoody shows that $\bar{N}_2 \oplus \mathbb{Z}G \simeq \bar{N}_1 \oplus \mathbb{Z}G \simeq \mathbb{Z}G \oplus \mathbb{Z}G$, whence $\bar{N}_2$ is projective, but he shows that $\bar{N}_2$ is not free, nor of the form $\bar{N}_2 \simeq \mathbb{Z}G \oplus M$ for any module M. Dunwoody shows also that for $G = (x, y; x^5)$ the relation module $\bar{N}$ can be generated by a single element that is not the image of any element r of N, thereby refuting a conjecture of Wall (1966).

We turn now to the kernel K_2 of d_2: $M_2 \to M_1$. The elements of M_2 are elements of the form $\mu = \sum \gamma_i \tilde{r}_i$ for $\gamma_i \in \mathbb{Z}G$ and $r_i \in R$. We have been using additive notation because we are dealing with modules, and operators on the left (rather than on the right) because we are using a formalism that arose in topology rather than in group theory. We retain the left operators, but pass to a multiplicative notation, writing $\mu = \prod {}^{\gamma_i}\tilde{r}_i$. The values μd_2 in $K_1 \simeq \bar{N}$ are then of the form $\mu d_2 \equiv \prod {}^{\gamma_i} r_i$, modulo $[N, N]$. (Here, for $c \in \mathbb{Z}$ and $g \in G$, one has ${}^{(cg)}r = g r^c g^{-1}$, with the meaning of ${}^{\gamma}r$ clear from linearity). Thus K_2 comprises those μ of this form such that $\mu d_2 = 1$, and correspond to the 'relations among relators' of the form $\prod {}^{\gamma_i} r_i \equiv 1$ (modulo $[N, N]$), or, more explicitly, of the form $\prod g_j \cdot r_{ij}^{e_j} \cdot g_j \equiv 1$ (modulo $[N, N]$), for $g_j \in G$, $e_j = \pm 1$. These are usually called *identities among relations*, and we shall return to them below.

We note that Ojanguren (1968) has studied the representation of G on $\bar{N}$, and also the induced complex representation, in the case that G is finite.

The free resolution given above, associated with a presentation, can be used to gain certain information about the cohomology and homology of a group. Among the most important general formulas is that of Hopf, $H^2(G, \mathbb{Z}) \simeq (N \cap [F, F])/[N, N]$ ((1942); see also Lyndon (1950); and for this and similar invariants, Oranguren (1966); Stallings (1966); Stammbach (1966)). This method provides information about the cohomology of a free product or an amalgamated product; see Lyndon (1950); Swan (1960, 1969).

If $G = 1$, one has a free resolution $0 \to \mathbb{Z}G = \mathbb{Z} \to \mathbb{Z}$ with $M_1 = 0$. If G is free, then one has a resolution $0 \to M_1 \to M_0 = \mathbb{Z}G \to \mathbb{Z}$ with $M_2 = 0$. Among the first calculations in the cohomology theory of groups, in the initial papers of Eilenberg and MacLane (1949), were those of cyclic groups. Using methods of Reidemeister (1934) and Magnus (1930), Lyndon (1950) extended their results to groups defined by a single relation, $G = (X; r)$. If r is not a proper power in F, that is, one does not have $r = s^n$, $n > 1$, then G has a resolution $0 \to M_2 \to M_1 \to M_0 = \mathbb{Z}G \to \mathbb{Z} \to 1$.

A group G has *cohomological dimension* cd $G = n$ if it possesses a free resolution such that all $M_i = 0$ for all $i > n$, but none with $M_n = 0$. The remarks above imply that if $G = 1$, then cd $G = 0$, that if G is free and non-trivial, then cd $G = 1$, and that if G is defined by a single relator that is not a proper power, then cd $G \leqslant 2$. (A more intrinsic definition of the condition cd $G = n$ is that n is the least integer such that $H^n(G, M) = 0$ for all $\mathbb{Z}G$-modules M.) It is trivial that, conversely, cd $G = 0$ implies $G = 1$. It was a famous conjecture of Eilenberg and Ganea (1957) that cd $G = 1$ implies that G is free; this was proved by Stallings (1968) for G finitely generated, and by Swan (1970) for arbitrary G. The groups G with cd $G = 2$ are not fully known. Lyndon (1950) shows that if G is defined by a single relator that is not a proper power, then the relation module $\bar{N}$ is free on the image of this relator, and (1962) extends this result. Serre (1971) asks whether, if cd $G \leqslant 2$, then G has a presentation such that $\bar{N}$ is free on the set of the images of the elements of R.

If $G = (X; r)$ with r a proper power, then cd $G = \infty$; Lyndon (1950) showed that in this case, extending the result of Eilenberg and MacLane for cyclic groups, G has periodic cohomology: $H^{n+2}(G, M) \simeq H^n(G, M)$, $n \geqslant 2$.

The *geometric dimension* gd G of a group G is defined to be the lowest dimension of an aspherical cell complex with fundamental group G. It is known that gd G = cd G provided that cd $G \neq 2$, and that cd $G = 2$ implies gd $G \geqslant 2$. Eilenberg and Ganea pose the problem whether cd $G = 2$ in fact implies gd $G = 2$; Dyer and Vasquez (1973) establish this conclusion for the case that G is a one-relator group.

We have observed earlier that the *multiplication table* for a group G yields a presentation in which X is in one-to-one correspondence with G and R consists of all valid relators of length 3. The free resolution arising naturally from this presentation is essentially the *standard resolution* of Eilenberg and MacLane. (This observation has also been used by Stallings (1968) to conclude that every group has a Cayley complex (see III) that is simplicial.)

A somewhat different resolution has been associated to a presentation by Gruenberg (1960, 1967, 1970). Let $G = F/N$ where F is free with basis X, and let Y be a basis for the free group N. Let $\mathscr{F}$ be the kernel of the augmentation map from $\mathbb{Z}F$ onto $\mathbb{Z}$, and let $\mathscr{R}$ be the kernel of the naturally induced map from $\mathbb{Z}F$ onto $\mathbb{Z}G$. We have observed that $\mathscr{F}$, as left $\mathbb{Z}F$-module, is free with a basis of all $x - 1$ for x in X; Gruenberg shows that $\mathscr{R}$, as $\mathbb{Z}F$-module, is free with a basis of all $y - 1$ for y in Y. He proves the following theorem.

Proposition 3.1 *If $G = F/N$, with $\mathscr{F}$ and $\mathscr{R}$ as above, then G has a free resolution as follows*:

$$\cdots \to \mathscr{R}^2/\mathscr{R}^3 \to \mathscr{F}\mathscr{R}\mathscr{F}\mathscr{R}/\mathscr{F}\mathscr{R}^2 \to \mathscr{R}/\mathscr{R}^2 \to \mathscr{F}/\mathscr{F}\mathscr{R} \to \mathbb{Z}G \to \mathbb{Z} \to 0. \quad \square$$

In this connection see also Hughes (1966), Gildenhuys (1976).

4. The Reidemeister-Schreier Method

An important result of Reidemeister (1932) and Schreier (1927) enables one, given a presentation of a group G, and suitable information about a subgroup H of G, to obtain a presentation for H. The original theorem of Reidemeister had a weaker hypothesis but a somewhat more complicated conclusion than the version we present here; on the other hand, Magnus, Karrass, and Solitar (p. 87) have presented further refinements of the results we present here. It has long been known (see, for example, Zieschang, Vogt, Coldewey (1970)) that these ideas have a natural geometric interpretation.

Recall (see I.3.8) that a Schreier transversal of a subgroup H of F, free with basis X, is a subset T of F such that, for distinct t in T, the cosets Ht are distinct, that the union of the Ht is F, and such that every initial segment of an element of T itself belongs to T.

Proposition 4.1. *Let $G = F/N$, F free with basis X and N the normal closure of R in F, and let ϕ be the canonical map from F onto G. Let H be a subgroup of G, with $\tilde{H}$ the inverse image of H under ϕ, and T a Schreier transversal for $\tilde{H}$ in F. For w in F we define $\overline{w}$ by the condition that*

$$Hw = H\overline{w}, \overline{w} \in T.$$

For $t \in T$ and $x \in X$ we define

$$\gamma(t, x) = tx(\overline{tx})^{-1}, \gamma(t, x^{-1}) = tx^{-1}(\overline{tx^{-1}})^{-1} = \gamma(tx^{-1}, x)^{-1}.$$

Then H has a presentation $H = (X_1^*; R_1^*)$, as follows.

Let X_1 consist of all elements $\gamma(t, x) \neq 1$ for $t \in T$, $x \in X$, let X_1^* be a set of elements $\gamma(t, x)^*$ in one-to-one correspondence with those of X_1, and let F_1 be the free group with basis X_1^*. Define a function τ from F into F_1 as follows if $w = y_1 \cdots y_n$, $y_i \in X \cup X^{-1}$, then

$$\tau(w) = \gamma(1, y_1)^* \cdots \gamma(\overline{y_1 \cdots y_{i-1}}, y_i)^* \cdots \gamma(\overline{y_1 \cdots y_{n-1}}, y_n)^*.$$

Then R^* consists of all $\tau(trt^{-1})$ for $t \in T$ and $r \in R$.

□ It was seen (I.3.7), by a direct application of Nielsen's method, that X_1 is a basis for a free subgroup F_1 of F. We may therefore without ambiguity simplify notation by identifying X_1^* with X_1 and F_1^* with F_1; thus we write $\gamma(t, x)^* = \gamma(t, x)$. Another routine calculation made earlier shows that $\tau(w) = w\overline{w}^{-1}$, whence, in particular, if $w \in \tilde{H}$, then $\tau(w) = w$. Now $N \subseteq \tilde{H}$, whence if $t \in T$, $r \in R$, then $trt^{-1} \in N$, and $\tau(trt^{-1}) = trt^{-1}$. It follows that $R_1 \subseteq N$ and hence the normal closure N_1 of R_1 in F_1 is contained in N. To complete the proof it will suffice to show that, conversely, $N \subseteq N_1$. Let $w \in N$; then w is a product of factors $p = uru^{-1}$ for $u \in F$, $r \in R^{\pm 1}$. Since $p \in N \subseteq \tilde{H}$, $\tau(p) = p$. We shall show that $p \in N_1$. If $\overline{u} = t$, then $Hu = Ht$, $u = ht$ for some $h \in \tilde{H}$. Then $p = uru^{-1} = \tau(uru^{-1}) = \tau(htrt^{-1}h^{-1}) = \tau(h)\tau(trt^{-1})\tau(h)^{-1} = h\tau(trt^{-1})h^{-1} \in N_1$. Thus $N \subseteq N_1$. □

The following observation (Magnus, Karrass, Solitar, p. 90) follows immediately from the argument just given.

Proposition 4.2. *Let H be a subgroup of finite index in a group G. If G is finitely generated, then H also is finitely generated. If G is finitely presented, then H also is finitely presented.* □

We conclude this brief discussion with the remark that the transformation τ, from F free with basis X into F^* free with basis X^*, is the prime example of what Magnus, Karrass, and Solitar call a *rewriting process*; they employ this process in a considerably more general context.

5. Groups with a Single Defining Relator

Groups with a single defining relator, $G = (X; r)$, have received much attention. A primary historical reason for this is that the fundamental groups of 2-manifolds fall within this class. They also present a natural extension of the class of free groups, with which they exhibit some similarities, and they have proved to some degree susceptible to explicit analysis.

The earliest results concerning the class of all one-relator groups were proved by Magnus, using a more or less uniform method. This method used an inductive argument, which required passing to a larger class of groups. We define a *staggered presentation* $G = (X; R)$ by the following conditions. First, let $I = \mathbb{Z}$ or $I = \{1, 2, \ldots, n\}$, and let Y be a subset of X that is the disjoint union of sets Y_i, $i \in I$. Let $R = \{r_j : j \in J\}$, where J is a linearly ordered set and each r_j is cyclically reduced and contains some generator from Y. For each r_j we denote by α_j the least i such that r_j contains a generator from Y_i, and by ω_j the greatest such i. For a staggered presentation we require that $j < k$ implies that $\alpha_j < \alpha_k$ and $\omega_j < \omega_k$.

Apart from the rôle of staggered presentations in carrying out inductive arguments concerning one-relator groups, one can extend to staggered presentations many properties that are known to be possessed by the one-relator groups $G_i = (X; r_i)$. See Lyndon, 1962, for this, and for further generalizations of the concept of staggered presentation.

The method of Magnus is powerful, but rather computational. Some of the results obtained by this method can be obtained, even in greater generality, by more perspicuous methods. But there remain results for which no alternative proof is known. For these reasons we state a number of results concerning one-relator groups, and groups with a staggered presentation, in this section, without giving proofs. In the following section we give two important examples, illustrating Magnus' method of proof.

The first general result concerning one-relator groups, and one of the most striking and most useful, is the Freiheitssatz, proposed by Dehn and proved by Magnus (1930); for a somewhat different proof, see Lyndon (1972). See also Schupp (1976). This theorem is the analog of an obvious fact in linear algebra; its name appears to come from the following formulation. Let $G = (X; r)$, and let r, which we may suppose cyclically reduced, contain an element x from X. Then (the image of) $X - x$ is a basis for a free subgroup of G. We give a formulation that is obviously equivalent.

Proposition 5.1. *Let F be a free group with basis X and r a cyclically reduced element of F that contains a certain generator x from X. Then every non-trivial element of the normal closure of r in F also contains x.* □

Magnus' proof established in fact the following more general result.

Proposition 5.2. *Let $(X; R)$ be a staggered presentation, in the notation introduced above. Suppose that a consequence w of R contains generators y in Y_i only for i in a certain interval $\alpha \leqslant i \leqslant \omega$. Then w is a consequence of those r_j that contain generators y in Y_i only for i in the same interval.* □

An immediate consequence of the Freiheitssatz is that the simple adjunction problem (see I.6) has a positive solution for free groups.

Proposition 5.3. *Let F be a free group, let $w_1, \ldots, w_n$ be non trivial elements of F, and let $a_1, \ldots, a_n$ be non zero integers. Then F can be embedded in a group G containing an element g such that $w_1 g^{a_1} \cdots w_n g^{a_n} = 1$.*

□ Let F be free with basis X; we may embed F in F_1 free with basis $X_1 = X \cup \{x\}$, where we may suppose $x \notin X$. Let $r = w_1 x^{a_1} \cdots w_n x^{a_n}$, in F_1, let N be the normal closure of r in F_1, and let ϕ be the canonical map from F_1 onto $G = F_1/N$. Now r is clearly cyclically reduced and involves the generator x of F_1. By the Freiheitssatz, we conclude that $N \cap F = 1$. But then ϕ maps F isomorphically into G, and the element $g = x\phi$ of G evidently satisfies the given equation. □

A typical example of the extensions of (5.2) obtained by Lyndon (1962) involves the case that the Y_i are indexed by points i in n-dimensional real space, and the interval mentioned in (5.2) is replaced by a convex set.

It is natural to seek a generalization of the Freiheitssatz to free products. Let $F = G_1 * G_2$ be a free product, and let r be a cyclically reduced element of F that is not contained in G_1; one might hope to show that the normal closure N of r in F was disjoint from G_1. This is false, with a simple counterexample, although all known counterexamples seem to be of essentially the same simple type. Let G_1 be generated by g_1 of order 2 and G_2 by g_2 of order 3; let $r = g_1 g_2$. It is easy to see that $N = F$. Schiek (1962, 1973) has studied additional hypotheses on r under which the desired conclusion holds.

A second basic result in the theory of one-relator groups is the solution by Magnus (1932) of the word problem for such groups.

Proposition 5.4. *Every presentation with a single defining relator has a solvable word problem.* □

In accordance with earlier remarks, the proof in fact establishes something stronger.

Proposition 5.5. *Every staggered presentation has a solvable word problem.* □

Magnus' proof in fact establishes a result that is stronger in a different and more interesting direction. This is the *extended word problem* or (a special case of) the *generalized word problem.*

Proposition 5.6. *Let $G = (X; r)$, with X_0 a recursive subset of X, and G_0 the subgroup of G generated by the image of X_0. Then it is decidable whether an arbitrary element of F represents an element of G_0.* □

B. B. Newman (1968) established the following generalization of this result, thereby answering a problem of Lyndon (1962).

Proposition 5.7. *Let F be a free group with basis X. Let X_1 and X_2 be recursive subsets of X, and let F_1 and F_2 be the subgroups of F that they generate. Let r be any element of F and N the normal closure of r in F. Then the subset F_1NF_2 is a recursive subset of F.* □

We remark that (5.5) is easily derivable from (5.6); it is also easily obtainable from more general results concerning free products with amalgamation.

An analysis of the exact logical force of Magnus' proof of (5.4) has been given by Cannonito and Gatterdam (1973).

B. B. Newman (1968) solves the conjugacy problem for one-relator groups with torsion, but it is not known whether every presentation with a single defining relator has a solvable conjugacy problem. The counterexamples of McCool-Pietrowski and of Zieschang mentioned above deprive us of the most obvious way of attacking the problem of isomorphism between groups given by one-relator presentations. It is not known if there exist two-relator groups with unsolvable word problem.

Another result proved by Magnus (1931) using the same basic method is the following.

Proposition 5.8. *If two elements r_1 and r_2 in a free group F have the same normal closure in F, then r_1 is conjugate to r_2 or to r_2^{-1}.* □

We give a version of Magnus' proof of this result in (II.6).

Greendlinger (1961) gives a generalization of (5.8) for certain small cancellation groups.

Magnus (1931) proved by the same method the following, which can also be obtained as a consequence of (5.17).

Proposition 5.9. *Let r_1 and r_2 be elements of a free group such that, for some positive integer n, r_1^n is in the normal closure of r_2^n. Then r_1 is in the normal closure of r_2.* □

Whitehead (1937) (see also Magnus-Karrass-Solitar, p. 167) proved the following.

Proposition 5.10. *If $G = (X; r)$ is a free group, then either $r = 1$ or r is a member of some basis for F.*

□ We may suppose that F has finite rank $n \geqslant 1$ and that $r \neq 1$. By (I.2.10), rank $G \leqslant n - 1$, while by abelianizing we see that rank $G \geqslant n - 1$. We can now apply the Grushko-Neumann Theorem (IV.1 below), or, more economically the result (I.2.11) of Federer-Jónsson, to conclude that F has a basis $y_1, \ldots, y_n$ such that the images of $y_1, \ldots, y_{n-1}$ form a basis for G. We conclude by Magnus' result (5.8) that, since r and y_n have the same normal closure in F, r is conjugate to y_n or to y_n^{-1}, and hence an element of a basis for F. (Alternatively we can invoke the Freiheitssatz to conclude, from the fact that y_n is in the normal closure of r, that r is conjugate to y_n^k for some k, and since G is torsion free we must have $k = \pm 1$.) □

Whitehead's proof was topological. That given above is based on one in Magnus-Karrass-Solitar (p. 288, Ex. 20) and a slightly different proof by Aust (1974).

Proposition 5.11. *$G = (X; r)$ cannot be generated by $n - 1$ elements unless r is a member of some basis for the free group F with basis X.* □

Shenitzer (1955) determined the possibilities for the free decomposition of a one relator group. He observes first that if w is an element of a free group F, of minimal length under $\text{Aut}(F)$, and if α is a Whitehead transformation other than a permutation of the letters such that $|w\alpha| = |w|$, then α cannot introduce into $w\alpha$ any generator that does not already occur in w. Using Whitehead's result (I.4.20) he deduces the following.

Proposition 5.12. *If r_1 and r_2 are elements of a free group F, of minimal length under $\text{Aut}(F)$, and equivalent under the action of $\text{Aut}(F)$, then the number of generators that actually occur in r_1 is the same as for r_2.* □

By the theorem of Grushko-Neumann (III.5), if $G = (X; r)$ is a proper free product, $G = G_1 * G_2$, then, after an automorphism of F, we may suppose that the basis X for F is the disjoint union of sets X_1 and X_2 whose images generate G_1 and G_2. But now r, cyclically reduced, must contain generators from only one of the sets X_1 and X_2. This, together with (5.12), yields the following.

Proposition 5.13. *Let $G = (x_1, \ldots, x_n; r)$ where r is of minimal length under $\text{Aut}(F)$ and contains exactly the generators $x_1, \ldots, x_k$ for some k, $0 \leqslant k \leqslant n$. Then $G \simeq G_1 * G_2$ where $G_1 = (x_1, \ldots, x_k; r)$ is freely indecomposable and G_2 is free with basis $x_{k+1}, \ldots, x_n$.* □

This proposition has an important corollary.

Proposition 5.14. *If G is a surface group, then G is not a proper free product.* □

We state next a result of Magnus (1931) and a related result of Steinberg (1971). Here an element of a free group is called *primitive* if it is a member of some basis.

Proposition 5.15. *If F is a free group and the normal closure in F of an element q contains some primitive element p, then q is conjugate to p or to p^{-1}, and thus is itself primitive.* □

Proposition 5.16. *Let q be any element of a free group F and p a primitive element. If the intersection of their normal closures is not contained in $[F, F]$, then q is conjugate to p or to p^{-1}.* □

Torsion in one-relator groups was studied by Karrass, Magnus, and Solitar (1960), using the basic method of Magnus. Every non-trivial element r of a free group F can be written in the form $r = s^m$ for some maximal m; s is then unique, and is the *root* of r. If $m = 1$, we say that r is not a *proper power*. They proved the following.

Proposition 5.17. *If $G = (X; r)$ where $r \neq 1$ and $r = s^m$ for m maximal, then the image $\bar{s}$ of s in G has order m, and every torsion element of G is conjugate to some power of $\bar{s}$.* □

Proposition 5.18. *If $G = (X; r)$ and r is not a proper power, then G is torsion free.* □

Gruenberg (1970) has given a cohomological proof of this result.

Proposition 5.19. *If $G = (X; r)$, with $r = s^m$, m maximal, and u is not a power of s, then the cyclic subgroups of G generated by the images of s and of $u^{-1}su$ have trivial intersection.* □

Magnus, Karrass, and Solitar note that (5.18) follows from a result of Lyndon (1950, see II.10 below). We remark that (5.17) and (5.19) are analogous to classical results for Fuchsian groups (see II.7 below). They prove also the following, which follows also from (5.18) together with a result of Schützenberger (1959, see I.6).

Proposition 5.20. *If $G = (X; r)$ where $r = [u, v]$ for some u and v, then G is torsion free.* □

Fischer, Karrass, and Solitar (1972) obtained another result for one-relator groups that is analogous to a classical result for Fuchsian groups (see III.7.11 below).

Proposition 5.21. *If $G = (X; r)$, then G has a torsion free normal subgroup of finite index.* □

They show also that if $G = (X; r)$, $r = s^m$, m maximal, then the subgroup of G generated by all torsion elements is the free product of all conjugates of the cyclic subgroup generated by the image of s.

The center of a group $G = (X; r)$ with a single defining relation has been studied by Murasugi (1964), who proved the following.

Proposition 5.22. *Let $G = (X; r)$. If $|X| \geqslant 3$, then G has trivial center. If $|X| = 2$ and G is non-abelian, then the center of G is infinite cyclic.* □

Baumslag and Taylor (1968) prove the following.

Proposition 5.23. *There is an algorithm for determining the center of a group with a single defining relation.* □

We give a proof of a result that is implicit in the proofs of the theorems cited above.

Proposition 5.24. *If $G = (X; r)$ is abelian, then $|X| \leqslant 2$. If $|X| = 2$, then F has a basis a, b such that either $r = b$ or $r = [a, b]$. Thus G is either cyclic or free abelian of rank* 2.

□ By (5.22), $|X| \leqslant 2$. So we may assume $|X| = 2$. By a change of basis we may suppose that $X = \{a, b\}$ and that r has exponent sum 0 in a. Thus r is in B, the normal closure of b in F, and B has a basis of elements $b_k = a^{-n}ba^n$. The normal closure N of r in F is then the normal closure in B of elements r_h, where r_0 is r rewritten in terms of the b_k, and r_h is obtained from r_0 by increasing all the subscripts on the b_k by h. We may suppose all the r_h cyclically reduced as words in the b_k.

The assumption that G is abelian implies that $p = b_0^{-1}b_1 = [b, a]$ is in N, hence, by (5.2), a consequence of those r_h that contain no b_k other than b_0 and b_1. Clearly $r_0 = r \neq 1$ contains some b_i, hence some least b_i and some greatest b_j, $j \geqslant i$. Since $p \neq 1$ is a consequence of those r_h that contain only b_0 and b_1, it is impossible that $j > i + 1$. If $j = i + 1$, there is a unique r_h containing only b_0 and b_1, and p is a consequence of this r_h. Since p is primitive in B, by (5.16), this implies that r_h is conjugate to $p = [a, b]$ or to p^{-1}, and hence r is conjugate in F to p or p^{-1}. The case remains that $j = i$. Here $r_h = b_k^m$ for some k and m, whence r is conjugate to b^m. But now the condition that G be abelian implies that $m = \pm 1$, that is, $r = b^{\pm 1}$, and G is infinite cyclic. □

Let Φ be a free group with basis $\xi_1, \ldots, \xi_n$ and let $w = w(\xi_1, \ldots, \xi_n)$ be an element of Φ. A group G is said to satisfy the *law*, or *identical relation*, $w = 1$ if $w(g_1, \ldots, g_n) = 1$ for all $g_1, \ldots, g_n$ in G; more precisely, if w is in the kernel of every homomorphism from Φ into G. The case that $w = 1$ (as word in Φ) gives the *trivial law*, satisfied by every group G. The general theory of laws in groups constitutes the subject of *varieties of groups*, which is developed extensively in the book of H. Neumann (1967). We mention these ideas here only in connection with the following theorem of Moldavanskii (1969).

Proposition 5.25. *Let G be a group defined by a single relation, and let H be a subgroup of H that satisfies some non-trivial law. If G is torsion free then H is either locally cyclic (that is, every finitely generated subgroup is cyclic) or else metabelian of the form $H = (x, y; x^{-1}yx = y^n)$. If G has torsion, then H is either cyclic or is the infinite dihedral group $H = (x, y; x^2 = y^2 = 1)$.* □

B. B. Newman (1968) proved the following.

Proposition 5.26. *Let G be a group with a single defining relation and H an abelian subgroup of G. Then H is either a locally cyclic group in which each non-trivial element is a p-th power for only finitely many primes p, or else H is free abelian of rank 2. If G is a group with with a single defining relation, and with torsion, and H is a solvable subgroup of G, then H is either cyclic or infinite dihedral.* □

Karrass and Solitar (1971) proved the following; see also Chebotar (1971).

Proposition 5.27. *Let G be a group with a single defining relation. Then every subgroup either contains a free group of rank 2 or is solvable. Moreover, if G has torsion, then every subgroup either contains a free subgroup of rank 2, is cyclic, or is infinite dihedral.* □

The following theorem is due to B. B. Newman (1968); a proof by McCool and Schupp (1973) will be given in (IV.5, below).

Proposition 5.28. *Let $G = (X; r)$ where $r = s^n$, $n > 1$. Let u and v be elements of F, free with basis X, that represent the same element of G, and suppose that some letter x from X occurs in u but not in v. Then there is a subword of u that is also a subword of r or of r^{-1}, and which has length greater than $(n - 1)|s|$.* □

The next result is due to Weinbaum (1972), whose proof is geometrical.

Proposition 5.29. *Let F be free with basis X and let r be a cyclically reduced element of F. Then the normal closure of r in F contains no non-trivial proper subword of r.* □

B. B. Newman (1968) proved the following.

Proposition 5.30. *If G is a one-relator group with torsion, then the centralizer of every non-trivial element is a cyclic group.* □

Baumslag and Gruenberg (1967) pose the following problem. Does every non-trivial subgroup, generated by two elements, of a one-relator group have a non-trivial finite quotient group?

Ree and Mendelsohn (1968) prove by matrix methods the following.

Proposition 5.31. *Let $G = (a, b; s^m)$ where $m > 1$ and s is not conjugate to a power of a or of b. Then, for all sufficiently large n, the pair a and b^n is a basis for a free subgroup of G.* □

Meskin (1972) has considered the question whether certain one-relator groups are residually finite.

A group G is called *SQ-universal* if every countable group is isomorphic to a subgroup of some quotient group of G. (This concept is discussed more fully in V.10 below.) Sacerdote and Schupp (1974) prove the following.

Proposition 5.32. *Every group G that has a presentation with at least 3 generators and a single defining relation is SQ-universal.* □

Results of Miller (1969, unpublished) and of Anshel and Stebe (1974) contain the solution of the conjugacy problem for groups of the from $G = (X, t; t^{-1}pt = q)$ where p and q are words over X and do not contain the generator t.

We mention here čertain extensions of properties of free groups to small cancellation groups (which of course contain a number of important one-relator groups). Seymour (thesis, Univ. of Illinois, 1974) and Truffault (1974) extended a result of Lipschutz (1972) to show that in a sixth-group the centralizer of every non-trivial element is cyclic. They also extend another result of Lipschutz (1972) to show that in a sixth-group, if g is an element of infinite order and $m \neq \pm n$, then g^m and g^n are not conjugate. (See also Anshel 1973, Lipschutz 1971.) The exceptional case that g and g^{-1} are conjugate in a small cancellation group has been studied exhaustively by Comerford (1974).

Shapiro and Sonn (1974) have examined the free factor groups of one-relator groups.

Lyndon (1950) determined the cohomology of one-relator groups, thereby extending results of Eilenberg and MacLane (1949) for cyclic groups. Using the method of Magnus, and also the ideas of Fox and of Reidemeister, he showed that if $G = (X; r)$ and r is not a proper power, then there is a free resolution

$$0 \to M_1 \to \mathbb{Z}G \to \mathbb{Z} \to 0,$$

where M_1 is a free $\mathbb{Z}G$ module of rank 1. This implies that G has cohomological dimension at most 2, and, in view of the result of Stallings (1968), exactly 2 unless

G is free. In this case the relation module $\bar{N} = N/[N, N]$ is a free cyclic $\mathbb{Z}G$ module. If r is a proper power there exists a resolution in which all the M_i are cyclic; the resolution is infinite, but has period 2. (See Swan 1969). In this case $\bar{N}$ is not free, but is cyclic and defined by a single relation. (We return to these matters in III.10.) In his paper Lyndon also sketched some ideas concerning resolutions connected with presentations of free products and amalgamated products, which were developed further by Swan (1969); see also Gildenhuys (1974, 1975).

6. Magnus' Treatment of One-Relator Groups

We have repeatedly mentioned the general method applied by Magnus to problems concerning one-relator groups. He and others have applied it to the solution of a large number of problems concerning such groups. It involves a reduction, which in practice is not always elegant, and some of the results obtained by this method are now available by more elegant, or more suggestive methods. Nonetheless, there remain important results that have not been obtained by any essentially different method. The method is more or less uniform, and we shall content ourselves here with two examples. The first of Magnus' results obtained by this method is the Freiheitssatz (5.1); two other important results obtained by this method are the positive solution of the word problem for one-relator groups (5.4; 5.5; 5.6), and Proposition (5.8). We shall give here what is essentially Magnus' original proof of the Freiheitssatz; for variant proofs, see Lyndon (1972; below), and Burns (1974). A modified version of his solution of the word problem is given in (IV.5) below. And we give also what is essentially Magnus' original proof of Proposition (5.8).

Two technical tools play an essential rôle in the argument. The first is the basic theorem of Schreier (1924) guaranteeing the existence of the amalgamated product of two groups with subgroups identified according to a specified isomorphism. Magnus became aware of this result only in time to acknowledge in a footnote to his paper on the Freiheitssatz that it could be used to simplify the presentation of his argument. The second is that a free group F with basis $x_1, \ldots, x_n$ can always be embedded in a free group F' with basis $y_1, x_2, \ldots, x_n$ in which $x_1 = y^m$ for arbitrary positive m; this is a consequence of Schreier's theorem, but can be obtained more easily from Nielsen's Subgroup Theorem. This has as consequence that if r is an element in a free group F of rank greater than 1, one can always embed F in a free group F', as above, such that r has exponent sum 0 in some element of a basis for F'.

Proof of the Freiheitssatz. The proof by induction requires that we prove the seemingly stronger result (5.2). It is clear that the Freiheitssatz (5.1) is contained as a special case in (5.2). To prepare the ground, we show that (5.2) is a consequence of (5.1). Since every consequence of an infinite set of relators is a consequence of some finite subset, it suffices to consider the case that I is finite, $I = \{1, \ldots, n\}$. The case $n = 1$ is (5.1), and we argue by induction on n. We may suppose the relators are $R = \{r_1, \ldots, r_m\}$, and that $\alpha_1 = 1$ and $\omega_m = n$. Let $X' = X - Y_n$,

$Y' = Y - Y_n$, $R' = R - \{r_m\}$. Then the presentation $G' = (X'; R')$ satisfies the hypothesis of (5.2) with $n' = n - 1$, and we may conclude by the inductive hypothesis that the normal closure N' of R' in F', free with basis X', contains no non-trivial relation among the generators $Z = (X - Y) \cup Y_1 \cup \cdots \cup Y_{n-1}$. Thus the image H' of $U = \text{Gp}\, Z$ in G' is free on the image of Z as basis. Similarly, let $X'' = X - (Y_1 \cup \cdots \cup Y_{n-1})$, let $Y'' = Y_n$, and let $R'' = \{r_m\}$. Then the presentation $G'' = (X''; R'')$ satisfies the hypothesis of (5.2) with $n'' = 1$, and we conclude similarly that the image H'' of U in G'' is free on the image of Z as basis. We now appeal to the theorem of Schreier to conclude that G is the free product of its subgroups G' and G'' with their subgroups H' and H'' amalgamated.

If, in the notation of (5.2), the interval $J = (\alpha, \ldots, \omega)$ does not contain n, then $w \in N \lhd F'$ and by Schreier's theorem $w \in N'$. In this case the desired conclusion follows by the induction hypothesis applied to $G' = (X'; N')$. The case that J does not contain 1 follows by symmetry. In the remaining case, $J = (1, \ldots, n)$, and the conclusion holds vacuously. This completes the proof that (5.1) and (5.2) are equivalent.

We now begin the proof of (5.1), arguing by induction on the length of r. We may suppose that $G = (X; r)$ where r is a non-trivial cyclically reduced word containing every generator in the set X. In order to reserve subscripts for another purpose, we write $X = \{t, a, b, \ldots, z\}$. The case that $X = \{t\}$ and F and G are cyclic is trivial, and we put it aside, noting that this case contains the initial case of our induction on $|r|$.

We treat first the case that some generator, say t, has exponent sum 0 in r, that is, that r lies in the normal closure F_1 of $a, b, \ldots, z$ in F. Then $N \lhd F_1$ and so $w \in F_1$. Now F_1 is generated by the set X_1 of elements $a_i = t^{-i}at^i, \ldots, z_i = t^{-i}zt^i$, $i \in \mathbb{Z}$. For, by conjugating all powers of t to the left, every element u of F can be written in the form $u = t^pu'$ where u' is a word over X_1; and if u is in F_1, then $p = 0$ and $u = u'$. By Nielsen's criterion, X_1 is a basis for F_1. If $s = u^{-1}ru$, where u, in F is written $u = t^pu'$ as above, then $s = u'^{-1}r_pu'$ where $r_p = t^{-p}rt^p$. It follows that N is the normal closure in F_1 of $R_1 = \{r_i = t^{-i}rt^i: i \in \mathbb{Z}\}$.

We note that r_i can be obtained from r_0 by increasing all subscripts on the $a_j, \ldots, z_j$ by i; thus we have a staggered presentation. Moreover, all the r_i have the same length; this is evidently the total number of occurrences in r of letters other than t and t^{-1}. In consequence the length $|r_0|$ of r_0 as a word over X_1 is less that the length of r as a word over X.

We must show that w contains t and also all of $a, \ldots, z$. For the first case we take $Y_i = \{a_i, \ldots, z_i\}$. Now r contains t, and some part $x^et^ky^f$ for $e, f = \pm 1$, $k \neq 0$, and x, y among $a, \ldots, z$. Then r_0, as a word over X_1, will contain x_{h+k} and y_h for some h; thus $\alpha_0 < \omega_0$. It is clear that all $\alpha_i < \omega_i$, and that $i < j$ implies $\alpha_i < \alpha_j$ and $\omega_i < \omega_j$. By (5.1), applied inductively, it follows that w, as a word over X_1, cannot contain letters from Y_0 only; but then w, as a word over X, must contain t. For the second case, to show that w contains, for example, a, we take $Y_i = \{a_i\}$. Since r contained a, r_0 must contain some a_i, and again applying (5.1) inductively, we conclude that w, as a word over X_1, must contain some a_i, and therefore, as a word over X, must contain a.

It remains to treat the case that no generator occurs in r with exponent sum 0.

We have assumed that X contains at least the two elements t and a. It will suffice to show that w contains, say, a. Let τ be the exponent sum of t in r and α the exponent sum of a. We embed F in a free group F' with basis $x, a, \ldots, z$ where $x^\alpha = t$. Since w is a consequence of r in F, it is also in F'. Now F' has another basis, $X^* = \{x, a^*, b, \ldots, z\}$ where $a^* = ax^{-\tau}$. As a word over this basis, r has exponent sum 0 in x. We pass as before to the subgroup F_1' of F' with basis $X' = \{a_i^* = x^{-i}a^*x^i, b_i = x^{-i}bx^i, \ldots, z_i = x^{-i}zx^i; i \in \mathbb{Z}\}$. The length of r relative to this basis is evidently the total number of occurrences in r, as a word over X, of letters other than t and t^{-1}, and is thus less than the length of r as a word over X. We may thus apply the inductive hypothesis as before to conclude that w, as a word over X', contains some a^*, and therefore, as a word over X, contains a. This completes the proof of the Freiheitssatz. □

Proof of (5.8). We assume that two elements r and s of the free group F with basis X have the same normal closure N in F, and we must show that r is conjugate to s or to s^{-1}. We may suppose r and s non-trivial and cyclically reduced. By the Freiheitssatz, since each is a consequence of the other, they contain exactly the same generators. We may suppose that $X = \{t, a, \ldots, z\}$ and that both r and s contain all these generators. The case of a single generator is trivial, and we put it aside. This disposes of the initial case of an induction on the length of r. As before, by embedding F in a larger group F' if necessary, we can suppose that t has exponent sum 0 in r. As before, we pass to F_1 with a basis $X_1 = \{a_i, \ldots, z_i\}$ and conclude that $N \lhd F_1$ is the normal closure in F_1 of $R_1 = \{r_i : i \in \mathbb{Z}\}$ and also of $S_1 = \{s_i : i \in \mathbb{Z}\}$.

Some r_p will contain a_0 as a_i of lowest index, and some a_m of highest index. Similarly, some s_q will contain a_0 as a_i of lowest index, and some a_n of highest index. If one had $n < m$, the Freiheitssatz applied to the presentation $(X_1 : R_1)$ would contradict the fact that s_q is a consequence of R_1. Thus $n \geqslant m$, and by symmetry we conclude that $n = m$. But now the Freiheitssatz implies that s_q is a consequence of r_p, and, symmetrically, r_p is a consequence of s_q. This means that r_p and s_q have the same normal closure in F_1. Since r_p as a word over X_1 is shorter than r as a word over X, we can apply the induction hypothesis to conclude that r_p is conjugate in F_1 to $s_q^{\pm 1}$. But then r_p is conjugate to $s_q^{\pm 1}$ in F; since r_p is conjugate to r and s_q to s, it now follows that r is conjugate to $s^{\pm 1}$ in F. This completes the proof of (5.8). □

Chapter III. Geometric Methods

1. Introduction

We have mentioned the strong influence of geometry, topology, and parts of analysis on the origin and development of combinatorial group theory, as well as the application of geometric and topological methods to abstract group theory. Here we develop some of the most elementary of these methods, partly because of the intrinsic interest of these connections, partly to present geometric proofs of some theorems that are proved by other means elsewhere, and partly to provide a basis for the geometric ideas that enter into our discussion of small cancellation theory in Chapter V. We have tried to include in this chapter everything of a geometric nature appropriate to our topic and accessible by our limited means, except for the systematic development of small cancellation theory.

Much of the material here has long been known, and is to an extent anonymous. For many of the ideas, although important, are very natural and appear to have been introduced separately by many workers. We mention only the early work of Cayley, Dyck, Fricke and Klein, Poincaré, and somewhat later of Dehn, Nielsen, Reidemeister, and Threlfall.

A number of concepts, proofs, and theorems in this chapter are taken more or less directly from Zieschang, Vogt, Coldewey (1970) and also from Zieschang (1966); and much of what follows does not differ greatly from their treatment. Zieschang's approach, following Reidemeister's, is to replace analytic by combinatorial geometric arguments so far as possible; that of Hoare, Karrass, Solitar (1972, 1973) is to replace geometric arguments by pure combinatorial group theory. We have tried to incorporate the results of Hoare, Karrass, Solitar into an approach similar to that of Zieschang. However, we have taken the Cayley complex (corresponding to a common topological approach) as the unifying theme, reverting to the dual *Fuchsian complex* (corresponding to the usual analytic approach) only when we felt there was a real advantage.

The use of geometric methods, in the present sense, and especially of covering space arguments and their generalizations, has long been wide spread. Among recent treatments in this spirit we mention, in addition to Zieschang-Vogt-Coldewey, the work of Chipman (1973), Crowell-Smythe (preprint), Griffiths (1967, 1967),

Higgins (1964, 1971), Ordman (1970, 1971), Rotman (1973, 1970), and Tretkoff (1975). Tretkoff (preprint), in particular, has put the theory of groups acting on trees, due to Serre (1968/69) and Bass, into the context of covering spaces.

2. Complexes

We begin with purely combinatorial definitions of 1-complexes and 2-complexes, which are perhaps a little broader than usual.

We shall take the terms *graph* and 1-*complex* as synonymous. We take a 1-*complex* C to consist of two sets V and E, together with three functions $\alpha: E \to V$, $\omega: E \to V$, and $\eta_1: E \to E$. We call the elements of V *vertices* (or *points*) and those of E *edges*. For e in E we call $\alpha(e)$ the *initial point* of e and $\omega(e)$ the *terminal point*, and say that e *runs from* $\alpha(e)$ *to* $\omega(e)$. We call $\eta_1(e)$ the *inverse* of e, or the *oppositely oriented* edge, and write $\eta_1(e) = e^{-1}$. We impose on these functions the conditions that η_1 should be an involution without fixed elements, and that e^{-1} run from $\omega(e)$ to $\alpha(e)$.

Since we require that C contain together with each edge its inverse, our concept of graph is essentially that of undirected graph. We shall sometimes speak of an *undirected edge*; this can be taken to be a pair $\{e, e^{-1}\}$ of inverse edges. At one point below we shall speak of orienting an undirected graph; this can be thought of as choosing one from each pair of inverse edges.

A *path* in C is a finite sequence of edges, for which we write $p = e_1 \cdots e_n$, $n \geqslant 1$ such that, for $1 \leqslant i < n$, e_{i+1} begins where e_i ends, that is, $\alpha(e_{i+1}) = \omega(e_i)$. The *length* of a path p is $|p| = n$. The path p *begins* at $\alpha(p) = \alpha(e_1)$ and *ends* at $\omega(p) = \omega(e_n)$; if these two points are the same p is a *loop*. It is convenient not to introduce a single empty path, but rather for each vertex v to postulate a path 1_v without edges, beginning and ending at v; then 1_v is a loop and has length 0. (Technically we could take $1_v = v$, defining $\alpha(v) = \omega(v) = v$ and $|v| = 0$.) The *inverse* p^{-1} to the path p is the path $p^{-1} = e_n^{-1} \cdots e_1^{-1}$.

If $p = e_1 \cdots e_n$ is a loop, then every cyclic permutation $p' = p_i \cdots p_n p_1 \cdots p_{i-1}$ of p is also a loop; we call the set of all cyclic permutations of p a *cyclic path* or *cycle*. A path is *reduced* if it contains no part ee^{-1}; a loop or the corresponding cycle is *cyclically reduced* if it is reduced and $e_1 \neq e_n^{-1}$. A path is *simple* if for $i \neq j$ one has $\alpha(e_i) \neq \alpha(e_j)$ and $\omega(e_i) \neq \omega(e_j)$.

A 2-*complex* C consists of a 1-complex C^1, its 1-*skeleton*, together with a set F of 2-*cells* or *faces*, and two functions ∂ and η_2 defined on F. To each D in F the function ∂ assigns a cyclically reduced cycle ∂D in C^1, the *boundary* of D, and the function η_2 assigns to D a second face $\eta_2(D) = D^{-1}$, the *inverse* of D; we require that $\partial(D^{-1})$ be the inverse to ∂D in the obvious sense. A vertex v is on a face D if it is the initial point of some edge in ∂D; then a *boundary path for D at v* is any loop in the cycle ∂D that begins at v. In the most interesting cases ∂D will be simple, whence there is a unique boundary path for D at each vertex on D.

We note that under our definition every 1-complex is also a 2-complex with an empty set of faces.

The intended geometric meaning of these definitions is clear, and we shall not hesitate to use intuitive geometrical language on occasion.

A path in a 2-complex C will mean a path in its 1-skeletion. The set $\Pi(C)$ of all paths in C has a certain amount of algebraic structure. We define the product pq of two paths, provided $\omega(p) = \alpha(q)$, by juxtaposition. This multiplication is associative: if either of $p(qr)$ and $(pq)r$ is defined, the other is also and the two are equal. One has $1_{\alpha(p)} \cdot p = p$ and $p \cdot 1_{\omega(p)} = p$, and, if pq is defined, $(pq)^{-1} = q^{-1}p^{-1}$. (One could describe $\Pi(C)$ as a category, or semigroupoid, with involutory anti-isomorphism.)

We define a relation of 1-*equivalence* between paths p and p', and write $p \underset{1}{\sim} p'$, which holds if and only if one can pass from p to p' by a succession of steps that consist of insertion or deletion of parts of the form ee^{-1}. This is clearly an equivalence relation and indeed a congruence on $\Pi(C)$ in the sence that if $p \underset{1}{\sim} p'$ and $q \underset{1}{\sim} q'$ and pq is defined, then $p'q'$ is defined and $pq \underset{1}{\sim} p'q'$, and that $p \underset{1}{\sim} p'$ implies $p^{-1} \underset{1}{\sim} p'^{-1}$. Thus we can pass to the quotient structure $\Pi^1(C)$ of $\Pi(C)$ by this relation. Since $pp^{-1} \underset{1}{\sim} 1_{\alpha(p)}$, $\Pi^1(C)$ is a structure with inverses, hence is a *groupoid* (or category with inverses).

It is easy to see, exactly as in treating reduced words in free groups, that every path is 1-equivalent to a unique reduced path. In particular, a nontrivial reduced loop in $\Pi(C)$ will not map into one of the neutral elements (idempotents) in $\Pi^1(C)$.

We define a relation of 2-*equivalence* among paths p and p', and write $p \sim p'$, if it is possible to pass from one to the other by a succession of insertions and deletions of parts of the form ee^{-1} or of the form q where q is a boundary path at some point for a face D. Evidently this too is a congruence on $\Pi(C)$, and the quotient of $\Pi(C)$ by this relation is again a groupoid, the *fundamental groupoid* $\pi(C)$ of the complex C. Evidently $\Pi^1(C) = \Pi^1(C^1) = \pi(C^1)$, the fundamental groupoid of the 1-skeleton C^1 of C, and $\pi(C)$ is naturally a homomorphic image of $\pi(C^1)$.

Observe that for any vertex v the subset $\Pi(C, v)$ of $\Pi(C)$ consisting of all loops at v is a semigroup and that its image $\pi(C, v)$ in $\pi(C)$ is a group, the *fundamental group* of C at the point v. It is familiar that in the interesting case where C is connected all its fundamental groups at various points are conjugate and hence isomorphic, although ordinarily not by any unique naturally given isomorphisms. This latter is one reason that fundamental groupoids are a more elegant tool in topology. We mention also that the theory of groupoids can be developed abstractly and applied with elegance and power to problems in combinatorial group theory; this has been done systematically by Higgins (1971) and we believe that his method might prove to be the natural tool for certain further matters that we treat below. However, in the interest of simplicity we shall make very sparing mention of groupoids. We note that a theory very close to Higgins' theory of groupoids has been developed by Crowell and Smythe (1974).

We now embark on a study of certain complexes associated with groups or presentations of groups.

Proposition 2.1. *If C is a* 1*-complex and v any vertex of C, then $\pi(C, v)$ is a free group.*

☐ Since $\pi(C, v)$ clearly coincides with $\pi(C_v, v)$ where C_v is the connected component of C containing v, we may as well assume C connected. A *tree* is a connected 1-complex without non trivial cycles. By Zorn's lemma, C contains a maximal tree T. Then T must contain every vertex x, together with a unique reduced path $\overline{vx}$ in T from v to x. With each edge e, running say from vertex x to vertex y, we associate the loop $\tilde{e} = \overline{vx} \cdot e \cdot \overline{vy}^{-1}$; let $\bar{e}$ be the equivalence class of e in $G = \pi(C, v)$ and let X be the set of all $\bar{e} \neq 1$. If $p = e_1 \cdots e_n$ is any loop at v, evidently $p \sim \tilde{e}_1 \cdots \tilde{e}_n$; thus X generates G. Moreover, since $e^{-1} = (\tilde{e})^{-1}$, $X^{-1} = X$. We shall show that G is a free group with X as symmetrized basis, that is, that if $w = \bar{e}_1 \cdots \bar{e}_n$, $n > 0$, with each $\bar{e}_i$ in X and no $\bar{e}_i\bar{e}_{i+1} = 1$, then $w \neq 1$. Let $p = \tilde{e}_1 \cdots \tilde{e}_n$; we must show that the reduced form of p as a word in the edges e_j is non-trivial. Now from the definition of the $\tilde{e}_i$ we see that after cancellation p takes the form $p = \overline{vx_i} \cdot e_1 \cdots e_n \cdot \overline{vy_n}^{-1}$. Now this is reduced, since $\bar{e}_i\bar{e}_{i+1} \neq 1$ implies $\tilde{e}_i\tilde{e}_{i+1} \neq 1$. From the uniqueness of reduced form in $\pi(C)$ we conclude that $p \nsim 1$ and so $w \neq 1$. ☐

Proposition 2.2. *Let C be a finite connected 1-complex and v any vertex. Let γ_0 be the number of vertices in C and γ_1 the number of undirected edges (that is, of unordered pairs $\{e, e^{-1}\}$ of inverse edges). Then $\pi(C, v)$ is a free group of rank $\gamma_1 - \gamma_0 + 1$.*

☐ We continue the notation of the preceding proof. Note that if the edge e is in T, then $\bar{e} \sim 1$, while otherwise $\tilde{e}$ is reduced and non-trivial. Thus X consists of the $\bar{e}$ in one to one correspondence with the edges e not in T, whence the rank of $\pi(C, v)$ is $\gamma_1 - \tau$, where τ is the number of undirected edges in T. Since T is a tree with γ_0 vertices, we have $\gamma_0 = \tau + 1$. The result follows. ☐

With every presentation $G = (X, R)$ where all r in R are cyclically reduced we associate a special complex $K(X; R)$ with a single vertex. First, K has a single vertex v, and an edge $\tilde{x}$ (from v to v) for each element x of X, together with its inverse $\tilde{x}^{-1}$. Now every path in K is a loop. Second, if $r = x_1^{e_1} \cdots x_n^{e_n}$ is in R where all $x_i \in X$, $e_i = \pm 1$, we introduce a face D with boundary path (at v) $\tilde{x}_1^{e_1} \cdots \tilde{x}_n^{e_n}$, together with D^{-1}.

Proposition 2.3. *If $G = (X; R)$ and $K = K(X; R)$ is associated with the presentation as above, then $\pi(K, v) \simeq G$.*

☐ Let ϕ be the map from F, free with basis X, into $\pi(K^1)$ carrying each x in X into the equivalence class of the loop $\tilde{x}$. Since $\{v\}$ is a maximal tree in K^1, the argument above shows that ϕ is in fact an isomorphism from F onto $\pi(K^1)$. Let K be the natural map from $\pi(K^1)$ onto $\pi(K)$. Clearly $R\phi$ is in the kernel of K. But on the other hand, it is easy to see from the definitions that if two loops p and p' are in the relation $p \sim p'$, then their equivalence classes in $\pi(K^1)$ are congruent modulo $R\phi$. ☐

If the presentation $G = (X; R)$ is finite, then $K(X; R)$ is finite. If $G = (X; R)$ is the multiplication table presentation in which every element of R has length 3, then every face of $K(X; R)$ is a triangle and K is simplicial. Any presentation $G = (X; R)$

can be converted to one where all relators have length 3, essentially by triangulating each face; if the original presentation was finite the new one will be also.

The complexes $K(X; R)$ are related to the complexes $K(\pi, n)$ of Eilenberg and MacLane (see MacLane (1963)). As we shall see below, they are closely related to the Cayley complexes.

3. Covering Maps

The exposition that follows is taken more or less directly from Zieschang, Vogt, and Coldewey (1970); a general and elegant, but very abstract, treatment of these matters is to be found in Higgins (1971).

We understand that a map f from one 2-complex C' into another 2-complex C should preserve dimension and incidence. We shall deal here only with *unbranched* coverings: we further require of a *covering* f that it be onto, and one-to-one on the set of edges and faces incident with each vertex.

Proposition 3.1. *If $f: C' \to C$ is a covering and v' a vertex of C', then f induces a monomorphism f^* from $\pi(C', v')$ into $\pi(C, v'f)$.*

□ If p' is a loop at v' in C', evidently its image $p = p'f$ in C is a loop at $v = v'f$ in C. Let p_1' and p_2' be immediately equivalent loops at v' in C', that is, $p_1' = u'q_1'v'$ and $p_2' = u'q_2'v'$, where $q_1'q_2'^{-1}$ is the boundary of a face D' in C'. Then the image $q_1q_2^{-1}$ is the boundary of a face D in C, and the images $p_1 = uq_1v$ and $p_2 = uq_2v$ of p_1' and p_2' are equivalent in C. Thus f induces a homomorphism f^* from $\pi(C', v')$ into $\pi(C, v)$. Now a covering map is one-to-one on the set of edges incident with any fixed vertex. It thus follows by induction on the length of a reduced path p, that if p begins at a vertex v, and $v'f = v$, then there is a unique reduced path p' in C' which begins at v' and has $p'f = p$. Suppose that p' is a loop in C' and that $p'f$ bounds a face D in C. Since f is onto, there is a face D' in C' with $D'f = D$. Then f maps the boundary of D' onto $p'f$, and by the uniqueness property noted above, it follows that p' must bound D'. This implies that f^* is in fact a monomorphism. □

The following proposition is essentially preliminary to (3.4), disposing of the 1-dimensional case.

Proposition 3.2. *Let C be a connected 1-complex, let v be a vertex of C, and let H be any subgroup of $\pi(C, v)$. Then there exists a connected 1-complex C', and a covering map $f: C' \to C$, carrying some vertex v' of C' onto v, and inducing an isomorphism f^* from $\pi(C', v')$ onto the subgroup H of $\pi(C, v)$.*

□ Let T be a maximal tree in C. Then, for each vertex x of C, there is a unique path $\overline{vx}$ in T from v to x. If e is any edge of C, running from a vertex x to a vertex y, let $\tilde{e}$ be the element of $\pi(C, v)$ determined by the loop $\overline{vx}.e.\overline{vy}^{-1}$ at v. Let W be the set of cosets Hg of H in $\pi(C, v)$. For the vertex set of C' we take the set $V' =$

$V \times W$, where V is the vertex set of C. For the edge set of C' we take the set $E' = E \times W$, where E is the edge set of C. If $e' = (e, Hg)$ is an edge in C', where the edge e in C runs from x to y, then we stipulate that e' run from the vertex $x' = (x, Hg)$ of C' to the vertex $y' = (y, Hg\tilde{e})$. It is easy to check that C' is a complex. Now the projections from V' onto V and from E' onto E evidently define a covering map $f: C' \to C$.

We choose as base point in C' the point $v' = (v, H)$; clearly $v'f = v$. We show next that the image of $\pi(C', v')$ under f^* is contained in H. Let $p' = e'_1 \cdots e'_n$ be a path in C' beginning at v'. If each $e'_i = (e_i, Hg_i)$ then $p'f = p = e_1 \cdots e_n$. The fact that p' is a path in C' requires that $Hg_{i+1} = Hg_i\tilde{e}_i$ for each i, $1 \simeq i < n$; thus p' ends at $y' = (y, H\tilde{e}_1 \cdots \tilde{e}_n)$ where y is the end point of p. If p' is closed we must have $y = v$ and $H\tilde{e}_1 \cdots \tilde{e}_n = H$, and consequently $\tilde{e}_1 \cdots \tilde{e}_n \in H$. This implies that the loop p in C represents the element $\tilde{e}_1 \cdots \tilde{e}_n$ of H. We have shown that if p' is a loop at v', representing an element g' of $\pi(C', v')$, then $p'f$ represents an element $g'f^*$ of $\pi(C, v)$ that lies in H.

It remains to show that the image of $\pi(C', v')$ under f^* is all of H. Let $p = e_1 \cdots e_n$ be a loop at v in C that represents an element g of H. Then $\tilde{e}_1 \cdots \tilde{e}_n$ also represents p. Since $\tilde{e}_1 \cdots \tilde{e}_n \in H$; the path $p' = e'_1 \cdots e'_n$ at v' in C', where $e'_i = (e_i, H\tilde{e}_1 \cdots \tilde{e}_i)$, is in fact a loop at v' in C', representing an element g' of $\pi(C', v')$ such that $g'f^* = g$. □

This provides one more proof, classical, and perhaps the most natural, granted the machinery, of the Subgroup Theorem of Nielsen and Schreier.

Proposition 3.3. *Every subgroup of a free group is free.*

□ Let $F = (X; \varnothing)$ be a free group and H a subgroup. Then there exists a 1-complex C (for example, $K(X; \varnothing)$) such that the fundamental group $\pi(C, v)$ at any vertex v is isomorphic to F. Thus we may take H to be a subgroup of $\pi(C, v)$. By the preceding theorem there exists a 1-complex C' such that $\pi(C', v')$ is isomorphic to H. Since C' is a 1-complex, by (2.1), $\pi(C', v')$ is a free group, whence H also is free. □

We now extend (3.2) to 2-complexes.

Proposition 3.4. *Let C be a connected 2-complex, let v be a vertex of C, and let H be any subgroup of $\pi(C, v)$. Then there exists a connected 2-complex C', and a covering map $f: C' \to C$, carrying some vertex v' of C' onto v, and inducing an isomorphism f^* from $\pi(C', v')$ onto the subgroup H of $\pi(C, v)$.*

□ By (3.1) we can construct a covering map f^1, from the 1-skeleton C'^1, of a space C' onto the 1-skeleton C^1 of C, such that f^1 maps $\pi(C'^1, v')$ onto the preimage H' of H in $\pi(C, v)$. We extend C'^1 to a 2-complex C', and f to a map from C' onto C, as follows. If p' is any closed path in C' whose image p in C bounds a face D of C, we introduce a face D' into C', with boundary p', and define $D'f = D$. This makes f a covering map from C' onto C.

Let p be a loop at v in C, representing an element h of the subgroup H of $\pi(C, v)$, and let p represent the element $\bar{h}$ of the preimage H^1 of H in $\pi(C^1, v)$. Then

f^{1*} maps some element h' of $\pi(C'^1, v')$ onto $\bar{h}$, whence f^* maps the image of h' in $\pi(C', v')$ onto the element h of H. This shows that f^* maps $\pi(C', v')$ onto H. By (3.1), f^* is a monomorphism. □

The following is a weak combinatorial version of the theorem of Seifert (1933) and van Kampen (1933) concerning the fundamental group of a union of spaces.

Proposition 3.5. *Let a 2-complex C be the union of subcomplexes C_i, for i ranging over an index set I, let a vertex v be common to the C_i, and let distinct C_i have only the vertex v in common. Then $\pi(C, v) = *_{i\in I}\pi(C_{i,v})$, a free product.*

□ Let T_i be a maximal tree in C_i, for each i in I. Then the T_i have only the point v in common, and their union T is a maximal tree in T. As before, there is a unique path $\overline{vx}$ in T to each vertex x of C, and with an edge e from a vertex x to a vertex y, we associate the element $\tilde{e} = \overline{vx}\cdot e\cdot \overline{vy}^{-1}$ of the group $F = \pi(C^1, v)$. If e is in T, evidently $e = 1$; the remaining $\tilde{e}$ evidently give a symmetrized basis $L = X \cup X^{-1}$ for the free group F. If L_i is the set of these $\tilde{e}$ for e in C_i, then L is evidently the disjoint union of the L_i, and each L_i is a symmetrized basis for $F_i = \pi(C^1, v)$, viewed as a subgroup of F.

It remains to show that the kernel N of the natural map from $F = \pi(C^1, v)$ onto $G = \pi(C, v)$ is the normal closure of a set R of elements of F each of which lies in one of the F_i. Now N is, by definition, the normal closure of the elements r of $\pi(C^1, v)$ determined by loops p at v of the form $p \simeq qsq^{-1}$ where q is a path from v to some vertex v', and s is the boundary, beginning at v', about some face D of C. Replacing r by a conjugate, we may suppose q minimal; then by our suppositions on C, p will lie entirely within some C_i. If $p = e_1 \cdots e_n$, then all the e_j lie in C_i, and $r = \tilde{e}_1 \cdots \tilde{e}_n$ where all the $\tilde{e}_j$ lie in L_i. This establishes that $G = \pi(C, v)$ is a free product, as described. □

We next give a proof of the Kurosh Subgroup Theorem taken directly from Zieschang-Vogt-Coldewey. The theorem is often stated in more detail (see, for example, MacLane 1958); these details can be recovered from the present proof.

Proposition 3.6. *Let G be the free product of groups G_i, where i runs over an index set I. Let H be a subgroup of G. Then H is the free product of a free group together with groups that are conjugates of subgroups of the free factors G_i of G.*

□ By (2.3), for each G_i there exists a connected complex C_i with a vertex v_i such that $G_i \simeq \pi(C_i, v_i)$. We form a complex C by adjoining to the disjoint union of the C_i edges e_i joining the v_i to a common vertex v. Now $G \simeq \pi(C_i, v_i)$ is obviously isomorphic to $\pi(C_i', v)$ where $C_i' = C_i \cup e_i$. By (3.5), $\pi(C, v) = *\pi(C_i', v)$, and we may suppose that $G = \pi(C, v)$ with each $G_i = \pi(C_i', v)$.

By (3.2), if H is a subgroup of G there is a covering map f from a complex $\tilde{C}$ onto C that induces an isomorphism f^* from $H = \pi(\tilde{C}, \tilde{v})$ onto H, where $\tilde{v}f = v$. The components K_j of the subcomplexes $C_i f^{-1}$ in C are disjoint, and $\tilde{C}$ is the union of these K_j together with a one-complex $L = \bigcup e_i f^{-1}$, having only vertices in common with the K_j. Let a maximal tree T_j be chosen in each K_j, and extend the union of the T_j to a maximal tree T in $\tilde{C}$. Let $\tilde{v}$ be a vertex in $\tilde{C}$ with $\tilde{v}f = v$.

As before, $F = \pi(\tilde{C}^{-1}, v)$ is a free group with a basis X of elements $x = \tilde{e}$ corresponding to the pairs $\{e, e^{-1}\}$ of edges of C not contained in T. Thus X can be partitioned into sets X_j together with a set X_L, according as e is in some K_j or e is in L.

Now $\tilde{H} = F/N$ where N is the normal closure of the set of all labels r on loops $p = sqs^{-1}$ at $\tilde{v}$ in $\tilde{C}$, where q is a boundary path for some face D of $\tilde{C}$. Replacing r by a conjugate, we may suppose that s is in T, whence r is a word in letters $x = \tilde{e}$ for edges e in the boundary path q of D. Since D must lie in some K_j, all these x must lie in X_j. Thus N is the normal closure of the union of sets R_j of wonds on the X_j. It follows that $\tilde{H}$ is the free product of groups $\tilde{H}_j = (X_j; R_j)$ together with a free group $\tilde{H}_L = (X_L; \varnothing)$.

It remains to identify the $\tilde{H}_j$. Let K_j be a component of $C_i f^{-1}$, and let s be a path in T from v to a vertex w in K_j such that $wf = v$. Then sf is a loop at v in C, representing some element h of G. Now each $x = \tilde{e}$ in X_j is represented by a loop $p = sqs^{-1}$ at $\tilde{v}$ in $\tilde{C}$ where q is a loop at w in K_j. Hence qf is a loop at v in C', representing some element g of G_i, and pf represents the element hgh^{-1} of hG_ih^{-1}. It follows that f^* maps $\tilde{H}_j$ isomorphically onto a subgroup of hG_ih^{-1}. Thus H, isomorphic to $\tilde{H}$, is the free product of such subgroups $\tilde{H}_j f^*$ of the hG_ih^{-1}, together with the free group $\tilde{H}_L f^*$. □

The Grushko-Neumann theorem, below, was proved independently by Grushko (1940) and Neumann (1943) and, in the infinitely generated case, by Wagner (1957); a somewhat more general result was proved by Higgins (1966) using groupoids; a proof in a more general context was given by Lyndon (1963); see also Lyndon (1965) and Cohen (1972). The proof we give below is essentially that of Stallings (1965) as revised by Massey (1967). (See Stallings, 1971, p. 1, for an historical remark.)

Proposition 3.7. *Let F be a finitely generated free group and α a homomorphism from F onto a free product $A = *A_\lambda$ of groups A_λ, $\lambda \in \Lambda$. Then F is a free product of groups F_λ, $F = *F_\lambda$, such that $F_\lambda\alpha = A_\lambda$ for each $\lambda \in \Lambda$.*

□ Let X be a basis for F and let H be the complex with a single vertex v, with edges e in one-to-one correspondence with the elements x of X, and with no 2-cells. If some $x\alpha = a_1 \cdots a_t$, normal form in $A = *A_\lambda$, we subdivide the corresponding edge, $e = e_1 \cdots e_t$. Let K° be the resulting complex, which we view as a 2-complex without 2-cells. We define a morphism ϕ from the edge groupoid of K° into A by setting, for x and e as above, $e_i\phi = a_i$.

We shall be concerned with finite connected 2-complexes K equipped with a designated vertex v and with a morphism ϕ from the edge groupoid into A. For each λ we define the subcomplex K_λ of K (not necessarily connected) to consist of all edges e with $e\phi$ in A_λ, and of all 2-cells bounded by a loop all of whose edges lie in K_λ. We consider the following properties:

(1) there is an isomorphism $\theta: \pi(K, v) \simeq F$ such that if p is a loop at v and $[p]$ its homotopy class, then $[p]\theta\alpha = p\phi$;

(2) $\bigcap K_\lambda$ is a disjoint union of trees.

Evidently K° is such a complex.

We show that given a complex K with these properties, and with $\bigcap K_\lambda$ not connected, we can modify K to obtain a new complex K' with the same properties and such that $\bigcap K'_\lambda$ has one component fewer than $\bigcap K_\lambda$. For this we make a definition and state a lemma. A *binding tie* is defined to be a path p in K connecting points in different components of $\bigcap K_\lambda$ and such that $p \subseteq K_\lambda$ for some λ and that $p\phi = 1$.

Lemma 3.8. *If $\bigcap K_\lambda$ is not connected, there exists a binding tie.*
We postpone the proof of the lemma.

Assume K as above, with $\bigcap K_\lambda$ not connected. By the lemma there exists a binding tie p. We form K' by adjoining to K an edge e with the same endpoints as p, and a 2-cell with boundary pe^{-1}. We extend ϕ by defining $e\phi = 1$. Inspection shows that K' satisfies (1) and (2) and that $\bigcap K_\lambda$ has one component fewer than $\bigcap K_\lambda$.

By iteration of this construction we arrive at a complex K satisfying (1) and (2) and such that $\bigcap K_\lambda$ is a tree. From the construction of K it can be seen that distinct K_μ and K_ν have no 2-cell in common, and only those edges that belong to $\bigcap K_\lambda$; thus $K_\mu \cap K_\nu = \bigcap K_\lambda$. It follows by the Seifert-van Kampen Theorem (III.3.5) that $\pi(K, v) = *\pi(K_\lambda, v)$. By (1) it follows that, if $F_\lambda = \pi(K_\lambda, v)\theta$, then $F = *F_\lambda$ and $F_\lambda\alpha \subseteq A_\lambda$; since α maps F onto A, it follows that $F_\lambda\alpha = A_\lambda$. □

We now prove the lemma. Since $\bigcap K_\lambda$ is not connected there is a path p in K connecting v to some vertex v' in a different component of $\bigcap K_\lambda$. Since α maps F onto A, there is a loop q at v in K with $q\phi = p\phi$. Let $r = q^{-1}p$; then r is a path from v to v' with $r\phi = 1$. Write $r = r_1 \cdots r_t$ where no successive r_i lie in the same K_λ; since $v' \neq v$, $r \neq 1$ and $t \geqslant 1$. We choose a point in each component of $\bigcap K_\lambda$ as 'base point', taking v and v' among them. For $1 \leqslant i < t$ we choose a path u_i in $\bigcap K_\lambda$ from the end point of r_i to the base point of that component of $\bigcap K_\lambda$ that contains it. Let $s = s_1 \cdots s_t$ where $s_1 = r_1u_1$, $s_2 = u_1^{-1}r_2u_2, \ldots, s_{t-1} = u_{t-2}^{-1}r_{t-1}u_{t-1}$, $s_t = u_{t-2}^{-1}r_t$; evidently $s\phi = r\phi = 1$.

We now delete any s_i that is a loop with $s_i\phi = 1$, and consolidate any successive s_i that lie in the same K_λ. We thus arrive a product $s' = s'_1 \cdots s'_{t'}$; it remains true that $s'\phi = s\phi = 1$, and that successive s'_i lie in different K_λ and therefore successive $s_i\phi$ lie in different A_λ. We iterate this construction to obtain a product $s'' = s''_1 \cdots s''_{t''}$ such $s''\phi = 1$, that successive $s''_i\phi$ lie in different A_λ, and that no s''_i is a loop with $s''_i\phi = 1$. Moreover, since s'' runs from v to v', $t \geqslant 1$. Now in the free product A, the relation $(s''_1\phi) \cdots (s''_{t''}\phi) = 1$ implies that some $s''_i\phi = 1$. Since we have eliminated all loops s''_i with $s''_i\phi = 1$, s''_i must begin and end at base points in different components of $\bigcap K_\lambda$. Thus s''_i is a binding tie, as required. □

4. Cayley Complexes

Before turning to precise definitions we make a few informal remarks. It is well known that Cayley (1878) showed that every abstract group, satisfying one of the usual sets of axioms, is isomorphic to a permutation group. Indeed, the right regular representation Δ carries a group G isomorphically onto a group of permutations of its own elements; each g in G corresponds to the permutation $g\Delta: h \mapsto hg$. We have no indication that Cayley viewed the permutations $g\Delta$ as sets of ordered couples, but this approach provides one path to another of Cayley's important discoveries (1878), the *colour group* or group diagram (Gruppenbild).

If we view $g\Delta$ as the set $\{(h, hg): h \in G\}$ of ordered couples, it is natural to represent $g\Delta$ by a graph with vertex set $V = G$ and with a (directed) edge from h to hg for each ordered couple (h, hg) in $g\Delta$. If one considers several different $g\Delta$ at once, it is natural to distinguish them by labeling the edges representing the various $g\Delta$ with different colors. This is essentially the *Cayley diagram* for G relative to the set X of all those g considered. The diagram is evidently connected just in case X generates G, and nothing is lost by confining attention to this case.

We prefer to change notation slightly, and suppose that G is given as a quotient group of a free group F with basis X. It will be convenient and unambiguous, for $h \in G$ and $w \in F$, to write hw for the product in G of h and the image of w. Now for each $h \in G$ and $x \in X$ we introduce an edge from h to hx, and label it, not with a color, but with the element x itself. Apart from supplying inverse edges, this brings the Cayley diagram into agreement with the 1-skeleton of the Cayley complex, which we now formally define.

Let $G = (X; R)$ where R is a set of cyclically reduced words in the free group F with basis X. We construct the *Cayley complex* $C = C(X; R)$ of the presentation. As the set of vertices we take the set $V = G$, as the set of edges we take $G \times L$ (cartesian product) where $L = X \cup X^{-1}$, and as set of faces the set $G \times (R \cup R^{-1})$. An edge (g, y) for $g \in G$, $y \in L$, runs by definition from g to gy; its inverse is (gy, y^{-1}). The Cayley complex will be equiped with a *labeling function* ϕ, and we describe this before discussing the faces. To each edge $e = (g, y)$ we attach the label $e\phi = y$; note that $(e^{-1})\phi = (e\phi)^{-1}$. We extend ϕ multiplicatively: to a path $p = e_1 \cdots e_n$ we attach as label the word $p\phi = (e_1\phi) \cdots (e_n\phi)$. Thus $p\phi$ is a reduced word if and only if p is a reduced path. Evidently ϕ induces a homomorphism from the fundamental groupoid $\pi(C^1)$ onto F; at any given vertex v, ϕ gives a one-to-one correspondence between the set of paths beginning at v and the set of all words. We shall sometimes write $p\phi$ also for the element of F or even of G determined by the word $p\phi$. Then we may observe that if p begins at v it ends at $v(p\phi)$; in particular, p is a loop if and only if $p\phi$ is in the normal closure N of R in F. We now attach the faces. Indeed, a face $D = (g, s)$, for $g \in G$ and $s \in R \cup R^{-1}$, will ordinarily have as boundary ∂D the cycle determined by the loop p at g with label $p\phi = s$. However, if $s = t^m$, m maximal, and $m \geqslant 2$, the method just described leads to redundant faces $(g, s), (gt, s), \ldots$, all with the same boundary; in this case we content ourselves with only one of them, taking $(g, s), (gt, s), \ldots, (gt^{m-1}, s)$ as all being the same face. The inverse of $D = (g, s)$ is $D^{-1} = (g, s^{-1})$.

A label on the boundary of a face D, beginning at any point, will be called a *boundary label*. We see that the set R^* of boundary labels consists of all cyclic permutations of the reduced words in R together with their inverses.

By an *automorphism* α of the Cayley complex we mean an automorphism of C as 2-complex that preserves labels: for every edge e, $(e\alpha)\phi = e\phi$. Evidently the automorphisms of C are precisely those of C^1. The next proposition is only a restatement of the fact that the centralizer of the right regular representation in the full symmetric group on the set of elements of G is the left regular representation.

Proposition 4.1. *The automorphisms of $C(X; R)$ are exactly those induced by left multiplication by an element h of G:*

$$g \mapsto hg, (g, y) \mapsto (hg, y), (g, r) \mapsto (hg, r). \quad \square$$

This has the important consequence that C is homogeneous in the sense that its automorphism group is transitive on vertices. It follows also that no non-trivial automorphism fixes a vertex or an edge. However, in view of our modified construction of faces, if $s = t^m$ in the notation above, any conjugate $h = gt^ig^{-1}$ of a power of t will fix the face (g, s) (see 6.1 below).

The following proposition is essentially true by construction.

Proposition 4.2. *$C(X; R)$ is simply connected, that is, $\pi(C(X; R)) = 1$.*

$\square$ Let p be any loop at a vertex v; we must show that $p \sim 1$. Since $p\phi \in N$, and N is the normal closure of R, we have $p\phi = f_1 \cdots f_n$ where each $f_i = u_i s_i u_i^{-1}$ for some $u_i \in F$ and $s_i \in R \cup R^{-1}$. Now each f_i is the label on a loop $p_i = v_i t_i v_i^{-1}$ where v_i runs from v to $v(u_i\phi)$ with label u_i, and t_i is the boundary label of the face $(v(u_i\phi), s_i)$ at $v(u_i\phi)$. Since $t_i \sim 1$, $p_i \sim 1$, and since $p \sim p_1 \cdots p_n$ with all $p_i \sim 1$, we have $p \sim 1$. $\square$

The following is now obvious.

Proposition 4.3. *$C(X; R)$ is the universal covering for $K(X; R)$ and $K(X; R)$ is the quotient complex of $C(X; R)$ by its automorphism group.* $\square$

5. Planar Cayley Complexes

Our treatment at the beginning of this section follows closely the ideas of Hoare-Karrass-Solitar (1971, 1972). Their goal was somewhat different, to prove a number of important results without appeal to even the most elementary geometry or topology. We quickly relax this constraint, reverting to an approach similar to that of Zieschang-Vogt-Coldewey. We take a middle path, utilizing the modest amount of geometry of 2-complexes set forth above. By accepting a slight modification in the definition of a Cayley diagram, one already suggested by Cayley himself, we are able (in III.8) to apply the same methods to groups of isometries of the hyperbolic plane that may contain reflections; these are the non-Euclidean crystallographic groups studied by Wilkie (1966), Macbeath (1967), and Hoare (preprint). Since the non-Euclidean crystallographic groups do not fall within the topic of this section without some modification of our definitions, we put them off to Section 8.

We now turn our attention to the question of what groups admit presentations $G = (X; R)$ such that the associated Cayley complex $C = C(X; R)$ can be embedded in a 2-manifold. The exact sense that should be attached to the word 'embedded' in this context will become clear. We shall call such a complex (locally) *planar*. In fact, because C is simply connected, if it can be embedded at all it can be embedded in the plane or sphere, and in the sphere in a locally finite way precisely in case G is finite. This problem for finite groups was settled by Maschke (1886); the groups G are then essentially the finite groups of isometries of the 2-sphere. For infinite groups the answer is also essentially well known (see for example Zieschang, 1966, also Zieschang, Vogt, and Coldewey, 1970). The groups are essentially the Fuchsian groups (including those with non-orientable quotient space) together with certain free products, of sufficiently small cardinality, of cyclic groups.

We suppose then that $G = (X; R)$ and that $C = C(X; R)$ is embeddable in a 2-manifold M; indeed we shall suppose that C is so embedded. The only assumption about the nature of the embedding is that a neighborhood of each vertex can be embedded in the plane. By a *geometric face* we shall mean a pair $\{D, D^{-1}\}$, that is an orientable region on the manifold with its two orientations. Suppose R contained two distinct conjugate elements, say $r = uv$ and $r' = vu$. Then for any vertex x, the two faces (x, uv) and (xu, vu) would have the same boundary cycle; since $r \neq r'$ we are not in the special case provided for in the construction of C, and the two faces are distinct. Thus there are two geometric faces with the same boundary, their union is a topological sphere, and hence is all of M. The same conclusion follows if one element of R is conjugate to the inverse of another. In either case, the 1-skeleton of C is the common boundary cycle, and it follows that G is a finite cyclic group, and has a presentation $G = (x; x^m)$. Thus, putting this case aside, we may assume that no element of R is conjugate to another element or its inverse.

As before, we let R^* be the set of all cyclic permutations of elements of R and
As before we let R^* be the set of all cyclic permutations of elements of R and their inverses. As before, we define the *root* s of an element $r \neq 1$ as the unique element such that $r = s^m$ with m maximal. We let S be the set of all roots of elements of R, and S^* the set of all conjugates of elements of S and their inverses; evidently S^* is the set of all roots of elements of R^*.

Proposition 5.1. *If C is planar, then S is quadratic over X.*

□ If $x \in X$ and $s \in S$ contains an occurrence of a letter x, as x^{+1} or x^{-1}, then there is a unique cyclic permutation s^* of $s^{\pm 1}$ that begins with this occurrence of x. Thus the occurrences of x, as x or x^{-1}, in elements of S correspond one-to-one with the elements of S^* beginning with x, and so with the elements of R^* beginning with x.

At a given vertex v there is, for each $r \in R^*$, exactly one loop p with label $p\phi = r$. There is exactly one edge e at v with $e\phi = x$, and this edge can begin at most two loops. It follows that there are at most two $r \in R^*$ beginning with x. □

We recall (see I.7) that the star graph $\Sigma(S)$ of a set S of words over X is a graph with vertex set $L = X \cup X^{-1}$ and with an undirected edge connecting elements y

and z of L whenever some element of S^* has a part $y^{-1}z$ or, in case $z = y^{-1}$, that y belongs to S^*.

The remaining piece of information that we derive from the geometrical hypothesis of planarity is the following.

Proposition 5.2. *Suppose that a finite subset S_0 of S is strictly quadratic over a finite subset X_0 of X. Then $S_0 = S$, $X_0 = X$, and $\Sigma(S)$ is a cycle.*

□ Choose a vertex v and an orientation of a neighborhood of v. Then the edges at v with labels in $L_0 = X_0 \cup X_0^{-1}$ occur, in the positive sense, in some cyclic order $e_1, \ldots, e_{2t}$ with $e_i\phi = y_i$, where $t = |X_0|$. By hypothesis each y_i occurs twice in S_0, whence by the argument above there are exactly two faces at v, with boundary paths p and p' at v beginning with e_i, and with labels powers of distinct elements s and s' of S^*. These boundary paths end with edges e^{-1} and e'^{-1} where e and e' are edges at v; the labels y and y' on e and e' occur in the elements s and s' of S^* and hence belong to X_0. It follows that e and e' are e_{i-1} and e_{i+1}.

We have shown that between consecutive edges e_i and e_{i+1} (in cyclic order) there is a face D_i with boundary label at v some $r_i = s_i^{m_i}$ for $s_i \in S_0^*$. But these edges e_i together with the faces D_i fill out an entire neighborhood of v, and are hence all the edges and faces at v. This implies that $X_0 = X$ and $S_0 = S$. Since the boundary cycle of D_i contains a segment $e_{i+1}^{-1}e_i$, it has a boundary label with a segment $y_{i+1}^{-1}y_i$, and thus y_i and y_{i+1} are connected in $\Sigma(S)$. This implies that $\Sigma(S)$ is a cycle. □

We now define an *F-group* to be a group with a finite presentation $G = (X; R)$ such that the set S of roots of elements of R is strictly quadratic over X and has cyclic star graph; a more explicit characterization of these groups is provided by Propositions (5.3) and (5.4). They are essentially the Fuchsian groups (with orientable or non-orientable quotient space) excluding those that are free products of cyclic groups.

Proposition 5.3. *Every F-group has a presentation of the form*

$$G = (x_1, \ldots, x_p, y_1, \ldots, y_n; x_1^{m_1}, \ldots, x_p^{m_p}, x_1 \cdots x_p q)$$

where $p, n \geqslant 0$, all $m_i > 1$, and either

$$q = [y_1, y_2] \cdots [y_{2g-1}, y_{2g}] \text{ for } n = 2g,$$

or

$$q = y_1^2 \cdots y_g^2 \text{ for } n = g.$$

□ By (I.7) we can transform S by an attached sequence of automorphisms of F to have the form $s_1 = x_1, \ldots, s_{p-1} = x_{p-1}, s_p = x_1 \cdots x_{p-1}q$ for some p and some q of one of the two forms above over some subset Y_0 of the set Y of remaining generators. Since $\Sigma(S)$ is connected, by (I.7.8.), S is minimal, and, since S is strictly quadratic over X, S has total length $2|X|$. It follows that the transform of

S has the same length, and hence contains all the generators. We have thus a presentation of G of the form

$$G = (X_1, \ldots, x_{p-1}, y_1, \ldots, y_n \colon x_1^{m_1}, \ldots, x_{p-1}^{m_{p-1}}, s_p^{m_p})$$

where each $m_i \geqslant 1$, $s_p = x_1 \cdots x_{p-1} q$ and q has one of the required forms. By a Tietze transformation we introduce a new generator x_p with a new relator $x_p s_p$. We may now introduce a redundant relator x^{m_p}; the relator s^{m_p} is now redundant and can be deleted. After deleting any x_i for which $m_i = 1$ and reindexing the x_i, the presentation now has the required form. □

It is clear by inspection that every group of one of the forms in (5.3) is an F-group.

Proposition 5.4. *Every group with a presentation whose Cayley complex is embeddable in a 2-manifold is either an F-group or a free product of cyclic groups.*

□ By (5.1) a planar group G has a presentation $G = (X; R)$ where the set S of roots of elements of R is quadratic over X. Now S falls into connected components S_i, and X can be partitioned into sets X_i such that each S_i is quadratic over X_i together with a set X_0 of generators that appear in no element of S. Let R_i be the set of elements of R with roots in S_i. Evidently G is the free product of $G_0 = (X_0; \varnothing)$ and groups $G_i = (X_i; R_i)$. By (5.2), if some S_i is finite and strictly quadratic over X_i, then $S_i = S$, $X_i = X$, $\Sigma(S)$ is connected, and, by definition, $G = G_i$ is an F-group. Otherwise, each S_i is either infinite or else finite but not strictly quadratic. By (I.7.4) or (I.7.5), after an automorphism of F that involves only the elements of X_i, we can suppose that $S_i \subseteq X_i$. Thus S_i is a free product of cyclic groups. Since G_0 is a free group, this implies that G is a free product of cyclic groups. □

Every F-group is clearly either finite or countably infinite. It is also clear that a planar group can have at most the cardinal of the continuum, and for a group of this cardinality the embedding of the Cayley complex presumably would have to be rather pathological. If we require the embedded complex to be locally finite, clearly the group must be finitely generated. We do not demand that, but in the next theorem confine attention to groups that are at most countably generated.

Proposition 5.5. *Let G be either an F-group or a free product of at most countably many cyclic groups. If G is finite is has a presentation with Cayley complex embeddable in the sphere, and if G is infinite it has one that is embeddable in the plane.*

□ Much more is known of course, on geometric and analytic grounds, but the present modest assertion admits a more elementary proof. First let G be an F-group or a free product with a presentation $G = (X; R)$ such that S, the set of roots of R, is strictly quadratic over X and has $\Sigma(S)$ cyclic. This implies that the edges and faces at a vertex v fill an entire neighborhood $N(v)$ of v; these $N(v)$ evidently cover C, whence every point (not necessarily a vertex) in the geometric realization of C has a neighborhood homeomorphic to a disc. It follows that C is a connected 2-manifold without boundary. Since by (4.2) C is simply connected, it must be a sphere or a plane. If G is finite, C has only finitely many faces, hence cannot exhaust the plane and must be a sphere. If G is infinite C must be a plane, for it is easy to see that C is the union of an infinite increasing sequence of topological discs, each with its boundary interior to the next, and such a union cannot be a sphere.

Next let G be a free product of cyclic groups, $G = (x_i : i \in I; x_i^{m_i}, i \in I)$, where the index set I is at most countable and each $m_i \geqslant 0$. If G is finite it is cyclic and an F-group, a case already treated; thus we may assume G infinite. We choose a vertex v in the plane and construct out of v a pair of edges e_i and e'_i for each i in I, arranged so that no edge lies between e_i and e'_i in the positive sense about v. If $m_i > 0$ we construct a loop l_i at v of length m_i with e_i as first edge and $e_i'^{-1}$ as last edge, and we assign to all the edges of l_i the label x_i. If D_i is the region enclosed by l_i then D_i has boundary label $x_i^{m_i}$. If $m_i = 0$ we choose two infinite paths l_i and l'_i out of v and otherwise disjoint, the first beginning with e_i and the second with e'_i and assign the label x_i to all edges of l_i and x_i^{-1} to all the edges of l'_i. We let D_i be the unbounded region between l_i and l'_i, clockwise about v. (All this can be done without singularities: for example we can take v at the origin of a coordinate system and each D_i in the upper right sector enclosed by the two lines out of v with slopes $1/2i$ and $1/(2i + 1)$). Call the complex formed so far C_0.

Now we suppose inductively that we have a complex C_n that contains C_0 and in which the star of each vertex v' is contained in a subcomplex $C(v')$ of C_n that is isomorphic to a subcomplex of C_0; we may suppose $C(v')$ maximal for this property. If $C(v')$ is not already isomorphic to all of C_0, we can extend $C(v')$ in the same way as we constructed C_0 until it is. We let C_{n+1} be the result of doing this to all $C(v')$ for v' in C_n, say in order of the length of the shortest path from v to v'. Then the union of all the C_n is clearly a Cayley complex for the given presentation. □

We shall give a more effective construction of the Cayley complex of a presentation with planar Cayley complex; this gives a very elementary solution of the word problem for such groups, although admittedly a less practical, less elegant proof, and one of less general application than others.

If C is any graph, we define the *distance* $d(v, v')$ between two vertices v and v' to be the least length of a path connecting them. Then, for any $n \geqslant 0$ and any vertex v, the *ball* of radius n at v is the subcomplex $B_n(C, v)$ whose vertex set is $V = \{v' : d(v, v') \leqslant n\}$ and whose edges and faces are all those of C that are incident with no vertices other than those in V.

Lemma 5.6. *If for any presentation $G = (X; R)$ the 1-skeleton B_n^1 of the ball $B_n(C, 1)$ in $C = C(X; R)$ is, for all n, finite and effectively constructible, then the word problem for the presentation is solvable.*

□ Let $w \in F$ be given; we must decide if $w \in N$. Let p be the path at 1 in C with label w; then $w \in N$ if and only if p is a loop. that is, ends at 1. Now clearly p is contained in B_n^1, for $n = |w|$. If B_n^1 can be constructed effectively, then we can decide by inspection whether p ends at 1. □

Proposition 5.7. *If the presentation $(X; R)$ has planar Cayley complex then the word problem for this presentation is solvable.*

□ We may assume that $G = (X; R)$ is an infinite F-group. We must show how to construct $B_n^1(C)$ for $C = C(X; R)$ and arbitrary n. Suppose that K is a 2-complex that is a combinatorial disc, with its edges labeled with elements of L in such a way that $(e^{-1})\phi = (e\phi)^{-1}$, and that ψ is a (label preserving) homomorphism of K into C that is injective on cells except possibly for vertices on the boundary ∂K. Clearly ψ cannot be an epimorphism, whence $\partial K \neq 0$. Let e be any edge in ∂K, incident with a face D of K. In C, the image $e\psi$ separates $D\psi$ from a second face D'. Let θ be the inclusion map D' into C, and let K' be the quotient space of the disjoint union $K \cup D'$ by the kernel of the map $\psi \cup \theta: K \cup D' \to C$, and let ψ' be the induced map from K' into C. (Ordinarily, K' is the union of K and D' with a segment p of boundary containing e identified; exceptionally, if p is identified with all of $\partial D'$, the two ends in K of p will become identified in K'.) Let ψ be the induced map from K' into C. It follows from the hypothesis on ψ together with the fact that θ is injective that ψ is injective except possibly on vertices in $\partial K'$. We have also an induced homomorphism σ from K into K' such that $\sigma\psi = \psi$.

By iteration of this construction, choosing the edge e at each stage in an obvious fashion, one can construct K^* and ψ^*, satisfying the same hypotheses as K and ψ, and a map $\sigma^*: K \to K^*$ such that $\sigma^*\psi^* = \psi$, with the additional condition that $K \subseteq (K^* - \partial K^*)$. We now start with K_0 consisting of a single vertex v_0 and ψ_0 mapping v_0 onto 1 in C. Taking successive $K_{n+1} = K_n^*$, we have maps $\psi_n: K_n \to C$ and maps $\sigma_n: K_n \to K_{n+1}$, such that each pair K_n, ψ_n satisfies the hypotheses on K, ψ, that $\sigma_n\psi_{n+1} = \psi_n$, and that $K_n \subseteq (K_{n+1} - \partial K_{n+1})$. Examination of the local structure shows that the direct limit K_∞ of this system is isomorphic to C under the induced map $\psi_\infty: K_\infty \to C$.

From the condition $K_n \subseteq (K_{n+1} - \partial K_{n+1})$ it follows inductively that $B_n(C) \subseteq K_n\psi_n$. Thus ψ_{n+1} maps $B_n(K_{n+1}, v_0)$ isomorphically onto $B_n(C, 1)$. Since we have seen how to construct K_{n+1} we have also $B_n(K_{n+1}, v_0)$ and so $B_n(C, 1)$, and with it $B_n^1(C, 1)$. □

It should be emphasized that here, in contrast to a similar construction in Zieschang (1966), we are assuming in advance that C lies in the plane; without this we would have no assurance that the ψ_n were injective. A more general construction for Cayley complexes is given in III.12 below.

We mention an extension of the preceding result. We say that an arbitrary connected 2-complex K satisfies the *maximum principle* if, whenever v_0 is a vertex of K and Q is any combinatorial (closed) disc in K, then the maximum value of $d(v_0, v)$ for all v in Q is attained for some v in ∂Q. Lyndon (1967) showed that every 2-complex of type $C(3, 6)$ or $C(4, 4)$, in the sense of Chapter V, satisfies the maximum principle; and from well known properties of F-groups it is not difficult to show that the Cayley complex of any strictly quadratic presentation of such a group also satisfies the maximum principle. In the following proposition we assume that the presentation is recursive; this is automatic if R is finite.

Proposition 5.8. *If the Cayley complex of a presentation satisfies the maximum principle, then the word problem for this presentation is solvable.*

□ If C is the Cayley complex, we must again show that the 1-skeleton B_n^1 of $B_n = B_n(C)$ is constructible for each n. We construct a 1-complex A, with labels in Y, as follows. The vertices of A will be all elements w of F of length at most n. If for some y in L both w and wy are in A, we introduce an edge e with label y from w to wy, together with its inverse. We introduce a relation $w \approx u$ on vertices of A, which holds just in case that there is a path in A from w to u that is a product of paths of the form zqz^{-1} where the label on q belongs to R^*. This is obviously an equivalence relation; moreover, it has an obvious extension to an equivalence on the edges of A that preserves incidence and labeling. Therefore we can form the quotient space B of A modulo this relation. We propose to show that B, which is evidently finite and constructible, is isomorphic to B_n^1.

We note first that B_n is simply connected. For this we must show that if p is a loop in B_n, then p is contractible in B_n. By an obvious reduction we may suppose p is a simple loop. Since C is simply connected, p is the boundary of a combinatorial disc Q in C. But now the maximum principle tells us that since the boundary p of Q lies in B_n, in fact Q itself lies in B_n.

To show B isomorphic to B_n^1 it suffices to show that if w is a vertex of A and the image of w in C under the obvious map is the vertex 1, then w and 1 have the same image in B, that is, that $w \approx 1$. This hypothesis implies that the path p in C with label w is a loop, and that p is in B_n. By a standard argument $p \underset{1}{\sim} p_1 \cdots p_t$ where each p_i is of the form zqz^{-1} for z, q in B_n and q with label in P^*. Since the path $\tilde{p}$ with label w in A is 1-equivalent to the product of paths $\tilde{p}_i$ in A, with the same label as the p_i, and $\tilde{p}_i$ leads from the vertex 1 to w, it follows from the definition that $1 \approx w$. □

6. F-Groups Continued

We propose now to establish certain well known facts about Fuchsian groups by methods based, for the most part, on Cayley complexes. In this we take a middle path between the classical metric or analytic arguments and the purely non-geometrical methods of Hoare, Karrass, and Solitar (1971, 1972). We borrow heavily from both sources. For some purposes it seems preferable to consider not the Cayley complex but a dual complex, borrowed from the usual analytic treatment, which we shall call a Fuchsian complex. But for our first few results we shall not need this. We continue to borrow heavily from Zieschang-Vogt-Coldewey.

We shall call a Cayley complex $C(X; R)$ *strictly planar* if it is planar but not a sphere, that is, if it is planar and infinite.

Proposition 6.1. *A non-trivial automorphism of a strictly planar Cayley complex C fixes no point and no geometric edge; if it leaves invariant any non-empty finite union of faces, then it fixes exactly one face.*

□ Let $G = (X; R)$ with planar Cayley complex $C = C(X; R)$. We have seen that all automorphisms of C are given by left multiplication by elements of G. Let α be the automorphism determined by left multiplication by an element $g \neq 1$ of G. Then α can fix no vertex h, else we would have $gh = h$. If α fixed a geometric edge $\{e, e^{-1}\}$, since it cannot fix its end points it would have to exchange them; but then

α would have to interchange e and e^{-1}, which is impossible since they have opposite labels. From this we conclude also that α can fix no simple arc, since if it did it would fix either a middle vertex or a middle edge of the arc.

We now suppose that α fixes some finite union E of faces. Since α must permute the finite set of vertices in E, some power of α must fix one of them and, by the above, this implies that g has finite order $n > 1$. We now choose a finite connected subcomplex S containing both E and αE. Then the union E' of all the $g^i S$ for $i = 0, 1, \ldots, n-1$ is finite, connected and invariant under α. If E'' is the union of E' with all the finite components of its complement, then E'' is finite, connected, simply connected, and invariant under α.

Simplifying notation we may suppose that a combinatorial disc E is invariant under α. We shall show by induction on the number of faces of E that α fixes a single face in E. If E has only one face, this assertion is tautologous. If E had exactly two faces, α would have to fix the geometric edge separating them, which we have seen is impossible. We may assume then that E has at least three faces. Now it is easy to see that there must be some face D of E such that the part of ∂D on the boundary of E is a simple arc. Since α cannot fix this arc it cannot fix D, nor can any non-trivial power of α. Thus the $\alpha^i D$ are n distinct faces, each meeting ∂E in a simple arc. If $\alpha^j D$ is the next after D in the positive sense along ∂E, then α^j must have order n and hence must generate the same group as α. After replacing α by α^j, we may suppose that $D, \alpha D, \ldots, \alpha^{n-1} D$ occur in cyclic order along ∂E. If the $\alpha^i D$ are disjoint, then $E' = E - \bigcup \alpha^i D$ is again a disc, invariant under α, and the conclusion follows by induction. It is easy to see that if D meets any other $\alpha^i D$, then it must meet αD and $\alpha^{-1} D$; moreover, if D met any $\alpha^i D$ beyond αD and $\alpha^{-1} D$, then $\bigcap \alpha^i D$ would be a point, fixed under α. Therefore we may suppose that D meets αD and $\alpha^{-1} D$, and no further $\alpha^i D$.

If $n = 2$, let V be the complement of the union of the interiors of D and αD, and let V_0 be the component of $V \cap E$ that contains $D \cap \alpha D$. Now V_0 is a chain of simple arcs and discs, and α reverses this chain. But α cannot leave a simple arc invariant; moreover, it cannot exchange two adjacent discs, else it would fix their common point. Therefore α must leave a disc in V_0 invariant, and the conclusion follows by induction.

Let $n > 2$. Let D' be the union of D with the closures of all bounded components of the complement of $D \cup \alpha D$. Then $D' \cap \alpha D' = \sigma$, where σ is either a point $p = q$ on ∂E, or a simple arc from p on ∂E to a point q interior to E. Since $D \cap \alpha^2 D = \varnothing$, $\alpha q \neq q$. Now $\partial D'$ consists of $\sigma, \alpha^{-1}\sigma$, an arc on ∂E from $\alpha^{-1} p$ to p, and an arc τ from $\alpha^{-1} q$ to q. Thus $\bigcup \alpha^i \tau$ is a simple closed curve, invariant under α, which therefore bounds a proper subdisc E' of E that is invariant under α. The conclusion again follows by induction.

This completes the inductive proof that an invariant combinatorial disc contains exactly one invariant face. It now follows that an automorphism α can leave at most one face invariant, since if it left two faces invariant, then by the argument above it would have finite order, and both these two faces could be included in an invariant combinatorial disc. □

Proposition 6.2. *Let $G = (X; R)$ have a planar Cayley complex $C = C(X; R)$ and* *let S be the set of roots of $R = \{s^{m(s)}: s \in S\}$. Then every non-trivial element of finite order in G is the image $us^b u^{-1}$ of a unique element $s \in S$, with b unique in the range $0 < b < m(s)$, and with u unique up to replacement by some $u' = us^i$.*

☐ Let g in G have finite order $n > 1$. If D is any face, then g fixes the finite union E of the faces $g^i D$, whence by the preceding proposition g fixes a unique face D_0. Now D_0 will have boundary label some r in R, beginning at some vertex u on ∂D_0, and since g fixes D_0, it follows that gu lies on ∂D_0 and D_0 has boundary label r beginning at gu. If t is the label on the arc of ∂D_0 from u to gu, then $r = t^n$, and hence $r = s^{m(s)}$ for some $s \in S$, with $t = s^b$ for some b, $0 < b < m(s)$ and $nb = m(s)$. Now by the definition of t, $gu = ut$, whence g is the image of $utu^{-1} = us^b u^{-1}$. The uniqueness of s follows from the uniqueness of D_0, and that of b from the choice of t. Moreover, the choice of u is unique up to replacing it by some us^i. ☐

It follows from the above that the images of the s in G have orders exactly $m(s)$, that the cyclic groups G_s generated by the images of those s with $m(s) > 1$ are a set of representatives of the conjugacy classes of maximal non-trivial finite cyclic subgroups in G, and that these groups G_s are self-normalizing. It follows in particular that if all $m(s) = 1$, in particular if G is a free group or the fundamental group of a closed 2-manifold (other than the projective plane), then G is without torsion.

The presentations described in (5.3) are canonical to the extent that, putting aside finite cyclic groups, and assuming $2 \leqslant m_1 \leqslant \cdots \leqslant m_p$, groups described by different presentations of this form are non-isomorphic. We give below only a sketch of the proof. First we observe that if $n = 0$ and $p \leqslant 2$ or if $n = 1$ (whence $q = y_1^2$) and $p \leqslant 1$, then C is finite cyclic; from the results below it is clear that these are the only cases in which G is finite cyclic. We exclude these from the considerations below.

The measure of G is defined to be $\mu(G) = n - 2 + \sum_{i=1}^{p}(1 - 1/m_i)$ (see 7.8 below). Inspection shows that $\mu(G) < 0$ implies that $n = 0$ and $p = 3$, and that, further, either $(m_1, m_2, m_3) = (2, 2, n)$ for some n, whence G is a dihedral group of order $2n$, or else $(m_1, m_2, m_3) = (2, 3, n)$ for $n = 3$, 4, or 5, whence G is one of the three rotation groups of the regular solids. These groups are all finite and non-isomorphic.

It follows from the general theory that if $\mu(G) \geqslant 0$ then G is infinite, but we give next a direct proof. If $n = 1$, hence $q = y_1^2$, then (excluding always the cyclic cases), G is obtained by adjoining a square root to an element in a free product of cyclic groups, and hence is infinite. In the remaining cases that $n \neq 0$, one can observe that $G/[G, G]$ is infinite. If $n = 0$, by passing to a homomorphic image it suffices to treat the case that $p = 3$ together with the cases $p = 4$ in which $(m_1, \ldots, m_4)$ is $(2, 2, 2, n)$ or $(2, 2, 3, n)$ for some $n \geqslant 2$. For $p = 3$, we consider a more economical presentation $G = (x^a, y^b, (xy)^c)$ and the associated Cayley complex C. We obtain a new complex C^* from C by contracting each face with boundary label y^b to a point. Then at each vertex of C^* there are $2b$ edges, separating faces that are alternately a-gons and c-gons. If we assume that C and therefore C^* are finite and so spherical, calculation of the characteristic implies that $1/a + 1/b + 1/c > 1$, whence G is one of the finite groups G with $\mu(G) < 0$ listed above. For the case

$(2, 2, 2, n)$ we use the presentation $G = (x^2, y^2, z^2, (xyz)^n)$ with Cayley complex C. We form C^* by contracting each digon with boundary label x^2, y^2, or z^2 to a single edge; then C^* is made up of $3n$-gons, 3 meeting at each vertex, which is impossible for a finite complex on the sphere. For $(2, 2, 3, n)$, $G = (x^2, y^2, z^3, (xyz)^n)$ we contract each digon with boundary label x^2 or y^2 to an edge, and each face with boundary label z^3 to a point. The complex C^* thus obtained is made up of $2n$-gons, 6 at each vertex, again impossible for a finite complex on the sphere.

To show that these groups are non-isomorphic it is enough to treat the infinite groups; for these (6.2) shows that the sequence $m_1 \leqslant \cdots \leqslant m_p$ is an invariant. If $n \neq 0$, we let T be the subgroup generated by all elements of finite order, let $G^* = G/T$, and let $G^{**} = G^*/[G^*, G^*]$. Evidently $G^* = (q)$, and G^{**} is free abelian of rank n if $q = [y_1, y_2] \cdots [y_{n-1}, y_n]$, while G^{**} is the direct product of a group of order 2 with a free abelian group of rank $n - 1$ if $q = y_1^2 \cdots y_n^2$.

We remark also that none of these groups is a free product of cyclic groups. This follows from (II.5.14), but we give here a direct proof. If G is a free product of cyclic groups of which some number r are infinite cyclic, the group $G^* = G/T$ defined as before is free of rank r; if $r > 0$, this shows G is not isomorphic to a group of type (5.3). If $n = 0$, from (3.6) we see that the m_i are the orders of the cyclic factors, and G could be isomorphic to a Fuchsian group H only in case G is a free product of a finite number of finite cyclic groups of orders $m_1, \ldots, m_p$, while H is the Fuchsian group with the same m_i and with $n = 0$. But now $H/[H, H]$ is obtained by imposing a non-trivial relation on the finite abelian group $G/[G, G]$, whence $H/[H, H]$ is not isomorphic to $G/[G, G]$, and hence G is not isomorphic to H.

7. Fuchsian Complexes

There is a classical construction (see Poincaré (1882); Macbeath (1963); Benson and Grove (1971)) for reading off a presentation for a discontinuous group from a tessellation of the space on which it acts into translates of a suitable fundamental region. For the groups that concern us here this amounts roughly to showing that the tessellation is, in a sense that will be explained, dual to a Cayley complex for the presentation. Since we want to use this connection without entering into analytic considerations, we give a purely combinatorial definition of a tessellation by fundamental regions, which we shall call a *Fuchsian complex*.

Most of the arguments below go through with minor variation for all planar groups, but we are primarily concerned with Fuchsian groups, and will consequently frequently put aside the finite planar groups, and will give somewhat less attention to those groups that are free products of cyclic groups.

The complexes we shall consider may then all be considered as embedded in the plane. As a technical convenience we will admit henceforth as faces all components of the complement of the 1-skeleton, including those that are unbounded; with this convention, all complexes to be considered are homeomorphic to the plane. It is known that the mentioned tessellations for Fuchsian groups can be chosen to be quite non-pathological, indeed polygonal, and the constructions given above for planar Cayley complexes share this property. Therefore for our discussion we shall understand that every complex is polygonal and, in particular, that every edge is homeomorphic to a segment (finite or infinite) of the real axis, that every face is homeomorphic to the closed disc or the closed half plane, and that the set of vertices has no accumulation points. We also assume that the intersection of two faces is empty, a single vertex, or a simple arc, finite or infinite. We call such complexes *planar*. An infinite planar group G has a presentation with Cayley complex C that is planar in the above sense, and G acts (on the left) as the automorphism group of C, as labeled complex. In particular, we have seen that G acts regularly on the set of vertices of C.

By a *Fuchsian complex* for G we mean a planar complex on which G acts (on the left) as a group of automorphisms, and regularly on the faces: that is, G is transitive on the set of faces and no non-trivial element fixes any face. As a matter of technical convenience we assume the intersection of two faces, if not empty, is a single vertex or a single edge, with the following exception: if an element g of G (necessarily an involution) exchanges two faces D and D' with intersection an arc p, and exchanges the two ends of p, then we require that p consist of two geometric edges, exchanged by g.

We call two planar complexes K and L *dual* if there is a one-to-one correspondence between their cells under which a face of the one corresponds to a vertex of the other, interior to that face, and an edge of the one corresponds to an edge of the other, crossing that edge exactly once and meeting no other edge.

It is almost true that, for the groups under consideration, each Fuchsian complex determines a dual Cayley complex and conversely. This is indeed true if one imposes on Fuchsian complexes the additional condition that they contain no *reflections*, that is, no edges left fixed by a non-trivial element of G. It is also true if one admits reflections in the Fuchsian complex but modifies the definition of a Cayley complex in a seemingly innocuous way that was indeed already suggested by Cayley (1878). We first define a *modified presentation*. Let F_1 be a free group with basis X, and F_2 the free product of two-element groups $\{1, x\}$ for x ranging over a set J. Let F be the free product of F_1 and F_2, let R be a subset of F, and N its normal closure in F. If $G = F/N$, we say that the triple $(X, J; R)$ is a modified presentation for G. The *modified Cayley complex* of such a presentation is defined exactly as the ordinary Cayley complex with one exception: given a vertex v and an element x in J, there is only one edge emamating from v with the label $x\ (= x^{-1})$ and in consequence there are no faces with boundary label x^2 for x in J. We remark that ordinary presentations and ordinary Cayley complexes may be subsumed under the case $J = \varnothing$ of the corresponding modified concepts.

We have introduced these concepts relating to reflections here in the interest of perspective and of a unified treatment of certain basic results. But the groups with Fuchsian complexes with reflections are what have been called the *non-Euclidean crystallographic groups* (Wilkie 1966) about which somewhat less is known than about the classical Fuchsian groups, and we put off what little special knowledge we have of them to a later section (III.8 below).

Proposition 7.1. *Let a group G have a Fuchsian complex K. Then G has a modified presentation $G = (X, J; R)$ whose modified Cayley complex $C = C(X, J; R)$ is dual to K. Moreover, if g in G carries a face D of K into a face gD, and v, v' are the vertices of C in D, gD, then $v' = gv$. If K is without reflections, then C can be taken as an ordinary Cayley complex.*

□ We choose a face D_0 of K, and let $\bar{L}$ be the set of elements g in G such that D_0 and gD_0 have an edge in common. Since $g^{-1}D_0 \cap D_0 = g^{-1}(D_0 \cap gD_0)$, if g is in $\bar{L}$ then g^{-1} is in $\bar{L}$. Let $\bar{J}$ be the set of reflections in $\bar{L}$, that is, those non-trivial elements that fix edges on the boundary of D_0. Let $\bar{X}$ be a set containing exactly one out of each pair $\{g, g^{-1}\}$ contained in $\bar{L} - \bar{J}$. We shall show that $\bar{X} \cup \bar{J}$ generates G; for this it suffices to show that $\bar{L}$ generates G. Let g be any element of G and choose a path in the plane from a point interior to D_0 to a point interior to gD_0. Since the vertex set of K has no accumulation point, p can pass through only finitely many vertices and, by deformations in the neighborhoods of these vertices, we can arrange that p passes through no vertex. Then p passes successively through faces $g_0D_0, \ldots, g_nD_0$ where $g_0 = 1$ and $g_n = g$, and successive faces have an edge in common. If for $0 \leqslant i < n$ we write $g_{i+1} = g_ih_{i+1}$ then, since g_iD_0 and $g_{i+1}D_0 = g_ih_{i+1}D_0$ have an edge in common, it follows that D_0 and $h_{i+1}D_0$ have an edge in common, and therefore h_{i+1} is in $\bar{L}$. But then $g = h_1 \cdots h_n$ lies in the subgroup generated by $\bar{L}$. We now take a group F generated by sets X and J as in the definition of a modified presentation, mapping one-to-one onto $\bar{X}$ and $\bar{J}$, and inducing a homomorphism θ from F onto G. These will be the X and J of our modified presentation; the set R will be determined automatically once we have constructed the 1-skeleton of the modified Cayley complex C.

We now mimic barycentric subdivision by choosing a point $v(D)$ interior to each face D of K, a point $v(e)$ interior to each edge, and, for each edge e on the boundary of a face D, a path $p(D, e)$ from $v(D)$ to $v(e)$; we may take these paths disjoint except at their endpoints, and with each $p(D, e)$ interior to D except at its endpoint $v(e)$. For the vertices of C we take the points $v(D)$; under the correspondence $v(gD_0) \leftrightarrow g$, the group G acts on them as required. Now, for a given face D, the faces having an edge e in common with D are precisely the gD for g in $\bar{L}$; for each of these we introduce an edge $e^* = p(D, e)p(gD, e)^{-1}$ from $v(D)$ to $v(gD)$, and assign to it as label the preimage of g in $L = X \cup X^{-1} \cup J$. This completes the construction of the 1-skeleton C^1 of C, and the faces are determined as the components of the complement of C^1. For R, we choose for each bounded face of C at $v(D_0)$, the boundary label r in the positive sense beginning at $v(D_0)$; then the faces and the elements of R correspond as they should in a Cayley diagram, and it is clear by a standard argument that the normal closure of R is the kernel N of the map θ from F onto G, whence $C = C(X, J; R)$ is indeed a modified Cayley complex for G. □

We now prove a converse.

Proposition 7.2. *If a group G has a finite modified presentation $G = (X, J; R)$ such that $C = C(X, J; R)$ is strictly planar, then G has a Fuchsian complex K that is dual to C. K will be without reflections if and only if the presentation is ordinary.*

□ We suppose C is in fact embedded in the plane as a planar complex; thus G, as vertex set of C, has been identified with a set of points in the plane. We subdivide C, choosing a point $v(D)$ interior to each face, finite or infinite, a point $v(e)$ interior to each edge, and for each D paths $p(D, e)$ from $v(D)$ to $v(e)$ for each edge e on ∂D, and such that they are interior to D except at their endpoints $v(e)$ and disjoint except at the point $v(D)$. Let Q be the 1-complex consisting of the 1-skeleton of C together with the new points and paths (each edge of C now counting, of course, as two in Q). Let C^* be the complex with Q as 1-skeleton and with faces all components of the complement of Q in the plane.

Each face of C^* will be part of some face D of C and will have on its boundary a single vertex g from C; we call such a face $f(D, g)$. The faces of C^* thus correspond one-to-one to the pairs (D, g) such that g lies on ∂D. Let $S(g)$ be the union of the $f(D, g)$ for all D incident with g. Because we have admitted unbounded faces D, the union of the D incident with g contains a neighborhood of g, and it is easy to see that $S(g)$ is a finite polygon with g in its interior. Evidently the $S(g)$ are disjoint except on their boundaries and their union is the entire plane. Let K be the complex with faces all $S(g)$ and as edges and vertices all those from C^* that lie on the boundary of some $S(g)$. Clearly the complex K is dual to C.

Now the action of G on C extends naturally to an action on C^*. For h in G one has $hf(D, g) = f(hD, hg)$, and thus $hS(g) = S(hg)$. Thus an action on K is induced under which K is clearly a Fuchsian complex for G.

Each geometric edge e^* of K separates a pair of faces $S(g)$ and $S(gx)$ for some x in $L = X \cup X^{-1} \cup J$, and crosses the edge e of C between g and gx. If nontrivial h in G leaves e^* fixed it must permute g and gx, and since it cannot fix either it must interchange them, and thus reverse the directed edge e. But then e and e^{-1} must have the same label, whence $x = x^{-1}$ in F, and x is in J. Since $hg = gx$, we have $h = gxg^{-1}$. Conversely, if h is of this form, then it fixes e^*. Thus K is without reflections if and only if $J = \emptyset$. □

The proof of the following theorem is patterned after a similar argument of Dyck (1882/3; see also Burnside 1955, Chapter 18).

Proposition 7.3. *If K is a Fuchsian complex for a group G and H is a subgroup of G, then H has a Fuchsian complex L each of whose faces is a union of faces of K.*

□ By Zorn's lemma, there exists a subcomplex E of K that is a union of faces of K, and that is maximal subject to the following properties:

(i) E is 2-connected: each pair of faces in E can be connected by a 2-chain in E, that is a chain in which successive members have an edge in common;

(ii) E contains no pair of congruent faces, D and hD, $h \in H$.

We show that

(iii) every face of K is congruent to some face of E.

Suppose (iii) false, hence that some face D in K is not congruent to any face in E. Clearly K is 2-connected, whence there exists a 2-chain $D_0, D_1, \ldots, D_n = D$ from some D_0 in E to D. We suppose D and this chain chosen to make n as small as possible. If we had $n > 1$, minimality of n would require that D_{n-1} be congruent to some hD_{n-1} in E, yielding hD_{n-1}, hD as a shorter chain with the same properties. We conclude that $n = 1$, whence $E' = E \cup D$ satisfies (i) and (ii), contradicting the maximality of E.

We show that

(iv) E is simply connected.

Suppose (iv) false, hence that the complement of E in K has a bounded component U. Then U contains a face D, and, by (iii), $D = hD'$ for some face D' of E, and $h \in H$, $h \neq 1$. Now by (i) E is 2-connected, whence hE is also. By (ii) hE is disjoint from E. Since $hD \subseteq hE$ is in U, we conclude that $hE \subseteq U$. Let $V = E \cup U$; then V is 2-connected and in enclosed by the outer boundary β of E. Since hV is 2-connected and enclosed by $h\beta \subseteq U$, we conclude that $hV \subseteq U < V$. Iteration gives $V > hV > h^2V \ldots$, contrary to the local finiteness of K. We may now take L to be the planar complex whose faces are the translates hE of E, for all $h \in H$. We remark that if E is finite its boundary is a simple closed curve, and E is a combinatorial disc. If E is infinite, its boundary will be a disjoint union of doubly infinite simple curves; in this case L is a complex in the extended sense, admitting unbounded faces. □

Our proof of the following classical theorem is patterned after that of Hoare, Karrass, and Solitar (1971, 1972), although they did not use geometry.

Proposition 7.4. *If G is an F-group, then every subgroup H of finite index is again an F-group, while every subgroup H of infinite index is a free product of cyclic groups.*

□ The finite F-groups are just the finite groups of isometries of the sphere; thus we may put them aside. Otherwise, we have seen in the proof of (5.5) that an infinite F-group possesses a Cayley complex whose (finite) faces fill the plane. We saw earlier (5.2) that conversely, a group with such a Cayley complex has a presentation with the set S of roots finite and strictly quadratic, and with connected star graph, and is therefore an F-group. We observe that if a planar complex is locally finite and has all its faces finite, then the same is true of its dual, since a vertex of the dual in contained in a face of the first and a face of the dual is contained in the star of a vertex of the first.

Thus G has a Cayley complex with all faces finite, hence a dual Fuchsian complex K with all faces finite. If H has finite index j in G, then H has a Fuchsian complex L in which each face is the union of j faces from K, and therefore in which each face is finite. But then H has a dual Cayley complex in which each face is finite, and is therefore an F-group. If H has infinite index, then it has a Fuchsian complex L in which each face is the union of an infinite number of faces from K, and therefore is infinite. Then H has a presentation $H = (X; R)$ such that $C(X; R)$ is dual to L, hence is planar, but does not have all its faces finite. Thus H is a planar group with a presentation that is not strictly quadratic, and thus must be a free product of cyclic groups. □

We turn to another classical theorem, with a proof again inspired by the work of Hoare, Karrass, and Solitar (1971, 1972). We present, after some preliminaries, a combinatorial version of the index formula of Riemann and Hurwitz. See Lyndon (1976).

We begin with a combinatorial definition of angle. If K is any planar complex, we define an *angle measure* on K to be a real valued function α, defined on tripies (v, e, e') where e and e' are edges emanating from the vertex v, and satisfying the following condition:

if $e_1, \ldots, e_n$, *for* $n \geqslant 1$, *are edges emanating in that order cyclically about a vertex* v, *then*

$$\alpha(v, e_1, e_2) + \cdots + \alpha(v, e_{n-1}, e_n) + \alpha(v\ e_n, e_1) = 2\pi.$$

In this notation, we write α_{ij} for $\alpha(v, e_i, e_j)$. Then the case $n = 2$ of the above axiom gives $\alpha_{12} + \alpha_{21} = 2\pi$, and the case $n = 3$ gives $\alpha_{12} + \alpha_{23} + \alpha_{31} = 2\pi$. In combination, these equations give the following:

if e_1, e_2, e_3 *are edges occurring in that order cyclically about a vertex* v, *then*

$$\alpha_{13} = \alpha_{12} + \alpha_{23}.$$

Given an angle measure α we define the *curvature* $\kappa(p)$ of a closed path $p = e_1 \cdots e_n$ to be

$$\kappa(p) = (\pi - \alpha_{12}) + \cdots + (\pi - \alpha_{n-1,n}) + (\pi - \alpha_{n,1}).$$

In analogy with the Gauss-Bonnet formula we define the *area* of a subcomplex S bounded by a simple closed path p to be $A(S) = \kappa(p) - 2\pi$.

Proposition 7.5. *Let* S_1 *and* S_2 *be two subcomplexes, with simple boundaries, of a planar complex* K, *let* α *be an angle measure on* K, *and* A *the associated area measure. Suppose that* S_1 *and* S_2 *intersect only in a common boundary arc. Then* $A(S_1 \cup S_2) = A(S_1) + A(S_2)$.

□ Let the common boundary arc a of S_1 and S_2 run from vertices u_1 to u_2. Let the angles on the boundary of S_1 at these two points be α_1 and β_1 and those on S_2 be β_2 and α_2. Then $S = S_1 \cup S_2$ has boundary angles $\alpha_1 + \alpha_2$ at u_1 and $\beta_2 + \beta_1$ at u_2. If v is any interior point of a, where S_1 and S_2 have angles γ_1 and γ_2, then $\gamma_1 + \gamma_2 = 2\pi$, and hence $(\pi - \gamma_1) + (\pi - \gamma_2) = 0$. Thus $\kappa(\partial S)$ differs from the sum of $\kappa(\partial S_1)$ and $\kappa(\partial S_2)$ only in the addition of the difference $[(\pi - (\alpha_1 + \alpha_2)) + (\pi - (\beta_1 + \beta_2))] - [(\pi - \alpha_1) + (\pi - \beta_1) + (\pi - \alpha_2) + (\pi - \beta_2)] = -2\pi$; in short $\kappa(\partial S) = \kappa(\partial S_1) + \kappa(\partial S_2) - 2\pi$. From this it follows that $A(S) = A(S_1) + A(S_2)$. □

Corollary 7.6. *Let a subcomplex* S *of a planar complex* K *be the union of faces* $D_1, \ldots, D_n$, *such that each union* $D_1 \cup D_n \cup \cdots \cup D_i$, *for* $1 \leqslant i \leqslant n$, *is bounded by a simple closed curve, let* α *be an angle measure on* K, *and let* A *be the associated area measure. Then* $A(S) = A(D_1) + \cdots + A(D_n)$. □

Proposition 7.7. *If* K *is a Fuchsian complex for a group* G, *then there exists an angle measure* α *on* K *that is invariant under* G. □

□ Let $M = K/G$, a combinatorial 2-manifold. (Clearly passage to the quotient space is logically eliminable.) We know that G has a presentation $G = (X; R)$ with Cayley complex $C = C(X; R)$ dual to K, and with $R = \{r = s^{m(s)}: s \in S\}$, where S is a finite set of words in F, with basis X, strictly quadratic over X. The orbits of the set $\mathscr{D}$ of faces of C under action of G are of the form $\mathscr{D}_r$, for all r in R, where $\mathscr{D}_r$ consists of all faces bearing a boundary label r. In consequence the orbits of the set $\mathscr{V}$ of vertices of K are of the form $\mathscr{V}_r$, consisting of all vertices of K dual to a face D in $\mathscr{D}_r$. Thus there is one vertex v_r in M corresponding to each r in R. If D is a face of C with boundary label $r = s^{m(s)}$, then we know that, under the action of G on C, the stabilizer G_D of D is cyclic, generated by a conjugate of s, and has order $m(s)$. If v is the dual vertex in M, it follows that v is a branch point of multiplicity $m(s)$ in the projection $K \to M$. Therefore if we have a pseudo angle measure on M such that the angle sum at each vertex v_r is $2\pi/m(s)$, then lifting it to K will give a genuine invariant angle measure on K; clearly every invariant angle measure on K is thus obtainable. □

At each vertex v_r of M, where $r = s^{m(s)}$, there are $|s|$ (length of s) edges and therefore the same number of minimal angles, and the measures on these angles are subject only to the condition that their sum be $2\pi/m(s)$. Moreover, the conditions at different vertices of M are independent. Thus we see that at a vertex v_r the set of angle measures is naturally homeomorphic (under an obvious topology) to $\mathbb{R}^{|s|-1}$, and hence that the set of all angle measures on K is homeomorphic to $\mathbb{R}^{\Sigma_{s\in S}(|s|-1)}$.

We next show that *the area measure A associated with an invariant angle measure α is essentially independent of α*. This is an immediate consequence of the following.

Proposition 7.8. *Let G be an F-group with presentation $G = (X; R)$, where $R = \{s^{m(s)}: s \in S\}$, in the notation of III.4. Let K be a Fuchsian complex for G and Δ a face of K. If α is any invariant angle measure on K and κ is the associated curvature, then*

$$\kappa(\partial\Delta) = 2\pi\left(|X| - \textstyle\sum_{s\in S} \dfrac{m(s)}{1}\right).$$

□ It will suffice to establish the formula for the face $\Delta(1)$ of K dual to the vertex 1 of C. Now C and K have a common barycentric subdivision B, and the action of G extends in an obvious way to B. If a vertex g of C lies on the boundary of a face D of C, then there are exactly two triangles of B contained in D and incident with g; we call the union of these two triangles $\Delta(D, g)$. Evidently the face $\Delta(g)$ of K dual to g is the union of these $\Delta(D, g)$ for all faces D of C incident with g.

The two edges of the boundary of $\Delta(D, g)$ at the vertex $v = D_v$ dual to D are segments of adjacent edges of K at v; let $\alpha(D, g)$ be the angle from one to the other in the order such that $\Delta(D, g)$ lies, locally, in the sector between. Then, by the definition of an angle measure, the sum of the $\alpha(D, g)$ for fixed D and all g on the boundary of g must be 2π. We note also that, again by definition, the contribution at v to the curvature of $\partial\Delta(g)$ is $\pi - \alpha(D, g)$, whence $\kappa(\partial\Delta(g))$ is the sum of $\pi - \alpha(D, g)$, summed over all D incident with g.

We shall calculate $\kappa(\Delta(1))$. There is one face D at 1 for each conjugate of an element r of R. We consider a fixed $r = s^{m(s)}$ in R, and a face D at 1 with boundary label r, beginning at 1. The distinct conjugates r' of r have the form $r' = u^{-1}ru$, where u runs over the proper initial segments of s. The corresponding $\Delta(D', 1)$ are then congruent under G to subcomplexes $\Delta(D, u)$ of D. The totality of $\Delta(D, g)$ corresponds one-to-one to the proper initial segments $g = s^i u$ of r; here $0 \leqslant i < m(s)$ and the u are as before. It follows that, with summations over the indicated ranges,

$$\sum \alpha(D', 1) = \sum \alpha(D, u) = \frac{1}{m(s)} \sum \alpha(D, g) = \frac{2\pi}{m(s)}.$$

Since there are $|s|$ faces D', that is, whose boundary labels at 1 are conjugates of r, one has

$$\sum[\pi - \alpha(D', 1)] = \pi|s| - \frac{2\pi}{m(s)}.$$

To obtain $\kappa(\partial\Delta(1))$ we must sum $\pi - \alpha(D, 1)$ over all faces at 1, that is, we must sum the above formula over all r in R, or, what comes to the same, over all s in S. We obtain thus

$$\kappa(\partial\Delta(1)) = \pi \sum_{s \in S} |s| - 2\pi \sum_{s \in S} \frac{1}{m(s)}.$$

Now, since S is strictly quadratic over X, $\sum_{s \in S}|s| = 2|X|$ whence

$$\kappa(\partial\Delta(1)) = 2\pi\left(|X| - \sum_{s \in S} \frac{1}{m(s)}\right). \quad \square$$

The quantity $\mu = |X| - \sum_{s \in S}(1/m(s)) - 1$ is evidently an invariant of an F-group $G = (X; R)$ under transformations attached to the presentation, and is known as the *measure* $\mu(G)$ of G. We state the formula of Riemann and Hurwitz in terms of this measure.

Proposition 7.9. *If G is an F-group and G' a subgroup of finite index j in G, then G' is an F-group and*

$$j = \frac{\mu(G')}{\mu(G)}.$$

$\square$ By (7.4) we know that G' is an F-group, and further that if K is a Fuchsian complex for G, then G' possesses a Fuchsian complex K' each of whose face Δ' is the union, in the sense of (7.3), of j faces Δ of K. By (7.6) it follows that, for any invariant angle measure α on K and the induced measure on K', the associated area measures satisfy $A(\Delta') = jA(\Delta)$. Cancellation of factors 2π then gives the conclusion. $\square$

The Riemann-Hurwitz formula was first stated for discontinuous (Fuchsian) groups with compact fundamental domain, where $\mu(G)$ was the hyperbolic measure of any fundamental domain. However, the formula above holds equally in the case that both groups are free products of finitely many cyclic groups (provided the case $\mu = 0$ of a cyclic or infinite dihedral group is interpreted properly), despite the fact that in this situation μ does not admit the usual metric interpretation. This phenomenon was noted by Singerman (1970). For G a free product of cyclic groups of orders $m_1, \ldots, m_p$, we find that $\mu(G) = \sum(1 - 1/m_i) - 1$. The Riemann-Hurwitz formula was established by Nielsen (1948; see also Lyndon 1973) in the case that G is a free product of finitely many finite cyclic groups G_i and H the cartesian subgroup, that is, the kernel of the natural map of G onto the direct product of the G_i. Lyndon (1973) noted that Nielsen's argument applies if the G_i are arbitrary finite groups of orders m_i, and conjectured that the formula applied for any subgroup H of finite index in G. The truth of this conjecture had apparently long been known to P. Hall; see also Levi (1940), Kuhn (1952), and Stebe (1970). Chiswell (1973), using methods of Serre (1969), has established an index formula that contains this conjecture, the Riemann-Hurwitz formula, and presumably more.

For other generalizations of the measure function and related matters, see Brown (to appear), Chiswell (1973, 1976), Serre (1969/70; 1971), Verdier (1973), Wall (1961). For the related formula of Kneser, see Zieschang-Vogt-Coldewey (1969, p. 50). (See discussion in II.2.)

The Riemann-Hurwitz formula imposes restrictions on the types of subgroups H of finite index that can occur in a Fuchsian group G. There are also obvious conditions on the possible orders of periodic elements in any subgroup H of G. However the question of what types of subgroups H actually occur in G, and how many conjugacy classes of each type occur, appears difficult. This has been investigated by Greenberg (1963), Millington (1969), Singerman (1970, 1972), and Hoare (1974); for the classical problem were G is the modular group see Rankin (1969). The question of normal subgroups of G, and corresponding quotient groups, especially the finite quotient groups, has received much attention; see Singerman (1962), and Hoare-Singerman (1974). For the modular group, $G = (a^2, b^3)$, this is the question already mentioned of what groups are generated by an element a of order 2 together with an element b of order 3. The group $G = (a^2, b^3, (ab)^7)$, that is, $G = (2, 3, 7)$, has been noted since Hurwitz (1891) as the Fuchsian group with the smallest (positive) value of $\mu(G) = 1/42$. We have mentioned Higman's result that almost all alternating groups are quotient groups of this group; its finite quotient groups are discussed further by Macbeath (1961); see also Leech (1965).

Griffiths (1967) shows that every F-group G is residually finite. Sah (1969) shows this, and that, if G is infinite, there exists a torsion free normal subgroup N such that G/N is finite and solvable; he shows further that such N can be chosen so that the finite group G/N has any finite simple group as a composition factor. He also considers homomorphisms from a triangle group (l, m, n) into $\mathbb{PSL}(2, K)$ for K an algebraically closed field of characteristic $p > 0$, such that the image is finite and that the images of the generators retain the orders l, m, n; he shows that typically there exist many normal subgroups N such that $G/N \simeq \mathbb{PSL}(2, p^f)$ for some f.

The following shows that, with finitely many exceptions, the abelian subgroups of planar groups are cyclic.

Proposition 7.10. *Every abelian subgroup of a planar group is either cyclic or free abelian of rank 2. The planar groups containing a free abelian subgroup of rank 2 are the following (for brevity, we list only the defining relators of the presentation):*

(1) $([y_1, y_2])$;
(2) $(y_1^2 y_2^2)$;
(3) $(x_1^2, x_2^2, x_1 x_2 y^2)$;
(4) $(x_1^2, x_2^2, x_3^2, x_4^2, x_1 x_2 x_3 x_4)$;
(5) $(x_1^2, x_2^3, x_3^6, x_1 x_2 x_3)$;
(6) $(x_1^2, x_2^4, x_3^4, x_1 x_2 x_3)$;
(7) $(x_1^3, x_2^3, x_3^3, x_1 x_2 x_3)$.

□ Let G be a planar group and H an abelian subgroup of G. If H is a free product of cyclic groups then, since H is abelian, H must be a cyclic group. Otherwise H is an F-group, of finite index in G. If $p > 0$, and x_1 has order m_1, we have seen that the cyclic group generated by x_1 is self-normalizing, whence it is all of H and H is again cyclic. It remains to study the case that $p = 0$, where H has a single defining relator q. If $q = [y_1, y_2]$, then H is free abelian of rank 2. If $q = y_1^2$, then H is cyclic of order 2. For any other non-trivial q, H cannot be abelian (by the Freiheitssatz (see IV), or because H is non-trivially a free product with amalgamation). We have shown that H is either cyclic or free abelian of rank 2.

We now examine which F-groups G can contain a free abelian subgroup H of rank 2. We have seen that G must be a planar F-group, and that H must have finite index in G. But calculation shows that H has measure $\mu(H) = 0$. It follows by the Riemann-Hurwitz formula that $\mu(G) = 0$ (in other terms, G must be a Euclidean group). Now $\mu(G) = 0$ implies $n \leqslant 2$. If $n = 2$ it requires that $p = 0$, so that we have case (1) or (2) of the proposition. In case (1), G itself is free abelian of rank 2. In case (2), the Cayley complex C is combinatorially a regular tessellation of the Euclidean plane by squares, and one can easily read off a pair of elements that (under left multiplication) effect orthogonal translations of C; alternatively one can appeal to the fact known on topological grounds (or by the Reidemeister-Schreier theorem; see Zieschang-Vogt-Coldewey (1970, p. 21) that the group (2) contains a group (1), indeed of index 2.

If $n = 1$, the condition $\mu(G) = 0$ implies that $p = 2$ and $m_1 = m_2 = 2$, whence we have case (3). If we now form the modified Cayley diagram (see III.4 above) with respect to the involutions x_1 and x_2, it is again a combinatorially regular tessellation of the plane by squares, and we can find H as before.

If $n = 0$, inspection shows that the condition $\mu(G) = 0$ is satisfied only in cases (4) through (7). For each of these we introduce a more economical presentation of the form

$$G = (x_1, \ldots, x_{p-1} : x_1^{m_1}, \ldots, x_{p-1}^{m_{p-1}}, (x_1 \cdots x_{p-1})^{m_p}).$$

For (4), modifying the Cayley diagram with respect to the involution x_1 yields a combinatorially regular tessellation of the Euclidean plane by hexagons, from which we can again read off two independent translations. The modified Cayley diagram C for (5) has each vertex of degree 3, while the faces are of two kinds: triangles with boundary label x_2^3, and 12-gons with boundary edges labeled alternately with x_1 and x_2. We extend Cayley's device by forming a new graph C', upon which G acts, by shrinking each of the triangular faces to a point; then C' is a regular tessellation of the plane by hexagons. A pair of elements effecting independent translations on C' are now easily found, and generate a free abelian subgroup of rank 2 in G.

The treatment of (6) is entirely analogous. In the modified Cayley diagram C we shrink each rectangular face with label x_2^4 to a point; the resulting graph C' is again a regular tessellation of the plane by squares. For (7), in the ordinary Cayley diagram, shrinking to a point each face with label x_2^3 yields a regular tessellation of the plane by triangles. □

We remark that methods similar to those used above can be used to show in simple cases that certain F-groups are infinite, for example the groups $G = (x_1^2, x_2^3, x_3^n, x_1x_2x_3)$ for $n \geqslant 6$ (see Lyndon (1974)).

We note that (7.10) implies that in every Fuchsian group (F-group with $\mu(G) > 0$), all centralizers are cyclic.

A celebrated theorem, conjectured by Fenchel (see Bungaard and Nielsen, 1951) and proved by Fox (1952; see also Mennicke 1968, and Feuer, 1971) asserts that every F-group contains a torsion free subgroup of finite index. Fox's proof relies on a detailed study of finite permutation groups. We do not know any proof entirely within the spirit of the present development; we present one that relies on the representation of such groups by matrices, but is otherwise in keeping with ideas that will be discussed later. This proof is essentially one we learned from Zieschang, and appears to have originated with Macbeath. We note that a related argument due to Selberg (1960) shows that in a finite extension of a torsion free F-group G the elements of infinite order are conjugacy separable in the sense that if two such elements are not conjugate in G, then there is a finite quotient group of G in which their images are not conjugate; Stebe (1972) establishes the latter result for all F-groups. In the present connection see also McCool (1969) and McCool and Schupp (1973).

For this proof we must make use of the classical fact, which lies beyond our present methods, that every infinite F-group is isomorphic to a finitely generated subgroup of the linear fractional group $\mathbb{PSL}(2, \mathbb{R})$.

To anticipate a concept that will be discussed more fully below (IV.4), we define a group G to be *residually finite* if for every non-trivial element g of G there is a homomorphism ϕ from G onto a finite group H such that $g\phi \neq 1$. Observe that in this case if $g_1, \ldots, g_n$ are finitely many non-trivial elements of G, and $\phi_1, \ldots, \phi_n$ homomorphisms from G onto finite groups $H_1, \ldots, H_n$ such that $g_1\phi_1, \ldots, g_n\phi_n \neq 1$, then the ϕ_i induce a homomorphism ϕ from G onto a (finite) subgroup H of the direct product $H_1 \times \cdots \times H_n$ such that $g_1\phi, \ldots, g_n\phi \neq 1$.

The central argument can be stated in more general form.

Proposition 7.11. *Every finitely generated subgroup of* $\mathbb{SL}(n, F)$*, for any* $n \geqslant 1$ *and any field* F*, is residually finite.*

□ Let G be a finitely generated subgroup of $\mathbb{SL}(n, F)$, with generators $a_1, \ldots, a_m$. Each a_h may be represented as a matrix $a_h = (\alpha_h(i, j))$ with entries in F. If P is the prime field for F, we may, without loss of generality, suppose F the extension of P generated by the finite set S of elements $\alpha = \alpha_h(i, j)$. A certain subset S_0 of S will be a base for a purely transcendental extension P_0 of P, and the remaining set S_1 will generate F as an algebraic extension of P_0. One can obtain a finite set of rational functions f in the elements of S over P such that every algebraic relation among the elements of S over P follows from the true equations $f_\nu = 0$ (for example, taking minimal polynomials of successive extensions); clearing of fractions one obtains a set of polynomials p_ν in the elements α of S with integer coefficients such that every relation among the α follows from the true equations $p_\nu = 0$ together with the equation $p = 0$ where p is the characteristic of P. In particular, every relation among the generators a_h of G will follow from these equations.

Let R be the ring generated over $\mathbb{Z}_p$ ($p \geqslant 0$) by the elements $\alpha \in S$, and let ϕ be any homomorphism from R onto a field K. Then ϕ induces a homomorphism ϕ^* from G onto a group $G\phi^*$ of matrices over K; in particular, if K is finite then $G\phi^*$ is finite.

Let g be any non trivial element of G, with matrix form $g = (\gamma(i, j))$, and let H be the matrix $g - I$; then some entry $\eta(i, j)$ of H is non zero. Now $\eta(i, j)$ is expressible as a non-zero polynomial h in the α, with integer coefficients, and we may suppose that no coefficient of h is divisible by p. In any case we may find a rational prime q that does not divide all the coefficients of h, and a prime ideal $\tilde{\mathfrak{p}}$ in the ring R that contains q. Let K be the field $R/\tilde{\mathfrak{p}}$; as a finite extension of $\mathbb{Z}_q$, K is finite. Let ϕ be the natural projection from R onto K. By the choice of q and $\tilde{\mathfrak{p}}$, $h\phi \neq 0$, whence $H\phi$ is not the zero matrix over K, and so $g\phi$ not the identity matrix over K. Thus, under the homomorphism ϕ^* from G onto the finite group $G\phi^*$, the element g is not mapped onto the trivial element. □

Proposition 7.12. *Every F-group contains a torsion free subgroup of finite index.*

□ If the F-group G is finite the assertion is trivial. Thus we may suppose that G is strictly planar, and, by the unproved remark made earlier, is isomorphic to a finitely generated subgroup of $\mathbb{PSL}(2, \mathbb{R})$, and indeed the quotient group of a subgroup $\tilde{G}$ of $\mathbb{SL}(2, \mathbb{R})$ by the group $\{1, -1\}$. By (7.10) $\tilde{G}$ is residually finite, whence it follows easily that G is residually finite. For G in its canonical presentation, let A be the finite set of all non-trivial powers of $x_1, \ldots, x_p$. Then there is a homomorphism ϕ from G onto a finite group H such that $a\phi \neq 1$ for all a in A. Let N be the kernel of ϕ. Then N has finite index in G, and contains no a from A. But we have seen (7.4) that every non-trivial element of finite order in G is conjugate to some a in A. It follows that N contains no non-trivial element of finite order. □

We may always take N to be a surface group, that is, the fundamental group of a closed 2-manifold, and thus (see Zieschang-Vogt-Coldewey), of a closed orientable 2-manifold. It is then clear that the number n for G must coincide with the number $n' = 2g$ for N. The question, given G and finite Γ, of the number of maps of G onto Γ with kernel isomorphic to N, has been examined by Lloyd (1972).

We have seen that every subgroup of finite index in an F-group is itself an F-group. One may, dually, enquire what groups contain F-groups as subgroups of finite index. Obvious examples show that one must impose some further limitations if one wants to avoid trivialities. It has been conjectured that if a group G contains a torsion free F-group (a 'surface group') of finite index, and if G itself is torsion free, then G also is an F-group. An argument of Zieschang (1971) to establish this was unfortunately vitiated by dependence upon an assertion of Kravetz (1959) for which no proof is known. However, this gap has been corrected in Zieschang (1974).

The following is a small generalization of a minor result from the paper of Zieschang.

Proposition 7.13. *If a torsion free group contains a central free abelian group of finite index then it is itself free abelian.*

□ Assume G is torsion free and that A is a central free abelian subgroup of finite index. Let A be embedded in a direct sum $\bar{A}$ of copies of the additive group of the rationals. Let $\bar{G}$ be the direct sum of G and $\bar{A}$ with the common subgroup A amalgamated. Then $\bar{A}$ is normal in $\bar{G}$ and $\bar{G}/\bar{A} \simeq G/A = H$, finite. Since $\bar{G}$ is a central extension of the divisible group $\bar{A}$ by the finite group H, the extension splits, and $\bar{G}$ is isomorphic to the direct sum of $\bar{A}$ and H; let α and β be the induced projections of $\bar{G}$ onto $\bar{A}$ and onto H with α the identity on $\bar{A}$. If g is in G and $g\alpha = 1$, then $\text{Gp}(g)\alpha = 1$ whence β maps $\text{Gp}(g)$ isomorphically into H; since H is finite and G is torsion free, this implies that $g = 1$. Thus α maps G isomorphically into $\bar{A}$, and α is the identity on A. If g is in G but not in A, then some g^n is in A, whence $(g\alpha)^n \in A$. Thus $G\alpha$ is generated by a finite set of such roots $g\alpha$ of elements in A, and so is free abelian. □

We make a few further remarks concerning those F-groups that are fundamental groups of 2-manifolds, that is, those of form (5.3) with $p = 0$; hence with presentation $G = (q)$. The automorphism groups of these groups have received much attention. By a basic result of Nielsen (1927; for this and the following see Magnus-Karrass-Solitar and Zieschang-Vogt-Coldewey), if $G = \pi(M)$, the fundamental group of a closed 2-manifold M, then the outer automorphism group of G, $\text{Out}G = \text{Aut}(G)/JA(G)$, where $JA(G)$ is the inner automorphism group of G, is isomorphic to the group $A(M)$ of all autohomeomorphisms of M modulo, the group of all isotopies (the component of 1 in $A(M)$). A second result of Nielsen (1927); see also Zieschang (1970), and Peczynski (1972)) establishes that every automorphism of $G = (q)$ is induced by an automorphism of F. It follows that $\text{Out}(G)$ is isomorphic to the stabilizer of N in $\text{Aut}(F)$, and by (II.5.8) to the subgroup $A\{(q), (q^{-1})\}$ stabilizing the set of cyclic words $\{(q), (q^{-1})\}$ in $\text{Out}(F)$. From Nielsen's work, or by (I.5.1), generators for $\text{Out}(G)$ (and so for $\text{Aut}(G)$) can be obtained. A concise set of generators with a simple topological meaning was obtained by Lickorish (1963, 1964), but we do not know any non topological proof of his result. As noted earlier (I.5.5), finite presentations for these groups Out G can be derived from a result of McCool. See also Birman (1969, 1970) and Birman-Hilden (1971). We note that Nielsen (1943) showed that every finite cyclic group in $\text{Out}(G)$ is the natural isomorphic image of one in $\text{Aut}(G)$; Kravetz (1959) attempted to prove that, in analogy with (I.4.14), every finite subgroup of Out(G) is the natural isomorphic image of one in Aut(G), but his argument is incomplete; see Zieschang (1974).

The rank (minimum cardinal of a set of generators) for an F-group G has been determined. First, if G is not finitely generated or is free, the answer is obvious. Next, if $p = 0$, whence $G = (X; q)$, then rank $G = |X|$. If $G = (s_1, \ldots, s_p, X; s_1^{m_1}, \ldots, s_p^{m_p}, s_1 \cdots s_p q)$, $q \neq 1$, then rank $G = |X| + p - 1$. If $G = (s_1, \ldots, s_p; s_1^{m_1} \cdots s_1^{m_1}, s_1 \cdots s_p)$, $p \geqslant 3$, then, with the exceptions noted below, rank $G = m - 1$. The above results are due to Zieschang (1970), who, however, overlooked the exceptional cases. Burns, Karrass, Pietrowski, and Purzitsky (unpublished) observed that the following cases are irregular. For G in the last mentioned form, if m is even and $m_1 = \cdots = m_{p-1} = 2$ while m_p is odd, then rank $G = p - 2$. A definitive treatment of these results (correcting certain errors in Zieschang (1970)) is given by Peczynski, Rosenberger, and Zieschang (1975).

The F-groups $G = (y_1, \ldots, y_n; q)$, as in (5.3) are the fundamental groups of the closed 2-manifolds. In analogy with (strictly) quadratic sets of words, Neuwirth (1969) calls a set S of words in F *n-ic* if each generator x from X occurs exactly n times in the elements of the set S. He shows that if G is the fundamental group of a closed n-manifold, then for some free group F_1, the free product $G * F_1$ has a presentation $(X; R)$ with R *n-ic*. Hoare (unpublished) has shown that for $n = 3$, G itself has such a presentation. Markov (1958; see Massey 1967, p. 143) has shown that every finitely presented group is the fundamental group of some closed n-manifold for each $n \geqslant 4$. Although considerable is known, there is no complete description of a set of presentations yielding precisely the fundamental groups of 3-manifolds; for these matters we refer to Stallings (1972).

We mention only two special results. First, Scott (1973) has shown that every finitely generated subgroup of a fundamental group of a 3-manifold has a finite presentation. Second, it is known that every closed 3-manifold M has a decomposition with a single 0-cell, a single 3-cell, and the same number of 1-cells and 2-cells. Since the fundamental group G of M is the same as that of its 2-skeleton, we conclude that G has a balanced presentation $G = (X; R)$, with $|X| = |R|$. Neuwirth (1968) has given a purely group theoretic procedure for deciding what, if any, manifolds are associated thus with a given balanced presentation. (We have noted earlier that the number L of components of the star graph enters essentially into his arguments.) For certain small presentations this algorithm has been simplified and applied by Stevens (to appear) and Osborne and Stevens (to appear).

For the cohomology of F-groups see Curran (1973).

8. Planar Groups with Reflections

We examine now a class of groups first studied by Wilkie (1966), and called by him (2-dimensional hyperbolic) *non-Euclidean crystallographic groups*, or *NEC groups*. These are discontinuous groups that differ from Fuchsian groups only in that they are permitted to contain reflections, or, analytically, transformations of the upper half plane of the form

$$z \mapsto \frac{a\bar{z} + b}{c\bar{z} + d}$$

for a, b, c, d real, $ad - bc = -1$, where $\bar{z}$ is the complex conjugate of z.

We limit ourselves to obtaining a class of presentations that includes all NEC groups and only such groups. For this see also Zieschang (1966) and Zieschang-Vogt-Coldewey. For the classification of NEC groups see Macbeath (1967), Tukia (1972), and Keller (1973). For a subgroup theorem and index theorem see Hoare-Karrass-Solitar (1974). For torsion in these groups see Zieschang-Vogt-Coldewey.

It should be remarked that we have already admitted to the class of F-groups elements that reverse orientation of their Cayley complex or Fuchsian complex; but, as we shall see, the groups now under consideration form a broader class. Quite simply, they are the discontinuous groups of isometries of the hyperbolic plane. For the purposes of our combinatorial approach, we define an *NEC group* to be a group G that acts on a 2-complex K, combinatorially a (hyperbolic) plane, and regularly on the faces of K. We emphasize that we have now dropped the earlier requirement that no non-trivial element of G leave an edge invariant.

We shall call an element of G *even* if it preserves orientation of K, and otherwise *odd*. Consider now a non-trivial element of G that fixes an edge e of K. It must in any case interchange the two faces of K separated by e, and hence must be an involution. If it interchanges the two end points of e, it is easy to see that it is even. In this case we may modify K by introducing a new vertex v, dividing e into two parts, and stipulating that g fix v while exchanging (with the obvious effect on orientation) the two parts of e. For each g, this can be done uniformly; moreover it can be done simultaneously for all g of the sort under consideration. Quite analogously to an assumption that we imposed on Fuchsian complexes for F-groups, we may thus assume, without loss of generality, that if an element of G leaves an edge invariant, then it fixes both its end points.

A non-trivial element of G, necessarily an involution, that leaves invariant an edge of K, will be called a *reflection* in this edge. If we now attempt to construct from the Fuchsian complex K a dual Cayley complex C, all goes well, as before, except that we find in the case of a reflection x, that there is at each vertex only a single edge e^* of C, claiming as label both x and x^{-1}. This situation was anticipated in the definition of a modified Cayley complex, where we admitted to F a set J of involutions. Thus we have a modified presentation $G = (X, J; R)$ with $C = C(X, J; R)$ dual to K, where J is the preimage in F of the set of reflections among the generators for G.

Our goal in this section is to use the ideas above to obtain something approaching a canonical form for the presentation $G = (X, J; R)$ for an NEC group. The arguments parallel those borrowed from Nielsen, Hoare-Karrass-Solitar, and Zieschang-Vogt-Coldewey in our discussion of F-groups. The result, (8.1), we obtain, although not new, is not perspicuous, and we prefer to postpone the statement of it until we have carried through an argument that should make it appear not only true but natural.

We suppose then that G is an NEC group with Fuchsian complex K and with modified presentation $G = (X, J; R)$ whose Cayley complex is dual to K. We shall give no further consideration to K, but shall modify the presentation, without changing J, to reduce it to a partially canonical form.

We repeat that at each vertex of the (modified) Cayley diagram C, there will emanate exactly one edge bearing each label from the set $L = X \cup X^{-1} \cup J$. At each vertex g, let $R(g)$ be the cyclically ordered set (in the positive sense) of positive boundary labels on the faces at g, starting at g. In particular, there will be exactly one element of $R(g)$ beginning with each element of L. Let $S(g)$ be the set of roots of the elements of $R(g)$. We note that if h is even, then $R(gh) = R(g)$, while if h is odd, $R(gh) = R(g)^{-1}$ (with inverted order). In particular, if pq is in $R(g)$ and p is even, then qp is in $R(gp) = R(g)$, while if p is odd $(qp)^{-1}$ is in $R(g)$.

Let $S = S(1)$. Then for each $x \in J$ there is exactly one element $t_x = xu$ of S beginning with x. Since x is odd, $(ux)^{-1} = xu^{-1} \in S$, whence $xu = xu^{-1}$, $u = u^{-1}$, and the involution u has the form $u = aya^{-1}$ for some $y \in J$. Thus

$$t_x = xaya^{-1} \text{ for some } y \in J \text{ and some } a.$$

Similarly, S contains exactly one element t'_x ending in x, and

$$t'_x = bzb^{-1}x \text{ for some } z \in J \text{ and some } b.$$

Note that both t_x and t'_x are conjugate to their own inverses. We now show that each t in S containing x is conjugate to t_x or to t'_x. If t in S contains x, we may write $t = uxv$. If u is even, then $xvu \in S$, whence $xvu = t_x$. If u is odd, then $(xvu)^{-1} = u^{-1}v^{-1}x \in S$, whence $u^{-1}v^{-1}x = t'_x$, t is conjugate to $xvu = t'^{-1}_x$, and, since t'^{-1}_x is conjugate to t'_x, t is conjugate to t'_x.

Suppose now that x occurs twice in t_x, thus t_x has the form $t_x = xuxv$ for some u and v. If xu is even, then $xvxu \in S$, whence $xvxu = t_x$; but $xuxv = xvxu$ implies that xu and xv are both powers of a common element w, whence t_x is a proper power of w, contrary to the fact that t_x is a root. Therefore xu is odd and $(xvxu)^{-1} = u^{-1}xv^{-1}x$ S, whence $u^{-1}xv^{-1}x = t'_x$, t_x^{-1} is conjugate to t'_x and hence t_x is conjugate to t'_x. In fact, we have seen that the cyclic permutation $xvxu$ of t_x is t'^{-1}_x. Since distinct cyclic permutations of the root t_x are distinct, t_x has the form $xuxv$ for unique u, which implies that t_x contains x only twice. Further, t_x has the form $t_x = xaya^{-1}$ and x cannot occur in a, else it would occur also in a^{-1} and so occur in t_x more than twice. It follows that $x = y$ and that $t_x = xaxa^{-1}$ and $t'_x = a^{-1}xax$.

We show that, in $t_x = xaya^{-1}$, a contains no letter $z \in J$. If z occurred in a, it would occur also in a^{-1}, whence $z \neq x, y$. Moreover, t_x would be conjugate to $t_z = zczc^{-1}$; since t_z contains x it must contain it twice, whence $y = x$ and $t_x = xaxa^{-1}$. Now a must have the form uzv and so $t_x = xuzvxv^{-1}zu^{-1}$. If xu is even, then $zvxv^{-1}zu^{-1}xu$ is in S, and is therefore t_z, which implies that $u^{-1}xu = (vxv^{-1})^{-1} = vxv^{-1}$ and $t'_z = (zvxv^{-1})^2$, impossible since t_z is a root. If xu is odd, we find similarly that $t_z = (vxv^{-1}z)^2$, again impossible.

We construct a graph Γ with J as vertex set and an undirected edge between elements x and y for each element $t_x = xaya^{-1}$. From what we have seen, if $t_x = xaxa^{-1}$, then there is a component of Γ consisting of a cycle of length 1 with sole vertex x. For each other x we have $t_x = xaya^{-1}$, and $t'_x = bzb^{-1}x$ conjugate to $t_z = zb^{-1}xb$, hence exactly two edges at x. It follows that Γ falls into cycles $\Gamma_j, j = 1, \ldots, m$.

With a cycle $\Gamma_j = (x_{j1}, \ldots, x_{jn_j})$ of length $n_j \geqslant 1$ we take T_j to consist of the set of all $t_{jh} = t_{x_{jh}}$, subscripts h being taken cyclically modulo n_j. Clearly the union T^* of the T_j comprises all the t_x; from what has been seen, every element of T is conjugate to some element of T^*.

We have established all but the last assertion of the following.

Proposition 8.1. *Let G be an NEC group. Then G has a presentation $G = (X \cup J; R_0 \cup R_1 \cup R_2)$ of the following form. J is the disjoint union of ordered sets $J_j = (x_{j1}, \ldots, x_{jn_j})$, $n_j \geqslant 1$. R_0 consists of all x_{jh}^2 for $x_{jh} \in J$. R_1 is the union of sets*

$$R_{1j} = (t_{j1}^{m_{j1}}, \ldots, t_{jn_j}^{m_{jn_j}}).$$

Here the m_{jh} are positive integers and $t_{jh} = x_{jh}a_{jh}x_{j,h+1}a_{jh}^{-1}$ (index h cyclically modulo n_j) where the a_{jh} are words containing only generators from X. R_2 is a set of words of the form $r_k = s_k^{m_k}$ where the m_k are positive integers and the s_k are words containing only letters from X. Finally, in the set of all a_{jh} together with all s_k, each generator from X occurs exactly twice.

□ It remains only to prove the last assertion. We know that for each z in X there is one element of $R(1)$ beginning with z and one beginning with z^{-1}. These give rise to distinct occurrences of z in the defining relators, whence it follows that z must occur at least twice. Conversely, an occurrence of z in an element of $R_1 \cup R_2$ gives rise to an element of $R(1)$ beginning with z or z^{-1}, distinct occurrences in R_1 give rise to distinct elements of $R(1)$, and occurrences in distinct relators give rise to distinct elements of $R(1)$. What remains to be shown is that an occurrence of z in some a_{jh}, which provides two occurrences in t_{jh}, gives rise to only a single element of $R(1)$ beginning with z or z^{-1}. Simplifying notation, let $t_{jh} = t = xaya^{-1}$ where $a = uzv$; thus $t = xuzvyv^{-1}z^{-1}u^{-1}$. Since x and y are odd and all other factors even, the cyclic permutation obtained by removing the initial segment xu to the end of t will not belong to $R(1)$; but rather its inverse, which ends in z^{-1}. However, moving the segment xuz to the end gives us an element $(vxv^{-1}z^{-1}u^{-1}xuz)^{-1} = z^{-1}u^{-1}xuzvxv^{-1}$ of $R(1)$. The other possibility of obtaining an element of $R(1)$ beginning with z or z^{-1} is by moving to the end an even segment, containing both letters x; for this we must move the segment $xuzvxv^{-1}$ to the end. But this gives us the same element of $R(1)$ as before. This shows that a given occurrence of z (or similarly z^{-1}) in some a_{jh} gives rise to only a single element of $R(1)$ beginning with z or z^{-1}, thereby completing the proof. □

9. Singular Subcomplexes

We define a *singular subcomplex* S of a 2-complex C to consist of a pair (S, f) where S is a 2-complex and f a map from S into C that preserves dimension and incidence.

We shall be concerned solely with singular subcomplexes of the Cayley complex $C = C(X; R)$ of a group G with presentation $G = (X; R)$. It seems on the whole more natural to work with the Cayley complex C, although there are points where it would be more advantageous to work with the quotient complex $K = K(X; R)$ (see 4.3). In any case, in view of the natural map from C onto K, every singular subcomplex of C can be viewed naturally as a singular subcomplex of K. If S is a singular subcomplex of C, as above, then the labels on C induce labels on S. For a singular subcomplex equipped with this induced labelling we shall often use the word *diagram*, referring to S with the induced labelling on its edges as a diagram over the presentation $(X; R)$. Note that a connected diagram S more or less uniquely determines the map f from S into C: given vertices v in S and v' in C, there is exactly one map f from S into C that preserves labels and carries v into v'.

We shall be concerned for the present with only two basic types of singular complexes S. The first is that S is a connected and simply connected proper subcomplex of a combinatorial sphere, which we shall call a *simple diagram* or *singular disc*; the second is that S is a full combinatorial sphere, which we shall call a *spherical diagram* or *singular sphere*. We shall also be concerned incidentally with diagrams S that are disjoint unions of finitely many subdiagrams S_i of these two types. If S_i is spherical, then its boundary ∂S_i is empty. If S_i is a non-empty singular disc, then ∂S_i is not empty, and, starting at any directed edge e_1 on ∂S_i, there is a unique directed edge e_2 on ∂S_i, beginning at the vertex v where e_1 ends, and such that there is no element of S_i incident with v and lying to the right of the segment e_1e_2. Proceeding thus we obtain a cycle of edges $e_1, \ldots, e_n$ on the boundary of S_i, each related to the preceding as indicated (in cyclic order), and exhausting ∂S_i. The loop $p = e_1 \cdots e_n$, which is not necessarily a simple loop, will then be called a *boundary path* or *boundary cycle* for S_i, and the label on p will be called a *boundary label*.

We have seen (4.2) that the Cayley complex $C = C(X; R)$ for a presentation $G = (X; R)$ is simply connected; but it is not true that every closed path in C bounds a singular combinatorial disc (S, f) in our present sense, since one cannot require f to preserve dimension. To remedy this we have, above, replaced the concept of a singular combinatorial disc by that of a simple diagram. In (9.2) below, we shall see that every closed path in C is the image of ∂S under a map of some simple diagram S into C. An example of this construction is given in (V.I).

We begin by describing certain modifications of a diagram or singular subcomplex S, in the sense above, in the case that some boundary label is not a reduced word. Suppose some component S_i of S has boundary path $p = e_1 \cdots e_n$ such that the corresponding boundary label is not reduced. Then two successive edges e_i and e_{i+1} will have opposite labels, and will therefore map into opposite edges in C. If e_i and e_{i+1} are opposite edges in S_i, then they constitute a spine on the boundary of S_i; deletion of these two edges and the vertex where e_i ends and e_{i+1} begins then yields a diagram S_i' with boundary path $p' = e_1 \cdots e_{i-1}e_{i+2} \cdots e_n$ that cannot be trivial; in fact S_i' is obtained from S_i by deleting a spine. If e_i and e_{i+1} are not opposite edges in S_i, and if e_ie_{i+1} is not a loop, then we can identify e_i and e_{i+1}^{-1} to obtain a new diagram S_i' with non-trivial boundary path p' as before. If $p = e_ie_{i+1}$ is a loop, bounding S_i, we again identify e_i and e_{i+1}^{-1}, but now obtain a spherical diagram S_i' with empty boundary. We call all of these operations *sewing up* the boundary of S.

There remains the possibility that $e_i e_{i+1}$ is a loop, but bounds only a part T of S_i. In this case T and the complement U of T in S_i have only a vertex v in common. We first separate them, that is, replace U and T by isomorphic complexes S_i' and T' that are disjoint; finally T' will have boundary path an isomorphic replica of the loop $e_i e_{i+1}$, and we sew up this loop as before, thus replacing T' by a spherical diagram S_i''. We refer to the operation of replacing S_i by two components S_i' and S_i'' as *detachment*, followed by sewing up.

Proposition 9.1. *If S is a singular subcomplex (in the sense above), then by successive detachment and sewing up we can obtain a singular subcomplex S' each of whose components $S_1, \ldots, S_n$ either is a singular disc with boundary label reduced (at whatever point one starts, that is, cyclically reduced) or is a singular sphere.*

□ This follows by induction on the total length of the boundary of S, using the definition of sewing up and detachment. □

An important consequence of the preceding is the following theorem of van Kampen (1933).

Proposition 9.2. *Let $G = (X; R)$ with w a reduced word representing an element of the normal closure N of R in F. Then there is a simple diagram S^* over the Cayley diagram $C = C(X; R)$ such that the boundary label on S^*, beginning at a vertex v, is w.*

□ We note that the case $w = 1$ is not excluded; in this case the argument to be given yields for S^* the trivial diagram consisting of the single point v. To exclude discussion of degenerate cases we now assume that $w \neq 1$ in the free group F. Since w is in N, w is the reduced form of an unreduced word w' of the form $w' = p_1 r_1 p_1^{-1} \cdots p_n r_n p_n^{-1}$ where each $r_i \in R \cup R^{-1}$. For each $w_i = p_i r_i p_i^{-1}$ we construct a diagram S_i consisting of a path p_i with label p_i beginning at a vertex v_i and running to a point v_i', followed by a loop at v_i' with label r_i, and by a path p_i^{-1} returning to v_i. Thus S_i is a diagram with boundary label w_i. If we choose a vertex $\bar{v}$ in C and demand that $v_i f_i = \bar{v}$, then a singular diagram (S_i, f_i) is unambiguously determined. Let S be the union of the S_i, with the vertices v_i identified, and otherwise disjoint; let f be the union of the f_i. Clearly S is a simple diagram. We now apply sewing up and detachment to S. At each stage we obtain a diagram with components $S_0, \ldots, S_K$ where S_0 has boundary label w_0 representing the same element of N as w, and the remaining S_i are spherical diagrams without boundary. By induction on the length of w_0, we arrive ultimately at the situation that w_0 is completely reduced, thus $w_0 = w$. Then $S_0 = S^*$, with the required properties. □

The consequences of this theorem of van Kampen will be developed extensively in Chapter V. We digress now only to give two illustrative examples that require no more machinery than is available at this point. The first, for which a different proof was offered by Lyndon (1962), is of some minor interest in its analogy with a result of Craig (1957) in mathematical logic.

Proposition 9.3. *Let F be a free group with basis X, let $Y, Z \subseteq X$, and $P \subseteq$ Gp(Y),*

$Q \subseteq \mathrm{Gp}(Z)$. *If* $Q \subseteq Ncl_F(P)$, *then there exists* $M \subseteq \mathrm{Gp}(Y \cap Z)$ *such that* $M \subseteq Ncl_F(P)$ *and* $Q \subseteq Ncl_F(M)$.

□ Without loss of generality we may suppose that $X = Y \cup Z$ and that Q consists of a single element q, non-trivial, cyclically reduced, and that P is finite and cyclically reduced. Then in the presentation $G = (X; P)$, the element q belongs to the normal closure N of P in F, the free group with basis X. By (9.2) there exists a simple diagram S over $(X; P)$ with boundary label q. Let S' be the result of deleting all interior edges of S. Then each face D' of S' is a union of faces D of S and since these faces D have boundary labels from $P \subseteq \mathrm{Gp}(Y)$, all the edges on the boundary of each face D' of S' lie in $Y \cup Y^{-1}$. On the other hand, the boundary of each face D' of S' is part of the boundary of S, hence has labels contained in q, and thus belonging to $Z \cup Z^{-1}$. Thus each face D' of S' has boundary label in $\mathrm{Gp}(Y \cap Z)$. If we take M to be the set of boundary labels on the faces D' of S', then the relation between S and S' implies that the conditions of the proposition are met. □

As a second consequence of the theorem (9.2.) of van Kampen we give a proof of the Freiheitssatz of Dehn and Magnus (see II.5.1). The present proof is a revision of one due to Lyndon (1972); a very similar argument was given by Weinbaum (1972).

Proposition 9.4. *Let r be a cyclically reduced element of a free group F with basis X, and let w be any nontrivial element in the normal closure of r in F. Then every $x \in X$ that occurs in r occurs also in w.*

Both Magnus' original proof and that to be given here proceed by induction, and, although the two inductions are different, they both establish a more general form of the Freiheitssatz. To state this, we define a presentation $G = (X; R)$ to be *staggered* if both R and a subset $X_0 \leqslant X$ are linearly ordered in such a way that

(1) each r in R is cyclically reduced and contains some $x \in X_0$;

(2) if r and r' are in R and $r < r'$, then r contains some $x \in X_0$ that precedes all $x \in X_0$ that occur in r', and r' contains some $x \in X_0$ that comes after all those in r.

Proposition 9.5. *Let $G = (X; R)$ be a staggered presentation, and let w lie in the normal closure of R in F. If $w \neq 1$, then w contains some $x \in X_0$. Let $w \neq 1$, let x_a be the least $x \in X_0$ in w, and let x_b be the greatest. Then w lies in the normal closure of R_0 in F, where R_0 consists of those $r \in R$ that contain $x \in X_0$ only for $x_a \leqslant x \leqslant x_b$.*

Proof of (9.4). To deduce (9.4) from (9.5) let $x \in X$ occur in r, and apply (9.5.) with $R = \{r\}$, $X_0 = \{x\}$. □

Proof of (9.5). In view of van Kampen's theorem (9.2), the preceding proposition is equivalent to the following. □

Proposition 9.6. *Let $G = (X; R)$ be a staggered presentation, and Δ a non-trivial diagram over this presentation. If x is the greatest element or the least element of X_0 occurring as label on an edge of Δ, then x occurs as label on an edge of $\partial\Delta$.*

The proof that will be given proceeds by contradiction, and applies equally to the case that Δ is a finite decomposition of the sphere. In that case it shows the following. We define a diagram to be *reduced* if it does not contain a subdiagram Δ' with exactly two faces such that the label on $\partial\Delta'$ reduces to the trivial element of F.

Proposition 9.7. *If $G = (X; R)$ is a staggered presentation, there exists no reduced spherical diagram over this presentation.* □

Proof of (9.6). The proof will go by induction on the number of faces of Δ. We introduce some simplifying assumptions. First, we may suppose Δ reduced. Second, we may suppose that Δ (if it is not a sphere) is a combinatorial disc. Third, we may suppose that X and R are finite, say $R = \{r_1, \ldots, r_m\}$, $m \geqslant 1$, with $r_1 < \cdots < r_m$, that each $x \in X$ occurs in some r_i, and that r_1 and r_m actually occur as boundary labels on faces of Δ.

We suppose Δ given, that the proposition holds for all diagrams with fewer faces than Δ, but that it fails for Δ. From this we derive a contradiction. We treat first the case that $m > 1$, and then reduce the case $m = 1$ to this case.

Let $m > 1$. Let K_1 be the subcomplex of Δ consisting of all the (closed) faces with boundary label r_m, and let K_2 consist of all faces with boundary label r_i for $i < m$. If any component of K_1 is not simply connected, it encloses a component of K_2; if this is not simply connected, it encloses another component of K_1. Continuing thus we arrive either at a simply connected component Δ_1 of K_1, or at a simply connected component Δ_2 of K_2 that is entirely enclosed in K_1, that is, with $\partial\Delta_2 \subseteq \partial K_1$. Clearly Δ_1 or Δ_2 is a diagram with fewer faces than Δ.

If we have a diagram Δ_1, we claim that no edge e of $\partial\Delta_1$ has label x_b, the greatest $x \in X_0$ occurring in r_m, and so the greatest on any edge of Δ_1. If e lies on $\partial\Delta$, this is true by hypothesis. Otherwise e separates Δ_1 from some face F with boundary label r_i, $i < m$, and $e\phi \neq x_b$ since x_b does not occur in r_i. This contradicts the induction hypothesis.

If we have a diagram Δ_2, let x_a be the least $x \in X_0$ occurring as label on an edge of Δ_2. Then x_a is the least $x \in X_0$ on some r_i for $i < m$, and does not occur in r_m. It follows that x_a does not occur on the boundary of any face with boundary label r_m, hence not on ∂K_1, and, since $\partial\Delta_2 \subseteq \partial K_1$, not on $\partial\Delta_2$. This (after reversal of order) contradicts the induction hypothesis.

We shall now reduce the case $m = 1$ to the case $m > 1$, already treated. In Magnus' argument the case $m = 1$, of a single relator r with normal closure N in a free group F, is reduced to the case of an infinite number of shorter relators r_i in a subgroup F_1, but having N as normal closure in F_1. In our context this amounts to a relabelling of the diagram Δ, possibly after subdivision of the edges. In general, in Δ, possibly after subdivision, there will be certain 'accidental' agreements of the labels on certain edges, in the sense that certain edges bear the same label although the hypotheses would all remain valid if the labels on these edges were taken as different. The rather technical argument below is aimed at eliminating these accidental agreements. Apart from a few easily handled cases, this leads to a relabelled diagram Δ' with $m' > 1$, such that the conclusion for Δ' implies the desired conclusion for Δ.

We assume henceforth that $m = 1$, and write $r = y_1 \cdots y_n$, $n > 1$, $y_i \in L$, cyclically reduced. We assume that all $x \in X$ occur in r, but that some x_0 does not occur as label on any edge of $\partial\Delta$. Clearly we may further assume that r is not a proper power. We may further assume that r contains x_0 more than once, since otherwise G has a basis $X - \{x_0\}$.

As names for the 'positions' on r (and their inverses) we take the set $P = \{1, \ldots, n\} \times \{+1, -1\}$; it will be convenient to write $(i, +1) = \eta_i$ and $(i, j)^{-1} = (i, -j)$. We define a function $\pi: P \to L = X \cup X^{-1}$ by setting $\eta_i^{\pm 1}\pi = y_i^{\pm 1}$; thus $\eta_i\pi$ is the letter occurring at position η_i in r. Since r is not a proper power, for each face F there is a unique *basic loop* γ_F, at a *base point* v_F on ∂F, describing ∂F in one sense or the other, and with $\gamma\phi = r$. If $\gamma_F = e_1 \cdots e_n$, we define $e_i^{\pm 1}\psi_F = \eta_i^{\pm 1}$. If an edge e lies between two faces F_1 and F_2, and $p_1 = e\psi_{F_1}, p_2 = e\psi_{F_2}$, we write $p_1 \sim p_2$. We write $p_1 \approx p_2$ for the transitive closure of this relation on P. From the definitions, $p_1 \sim p_2$ implies $p_1^{-1} \sim p_2^{-1}$ and $p_1\pi = p_2\pi$. It follows that $p_1 \approx p_2$ implies $p_1^{-1} \approx p_2^{-1}$ and $p_1\pi = p_2\pi$. Since $y \neq y^{-1}$ for $y \in L$, it follows that $p \not\approx p^{-1}$.

Let $\tilde{L}$ be the set of equivalence classes $[p]$ of elements of P under the relation $p_1 \approx p_2$. Let $\tilde{X}$ be the set of $[p]$ such that $p\pi \in X$, and let $[p]^{-1} = [p^{-1}]$. Then $\tilde{L} = \tilde{X} \cup \tilde{X}^{-1}$, and $\tilde{X} \cap \tilde{X}^{-1} = \varnothing$. Let $\tilde{F}$ be the free group with basis $\tilde{X}$. Now $\pi: P \to L$ induces a map which we still denote as π from $\tilde{L}$ onto L, carrying $\tilde{X}$ onto X, and this extends to a homomorphism π from $\tilde{F}$ onto F. We define a function $\tilde{\phi}$ assigning to the edges of Δ labels in $\tilde{L}$ by setting $e\tilde{\phi} = [e\psi_F]$ where e lies on ∂F; this is justified by the definitions. Then Δ with this new labeling function is a diagram over the presentation $(\tilde{X}; \tilde{r})$, where $\tilde{r} = \tilde{y}_1 \cdots \tilde{y}_n$, $\tilde{y}_i = [\eta_i]$. Observe that $\phi = \tilde{\phi}\pi$ and that, if $\tilde{x}_0 \in \tilde{X}$ with $\tilde{x}_0\pi = x_0$, then $\tilde{x}_0$ occurs as the label on an edge of Δ but on no edge of $\partial\Delta$.

We may now drop tildes, having gained the further hypothesis that if some $y_i = y_j^{\pm 1}$, then $\eta_i \approx \eta_j^{\pm 1}$.

Let μ be any homomorphism from F into $\mathbb{Z}_+$, the additive group of integers, such that $r\mu = 0$. It follows for each of the basic loops γ_F, and hence for any loop γ in Δ, that $\gamma\phi\mu = 0$. Thus if δ_1, δ_2 are two paths from one vertex to another, then $\delta_1\phi\mu = \delta_2\phi\mu$. Choose a face F_0, with base point v_{F_0}, and, for all vertices v of Δ, define $v\sigma$ to be the common value of $\delta\phi\mu$ on all paths δ from v_{F_0} to v.

Let $X^* = X \times \mathbb{Z}$, let F be free with basis X^*, and let $L^* = X^* \cup X^{*-1}$. If $y \in L$, $y = x^{\pm 1}$, $x \in X$, we write $y(i) = (x, i)^{\pm 1} \in L^*$. Define a new function ϕ^* assigning to the edges of Δ values in L^* by setting $e\phi^* = y(i)$ where $e\phi = y = x^{\pm 1}$ and $i = v\sigma$ for v the initial vertex of $e^{\pm 1}$. Now

$$\gamma_{F_0}\phi^* = r(0) = y_1(i_1) \cdots y_n(i_n)$$

Where

$$i_k = (y_1 \cdots y_{k-1})\sigma \quad \text{if } y_k \in X$$

and

$$i_k = (y_1 \cdots y_k)\sigma \quad \text{if } y_k \in X^{-1}$$

It follows that for each face F,

$$\gamma_F\phi^* = r(h) = y_1(i_1 + h) \cdots y_n(i_n + h)$$

where $h = v_F\sigma$. Now Δ, with ϕ^*, is a diagram over $R^* = \{r(h): h \in \mathbb{Z}\}$, and if $X_0^* = \{x_0(h): h \in \mathbb{Z}\}$, both with the order induced from $\mathbb{Z}$, then the presentation (X^*, R^*) is staggered. Moreover, no $x_0(h) \in X_0^*$ in fact occurs as label on an edge of Δ. If the faces of Δ have boundary labels $\gamma_F\phi^* = r(h)$ for more than one value of h, then we are in the case $m > 1$, with the number of faces in Δ unchanged, and the proof is complete.

The above argument fails only if $v_F\sigma = 0$ for the base point v_F of each face F. Suppose this is the case. Suppose $p_1 \approx p_2$; this corresponds to two indicated occurrences of some y in r in one of the following forms: $r = uywyz$ or $r = uywy^{-1}z$. We define the value of μ on the interval between corresponding points of the two positions of occurrence of y to be $J(p_1, p_2) = (yw)\mu$ in the first case and $J(p_1, p_2) = (ywy^{-1})\mu = (w)\mu$ in the second. Observe that if $p_1 \approx p_2 \approx p_3$, then $J(p_1, p_3) = J(p_1, p_2) + J(p_2, p_3)$; it follows that if $p_1 \sim p_2$ implies $J(p_1, p_2) = 0$, then $p_1 \approx p_2$ implies $J(p_1, p_2) = 0$.

Let $p_1 \sim p_2$ with $p_1\pi = p_2\pi = y$, and $p_1 = e\psi_{F_1}$, $p_2 = e\psi_{F_2}$ as before. There are two cases according as γ_{F_1} and γ_{F_2} have the same or opposite orientations. If the orientations are the same, then $r = uywy^{-1}z$ with e corresponding to the indicated occurrence of y in $\gamma_{F_1}\phi$ and to that of y^{-1} in $\gamma_{F_2}\phi$. Let v be the initial point of e; then, on γ_{F_1}, $u\mu = v\sigma - v_1\sigma$, while, on γ_{F_2}, $(uywy^{-1})\mu = v\sigma - v_2\sigma$. If $v_1\sigma = v_2\sigma = 0$ then $u\mu = (uywy^{-1})\mu$ and $J(p_1, p_2) = (w)\mu = 0$. If the orientations are opposite, then $r = uywyz$ with e corresponding, say, to the first occurrence of y in $\gamma_{F_1}\phi$ and to the second in $\gamma_{F_2}\phi$. If $v_1\sigma = v_2\sigma = 0$, we conclude now that $u\mu = (uyw)\mu$ and again that $J(p_1, p_2) = 0$. Thus the assumption that all $v_F\sigma = 0$ implies that $p_1 \sim p_2$ implies $J(p_1, p_2) = 0$, and therefore that $p_1 \approx p_2$ implies $J(p_1, p_2) = 0$.

To complete the proof it suffices to show that μ can be chosen so that, for some $p_1 \approx p_2$, we have $J(p_1, p_2) \neq 0$. That is, we must show that r (or some cyclic permutation of $r^{\pm 1}$) has a part ywy with $(yw)\mu \neq 0$ or a part ywy^{-1} with $w\mu \neq 0$.

Now μ is determined by its values $\mu_i = x_i\mu$, and these are subject to a single constraint, that $\Sigma a_i\mu_i = 0$, where a_i is the exponent sum of x_i in r. Suppose first that some $a_i = 0$. If $r^{\pm 1}$ had a part x_iux_i where u did not contain x_i, then we could choose $(x_iu)\mu = x_i\mu + u\mu$ arbitrarily, and would be done. Otherwise, since x_i must occur at least twice, r (or a cyclic permutation of $r^{\pm 1}$) must have the form $r = x_iu_1x_i^{-1}v_1 \cdots x_iu_kx_i^{-1}v_k$, where x_i does not occur in the u_h, v_h. If a letter y occured in u_1 and v_1, we would have a part $ywy^{\pm 1}$ of $u_1x_i^{-1}v_1$ in which w contained x_i only once, whence $(yw)\mu$ (or $w\mu$) could be taken arbitrary. Thus we may suppose u_1 and v_1 have no x_j in common. Now if either, say, v_1 contained any x_j with $a_j \neq 0$, we could take $v_1\mu \neq 0$ unless v_1 contained all such x_j; thus we may suppose in any case that u_1 contains x_j only for $a_j = 0$. Now if we choose a part $x_j^ewx_j^f$ $(e, f = \pm 1)$ of $x_iu_1x_i^1$ with w as short as possible, then w will contain some x_h only once, and since $a_h = 0$, we can choose $w\mu$ arbitrary.

The case remains that no $a_i = 0$. If r (or a cyclic permutation of $r^{\pm 1}$) had a part $x_iux_i^{-1}$ where u did not contain x_i, then we could choose $u\mu \neq 0$. Thus we may suppose each x_i occurs in r always with the same exponent, say $+1$. Now, if r contains a part x_iux_i, we can choose $(x_iu)\mu \neq 0$ unless all $x_j \neq x_i$ occur in u. Thus we may suppose further that, between any two occurrences of any x_i there is an occurrence of each other x_j. But this implies that, for some permutation π of the indices,

$$r = (x_{\pi(1)} \cdots x_{\pi(n)})^t, t \geqslant 1.$$

Since r is not a proper power, $t = 1$. But then r contains x_0 only once, contrary to hypothesis. This completes the proof of (9.6.). □

10. Spherical Diagrams

In the previous section we have discarded spherical diagrams as an unavoidable nuisance; but they have their group-theoretical significance, which we shall develop now. Before entering into this we should mention that other types of singular subcomplexes, or diagrams, in addition to singular discs and singular spheres, have proved useful. Singular annuli, or annular diagrams, have been used by Schupp (1968; see V.5) in connection with the conjugacy problem. Schupp (unpublished) has also used diagrams on 2-manifolds in studying the solutions of quadratic equations in groups, and to obtain a proof of the result of Nielsen that, for the canonical presentation $G = (X; r)$ of a surface group, every automorphism of G is induced by an automorphism of the free group F with basis X.

To recapitulate, we define a *spherical diagram* over a presentation $G = (X; R)$ to be a pair (S, f), where S is a finite combinatorial sphere, and f a dimension preserving map from S into $C = C(X; R)$. We shall call a spherical diagram S *reduced* if it does not contain any singular subdisc S_0 with only two faces such that a boundary label of S_0 represents the trivial element of F. If S does contain such a subcomplex, but it is not all of S, then after deleting this subcomplex and sewing up the resulting diagram, one obtains a new spherical diagram S' with two fewer faces; if the two faces are all of S, we take S' to be the empty diagram. In either case, we call the passage from S to S' *reduction*. A spherical diagram will be called *trivial* if it can be reduced to the empty diagram. A presentation $G = (X; R)$, and the associated Cayley complex $C(X; R)$, will be called *aspherical* if there are no non-trivial spherical diagrams over $(X; R)$.

The problem of identities among relations, which has been studied by Peiffer (1949), Reidemeister (1949), and Lyndon (1950), is closely related to that of spheres. As a first approximation, an identity among the relators in a presentation $(X; R)$ is an equation $u_1 r_1^{e_1} u_1^{-1} \cdots u_n r_n^{e_n} u_n^{-1} = 1$, where each $r_i \in R$, $u_i \in F$, $e_i = \pm 1$, that holds in F. However, there are certain trivial equations of this sort that always hold, and to take these into account we introduce the concept of a Peiffer transformation.

Let $\pi = (p_1, \ldots, p_n)$ be any sequence of elements in a group G. A *Peiffer transformation of the first kind* consists of replacing π by $\pi' = (p'_1, \ldots, p'_n)$ where, for some i, $1 \leqslant i < n$, either

$$p'_i = p_{i+1} \text{ and } p'_{i+1} = p_{i+1}^{-1} p_i p_{i+1}$$

or

$$p_i' = p_i p_{i+1} p_i^{-1} \text{ and } p_{i+1}' = p_i,$$

where in either case $p_j' = p_j$ for $j \neq i, i+1$. A *Peiffer transformation of the second kind* consists of replacing π by $\pi' = (p_1, \ldots, p_{i-1}, p_{i+2}, \ldots, p_n)$, where $p_i p_{i+1} = 1$. It is clear that in either case the products $p_1 \cdots p_n$ and $p_1' \cdots p_n'$ represent the same element of the group G. (Transformations of this sort were considered, in a slightly different context, by Greendlinger (1960).)

If $G = (X; R)$ and $p_1, \ldots, p_n$ are conjugates of elements of $R \cup R^{-1}$ such that $p_1 \cdots p_n = 1$ in F, then we call $\pi = (p_1, \ldots, p_n)$ an *identity among the relations* of the given presentation. We call π *reduced* if it cannot be shortened by Peiffer transformation, and *trivial* if a sequence of Peiffer transformations carries it into the empty sequence π' (with $n' = 0$).

Proposition 10.1. *A presentation is aspherical if and only if there are no non-trivial identities among relations.*

□ In the proof of (9.2.) we showed that for any sequence $\pi = (p_1, \ldots, p_n)$ of conjugates p_i of elements of $R \cup R^{-1}$ there is a singular disc with boundary label, at a certain vertex v_0, the unreduced word $p_1 \cdots p_n$; we shall denote this singular disc by $S(\pi)$. If π is an identity among relations of the presentation $G = (X; R)$ then the boundary label on $S(\pi)$ represents the trivial element of F, whence by sewing up the boundary of $S(\pi)$ we obtain a spherical diagram S'. We shall show that conversely every spherical diagram is obtainable in this way. Let S be a non-trivial spherical diagram; S must have more than one face. We choose a face D_1 of S and a vertex v_0 of D_1; then $S - D_1$ is a singular disc and hence is isomorphic to a singular disc E_1 in the plane. We let S_1 be the singular disc in the plane consisting of (a replica of) D_1 together with E_1, embedded in such a way that they have only (the images of) v_0 in common. Evidently S can be obtained by sewing up and detachment (in the case that E_1 has trivial boundary label) from S_1, and D_1 has a certain label p_1 in $R \cup R^{-1}$ and E_1 a label q in N, beginning at v_0. If E_1 consists of a single face we are done, for then q is a conjugate of an element of $R \cup R^{-1}$ and S_1 is (isomorphic to) $S(\pi)$ for $\pi = (p_1, q)$. Otherwise E_1 has more than one face, and we choose a face D_2 on the boundary of E_1 and a simple are α in ∂E_1 from v_0 to a point v on D_2; this can be done so that $E_1 - D_2$ contains v_0. It is evident that E_1 can be obtained by sewing up from a diagram E_2 consisting of two parts E_2' and E_2'' with only a vertex v_0 in common, where E_2' is isomorphic to $D_2 \cup \alpha$ and E_2'' is isomorphic to $E_1 - D_2$. Now E_2 has one face fewer than E_1, whence by iteration of this argument we can arrive at singular disc E, consisting of subcomplexes $E_2', \ldots, E_n'$ with only the vertex v_0 in common to any two, such that E_1 can be obtained by sewing up E, that each E_i' has boundary label p_i conjugate to an element of $R \cup R^{-1}$, and hence that E is (isomorphic to) $S(\rho)$ for $\rho = (p_2, \ldots, p_n)$. But now the union of D_1 and E, with only the point v_0 identified, is isomorphic to $S(\pi)$ for $\pi = (p_1, \ldots, p_n)$, and S can be obtained by sewing up this complex.

If S is a spherical diagram obtained by sewing up and detachment from $S(\pi)$, then it is easy to see that S is reduced if and only if $S(\pi)$ is reduced. Thus to complete the proof it suffices to show that $S(\pi)$ is reduced if and only if π is reduced.

If π' is obtained from π by a transformation of the first kind, then inspection shows that the reduced diagrams obtainable from $S(\pi)$ and $S(\pi')$ by sewing up and detachment are the same; thus $S(\pi)$ is reduced if and only if $S(\pi')$ is reduced. Now suppose that $S(\pi)$ is not reduced; then it contains a subdisc with faces D_i and D_j and trivial boundary label. If, say, $i < j$, then by transformations of the first kind, conjugating p_i by $p_{i+1}, \ldots, p_{j-1}$ in turn, we can arrive at the position that $j = i + 1$, whence we conclude that $p_i p_{i+1} = 1$, and thus that π is not reduced. Conversely, if π is not reduced, then after transformations of the first kind we can suppose that some $p_i p_{i+1} = 1$. But then $S(\pi)$ contains a subcomplex $S_0 = S(\pi_0)$, where $\pi_0 = (p_i, p_{i+1})$, with trivial boundary label, whence $S(\pi)$ is not reduced. □

We next show that asphericity implies a condition (I.1 below) that was considered by Lyndon (1950).

Proposition 10.2. *If $G = (X; R)$ is aspherical, and no element of R is conjugate to another or to its inverse, then the following condition holds*:

(I.1) *Let $p_1 \cdots p_n = 1$ where each $p_i = u_i r_i^{e_i} u_i^{-1}$ for some $u_i \in F$, $r_i \in R$, and $e_i = \pm 1$. Then the indices fall into pairs (i, j) such that $r_i = r_j$, $e_i = -e_j$, and $u_i \in u_j N C_i$ where C_i (the centralizer of r_i) is the cyclic group generated by the root s_i of $r_i = s_i^{m_i}$.*

□ We argue by induction on n, the initial case when $n = 0$ being trivial. By (10.1), asphericity of the presentation implies that the identity $\pi = (p_1, \ldots, p_n)$ is reducible. Since neither the hypothesis nor the conclusion is altered by application of Peiffer transformations of the first kind, we may suppose that some $p_i p_{i+1} = 1$. It follows that r_i and $r_{i+1}^{\pm 1}$ are conjugate and therefore that $r_i = r_{i+1}$ and $e_i = -e_{i+1}$, with $c = u_i^{-1} u_{i+1}$ centralizing r_i. But then $c \in C_i$, and the conclusion follows. □

The condition (I.1) can be formulated more elegantly. Recall that with a presentation $G = (X; R)$ is associated a natural G-module $\overline{N} = N/[N, N]$, the *relation module* of the presentation. For n in N, we write $\bar{n}$ for its image in $\overline{N}$; for w in F, we write, with harmless ambiguity, $\bar{n} \cdot w$ for the transform of $\bar{n}$ by the image of w in G, that is, for the element $\overline{w^{-1}nw}$ of $\overline{N}$.

Proposition 10.3. *Condition* (I.1) *is equivalent to the condition that $\overline{N}$ is the direct sum of cyclic G-modules $\overline{N}_i$ generated by the images $\bar{r}_i$ of the elements r_i of R, each defined by a single relation $\bar{r}_i \cdot s_i = \bar{r}_i$, where s_i is the root of r_i.*

□ To match the notation already established, which has become standard, we view $\overline{N}$ as a left, rather than right, G-module; thus we write $w \cdot \bar{n} = \overline{wnw^{-1}}$. We assume (I.1). Suppose a relation $\sum e_i u_i \cdot \bar{r}_i = 0$ holds in $\overline{N}$ among the elements r_i, where the $e_i = \pm 1$ and the u_i are elements of F. Then in N a relation

$$\prod u_i r_i^{e_i} u_i^{-1} = k$$

holds, where k is in $[N, N]$. Now k is a product of commutators $[p, q]$ of conjugates of elements of $R \cup R^{-1}$, hence is a product of factors of the form $p^{-1} q^{-1} pq$;

thus k^{-1} is a product of factors p'_j that fall into pairs related as in (I.1). Now if $p_i = u_i r_i^{e_i} u_i^{-1}$, we have a relation $p_1 \cdots p_n k^{-1} = p_1 \cdots p_n p'_1 \cdots p'_m = 1$. By (10.2) these factors pair up, and we have seen that the p'_j pair among themselves; it follows that the p_i pair among themselves. Now if p_i and p_j pair together it follows that $r_i = r_j$, that $e_i = -e_j$, and that $u_i = u_j c$ for some c in C_i. Thus in $\bar{N}$ one has $e_i u_i \bar{r}_i + e_j u_j \bar{r}_j = \pm u_i(r_i - c \cdot \bar{r}_i)$ where $c = s_i^h$ for some h. It follows that the given relation in $\bar{N}$ is a consequence of relations of the form $s_i \cdot \bar{r}_i = \bar{r}$. This shows that $\bar{N}$ has the structure asserted by the proposition. □

Corollary 10.4. *If $G = (X; R)$ is aspherical and no element of R is a proper power, then the relation module $\bar{N}$ is a free G-module.*

□ After possibly deleting redundant elements from R, we may suppose that no element of R is conjugate to another or to its inverse. Now (10.3) applies, and, since each $s_i = r_i$ represents the trivial element of G, the defining relations $\bar{r}_i \cdot s_i = \bar{r}_i$ are all tautologous. □

In view of remarks in (II.3), $G = (X; R)$ has a free resolution of the form

$$\cdots \longrightarrow M_3 \xrightarrow{d_3} M_2 \xrightarrow{d_2} M_1 \xrightarrow{d_1} M_0 \xrightarrow{\varepsilon} 1,$$

where $M_2/\text{Ker}\, d_2 \simeq \bar{N}$. If $\bar{N}$ is a free G module, we can choose $M_2 = \bar{N}$ and $M_3, M_4, \ldots = 0$, obtaining a free resolution of the form

$$\cdots \longrightarrow 0 \xrightarrow{d_3} \bar{N} \xrightarrow{d_2} M_1 \xrightarrow{d_1} M_0 \xrightarrow{\varepsilon} 1.$$

In the established language this is expressed as follows.

Corollary 10.5. *If $G = (X; R)$ is aspherical and no element of R is a proper power, then G has cohomological dimension at most* 2. □

We remark that in view of the results of Stallings (1968) and Swan (1970; see also Cohen, 1972), G has cohomological dimension exactly 2 unless G is free. We remark also that if some elements of R are proper powers, then the cohomological dimension of G is infinite, but the cohomology of G has period 2, in that one can obtain a resolution in which $M_2 = M_4 = \ldots$, $M_3 = M_5 = \ldots$, $d_3 = d_5 = \ldots$, and $d_4 = d_6 = \ldots$. (For these matters see Lyndon 1950). We mention also a paper of Dyer and Vasquez (1973) that discusses asphericity of Cayley complexes.

We turn now to a condition that implies asphericity. If $G = (X; R)$ then the normal closure N of R in the free group F with basis X is free, as a subgroup of the free group F, and it is generated by conjugates of elements of R. It is natural to ask (see Lyndon, 1960) whether N has a basis B consisting of conjugates of elements of R.

Suppose that N has such a basis B. Then B is of the form $B = \{uru^{-1} : r \in R, u \in U(r)\}$ for certain subsets $U(r)$ of F. If, for a given r, B contains elements $b = uru^{-1}$ and $b' = u'ru'^{-1}$ where $u' = wu$ for some $w \in N$, then $b' = wbw^{-1}$ and the two basis elements b and b' are conjugate in N, whence they must coincide. It follows that we may choose each $U(r)$ within a transversal $V(r)$ for N in F, in the sense that the cosets $uN = Nu$ for $u \in U(r)$ are disjoint. Moreover, if c is in the centralizer $C(r)$ of r in F, and $u' = uc$, then $uru^{-1} = u'ru'^{-1}$; thus we may suppose that each $U(r)$ is contained in a left transversal $V(r)$ for $NC(r)$ in F, in the sense that all $uNC(r)$ for $u \in U(r)$ are disjoint.

We now examine the case that each $U(r)$ is a full left transversal for $NC(r)$ in F.

Proposition 10.6. *Assume that the presentation $G = (X; R)$ satisfies the following condition*:

(I.2) *N has a basis $B = \{uru^{-1}: r \in R,\ u \in U(r)\}$ where, for each $r \in R$, $U(r)$ is a full left transversal for $NC(r)$ in F.*

Then $(X; R)$ is a aspherical.

□ In view of (10.1) it will suffice to show that (I.2) implies there are no non-trivial identities among relations. Suppose then that $\pi = (p_1, \ldots, p_n)$ is a reduced identity among relations, with $n \geqslant 1$. Now each $p_i = u_i r_i^{e_i} u_i^{-1}$ for some $u_i \in F$, $r_i \in R$, and $e_i = \pm 1$. Since $U(r_i)$ is a left transversal for $NC(r)$, and since N is normal in F, we can write each u_i in the form $u_i = n_i v_i c_i$ with $n_i \in N$, $v_i \in U(r_i)$, and $c_i \in C(r)$. Now $p_i = n_i q_i^{e_i} n_i^{-1}$ where $q_i = v_i r_i v_i^{-1} \in B$. We express each n_i as a word over the basis B; then the expression for p_i in the form $p_i = n_i q_i^{e_i} n_i^{-1}$ will not be a reduced word over B if n_i ends in a power of q_i, say $n_i = n_i' q_i^m$ for m maximal; but then we may replace n_i by n_i' without effect on our argument. Thus we may suppose each $p_i = n_i q_i^{e_i} n_i^{-1}$ reduced without cancellation.

By hypothesis, $p_1 \cdots p_n = 1$. By (I.2.2), since all the p_i are of odd length, some must cancel more than half into an adjacent factor; we may suppose that p_i cancels more that half in the product $p_i p_{i+1}$, and hence that the part $q_i^{e_i} n_i^{-1}$ of p_i cancels. If it cancels exactly against the part $n_{i+1} q_{i+1}^{e_i+1}$, then $p_i p_{i+1} = 1$, contrary to the assumption that π is reduced. If it cancels wholly into n_{i+1}, then $p_{i+1}' = p_i p_{i+1} p_i^{-1}$ is shorter than p_{i+1}, and by a Peiffer transformation of the first kind we can replace π by a sequence π' with the sum of the lengths of the p_i' smaller than that of the p_i; in this case we are done by an induction on this sum. Finally, if it cancels against a part of p_{i+1} that is greater than $n_{i+1} q_{i+1}^{e_i+1}$, then this latter part of p_{i+1} cancels wholly into n_i, whence $p_{i+1}^{-1} p_i p_{i+1}$ is shorter than p_i and, again applying a Peiffer transformation of the first kind we are done by induction on the sum of the lengths of the p_i. □

We can offer only a partial converse to Proposition 10.6.

Proposition 10.7. *If $G = (X; R)$ is aspherical and no element of R is conjugate to another or to its inverse, and if B is any basis for N consisting of conjugates of elements of R, then B satisfies* (I.2).

□ It is enough to show that for each u in F and r in R there is some v in uN such that vrv^{-1} is in B. Since uru^{-1} is in N, and N has basis B, uru^{-1} is equal to a product p of elements $p_i^{e_i}$ where $p_i = v_i r_i v_i^{-1}$ is in B. Now (10.2) applied to the equation $(uru^{-1})p^{-1} = 1$ implies that, for some i, $r = r_i$, $e_i = 1$, and $v_i \in uNC_i$; thus $v_i = vc$ for some $v \in uN$ and $c \in C_i$, and $v_i r v_i^{-1} = vrv^{-1}$ is in B. □

Combining (10.6) and (10.7) we have the following.

Corollary 10.8. *If $G = (X; R)$ and N has some basis consisting of conjugates of elements of R that satisfies* (I.2), *then every such basis satisfies* (I.2). □

Relation modules $\bar{N}$ for finite groups $G = F/N$ have been studied by Ojanguren (1968) who examined the complex representation induced by the action of G on $\bar{N}$. They have also been studied by Williams (1973). He showed that for $|X|$ sufficiently large, $G = (X; R_1) = (X; R_2)$ implies that $\bar{N}_1 \simeq \bar{N}_2$; whether this remains true for $|X|$ minimal remains open. He gave also conditions for N to have a projective summand.

11. Aspherical Groups

We turn now to the question of what groups admit aspherical presentations. In view of (10.6), if a group has a presentation satisfying (I.2), then this presentation is aspherical. The property (I.2) was first established by Cohen and Lyndon (1963) for presentations with a single defining relator, and also more generally for staggered presentations (see 9.5). From this one obtains the following.

Proposition 11.1. *If $G = (X; R)$ where R consists of a single relator, or more generally, if the presentation is staggered, then the presentation is aspherical.* □

We do not prove this here, but note that Karrass and Solitar (1970) have given a proof that is at the same time simpler and more comprehensive than that of Cohen and Lyndon. In view of results in (III.10), Proposition 11.1 implies the results of Lyndon (1950) that, in the case at hand, there are no non-trivial identities among relators, and that the cohomology is as described in (III.10). A geometric proof, contained in Lyndon's (1973) proof of the Freiheitssatz, is given in (9.7).

Schiek (1953) proved a special case of (11.1).

Cohen and Lyndon (1963) proved also the following result, which applies to most of the groups whose word problem is solvable by means of Dehn's algorithm (see V.4).

Proposition 11.2. *Let $G = (X; R)$ and assume that every reduced word for a non-trivial element w of N contains a segment that constitutes more than one half of the reduced word for some element of R^*. Then N has a basis B consisting of conjugates of elements of R.*

□ By (I.2.7) there exists a basis U of N such that N is well ordered by a relation $u \prec v$ such that $|u| < |v|$ implies $u \prec v$ and that $w \in N$, $u \in U$, and $w \prec u$ implies that $w \in N_u = \mathrm{Gp}\{v: v \in U,\ v \prec u\}$. We argue by induction, assuming that N_u has a basis B_u consisting of conjugates of elements of R; for the induction we must show that $N_u' = \mathrm{Gp}\{N_u, u\}$ has such a basis B_u'. Now by hypothesis $u = aqb$ where q is more than half of some element $r = pq$ in R^*. Now $u' = u(b^{-1}r^{-1}b) = apb$ is shorter than u, whence $u' \in N_u$. But the facts that $B_u \cup \{u\}$ is a basis for B_u, that $u' \in N_u$, and that $u = u'(b^{-1}rb)$ imply that $B_u' = B \cup \{b^{-1}rb\}$ is a basis for N_u'. □

With a few exceptions it follows from small cancellation theory that the strictly planar F-groups satisfy the hypothesis and therefore the conclusion of (11.2). However, Zieschang (1965) has supplied a direct geometric proof of this.

Proposition 11.3. *If $G = (X; R)$ with $C(X; R)$ planar and filling the plane, then N has a basis of conjugates of elements of R.*

□ It is easy to see that, choosing a base point v_0, C is the union of a chain $C_1 \leqslant C_2 \leqslant \cdots$ where each C_i is a topological disc, where C_0 is a single face D_0 containing v_0, and each C_{n+1} is obtained from C_n by adding a face D_n. For each face D_n we choose a simple arc γ_n in C_{n-1} running from v_0 to a point v_n on $D_n \cap C_{n-1}$, and meeting D_n nowhere else. Let $\Delta_n = D_n \cup \gamma_n$; then the boundary δ_n of Δ_n has label at v_0 a conjugate p_n of an element in $R^{\pm 1}$. These p_n are a basis for a subgroup N' of N, since the corresponding boundary paths δ_n represent a basis for the fundamental group of the 1-skeleton C^1 of C, and any relation among the p_n would imply one among the (homotopy classes of the) δ_n.

It remains to show that $N' = N$; for this it suffices to show that every closed path λ in C is a product of the $\delta_n^{\pm 1}$. Now λ lies in some C_n, and we argue by induction on n. Clearly we may suppose that λ is a loop at v_0 consisting of a segment λ_1 within C_{n-1} to a point on ∂D_n, a segment α contained in ∂D_n, and then a segment λ_2 within C_{n-1} returning to v_0. The inductive hypothesis permits us to suppose first that λ_1 runs from v_0 to v_n, that α is a boundary path for D_n at v_n, and that λ_2 runs from v_n back to v_0; it further permits us to assume that $\lambda_1 = \gamma_n$ and $\lambda_2 = \gamma_n^{-1}$. But then $\lambda = \delta_n$. □

One might hope to extend this kind of geometrical argument to further cases where a basis of conjugates of elements of R is already known by other means to exist, and perhaps to some other presentations known to be aspherical.

Some presentations are known to be aspherical on topological grounds. For tame knot groups this follows from deep results of Papakyriakopoulos (1957). For alternating knot groups it was established by Aumann (1956), and also follows on combinatorial grounds from results of Weinbaum (1971) and Appel and Schupp (1972). More trivially, all planar presentations are aspherical. For, if (Δ, δ) is a reduced singular sphere over any Cayley complex $C = C(X; R)$, then there are no *foldings*: if D_1 and D_2 are distinct faces of Δ abutting along an edge e, then $D_1\delta$ and $D_2\delta$ are distinct faces of $\Delta\delta$ abutting along the edge $e\delta$. It follows in particular that the geometric subcomplex $\Delta\delta$ of C has empty boundary. Now a planar complex cannot contain a non-empty finite subcomplex without boundary.

The last argument can be refined. In general (Δ, δ) can have 'branch points': the punctured star of a vertex v in Δ may map n-to-one onto the punctured star of $v\delta$ for any $n \geqslant 1$. It follows however that the multiplicity of δ is the same for adjacent faces of Δ, and hence for all faces. In this case we call δ *n-to-one*, referring to its multiplicity on faces; it may well have different multiplicities on vertices and edges. If D_1 in Δ maps onto $D_1\delta$ in C, one can find Δ_1 in Δ, containing D_1 and connected and simply connected and mapping 1-to-1 under δ onto $\Delta_1\delta$. If $\Delta_1 = \Delta$, then δ is 1-*to*-1 and $\Delta\delta$ is a (non-singular) spherical subcomplex of C. Otherwise (Δ_1, δ_1), where δ_1 is the restriction of δ to Δ_1, is a singular disc with boundary label representing 1, and sewing up Δ_1 yields a singular sphere Δ' mapping 1-to-1 onto $\Delta'\delta'$, whence again (Δ', δ') is a sphere in C. One concludes again that if C is not aspherical then it contains spheres.

The argument just given shows that if (Δ, δ) is *strongly reduced* in that it contains no (necessarily proper) singular disc with at least one face that has boundary label representing 1 —in particular if (Δ, δ) is a singular sphere with the least possible number of faces —, then δ maps Δ 1-to-1 onto a sphere $\Delta\delta$ in C. It shows also that every singular sphere (Δ, δ) is a sum of spheres in C in the sense that, for certain spheres $S_1, \ldots, S_n$ at a common vertex v in C, Δ is the result of sewing up singular discs $\Delta_1, \ldots, \Delta_n$ with a common vertex $\tilde{v}$ such that δ maps each Δ_i 1-to-1 onto S_i and maps $\tilde{v}$ onto v. In particular, if there is in C only a single sphere S at each vertex — for example, if C is a sphere itself—then every singular sphere is a sum of 1-to-1 coverings of some such S. In this case, every identity among relations is a consequence of the single such identity associated with S; and $\bar{N}$, with the images $\bar{x}$ of the x in X as generators, is defined by a possible relation $\bar{s} \cdot \bar{r} = 0$ for each image $\bar{r}$ of an r in R, together with one further relation derived from the identity associated with the sphere S.

We note that a proof by combinatorial geometry of the asphericity of certain presentations with 'small cancellation' was given by Lyndon (1966); he treated certain analogous results for quotients of free products, and Schupp (1971) for quotients of free products with amalgamation. The same arguments would yield a further result of Cohen and Lyndon, analogous to theorems in logic concerning 'rearrangement of proof'.

Proposition 11.4. *Let $G = (X; R)$ be a staggered presentation, as in (9.5). For $p_i = u_i r_i^{e_i} u_i^{-1}$, $u_i \in F$, $r_i \in R$, $e_i = +1$, let the reduced form of $w = p_1 \cdots p_n$ contain the special generators x_i only for $a \leqslant i \leqslant b$. Then by Peiffer transformations the formal product $(p_1, \ldots, p_n)$ can be carried into a formal product $(q_1, \ldots, q_m)$ such that (of course) $q_1 \cdots q_m$ represents the same element of N as w, and that each $q_j = v_j r_j^{f} v_j^{-1}$ for some r_j that contains generators x_i only for $a \leqslant i \leqslant b$.* □

12. Coset Diagrams and Permutation Representatians

It is a basic and elementary fact in the theory of permutation groups that if a group G acts transitively, say on the right, on a set Ω, and if H is the subgroup fixing a given element ω of Ω, then Ω, as a set with operators from G, is isomorphic to the family of cosets Hg, under the correspondence that carries ωg into Hg. The same ideas that we proposed as motivation for constructing Cayley diagrams now lead to their generalization to *coset diagrams.* More precisely, let G be a group, H a subgroup of G, and X a subset of G (which in the most interesting cases generates G). We define the corresponding coset diagram to be a labeled graph Γ, as follows. The set of vertices of Γ is the set Ω of cosets Hg, for g in G. The edges are in one-to-one correspondence with $\Omega \times (X \cup X^{-1})$; with each pair (Hg, x) for $g \in G$ and $x \in X \cup X^{-1}$, we associate an edge $e = e(g, x)$ leading from Hg to Hgx, and with label $e\phi = x$; the inverse edge is $e^{-1} = e(gx, x^{-1})$. These diagrams have been used extensively, but we content ourselves here with a reference to Coxeter and Moser (1965), where a thorough discussion can be found, together with one or two particular topics that seem especially germane to our treatment.

First, we give a proof of a well known consequence of Schreier's formula (I.3.9); this is an easy consequence of that formula, but the present argument seems more revealing.

Proposition 12.1. *If G is a group generated by a finite set of n elements and H is a subgroup of finite index j in G, then H is generated by a set of no more than m elements, where* $m - 1 = j(n - 1)$.

□ If w is any word in the generating set X for G, then from the vertex H of Γ there is a unique path p with label w, ending at Hw. In particular, p is a loop at H if and only if $Hw = H$, that is, if $w \in H$. Since H is of finite index, Ω is finite, there is a finite basis $p_1, \ldots, p_m$ for the loops at H, $\pi(\Gamma)$ is generated freely by the elements determined by these p_i, and H is generated by their images in G. Thus H is generated by a set of no more than m elements. But, as we have seen earlier (2.2), $\pi(\Gamma)$ is free of rank m where $m = \gamma_1 - \gamma_0 + 1$, for γ_0 the number of vertices of Γ and γ_1 the number of undirected edges. Now there are at most $2n$ directed edges at each vertex, and since each directed edge is counted thus twice, it follows that $\gamma_1 \leqslant nj$, where $j = \gamma_0$ is the number of vertices. Thus we have that $m = nj - j + 1$, and the conclusion follows. □

We sketch the connection between Cayley diagrams and the Todd-Coxeter method of coset enumeration. The Cayley diagram $C = C(X; R)$ for a symmetrized presentation $G = (X; R)$ can be constructed inductively, as the limit C_∞ of a sequence of diagrams C_α under mapping $\gamma_{\alpha\beta}\colon C_\alpha \to C_\beta$ for all $\alpha < \beta$. We confine attention to the case that the presentation is finite, where C_∞ is the limit of a sequence $C_0, C_1, C_2, \ldots$ of finite diagrams under maps γ_{kl} determined by maps $\gamma_k\colon C_k \to C_{k+1}$. It is convenient to suppose the sets X and R are ordered, and at each stage to impose an order on the vertices of C_k.

We begin by taking C_0 to consist of a single vertex v. We now suppose C_k given and construct C_{k+1}, together with γ_k and an order on the vertices of C_{k+1}. There are three cases.

Case 1. At some vertex v of C_k there is a path p that is not a loop, but with label r in R. We choose the first such v, and, for this v, the unique path with first such r in R. Suppose p runs from v to v'. We define an equivalence relation on the vertices of C_k by setting $u \equiv u'$ if and only if there are paths q from v to u and q' from v' to u' with the same label. It is easy to verify that this is in fact an equivalence relation, and that it induces an equivalence on edges that preserves incidence and labeling. We take C_{k+1} to be the quotient of C_k by this equivalence relation, with γ_k the projection. We order the vertices of C_{k+1} according to the order in C_k of their earliest ranking preimages.

Case 2. The situation of Case 1 does not occur, but there is some vertex v and some $y = x^{\pm 1}$ for x in X such that there is no edge at v with label y. We choose the first such v, and, for this chosen v, the first such x. We choose $y = x$ if there is no edge with label x at v, otherwise $y = x^{-1}$. We obtain C_{k+1} from C_k by adjoining a new vertex u together with an edge from v to u with label y. We take γ_k to be the inclusion map. The vertices of C_k are ordered as before, with the new vertex u coming after all of them.

Case 3. Neither the situation of Case 1 nor that of Case 2 occurs. Then we take $C_{k+1} = C_k$ with γ_k the identity.

If C_∞ is the limit of the C_k under the maps γ_k, it is easy to see that C_∞ is (isomorphic to) the Cayley diagram C. If C_k falls under Case 3 for some k it is easy to see that $C_\infty = C_k$, and, since the Cayley diagram C_∞ for the presentation is finite, the group G must be finite. It is a little more difficult to see that, conversely, if G is finite, then for some k one has C_k in Case 3 and hence $C_\infty = C_k$.

We examine now the method of coset enumeration for the special case of cosets of the trivial subgroup $H = 1$. We are interested in discovering, given the presentation $G = (X; R)$, whether G is finite, obtaining its order, and obtaining a permutational representation of it (in fact the regular representation) in case it is finite. We assume that every generator x in X occurs (as x or x^{-1}) in some relator r in R; if this is not the case then G is surely infinite. We do not require any longer the hypothesis that R be symmetrized. The method now consists of arranging a variant of the above construction in a tabular form suited to efficient computation.

Intuitively, the successive steps in constructing the C_k are recorded by listing in order names for the vertices, in order, on each loop with label r, where $r \in R$. For each $r \in R$ we make a table of these lists, and, at certain stages (corresponding roughly to the constructions under Case 2 above) we add further lists to these tables. At other steps (corresponding to Case 1 above) we record certain equivalences between names in our table, indicating that they are names for the same vertex.

Let $r \in R$, say $r = y_1 \ldots y_n$ reduced, with each $y_i \in X \cup X^{-1}$. We make for r a table as shown below, marking the internal vertical dividing lines with $y_1, \ldots, y_n$.

	y_1	y_2	$\cdots$	y_{n-1}	y_n
v_1		v_2	$v_3 \cdots v_{n-1}$	v_n	v_{n+1}

A row in this table, as shown, is intended to indicate that $v_1, v_2, \ldots, v_n, v_{n+1}$ are in order the vertices of a loop with label r, and that v_{n+1} is in fact the same vertex as v_1.

In addition to these tables it is convenient to think of a separate record of relations among the v_i, although all this information is in fact implicit in the tables. Specifically, for each row $v_1, v_2, \ldots, v_{n+1}$ as above, we record the following relations:

$$v_1y_1 = v_2, v_2y_2 = v_3, \ldots, v_{n-1}y_{n-1} = v_n, v_ny_n = v_{n+1}$$

and also the equation $v_{n+1} = v_1$. Moreover, with each relation $v_iy_j = v_k$ we record also the relation $v_ky_j^{-1} = v_i$; also, given an equation $v_i = v_j$, with $v_iy_k = v_l$ we record also $v_jy_k = v_l$, with $v_ly_k = v_i$ also $v_ly_k = v_j$, and with $v_i = v_k$ also $v_j = v_k$. In practice, we replace the entries v_i by their indices $i = 1, 2, \ldots$.

The algorithm begins by entering a first row $1, 2, \ldots, n, 1$ in the first table, where n is the length of the first $r \in R$. All the derived information is recorded, as indicated above. Thereafter it proceeds as follows. Suppose that some number k_1 appears in the tables, but does not begin a row in each table. We choose the first such k_1, and let $r = y_1 \ldots y_n$ be the first $r \in R$ such that k_1 does not begin a row in the table for r nor any k_1' for which we have recorded an equation $k_1 = k_1'$. We put k_1 in the first place in a new row in the table for r. If we have on record an equation $k_1y_1 = k_2$, for some least k_2, we put k_2 in the second place in the row. Continuing thus it may happen that we complete the row, putting some k_{n+1} in the last place; in this case we record the equation $k_1 = k_{n+1}$ together with its consequences, as indicated above. Otherwise we arrive at some k_h in the h-th place, $1 \leqslant h \leqslant n$, and no recorded equation $k_hy_h = k_j$. We then complete the row to give it the form $k_1, k_2, \ldots, k_h, l, l + l, \ldots, m, k_1$, where $l, l + l, \ldots, m$ are in order the first numbers not already appearing in the table; again we record the appropriate equations. The possibility remains that at some stage for every number k that appears in the tables either k, or some k' for which we have recorded the equation $k = k'$, begins a row in each table; in this case the algorithm terminates.

If G is finite, reference to the Cayley diagram shows that the algorithm must terminate. The usefulness of the algorithm lies in the fact that, conversely, if the algorithm terminates, then G is finite. Suppose in fact that it terminates. We may replace each k by the least k' for which an equation $k = k'$ is recorded. Then the set of numbers appearing in the tables will be $\Omega = \{1, 2, \ldots, N\}$ for some N, and each such number will begin exactly one row in each of the tables, and ends the same row. Moreover, for each $h \in \Omega$ and $y \in X \cup X^{-1}$, the information $hy = k$ is recorded for exactly one $k \in \Omega$. Now the first column of the table for $r = y_1 \ldots y_n$ is a permutation of Ω, whence the second column of this table is also a permutation of Ω, and it follows that the map $h \to hy_1$ is a permutation. Now the tables give a finite Cayley diagram for G with N vertices, whence G has order N, and the maps $h \to hy$ define a regular representation of G.

If H is any subgroup of G, one proceeds in the same way to enumerate the cosets Hg of H in G. The entries in the tables now represent cosets, and, for the algorithm to be effective, we must be able to recognize when two cosets Hg and Hg' are the same. Otherwise everything goes as before, and the algorithm terminates just in case H has finite index $[G: H] = N$ in G, in which case it provides a complete coset diagram, or, alternatively, a representation of G by its action on the cosets of H in G.

With infinite groups as with finite groups, much knowledge of the structure of a group G can often be obtained from what appears to be rather modest knowledge of its action on a set Ω. The essential connection is always that Ω, as G-set, is isomorphic to a direct sum of G-sets consisting of coset diagrams for subgroups of G. The foremost example of this is perhaps the argument by which Poincaré (1882) obtains a presentation for a Fuchsian group from a knowledge of its action on the translates of a fundamental region, and (1882) the analogous result for Kleinian groups acting on hyperbolic 3-space; for these matters we refer to Maskit (1973).

Our interest here is in theorems of this sort that are of a more primitive nature, in that the set Ω is endowed with no additional structure. The prototype for such theorems seems to be the *combination theorem* of Klein (1883; see also Ford 1929) giving conditions for a Fuchsian group to be a free product of certain subgroups. It seems to have been noticed first by Macbeath (1963) that the validity of this theorem is independent of any structure, analytic or otherwise, on the set Ω. Somewhat similar ideas are contained in Tits (1969); see also Dixon (1974). In the interest of simplicity, we present Macbeath's result in its most elementary form (see Lyndon and Ullman, 1968).

Proposition 12.2. *Let a group G of permutations of a set Ω be generated by two subgroups G_1 and G_2, and let Ω_1 and Ω_2 be disjoint non-empty subsets of Ω such that*

$$1 \neq g_1 \in G_1 \quad \textit{implies} \quad \Omega_1 g_1 \subseteq \Omega_2,$$
$$1 \neq g_2 \in G_2 \quad \textit{implies} \quad \Omega_2 g_2 \subseteq \Omega_1.$$

Then either G is the free product $G = G_1 * G_2$, without amalgamation, or else $|G_1| = |G_2| = 2$ and G is a dihedral group.

□ Assume first that, say, $|G_1| > 2$, and that $1, g_1', g_1$ are distinct elements of G_1. Since $\Omega_1 g_1 g_1'^{-1} \cap \Omega_1 = \varnothing$, $\Omega_1 g_1$ and $\Omega_1 g_1'$ are disjoint non-empty subsets of Ω_2; it follows that $1 \neq g_1 \in G_1$ implies $\Omega_1 g_1 < \Omega_2$. It suffices to show that if $w = g_1 g_2 \cdots g_{2n}$ with $1 \neq g_1, g_3, \ldots, g_{2n-1} \in G_1$ and $1 \neq g_2, g_4, \ldots, g_{2n} \in G_2$, for $n \geqslant 1$, then $w \neq 1$. But now we have $\Omega_1 g_1 g_2 < \Omega_2 g_2 \subseteq \Omega_1$, and $\Omega_1 g_{2i-1} g_{2i} < \Omega_1$, whence it follows by induction that $\Omega_1 w < \Omega_1$ and $w \neq 1$. If $|G_1| = 1$ or $|G_2| = 1$, the assertion is trivial. The case remains that $G_1 = \{1, a\}$ and $G_2 = \{1, b\}$, with $a^2 = b^2 = 1$. Any further relation n can be supposed of the form $(ab)^n = 1$. If no such relation occurs $G = C_2 * C_2$, the infinite dihedral group. If $(ab)^n = 1$ for some least $n \geqslant 1$, G is the finite dihedral group of order $2n$. □

We remark that, as a converse to (12.2), if $G = G_1 * G_2$, then, under the regular representation of G by right multiplication on $\Omega = G$, sets satisfying the condition of this proposition can be found. Indeed, we can take Ω_1 to consist of all non-trivial elements w of G whose normal form ends in a factor from G_2, and Ω_2 that of all $w \neq 1$ ending in a factor from G_1. Similar remarks apply to the generalizations of (12.2) mentioned below.

To illustrate the application of this theorem, we derive a theorem of Sanov (1947).

Proposition 12.3. *The matrices $A = \begin{pmatrix} 1 & 2 \\ 0 & 1 \end{pmatrix}$ and $B = \begin{pmatrix} 1 & 0 \\ 2 & 1 \end{pmatrix}$ over $\mathbb{Z}$ are a basis for a free group.*

□ The group $G = \mathrm{Gp}\{A, B\}$ is a subgroup of $H = \mathrm{Gp}\{A, J\}$ where $J = \begin{pmatrix} 0 & 1 \\ 1 & 0 \end{pmatrix}$, and $B = JAJ$. We must show that $A^{m_1}B^{n_1} \cdots A^{m_k}B^{n_k} \neq 1$ provided that $k \geqslant 1$ and all $m_i, n_i \neq 0$. This comes to showing that $A^{p_1}JA^{p_2}J \cdots JA^{p_n} \neq 1$ provided $n \geqslant 1$ and all $p_i \neq 0$. Let H act as a group of linear fractional transformations on the Riemann sphere $\mathbb{C}^* = \mathbb{C} \cup \{\infty\}$, with $zA = z + 2$ and $zJ = 1/z$. Let $\Omega_1 = \{z: |z| < 1\}$ and $\Omega_2 = \{z: |z| > 1\}$. Then $\Omega_1 A^p \leqslant \Omega_2$ for $p \neq 0$, and $\Omega_2 J \leqslant \Omega_1$. By (12.2), H is the free product of the infinite cyclic group H_1 generated by A and the group $H_2 = \{1, J\}$. The conclusion follows. □

The argument just given serves as well to show that $G(\lambda)$ generated by $A = \begin{pmatrix} 1 & \lambda \\ 0 & 1 \end{pmatrix}$ and $B = \begin{pmatrix} 1 & 0 \\ \lambda & 1 \end{pmatrix}$, for any $\lambda \in \mathbb{C}$ such that $|\lambda| \geqslant 2$, has a basis of the two elements A and B. Beginning with the result of Sanov, arguments of this sort were refined successively by Brenner (1955), Chang, Jennings, and Ree (1958), and Lyndon and Ullman (1969) to show that the same conclusion holds for λ in a substantially larger region in $\mathbb{C}^*$, although the regions obtained are clearly not best possible. It follows immediately from (12.3) that $G(\lambda)$ is free if λ is transcendental, or algebraic with a conjugate λ' such that $|\lambda'| \geqslant 2$; on the other hand, a few algebraic numbers λ are known for which $G(\lambda)$ is not free. But it is not known, for example, if there exists any rational λ, with $0 < |\lambda| < 2$, such that $G(\lambda)$ is free. The values $\lambda = 3/2, 4/3, 5/3, 5/4$ (and their submultiples) were excluded by Lyndon and Ullman (1969), the value 7/4 by Conway and Brenner independently, the value 8/5 by Brenner (all unpublished).

The question of which pairs of elements of $\mathbb{PSL}(2, \mathbb{R})$ generate discontinuous groups, free products, or free groups has been examined also by Fouxe-Rabinovitch (1949), Newman (1966), Purzitsky-Rosenberger (1972), Rosenberger (1972), Wamsley (1973), Charnow (1974). For free subgroups of linear groups see Doniakhi (1940), De Groot (1956), Swierczkowski (1958), Tits (1972), Wehrfritz (1973). For free subgroups of small cancellation groups see Collins (1973).

Macbeath's result (12.2) as well as analogous results for free products with amalgamation and for HNN-extensions seems to have been found independently by Maskit (1965, 1968; see 1971). His theorems have topological conditions in both hypothesis and conclusion; we state below versions in which these considerations have been omitted.

Proposition 12.4. *Let a group G be generated by two of its subgroups, G_1 and G_2, with intersection $G_1 \cap G_2 = H$. We assume that H is a proper subgroup of both G_1, and G_2, and does not have index 2 in both. Let G act on a set Ω, and let Ω_1 and Ω_2 be disjoint non-empty subsets of Ω. We assume that*

(1) $\Omega_1(G_1 - H) \subseteq \Omega_2, \quad \Omega_2(G_2 - H) \subseteq \Omega_1;$
(2) $\Omega_1 H \subseteq \Omega_1, \quad \Omega_2 H \subseteq \Omega_2.$

Then $G = G_1 \ast_H G_2$, the free product of G_1 and G_2 with H amalgamated.

□ Suppose that $|G_1 : H| > 2$. If $g \in G_1 - H$, then there exists $f \in G_1$ such that the cosets H, Hg, Hf, are distinct, and hence $gf^{-1} \in G_1 - H$. By (1), $\Omega_1 g, \Omega_1 f, \Omega_1 gf^{-1} \subseteq \Omega_2$, whence $\Omega_1 g \subseteq \Omega_2 f$. Since $\Omega_1 \cap \Omega_2 = \emptyset$, $\Omega_1 f \cap \Omega_1 f = \emptyset$, and therefore $\Omega_1 g \cap \Omega_1 f = \emptyset$. Since $\Omega_1 f \neq \emptyset$, $\Omega_1 g < \Omega_2$. If $|G_2 \colon H| > 2$ we reason similarly. We conclude thus that either $g \in G_1 - H$ implies $\Omega_1 g < \Omega_2$ or $g \in G_2 - H$ implies $\Omega_2 g < \Omega_1$.

It suffices to show that if $w = hg_1 g_2 \cdots g_n$ where $h \in H$ and the g_i are alternately from $G_1 - H$ and $G_2 - H$, with $h \neq 1$ if $n = 0$, then $w \neq 1$. The case $n \leqslant 2$ follows from the definition of H. We assume $n \geqslant 2$ and, without loss of generality, that $g_1, g_3, \ldots \in G_1 - H$ and $g_2, g_4, \ldots \in G_2 - H$. By (1) and (2) we have $\Omega_2 H \subseteq \Omega_2$, $\Omega_2 g_1 \subseteq \Omega_1$, $\Omega_1 g_2 \subseteq \Omega_2$, where one of the latter two inclusions is proper; thus we have $\Omega_2 hg_1 g_2 < \Omega_1$. Inductively, if $\Omega_2 hg_1 \cdots g_{2m} < \Omega_1$ then $\Omega_2 hg_1 \cdots g_{2m+1} < \Omega_2$, and if $\Omega_2 hg_1 \cdots g_{2m+1} < \Omega_2$ then $\Omega_2 hg_1 \cdots g_{2m+2} < \Omega_1$. Thus $\Omega_2 w < \Omega_1$ or $\Omega_2 w < \Omega_2$; in either case $\Omega_2 w \neq \Omega_2$, whence $w \neq 1$. □

Proposition 12.5. *Let G be a group of permutations of a set Ω, generated by a subgroup G_0 of G together with an element f of G. Let H_{+1} be a subgroup of G_0 such that $H_{-1} = fH_{+1}f^{-1}$ is also contained in G_0. Assume that Ω is the disjoint union of non-empty sets Ω_{-1}, Ω_0, and Ω_{+1}, such that*

(1) $(\Omega_0 \cup \Omega_\sigma)f^\sigma \subseteq \Omega_\sigma$, $\sigma = \pm 1$
(2) *$g \in G_0$ and $g \notin H_\sigma$ implies $\Omega_\sigma g \subseteq \Omega_0$, $\sigma = \pm 1$.*

Then G is an HNN-extension of G_0 by the isomorphism from H_{+1} to H_{-1} effected by conjugation by f.

□ (We remark that either of the two cases of (1) implies the other.) Let $\tilde{G}$ be the indicated HNN-extension; then $\tilde{G}$ maps onto G and so acts on Ω, and we must show that $\tilde{G}$ acts faithfully. Now every non-trivial element of G is conjugate to a word w of one of the forms $w = g \in G_0$, $w = f^a$, or $w = f_1^{a_1} g_1 \cdots f_n^{a_n} g_n$ for $n \geqslant 1$, $a_1 \neq 0$, and $g_i \in G_0$, $g_i \notin H_{\sigma_i}$ where $\sigma_i = a_i/|a_i| = \mathrm{Sgn}(a_i)$.

If $w = g \neq 1$, then w acts faithfully since G_0 acts faithfully. We observe next that if $a \neq 0$, and $\sigma = \mathrm{Sgn}(a)$, then $\emptyset \neq \Omega_0 f^\sigma$, $\Omega_\sigma f^\sigma \subseteq \Omega_\sigma$, and $\Omega_0 f^\sigma \cap \Omega_\sigma f^\sigma = \emptyset$, whence $\Omega_0 f^\sigma < \Omega_\sigma$. Thus $\Omega_0 f^a = \Omega_0 f^\sigma f^{a-\sigma} < \Omega_\sigma f^{a-\sigma} \subseteq \Omega_\sigma$. If $w = f^a$, this proves that w does not act trivially on Ω. In the remaining case, $\Omega_0 f^{a_i} < \Omega_{\sigma_i}$ and, by (2), $\Omega_0 f^{a_i} g_i < \Omega_i g_i \subseteq \Omega_0$. By induction $\Omega_0 w < \Omega_0$, whence w does not act trivially. □

We remark that similar ideas appear in Kalme (1969) and Tits (1969); see also Tukia (1972). The concept of bipolar structure (see IV.6 below) introduced by Stallings (1965; see also 1971) is closely related. In view of (12.4) and (12.5) on the one hand and Stallings' result (1968; 1971) on the other, it is not difficult in the two cases of a free product with amalgamation and of an HNN-extension to define the sets occurring in the hypotheses of (12.4) and (12.5) in terms of those appearing in the definition of a bipolar structure, and conversely. The chief virtue of the concept of bipolar structure seems then to be that it treats the naturally related cases of free product with amalgamation and HNN-extension uniformly.

Swan (1971) uses fundamental regions to obtain generators and relations for groups $\mathbb{SL}(2, \mathbb{Q}\sqrt{-m})$.

13. Behr Graphs

Behr (1962) has given a graph-theoretic method for studying the structure of groups which is closely related to coset diagrams, and in its main applications, comes to a study of coset diagrams. It is very closely related to ideas of Serre (1969). After presenting Behr's general result, we shall describe his chief application, and shall mention its use by Behr (1967), Behr and Mennicke (1968), and Serre (1969) in the study the general linear groups $\mathbb{GL}(n, R)$ over certain rings R.

The concept of a *distance function* or metric on a set V is standard; d is a function $d: V \times V \to \mathbb{R}$ satisfying the following axioms:

(1) $d(u, v) \geqslant 0$ with $d(u, v) = 0$ iff $u = v$;
(2) $d(u, v) = d(v, u)$;
(3) $d(u, v) + d(v, w) \geqslant d(u, w)$.

For $v \in V$ and $r \in \mathbb{R}$, the *ball* at v with radius r is $S_r(v) = \{u: d(u, v) \leqslant r\}$.

We now state Behr's (1962) basic result.

Proposition 13.1. *Let V be a set and d an integer valued distance function on V. We assume the following*

(I) *for all $v \in V$ and all $l \geqslant 1$, the ball $S_l(v)$ is finite;*

(II) *there exists $k \geqslant 1$ such that for all $v \in V$ and all $l \geqslant 1$, if $p, q \in S_l(v)$ then for some n there exist $p_0 = p, p_1, \ldots, p_n = q$ in $S_l(v)$ such that $d(p_0, q) > d(p_1, q) > \cdots > d(p_n, q) = 0$, and that $d(p_0, p_1), d(p_1, p_2), \ldots, d(p_{n-1}, p_n) \leqslant k$.*

Let G be a group acting transitively on V and preserving distance: for $u, v \in V$ and $g \in G$, $d(ug, vg) = d(u, v)$. Then if the stabilizer H in G of some vertex v has a finite presentation, G itself has a finite presentation.

Before proving this proposition we try to clarify the ideas by stating an important special case. Let C be a graph. We will assume that C is *locally finite*, that is, there are only finitely many edges at each vertex. We define the *distance* $d(u, v)$ between two vertices to be the length of the shortest path between them, and we call such a path of shortest length a *geodesic*. We call C *locally convex* if every ball $S_n(v)$ about a vertex v with radius n has the property that every pair of points in $S_n(v)$ is joined by some geodesic contained in $S_n(v)$.

Proposition 13.2. *Let C be a locally finite and locally convex graph and G a group acting on the vertices and edges of C in a manner that preserves incidence and is transitive on the vertices. Then, if the stabilizer of a vertex in G has a finite presentation, G itself has a finite presentation.* □

□ We turn now to a proof of (13.1). We choose a vertex $o \in V$, and let H be the stabilizer of o. We assume that H has a finite presentation $H = (X_0; R_0)$ where $X_0 = X_0^{-1}$ is a symmetrized basis for a free group F_0. Now $S_k(o)$ is finite, and, since G acts transitively, there is a finite set of g carrying o into all $og = v$ in $S_k(o)$. We take X_1 to consist of such a set of g together with their inverses, and containing 1. We next prove three lemmas and a corollary.

Lemma A. *$X = X_0 \cup X_1$ generates G.*

□ We must show, for arbitrary $g \in G$, that $g \in G_0 = \mathrm{Gp}(X)$. Without invoking the full force of (II) we conclude that there exist $p_0 = o, p_1, \ldots, p_n = og$ such that all $d(p_i, p_{i+1}) \leqslant k$. By transitivity of G, we may write each $p_i = og_i$ with $g_0 = 1$ and $g_n = g$. Now $d(og_i, og_{i+1}) \leqslant k$ implies, by invariance of distance, that $d(o, og_{i+1}g_i^{-1}) \leqslant k$, whence $og_{i+1}g_i^{-1} \in S_k(o)$; now $og_{i+1}g_i^{-1} = ox$ for some $x \in X_1$, and $g_{i+1}g_i^{-1} = hx$ for some h in the stabilizer H of o. Thus $g_{i+1}g_i^{-1} \in G_0$. It follows that $(g_0g_1^{-1}) \cdots (g_{n-1}g_n^{-1}) = g_0g_n = g$ lies in G_0. This establishes Lemma A. □

Let w be a word of length $|w| \leqslant 3k + 3$ in X that represents an element $h \in H$. We choose a word w_0 in X_0 representing h. Let R_1 consist of a finite set of words ww_0^{-1} associated thus with the finite set of such words w. Let $R = R_0 \cup R_1$. We shall show that $G = (X; R)$.

Lemma B. *For $v \in V$ and $g_1, \ldots, g_n \in G$,*

$$d(v, vg_1 \cdots g_n) \leqslant \textstyle\sum_{i=1}^n d(v, vg_i).$$

□ To prove this we observe first that $d(v, vg_1 \cdots g_n) \leqslant d(v, vg_n) + d(vg_n, vg_1 \cdots g_n)$, and that $d(vg_n, vg_1 \cdots g_n) = d(v, vg_1 \cdots g_{n-1})$. By induction on n we may suppose that $d(v, vg_1 \cdots g_{n-1}) \leqslant \sum_{i=1}^{n-1} d(v, vg_i)$, which establishes the result. □

Lemma C. *Let g be a word in X of length s, let $v \in V$, and $u = vg$. Then there exist, for some n, elements $x_i, \ldots, x_n \in X$, such that $gx_1 \cdots x_n = 1$, that $x_i \in X_0$ for $i > sk$, and such that, for $0 \leqslant i \leqslant n$, $d(o, ux_1 \cdots x_i) \leqslant \max\{d(o, v), d(o, u)\}$.*

□ To begin the proof we let $p = og$ and $l = \max\{d(o, v), d(o, u)\}$. Then o and p lie in $S_l(u)$, and by (II) there exist $p_0 = o, p_1, \ldots, p_m = p$ in $S_l(u)$, for some $m \leqslant d(o, p)$, such that all $d(p_i, p_{i+1}) \leqslant k$. We propose to choose inductively elements $g_0 = 1, g_1, \ldots, g_m$ such that $p_i = og_i$ and that $g_i^{-1} = g_{i-1}^{-1}x_i$ with $x_i \in X_1$. To show this possible, suppose $g_0, \ldots, g_{i-1}$ already chosen for some $i \leqslant m$. Now $p_i = og'$ for some $g' \in G$, with $d(o, og'g_{i-1}^{-1}) = d(og_{i-1}, og') = d(p_{i-1}, p_i) \leqslant k$. Thus $og'g_{i-1}^{-1} \in S_k(o)$ and hence $og'g_{i-1}^{-1} = ox_i^{-1}$ for some $x_i \in X_1$. Thus $g'g_{i-1}^{-1} = hx_i^{-1}$ for some $h \in H$. Let $g_i = h^{-1}g'$. Then $og_i = og' = p_i$ and, from $g'g_{i-1} = hx_i^{-1}$ together with $g_i^{-1} = g'^{-1}h$ we have $g_ig_{i-1}^{-1} = x_i^{-1}$.

Now, for each i, $g_i^{-1} = x_1 \cdots x_i$, and in particular, $g_m^{-1} = x_1 \cdots x_m$. Thus $og = p = p_m = og_m$ and $ogg_m^{-1} = o$, whence $gg_m^{-1} = h \in H$ and $gx_1 \cdots x_m = h$. Now $h^{-1} = x_{m+1} \cdots x_n$ for some $x_{m+1}, \ldots, x_n \in X_0$, and we have $gx_1 \cdots x_n = 1$. If $g = y_1 \cdots y_s$ for some $y_i \in X$, each $d(o, oy_i) \leqslant k$, and, by the preceding lemma we have $d(o, p) = d(o, oy_1 \cdots y_s) \leqslant \sum_{i-1}^s d(o, oy_i) \leqslant ks$; thus $m \leqslant ks$ and thus $i > ks$ implies $x_i \in X_0$.

Since $d(o, v) = d(og, vg) = d(p, u)$, we have $\max\{d(o, v), d(o, u)\} = l$, and it remains to show that all $d(o, ux_1 \cdots x_i) \leqslant l$. If $o \leqslant i \leqslant m$, then $d(o, vx_1 \cdots x_i) = d(o, vg_i^{-1}) = d(og_i, v) = d(p_i, r) \leqslant l$ since $p_i \in S_l(v)$. If $m \leqslant i \leqslant n$, then $x_1 \cdots x_i = (x_1 \cdots x_m)(x_{m+1} \cdots x_i) = g_m^{-1}h$ for some $h \in H$, and $d(o, vx_1 \cdots x_i) = d(o, vg_m^{-1}h) = d(oh^{-1}, vg_m^{-1}) = d(o, vx_1 \cdots x_m) \leqslant l$. □

Corollary D. *Let g be a word in X of length $|g| = s \leqslant 3$, let $v \in V$ and $u = vg$. Then, modulo the normal closure N of R in F, free with basis X, there holds a relation $g = x_1 \cdots x_n$, $x_i \in X$, such that all $d(o, vx_1 \cdots x_i) \leqslant \max\{d(o, v), d(o, u)\}$.* □

We turn now to complete the proof of Proposition (13.1). Let $w = a_1 \cdots a_n$ be a word in X that represents the element 1 of G. We must show that $w \in N$. With w we associate a sequence W of points, $p_0 = 0, p_1 = oa_1, \ldots, p_i = oa_1 \cdots a_i, \ldots, p_n = 0$. We argue by induction on $\delta = \max\{d(o, p_i), 0 \leqslant i \leqslant n\}$.

Case 1. $\delta \leqslant k$. For each i, $d(o, p_i) \leqslant k$ implies that $p_i = ox_i$ for some $x_i \in X_1$, where we may choose $x_0 = 1$ and $x_n = 1$. Let $b_i = x_{i-1}a_ix_i^{-1}$: then $ob_i = oa_1 \cdots a_{i-1}a_i = p_i = o$ implies that $ou_i = o$, whence $u_i \in H$. Since $R_0 \leqslant N$, modulo N we have $u_i \equiv \bar{u}_i$ for some $\bar{u}_i$ a word in X_0; thus $w = u_1 \cdots u_n \equiv \bar{u}_1 \cdots \bar{u}_n$. But if w represents 1 in G so does $\bar{u}_1 \cdots \bar{u}_n$, whence $\bar{u}_1 \cdots \bar{u}_n$ as a relator among the generators X_0 for H, is a consequence of R_0, and therefore $\bar{u}_1 \cdots \bar{u}_n \equiv 1$ (modulo N) and so $w \equiv 1$ (modulo N).

Case 2. $\delta > k$. With each p_i we associate some $x_i \in X_1$ and $p_i' = p_ix_i^{-1}$ such that $d(o, p_i') < \delta$. If $d(o, p_i) < \delta$, we simply take $p_i = 1$ and $p_i' = p_i$. Otherwise $d(o, p_i) = \delta$, and, by (II), there exists some q with $d(o, q) \leqslant k$ and $d(q, p_i) < d(o, p_i)$. Now $q = ox_i$ for some $x_i \in X_1$; define $p_i' = p_ix_i^{-1}$. Then $d(o, p_i') = d(o, p_ix_i^{-1}) = d(ox_i, p_i) = d(q, p_i) < d(o, p_i) = \delta$, whence $d(o, p_i') < \delta$.

By the corollary, since each $p_i' = p_{i-1}'x_{i-1}a_ix_i^{-1}$, writing $g_i = x_{i-1}a_ix_i^{-1}$, we have, modulo N, a relation $g_i = x_{i1} \cdots x_{it_i}$ with all $x_{ij} \in X$ and all $d(o, p_{i-1}'x_{i1} \cdots x_{ij}) \leqslant \max\{d(o, p_{i-1}'), d(o, p_i')\} < \delta$. If we write $y_1, \ldots, y_m$ for the sequence $x_{11}, \ldots, x_{1t_1}, \ldots, x_{n1}, \ldots, x_{nt_n}$ then we have $w \equiv w'$ (modulo N) where $w' = y_1 \cdots y_m$. But, by the above construction, all the $d(o, oy_1 \cdots y_j) < \delta$, whence it follows by the induction on δ that $w' \equiv 1$ (modulo N). □

We now describe one of Behr's principal applications of this method, simplified, however, by restriction to the case of the ring $\mathbb{Z}$ of integers in the particular field $\mathbb{Q}$, and of a single prime $p \in \mathbb{Z}$, and to the particular algebraic group $\mathbb{SL}(n, R)$ where R is the ring of all rationals of the form a/p^k, for $a, k \in \mathbb{Z}$. Let $M = R^n$, and $o = \mathbb{Z}^n$, viewed as $\mathbb{Z}$-submodule of M. Now $G = \mathbb{SL}(n, R)$ acts naturally on M, and for each $g \in G$, og is a $\mathbb{Z}$-submodule of M, isomorphic to o. We let V be the set of these og for all $g \in G$. By this definition G acts transitively on V, and V is the set of all $\mathbb{Z}$-submodules of M of rank n. The stabilizer of o in G is evidently $H = \mathbb{SL}(n, \mathbb{Z})$, viewed as a subgroup of G.

For each pair of elements u and v in V, it is easy to see that there is a least $e \geqslant 0$ such that $p^eu \leqslant v$; we take this e for $d_1(u, v)$. If $n > 2$, we need not have $d_1(u, v) = d_1(v, u)$; to remedy this we define $d(u, v) = \min\{d_1(u, v), d_1(v, u)\}$. It is clear that d is a distance function of V, invariant under G, and that (I) holds; Behr shows also that (II) holds, with $k = 1$.

For $n = 2$, H is well known to have a finite presentation, $H = (a, b; a^2 = b^3, a^4 = 1)$ (see I.4.5), and it follows that G has a finite presentation. Moreover, it is in principal possible to calculate the generators and relators for G given by the proof of (13.1). Even in the simplest cases this calculation, followed routinely, becomes unwieldy, but, by ingenuity, Behr and Mennicke (1968) have used it to obtain reasonably simple presentations of these groups.

The case $n = 2$ has been extensively studied, especially by Serre (1969). An immediate simplification is that d_1 is already symmetric, whence $d = d_1$; this comes from the fact that by change of basis for both u and v we can always arrive at the case that u has a basis $\{\alpha, \beta\}$ and v a basis $\{p^d\alpha, p^{-d}\beta\}$ for $d = d(u, v)$. One has also then that the sequence $u_0 = u, u_1, \ldots, u_d = v$; where u_i has basis $\{p^i\alpha, p^{-i}\beta\}$, is a geodesic from u to v; this shows that V is connected.

Serre makes slightly different definitions, using $\mathbb{GL}(2, R)$ where we have used $\mathbb{SL}(2, R)$ above, using a vertex set V^* consisting of equivalence classes o^* of modules $o\lambda$ where λ runs through the non-zero scalars, and defining the distance between u^* and v^*, where u has basis $\{\alpha, \beta\}$ and v basis $\{p^a\alpha, p^b\beta\}$ to be $d^*(u^*, v^*) = |a - b|$. With these definitions he shows that V^* is a tree, with d^* the path distance on V^*. He goes on to study V^* and the action of G^*, showing that the induced action of certain subgroups of G^*, including $\mathbb{SL}(2, R)$, on V^* is in accordance with his general theory of groups acting on trees. For such groups he deduces from his general theory that, if u^*, v^* are two vertices of V^* joined by an edge u^*v^*, then G^* is the free product of the two vertex stabilizers G_{u^*} and G_{v^*} with the edge stabilizer $G_{u^*v^*}$ amalgamated.

Serre uses this in the cases $p = 2$ and $p = 3$ to recover the finite presentations for $\mathbb{SL}(2, R)$ obtained by Behr and Mennicke (1968).

This can be viewed as a generalization of the fact that $\mathbb{SL}(2, \mathbb{Z})$ is the free product of cyclic groups C_4 and C_6 with a cyclic group C_2 amalgamated. Serre's result, in the special case to which we have confined attention, is contained in one due to Ihara (1966).

Proposition 13.3. *Let p be a prime and R be the ring of rationals of the form a/p^k, for $a, k \in \mathbb{Z}$. Let H be the group of all matrices $\begin{pmatrix} a & b \\ c & d \end{pmatrix}$ with integer entries, determinant* 1, *and with $c \equiv 0$ (modulo p), viewed as a subgroup of $\mathbb{SL}(2, \mathbb{Z})$. Then $\mathbb{SL}(2, R)$ is the free product of two replicas of $\mathbb{SL}(2, \mathbb{Z})$ with corresponding subgroups H amalgamated.* □

A related result obtained by Serre using these methods is due to Nagao (1959).

Proposition 13.4. *Let F be a field and $F[t]$ the ring of polynomials in one indeterminate t over F. Let $T(F)$ be the group of all nonsingular matrices $\begin{pmatrix} a & b \\ c & d \end{pmatrix}$ over F with $c = 0$, viewed as a subgroup of $\mathbb{GL}(2, F)$ and also of $\mathbb{GL}(2, F[t])$. Let $T(F[t])$ be the analogous subgroup of $\mathbb{GL}(2, F[t])$. Then $\mathbb{GL}(2, F[t])$ is the free product of replicas of $\mathbb{GL}(2, F)$ and $T(F[t])$ with the corresponding subgroups $T(F)$ identified.* □

For a brief exposition of $\mathbb{SL}_2$ of local fields, and one of Serre's treatment of groups acting on trees, see Bass (1973). For a result related to (13.3) and (13.4), see (IV.6.9) below.

Chapter IV. Free Products and HNN Extensions

1. Free Products

In this chapter we will study the definitions, properties, and applications of the products of groups which are basic to doing combinatorial group theory. We begin with a study of free products.

Definition. Let A and B be groups with presentations $A = \langle a_1, \ldots ; r_1, \ldots \rangle$ and $B = \langle b_1, \ldots ; s_1, \ldots \rangle$ respectively, where the sets of generators $\{a_1, \ldots\}$ and $\{b_1, \ldots\}$ are disjoint. The *free product*, $A * B$, of the groups A and B is the group

$$(1) \qquad A * B = \langle a_1, \ldots, b_1, \ldots ; r_1, \ldots, s_1, \ldots \rangle.$$

The groups A and B are called the *factors* of $A * B$. We next see that the free product is independent of the choice of the presentations chosen for A and B.

Lemma 1.1. *The free product $A * B$ is uniquely determined by the groups A and B. Also, $A * B$ is generated by subgroups $\bar{A}$ and $\bar{B}$ which are isomorphic to A and B respectively, and such that $\bar{A} \cap \bar{B} = 1$.*

□ Let $A' = \langle a'_1, \ldots ; r'_1, \ldots \rangle$ and $B' = \langle b'_1, \ldots ; s'_1, \ldots \rangle$ also be disjoint presentations of A and B respectively, and let

$$(2) \qquad A' * B' = \langle a'_1, \ldots, b'_1, \ldots ; r'_1, \ldots, s'_1, \ldots \rangle.$$

Let $\psi : A \to A'$ and $\chi : B \to B'$ be isomorphisms. The map $\psi * \chi : A * B \to A * B'$ defined by $a_i \mapsto \psi(a_i)$ and $b_j \mapsto \chi(b_j)$ is a homomorphism since relators go to relators. The map $\psi^{-1} * \chi^{-1}$ defined by $a'_i \mapsto \psi^{-1}(a'_i)$ and $b'_j \mapsto \chi^{-1}(b'_j)$ is the inverse of $\psi * \chi$, establishing $A' * B' \simeq A * B$. Let $\bar{A}$ be the subgroup of $A * B$ generated by the a_i, and let $\bar{B}$ be the subgroup of $A * B$ generated by the b_j. Certainly, $A * B$ is generated by $\bar{A}$ and $\bar{B}$. To show $A \simeq \bar{A}$, map A to $\bar{A}$ by $\eta : a_i \mapsto a_i$. The *projection* π_A of $A * B$ onto A defined by $a_i \mapsto a_i$, $b_j \mapsto 1$ has $\pi_A \eta$ the identity on A. Hence, $A \simeq \bar{A}$, and similarly, $B \simeq \bar{B}$. Since $\pi_A \eta$ maps all elements of $\bar{B}$ to 1, we have $\bar{A} \cap \bar{B} = \{1\}$. In view of the above isomorphisms, we identify A with $\bar{A}$ and B with $\bar{B}$ and consider A and B as subgroups of $A * B$. □

We have chosen to work with two factors simply for convenience of notation. If $\{A_i: i \in I\}$ is any family of groups, we define the free product of the A_i, written $*A_i$, to be the group with presentation the union of disjoint presentations of the A_i. As above, the free product $P = *A_i$ is independent of the presentations chosen, and the other conclusions of Lemma 1.1 hold.

From the theorem on defining homomorphisms on presentations, it follows immediately that the free product $P = *A_i$ has the following mapping property.

1. There is a fixed family of homomorphisms $\{\eta_i: i \in I\}$ where $\eta_i: A_i \to P$ such that the $\bigcup_{i \in I} \eta_i(A_i)$ generates P.

2. For any group G and any family $\{f_i: i \in I\}$ of homomorphisms where $f_i: A_i \to G$, there is a homomorphism $\psi: P \to G$ such that the diagram

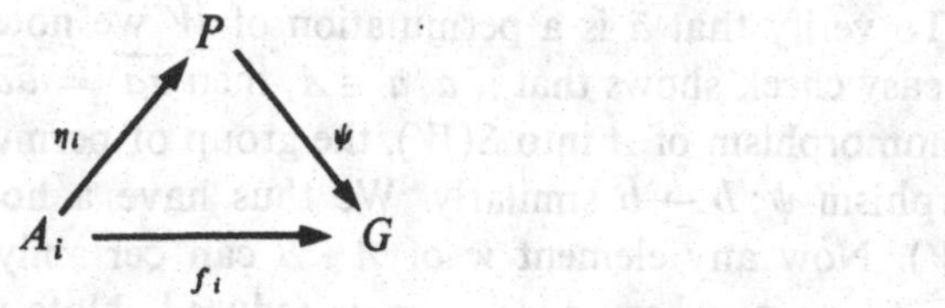

commutes for all $i \in I$.

It follows from general principles that any two groups possessing the above mapping property are isomorphic. The mapping property is thus often taken as the definition of the free product. In the language of category theory, the free product is the coproduct in the category of groups.

We turn to the basic theorem about free products.

Definition. A *reduced sequence* (or *normal form*) is a sequence $g_1, \ldots, g_n$, $n \geqslant 0$, of elements of $A * B$ such that each $g_i \neq 1$, each g_i is in one of the factors, A or B, and successive g_i, g_{i+1} are not in the same factor. (We allow $n = 0$ for the empty sequence).

Example. If $A * B = \langle a, b; a^7, b^5 \rangle$, the sequence a^5, b^3, a^2, b is reduced while the sequences a, b^5, a and a^2, a^3, b^3 are not reduced.

The basic theorem about free products is

Theorem 1.2. (The Normal Form Theorem for Free Products)

Consider the free product $A * B$. Then the following two equivalent statements hold.

(I) *If $w = g_1, \ldots, g_n$, $n > 0$, where $g_1, \ldots, g_n$ is a reduced sequence, then $w \neq 1$ in $A * B$.*

(II) *Each element w of $A * B$ can be uniquely expressed as a product $w = g_1 \cdots g_n$ where $g_1, \ldots, g_n$ is a reduced sequence.*

□ First of all, we show that statements (I) and (II) are equivalent. In statement (II), it is understood that 1 is the product of the elements in the empty sequence. Hence, (II) implies (I) is immediate. Assume that statement (I) holds. Let $w = g_1 \cdots g_n$ and $w = h_1, \ldots, h_m$ be reduced. Then $1 = g_1 \cdots g_n h_m^{-1} \cdots h_1^{-1}$. In order for the sequence $g_1, \ldots, g_n, h_m^{-1}, \ldots, h_1^{-1}$ not to be reduced, it is necessary that h_m be in the same factor as g_n. For the sequence $g_1, \ldots, g_{n-1}, g_n h_m^{-1}, h_{m-1}^{-1}, \ldots, h_1^{-1}$

not to be reduced it is necessary that $g_n h_m^{-1} = 1$, i.e., $h_m = g_n$. An induction argument gives $m = n$ and $h_i = g_i$, $i = 1, \ldots, n$.

We prove the theorem by using a homomorphism into a permutation group. (This idea is due to Artin (1947) and van der Waerden (1948).) Let W be the set of all reduced sequences from $A * B$. For each element $a \in A$, define a permutation $\bar{a}$ of W as follows. If $a = 1$, $\bar{a}$ is the identity. If $a \neq 1$ and $(g_1, \ldots, g_n)$ is a reduced sequence then

$$\bar{a}((g_1, \ldots, g_n)) = \begin{cases} (a, g_1, \ldots, g_n) & \text{if } g_1 \in B \\ (ag_1, \ldots, g_n) & \text{if } g_1 \in A, ag_1 \neq 1 \\ (g_2, \ldots, g_n) & \text{if } g_1 = a^{-1}. \end{cases}$$

To verify that $\bar{a}$ is a permutation of W we note that $\overline{a^{-1}}$ is the inverse of $\bar{a}$. An easy check shows that if $a, a' \in A$, then $\overline{aa'} = \bar{a}\bar{a}'$. The map $\phi: a \to \bar{a}$ is thus a homomorphism of A into $S(W)$, the group of permutations of W. Define a homomorphism $\psi: b \to \bar{b}$ similarly. We thus have a homomorphism $\phi * \psi: A * B \to S(W)$. Now any element w of $A * B$ can certainly be written as some product $w = g_1 \cdots g_n$ where $g_1, \ldots, g_n$ is reduced. Note that the permutation $\phi * \psi(w)$ sends the empty sequence to the sequence $(g_1, \ldots, g_n)$. Thus $w \neq 1$ if $n > 0$. □

The Normal Form Theorem allows us to define a length for elements of free products. If an element w of $G = A * B$ has normal form $g_1 \cdots g_n$ then the *length* of w, written $|w|$, is defined to be n. If $u(a_i, b_j)$ is a non-empty word on the a_i's and b_j's we can write $u = u_1 \cdots u_k$ where each u_i is a word on the a_i's alone or the b_j's alone, no u_i is empty (although it may equal 1 in G), and u_i and u_{i+1} are not both in the same factor of G. The subwords $u_1, \ldots, u_k$ are called the *syllables* of u. Clearly, $k \geqslant |u|$.

As an immediate corollary of the Normal Form Theorem we have

Corollary 1.3. *If A and B are both finitely generated groups with solvable word problem, then $A * B$ has solvable word problem.* □

Let u and v be elements of $A * B$ with normal forms $u = g_1 \cdots g_n$ and $v = h_1 \cdots h_k$. If g_n and h_1 are in different factors, the product uv has normal form $g_1 \cdots g_n h_1 \cdots h_k$. If $h_1 = g_n^{-1}$ we say that h_1 and g_n are *cancelled* in forming the product uv. After some number of cancellations we may arrive at $g_1 \cdots g_i h_j \cdots h_k$ where g_i and h_j are in the same factor but $h_j \neq g_i^{-1}$. We say that g_i and h_j are *consolidated* in forming the normal form of uv.

An element w of $A * B$ with normal form $w = g_1 \cdots g_n$ is called *cyclically reduced* if g_n and g_1 are in different factors or if $n \leqslant 1$. "Cyclically reduced" requires that there is neither cancellation nor consolidation between g_n and g_1 if $n > 1$. We call $g_1 \cdots g_n$ *weakly cyclically reduced* if $g_n \neq g_1^{-1}$ or $n \leqslant 1$. This definition allows g_n and g_1 to be in the same factor but requires that they do not cancel if $n > 1$.

The situation regarding conjugacy in free products is very similar to that in free groups. We have

Theorem 1.4. (The Conjugacy Theorem for Free Products) *Each element of $A * B$*

is conjugate to a cyclically reduced element. If $u = g_1 \cdots g_n$ and $v = h_1 \cdots h_m$ are cyclically reduced elements which are conjugate in $A * B$ and $n > 1$, then $m = n$ and the sequences $g_1, \ldots, g_n$ and $h_1, \ldots, h_m$ are cyclic permutations of each other. If $n \leqslant 1$, then $m = n$, and u and v are in the same factor and are conjugate in that factor.

□ It is clear that any element is conjugate to a cyclically reduced element. If u and v are conjugate cyclically reduced elements, let $u = cvc^{-1}$ and argue by induction on $|c|$. If $|c| = 0$, the result follows from the Normal Form Theorem. Suppose $c = c_1 \cdots c_k$ in reduced form, $k \geqslant 1$. Note that the equation

$$g_1 \cdots g_n = c_1 \cdots c_k h_1 \cdots h_m c_k^{-1} \cdots c_1^{-1}$$

cannot hold if there is not cancellation between either c_k and h_1 or between h_m and c_k^{-1}. (Otherwise $g_1 \cdots g_n$ cannot be cyclically reduced.) Thus if there is cancellation, say between c_k and h_1, we have

$$g_1 \cdots g_n = c_1 \cdots c_{k-1} h_2 \cdots h_m h_1 c_{k-1}^{-1} \cdots c_1^{-1}$$

and the result follows by induction. □

Corollary 1.5. *If A and B are finitely generated groups with solvable conjugacy problem, then $A * B$ has solvable conjugacy problem.* □

Theorem 1.6. (The Torsion Theorem for Free Products) *An element u of finite order in $A * B$ is a conjugate of an element of finite order in a factor of $A * B$.*

□ Let $v = g_1 \cdots g_n$ be a cyclically reduced conjugate of u. If $n > 1$, v^k has normal form $g_1 \cdots g_n \cdots g_1 \cdots g_n \neq 1$. □

The following lemma is similar to the corresponding lemma for direct products.

Lemma 1.7. *Let A and B be subgroups of a group G such that $A \cup B$ generates G, $A \cap B = \{1\}$, and if $g_1, \ldots, g_n$ is a reduced sequence with $n > 0$, then $g_1 \cdots g_n \neq 1$. Then $G \simeq A * B$.*

□ The hypotheses insure that the homomorphism $\phi: A * B \to G$ defined by $a \to a$ and $b \to b$ is an isomorphism. □

Remark. Let $G = A * B$. The set $\{aba^{-1}b^{-1}: 1 \neq a \in A, 1 \neq b \in B\}$ is a basis for a free subgroup of G.

This is easily checked by noting that not too much cancellation can occur. Thus if A has at least two non-trivial elements and $B \neq \{1\}$, the free product $A * B$ contains free subgroups of rank 2 and thus all countable ranks.

The proof we give of the following observation is due to P. M. Neumann. (See D. E. Cohen (1972).)

Observation. *No group G is both a non-trivial free product and a non-trivial direct product.*

□ Suppose that $G = A * B$ where $A \neq \{1\}$ and $B \neq \{1\}$. Let $g = ab$ where

$1 \neq a \in A$ and $1 \neq b \in B$. An easy induction on the length of c shows that if c commutes with g, then c is a power of g. Thus the centralizer C of g is infinite cyclic.

Now suppose that $G = D \times E$ where $D \neq \{1\}$ and $E \neq \{1\}$. Write $g = de$ where $d \in D$ and $e \in E$. The centralizer of g is $H \times K$, where H is the centralizer of d in D and K is the centralizer of e in E. Thus the centralizer C of g is a non-trivial direct product. This is a contradiction since an infinite cyclic group is not a non-trivial direct product. □

Two of the most important theorems about free products are the theorems of Grushko (1940) and Neumann (1943) and that of Kurosh (1934). These theorems are best proved by graph-theoretic arguments. Proofs are given in III.3..

Theorem 1.8. (Grushko-Neumann Theorem) *Let F be a free group, and let ϕ: $F \to *A_i$ be a homomorphism of F onto $*A_i$. Then there is a factorization of F as a free product, $F = *F_i$, such that $\phi(F_i) = A_i$.* □

What one most often uses is the following corollary.

Corollary 1.9. *If $G = A_1 * \cdots * A_n$ and the rank (minimum number of generators) of A_i is r_i, then the rank of G is $r_1 + \cdots + r_n$.*

□ Let $r = \text{rank } G$. Then there is a homomorphism ϕ from the free group F of rank r onto G. By the Grushko-Neumann Theorem, $F = *F_i$ where $\phi(F_i) = A_i$. Hence the rank of each F_i is at least r_i. Since the union of sets of free generators for the F_i is a set of free generators for F, we have $r \geqslant r_1 + \cdots + r_n$. On the other hand, since the A_i generate G, we clearly have $r \leqslant r_1 + \cdots + r_n$. □

Theorem 1.10. (Kurosh Subgroup Theorem) *Let $G = *A_i$, and let H be a subgroup of G. Then H is a free product, $H = F * (*H_j)$ where F is a free group and each H_j is the intersection of H with a conjugate of some factor A_i of G* □

2. Higman-Neumann-Neumann Extensions and Free Products with Amalgmation

In this section we introduce two constructions which are basic to combinatorial group theory. These constructions are the free product with amalgamated subgroup (introduced by Schreier in 1926) and Higman-Neumann-Neumann extensions (introduced by G. Higman, B. H. Neumann, and H. Neumann in 1949). We stress from the outset that these two constructions are very parallel, and are best viewed as each being half of a single basic concept. Indeed, we shall later give a single axiomatization (Stallings' concept of a bipolar structure) of both constructions.

We now define the constructions. Let

$$G = \langle x_1, \ldots; r_1, \ldots \rangle \quad \text{and} \quad H = \langle y_1, \ldots; s_1, \ldots \rangle$$

be groups. Let $A \subseteq G$ and $B \subseteq H$ be subgroups, such that there exists an isomorphism $\phi: A \to B$. Then the *free product of G and H, amalgamating the subgroups A and B by the isomorphism ϕ* is the group

$$\langle x_1, \ldots, y_1, \ldots ; r_1, \ldots, s_1, \ldots, a = \phi(a), a \in A \rangle.$$

We introduce the following convention on notation. If G is a group for which a presentation has been chosen, then by the notation

$$\langle G, z, \ldots ; u, \ldots \rangle$$

we mean the generators and defining relators of G together with whatever additional generators and relators are indicated. Any additional generators are understood to be disjoint from the generators of G. Thus we can write the free product with amalgamation as

$$\langle G * H ; a = \phi(a), a \in A \rangle.$$

We will sometimes write this even more simply as

$$\langle G * H ; A = B, \phi \rangle.$$

The basic idea of the free product with amalgamation is that the subgroup A is identified with its isomorphic image $\phi(A) \subseteq H$. The free product with amalgamation depends on G, H, A, B and the isomorphism ϕ. The groups G and H are called the *factors* of the free product with amalgamation, while A and B are called the *amalgamated subgroups*.

From now on, we shall shorten the term Higman-Neumann-Neumann extension to *HNN extension*. We now turn to the definition. Let G be a group, and let A and B be subgroups of G with $\phi: A \to B$ an isomorphism. *The HNN extension of G relative to A, B and ϕ* is the group

$$G^* = \langle G, t ; t^{-1}at = \phi(a), a \in A \rangle.$$

The group G is called the *base* of G^*, t is called the *stable letter*, and A and B are called the *associated subgroups*.

Note that both the free product with amalgamation and HNN constructions involve two subgroups and an isomorphism between them. In very loose language, the two constructions might be called the "disconnected case" and the "connected case" of one basic idea. In the free product with amalgamation, A and B are subgroups of separate groups G and H. In the HNN extension, A and B are already contained in a single group G.

As an aside for the reader familiar with fundamental groups, we discuss a topological situation which is often used as motivation for studying free products with amalgamation. All the spaces and subspaces which we mention are assumed to be arcwise connected. If X is a topological space, $\pi_1(X)$ will denote the fundamental group of X. Let X and Y be spaces, and let U and V be open arcwise connected subspaces of X and Y respectively such that there is a homeomorphism $h: U \to V$. Choose a basepoint $u \in U$ for the fundamental groups of U and X. Similarly, choose as basepoint $h(u) = v \in V$. There is a homomorphism $\eta: \pi_1(U) \to \pi_1(X)$ defined by simply considering a loop in U as a loop in X. Suppose that η and the similarly defined homomorphism $\delta: \pi_1(V) \to \pi_1(Y)$ are both injections. The homeomorphism h induces an isomorphism $h^*: \pi_1(U) \to \pi_1(V)$. Suppose we identify U and V by the homeomorphism h to obtain a new space Z. Under the assumptions made, the Seifert-van Kampen Theorem (cf. Massey (1967)) says that

$$\pi_1(Z) = \langle \pi_1(X) * \pi_1(Y); \pi_1(U) = \pi_1(V), h^* \rangle.$$

The HNN extension has a similar topological interpretation. Suppose that U and V are both subspaces of the arcwise connected space X. Assume the same hypothesis on U and V as above. Let I be the unit interval, and let $C = U \times I$. Identify $U \times \{0\}$ with U and identify $U \times \{1\}$ with V by the homeomorphism h. Let Z be the resulting space. (What we have done is to attach a handle to X.) The Seifert-van Kampen Theorem can be used to show that

$$\pi_1(Z) = \langle \pi_1(X), t; t^{-1}\pi_1(U)t = \pi_1(V) \rangle$$

For notational convenience, we will discuss the case of HNN extensions with a single stable letter. The general situation is as follows. Let G be a group, and let I be an index set. Let $\{A_i: i \in I\}$ and $\{B_i: i \in I\}$ be families of subgroups of G with $\{\phi_i: i \in I\}$ a family of maps such that each $\phi_i: A_i \to B_i$ is an isomorphism. Then the *HNN extension with base G, stable letters t_i, $i \in I$, and associated subgroups A_i and B_i, $i \in I$*, is the group

$$G^* = \langle G, t_i\ (i \in I); t_i^{-1} a_i t_i = \phi_i(a_i), a_i \in A_i \rangle$$

Similarly, let $\{G_i: i \in I\}$ be a family of groups. Suppose that A is a group, and $\{\phi_i: i \in I\}$ is a family of maps such that each $\phi_i: A \to G_i$ is a monomorphism. Then *the free product of the G_i, amalgamating the subgroups $\phi_i(A)$*, is the group

$$P = \langle *G_i; \phi_i(a) = \phi_j(a), a \in A, i, j \in I \rangle.$$

It is customary to first develop the basic properties of free products with amalgamation, and then to study HNN extensions. Since we feel that there are very good reasons for doing things the other way around, we take the HNN construction as basic.

Let $G^* = \langle G, t; t^{-1} a\, t = \phi(a), a \in A \rangle$ be an HNN extension. We consider two definitions which will allow us to formulate a normal form theorem for HNN extensions. For the rest of this section, the letter g, with or without subscripts, will denote an element of G. If g is thought of as a word, it is a word on the generators of G; that is, g contains no occurrences of $t^{\pm 1}$. The letter ε, with or without subscripts, will denote 1 or -1.

Definition. A sequence $g_0, t^{\varepsilon_1}, g_1, \ldots, t^{\varepsilon_n}, g_n, (n \geqslant 0)$ is said to be *reduced* if there is no consecutive subsequence t^{-1}, g_i, t with $g_i \in A$ or t, g_j, t^{-1} with $g_j \in B$.

In their original paper, Higman, Neumann, and Neumann proved that G is embedded in G^* by the map $g \to g$. The rest of the Normal Form Theorem for HNN Extensions was proved by J. L. Britton (1963) and is usually referred to as Britton's Lemma.

Britton's Lemma. *If the sequence* $g_0, t^{\varepsilon_1}, \ldots, t^{\varepsilon_n}, g_n$ *is reduced and* $n \geqslant 1$, *then* $g_0 t^{\varepsilon_1} \cdots t^{\varepsilon_n} g_n \neq 1$ *in* G^*. □

The products of the elements in two distinct reduced sequences may be equal in G^*. To actually get normal forms we need a further refinement. Choose a set of representatives of the right cosets of A in G, and a set of representatives of the right cosets of B in G. We shall assume that 1 is the representative or both A and B. The choice of coset representatives is to be fixed for the rest of the discussion. If $g \in G$, $\bar{g}$ will denote the representative of the coset Ag, and $\hat{g}$ will denote the representative of the coset Bg.

Definition. A *normal form* is a sequence $g_0, t^{\varepsilon_1}, \ldots, t^{\varepsilon_n}, g_n$ $(n \geqslant 0)$ where

(i) g_0 is an arbitrary element of G,
(ii) If $\varepsilon_i = -1$, then g_i is a representative of a coset of A in G,
(iii) if $\varepsilon_i = +1$, then g_i is a representative of a coset of B in G, and
(iv) there is no consecutive subsequence $t^{\varepsilon}, 1, t^{-\varepsilon}$.

The following discussion and example will explain our definition of a normal form. The defining relations

$$t^{-1} a\, t = \phi(a),\ a \in A \tag{1}$$

of the HNN extension, can be written as

$$t^{-1} a = \phi(a) t^{-1}. \tag{2}$$

By conjugating both sides of (1) by t, the relations (1) can also be written as

$$tbt^{-1} = \phi^{-1}(b),\ b \in B, \tag{3}$$

which are equivalent to

$$tb = \phi^{-1}(b) t. \tag{4}$$

We can view (2) and (4) as *quasi-commuting* relations. These relations allow us to move an element $a \in A$ to the left of a t^{-1} by changing a to $\phi(a)$. Similarly, we can move $b \in B$ to the left of a t, changing b to $\phi^{-1}(b)$. By working from right to left, we can show that every element of G^* is equal to a product $g_0 t^{\varepsilon_1} \cdots t^{\varepsilon_n} g_n$ where $g_0, t^{\varepsilon_1}, \ldots, t^{\varepsilon_n}, g_n$ is a normal form.

Example. Let $F = \langle c, d \rangle$, and let $F^* = \langle c, d, t;\ t^{-1} c\, t = d^2 \rangle$. Since c and d^2

have infinite order in F, F^* is an HNN extension of F. As representatives of cosets of $A = \langle c \rangle$, choose all freely reduced words on c and d which do not begin with c. As representatives cosets of $B = \langle d^2 \rangle$, choose all freely reduced words on c and d which do not begin with a power of d except possibly d^1.

Let

$$w = cd\,t^{-1}c^3t\,d^5cd\,t^{-1}c^3d^3.$$

We calculate the normal form of w by working from right to left. Since the representative of Ac^3d^3 is d^3 and $t^{-1}c^3 = d^6t^{-1}$, we have

$$w = cd\,t^{-1}c^3t\,d^5c\,d^7t^{-1}d^3.$$

Since the representative of Bd^5cd^7 is dcd^7, and $td^4 = c^2t$, we have

$$w = cd\,t^{-1}c^5t\,dc\,d^7t^{-1}d^3.$$

Since $t^{-1}c^5t = d^{10}$, we have

$$w = cd^{12}c\,d^7t^{-1}d^3$$

and $cd^{12}cd^7, t^{-1}, d^3$ is a normal form.

The Normal Form Theorem has two equivalent statements (I) and (II) below. Note that (I) is the combination of the theorem of Higman, Neumann, and Neumann and Britton's Lemma.

Theorem 2.1. (The Normal Form Theorem for HNN Extensions) *Let $G^* = \langle G, t; t^{-1}a\,t = \phi(a), a \in A \rangle$ be an HNN extension. Then*

(I) *The group G is embedded in G^* by the map $g \to g$. If $g_0t^{\varepsilon_1} \cdots t^{\varepsilon_n}g_n = 1$ in G^* where $n \geqslant 1$, then $g_0, t^{\varepsilon_1}, \ldots, t^{\varepsilon_n}, g_n$ is not reduced.*

(II) *Every element w of G^* has a unique representation as $w = g_0t^{\varepsilon_1} \cdots t^{\varepsilon_n}g_n$ where $g_0, t^{\varepsilon_1}, \ldots, t^{\varepsilon_n}, g_n$ is a normal form.*

□ We first prove that statements (I) and (II) are equivalent. Assume that (II) holds. Then it is clear that G is embedded in G^* by $g \to g$ since the normal form of g is the sequence g. Suppose that $g_0, t^{\varepsilon_1}, g_1, \ldots, t^{\varepsilon_n}, g_n$ is a reduced sequence with $n \geqslant 1$. Then the process of working from right to left yields a normal form $g_0', t^{\varepsilon_1}, g_1', \ldots, t^{\varepsilon_n}, g_n'$ with the same number of t symbols. Thus $g_0t^{\varepsilon_1} \cdots t^{\varepsilon_n}g_n \neq 1$.

Next assume that (I) holds. Suppose that

$$g_0t^{\varepsilon_1}g_1 \cdots t^{\varepsilon_n}g_n = h_0t^{\delta_1}h_1 \cdots t^{\delta_m}h_m$$

where both corresponding sequences are normal forms. If $n = m = 0$, then $g_0 = h_0$ by the first part of (I). Suppose $m > 0$. Now

$$1 = g_0t^{\varepsilon_1} \cdots t^{\varepsilon_n}g_nh_m^{-1}t^{-\delta_m} \cdots t^{-\delta_1}h_0^{-1}.$$

The only way that the corresponding sequence can fail to be reduced is for $\varepsilon_n = \delta_m$ and for $g_n h^{-1}$ to be in the appropriate subgroup. If, for example, $\varepsilon_n = \delta_m = -1$, both g_n and h_m are representatives for cosets of A in G, while $g_n h^{-1} \in A$. Thus $g_n = h_m$. We then have

$$g_0 t^{\varepsilon_1} \cdots t^{\varepsilon_{n-1}} g_{n-1} = h_0 t^{\delta_1} \cdots t^{\delta_{m-1}} h_{m-1}$$

and the result follows by induction on m.

In order to prove the theorem, we follow the Artin-van der Waerden idea of making G^* permute normal forms. Intuitively, the action of G^* will be "multiply on the left and then reduce to normal form." Let W be the set of all normal forms from G^*, and let $S(W)$ denote the group of all permutations of W. In order to define a homomorphism $\Psi: G^* \to S(W)$, it suffices to define Ψ on G and t, and then show that all defining relations go to 1.

If $g \in G$, define $\Psi(g)$ by

$$\Psi(g)(g_0, t^{\varepsilon_1}, \ldots, t^{\varepsilon_n}, g_n) = gg_0, t^{\varepsilon_1}, \ldots, t^{\varepsilon_n}, g_n.$$

Thus $\Psi(g)$ simply multiplies the first element of the sequence by g. Clearly, $\Psi(g'g) = \Psi(g')\Psi(g)$. In particular, $\Psi(g)\Psi(g^{-1}) = 1_W = \Psi(g^{-1})\Psi(g)$. Hence, $\Psi(g)$ is a permutation of W and Ψ is a homomorphism from G into $S(W)$.

Define $\Psi(t)$ as follows. Let $g_0, t^{\varepsilon_1}, g_1, \ldots, t^{\varepsilon_n}, g_n$ be a normal form. If $\varepsilon_1 = -1$ and $g_0 \in B$,

$$\Psi(t)(g_0, t^{-1}, \ldots, t^{\varepsilon_n}, g_n) = \phi^{-1}(g_0)g_1, t^{\varepsilon_2}, g_2, \ldots, t^{\varepsilon_n}, g_n.$$

Otherwise,

$$\Psi(t)(g_0, t^{\varepsilon_1}, \ldots, t^{\varepsilon_n}, g_n) = \phi^{-1}(b), t, \hat{g}_0, t^{\varepsilon_1}, g_1, \ldots, t^{\varepsilon_n}, g_n$$

where $g_0 = b\hat{g}_0$ with $b \in B$.

It is necessary to verify that $\Psi(t)$ is actually a permutation of W. We will show that $\Psi(t)$ has inverse $\Psi(t^{-1})$ defined as follows. Let $g_0, t^{\varepsilon_1}, \ldots, t^{\varepsilon_n}, g_n$ be a normal form. If $\varepsilon_1 = +1$ and $g_0 \in A$, then

$$\Psi(t^{-1})(g_0, t^1, \ldots, e^{\varepsilon_n}, g_n) = \phi(g_0)g_1, t^{\varepsilon_2}, g_2, \ldots, t^{\varepsilon_n}, g_n.$$

Otherwise,

$$\Psi(t^{-1})(g_0, t^{\varepsilon_1}, \ldots, t^{\varepsilon_n}, g_n) = \phi(a), t^{-1}, \bar{g}_0, t^{\varepsilon_1}, \ldots, t^{\varepsilon_n}, g_n$$

where $g_0 = a\bar{g}_0$ with $a \in A$.

In checking that $\Psi(t^{-1})\Psi(t) = 1_W$, there are two cases. Let $g_0, t^{\varepsilon_1}, \ldots, t^{\varepsilon_n}, g_n$ be a normal form. If the first clause in the definition of $\Psi(t)$ applies, then $\varepsilon_1 = -1$ and $g_0 \in B$. Note that it is then impossible to have $\varepsilon_2 = +1$ and $g_1 \in A$, since the sequence is a normal form. Now

$$\Psi(t)(g_0, t^{-1}, \ldots, t^{\varepsilon_n}, g_n) = \phi^{-1}(g_0)g_1, t^{\varepsilon_2}, g_2, \ldots, t^{\varepsilon_n}, g_n.$$

By the preceeding remark, the second clause of the definition of $\Psi(t^{-1})$ applies. Since g_1 is a coset representative and $\phi^{-1}(g_0) \in A$, the coset representative of $A\phi^{-1}(g_0)g_1$ is g_1. Therefore,

$$\Psi(t^{-1})(\phi^{-1}(g_0)g_1, t^{\varepsilon_2}, g_2, \ldots, t^{\varepsilon_n}, g_n) = g_0, t^{-1}, g_1, t^{\varepsilon_2}, \ldots, t^{\varepsilon_n}, g_n.$$

If the second clause of the definition of $\Psi(t)$ applies, it is immediate that

$$\Psi(t^{-1})\Psi(t)(g_0, t^{\varepsilon_1}, \ldots, t^{\varepsilon_n}, g_n) = g_0, t^{\varepsilon_1}, \ldots, t^{\varepsilon_n}, g_n.$$

Thus $\Psi(t^{-1})\Psi(t) = 1_W$. A similar check shows that $\Psi(t)\Psi(t^{-1}) = 1_W$ and that if $b \in B$, $\Psi(b) = \Psi(t^{-1})\Psi(\phi^{-1}(b))\Psi(t)$. Thus Ψ is indeed a homomorphism from G^* into $S(W)$.

To finish the proof it is necessary only to note that if $g_0, t^{\varepsilon_1}, \ldots, t^{\varepsilon_n}, g_n$ is a normal form, then

$$\Psi(g_0t^{\varepsilon_1} \cdots t^{\varepsilon_n}g_n)(1) = g_0, t^{\varepsilon_1}, \ldots, t^{\varepsilon_n}, g_n.$$

Thus the products of the elements in distinct normal forms represent distinct elements of G^*. □

For most purposes, there is no need to choose coset representatives. Thus we shall almost exclusively use statement (I) of the Normal Form Theorem. What is important is that G is embedded in G^* and that we have a criterion for telling when words of G^* do not represent the identity.

From now on we shall be rather sloppy in formally distinguishing between a sequence $g_0, t^{\varepsilon_1}, \ldots, t^{\varepsilon_n}, g_n$ and the product $g_0t^{\varepsilon_1} \cdots t^{\varepsilon_n}g_n$. It will be clear from the context which is actually meant. If w is a word of G^* we can write

$$w = g_0t^{\varepsilon_1} \cdots t^{\varepsilon_n}g_n$$

where the above sequence is not necessarily reduced. Consider operations, called *t-reductions*, of the form

(i) replace a subword of the form $t^{-1}gt$, where $g \in A$, by $\phi(g)$, or
(ii) replace a subword of the form tgt^{-1}, where $g \in B$, by $\phi^{-1}(g)$.

A finite number of t-reductions leads from w to a word

$$w' = g'_0t^{\delta_1} \cdots t^{\delta_k}g'_k$$

where the indicated sequence is reduced. If $k > 0$, Britton's Lemma says that w', and thus w, is not equal to 1 in G^*. If $k = 0$, then the theorem of Higman, Neumann, and Neumann says that $w' = 1$ in G^* only if $w' = 1$ in G. The process of performing t-reductions is effective if we can tell what words of G represent elements of A or B, and if we can effectively calculate the functions ϕ and ϕ^{-1}. (This later condition will always be satisfied if A and B are finitely generated.) Thus we have

Corollary 2.2. *Let $G^* = \langle G, t; t^{-1}At = B, \phi\rangle$ be an HNN extension. If G has solvable word problem and the generalized word problems for A and B in G are solvable, and ϕ and ϕ^{-1} are effectively calculable, then G^* has solvable word problem.* □

If a word w has the form $g_0t^{\varepsilon_1}\cdots t^{\varepsilon_n}g_n$ we say that w is *reduced* if the sequence $g_0, t^{\varepsilon_1}, \ldots, t^{\varepsilon_n}, g_n$ is reduced.

Lemma 2.3. *Let $u = g_0t^{\varepsilon_1}\cdots t^{\varepsilon_n}g_n$ and $v = h_0t^{\delta_1}\cdots t^{\delta_m}h_m$ be reduced words, and suppose that $u = v$ in G^*. Then $m = n$ and $\varepsilon_i = \delta_i$, $i = 1, \ldots, n$.*

□ Since $u = v$, we have

$$1 = g_0t^{\varepsilon_1}\cdots t^{\varepsilon_n}g_nh_m^{-1}t^{-\delta_m}\cdots t^{-\delta_1}h_0^{-1}.$$

Since u and v are reduced, the only way the indicated sequence can fail to be reduced is that $\varepsilon_n = \delta_m$ and $g_nh_m^{-1}$ is in the appropriate subgroup A or B. Making successive t-reductions we see that each $\varepsilon_i = \delta_i$ and $n = m$. □

We assign a length to each element z of G^* as follows. Let w be any reduced word of G^* which represents z. If $w = g_0t^{\varepsilon_1}\cdots t^{\varepsilon_n}g_n$, the *length* of z, written $|z|$, is the number n of occurrences of $t^{\pm 1}$ in w. In view of the above lemma, $|z|$ is well-defined. Under this definition, all elements g of the base G of G^* have length 0.

There is a natural notion of "cyclically reduced" in HNN extensions. An element $w = g_0t^{\varepsilon_1}\cdots t^{\varepsilon_n}$ is *cyclically reduced* if all cyclic permutations of the sequence $g_0, t^{\varepsilon_1}, \ldots, t^{\varepsilon_n}$ are reduced. Clearly, every element of G^* is conjugate to a cyclically reduced element.

Theorem 2.4. (The Torsion Theorem for HNN Extensions) *Let $G^* = \langle G, t; t^{-1}At = B, \phi\rangle$ be an HNN extension. Then every element of finite order in G^* is a conjugate of an element of finite order in the base G. Thus G^* has elements of finite order n only if G has elements of order n.*

□ The proof is the same as the proof of the corresponding theorem for free products. If u is an element of G^*, let $v = g_0t^{\varepsilon_1}\cdots t^{\varepsilon_n}$ be a cyclically reduced conjugate of u. If $n \geqslant 1$, then

$$v^m = g_0t^{\varepsilon_1}\cdots t^{\varepsilon_n}g_0t^{\varepsilon_1}\cdots t^{\varepsilon_n}\cdots g_0t^{\varepsilon_1}\cdots t^{\varepsilon_n} \neq 1.$$

by Britton's Lemma. □

The conjugacy theorem for HNN extensions is due to D. J. Collins (1969), and is usually called Collins' Lemma.

Theorem 2.5. (The Conjugacy Theorem for HNN Extensions) *Let $G^* = \langle G, t; t^{-1}At = B, \phi\rangle$ be an HNN extension. Let $u = g_0t^{\varepsilon_1}\cdots t^{\varepsilon_n}$, $n \geqslant 1$, and v be conjugate cyclically reduced elements of G. Then $|u| = |v|$, and u can be obtained from*

v by taking a suitable cyclic permutation v^* of v, which ends in t^{ε_n}, and then conjugating by an element z, where $z \in A$ if $\varepsilon_n = -1$, and $z \in B$ if $\varepsilon_n = 1$.

□ We will prove by induction on $|c|$ that if v^* is any cyclic permutation of v which ends in a t-symbol and $cv^*c^{-1} = u$, then the conclusion of the theorem holds. If $|c| = 0$, we have

$$g_0 t^{\varepsilon_1} \cdots t^{\varepsilon_n} = c h_0 t^{\delta_1} \cdots t^{\delta_m} c^{-1}, \quad \text{or}$$

$$1 = g_0 t^{\varepsilon_1} \cdots t^{\varepsilon_n} c\, t^{-\delta_m} \cdots t^{-\delta_1} h_0^{-1} c^{-1}.$$

Since the only possible t-reduction is $t^{\varepsilon_n} c t^{-\delta_m}$, we must have $c \in A$ if $\varepsilon_n = -1$, and $c \in B$ if $\varepsilon_n = 1$. By considering successive t-reductions, we have, exactly as in the proof of Lemma 2.2, that $n = m$ and, indeed, that $\delta_i = \varepsilon_i$, $i = 1, \ldots, n$.

Now suppose that c has reduced form $c = c_0 t^{\gamma_1} \cdots t^{\gamma_{k-1}} c_{k-1} t^{\gamma_k} c_k$ where $k \geqslant 1$. We have

$$(*) \quad u = c_0 t^{\gamma_1} \cdots t^{\gamma_{k-1}} c_{k-1} t^{\gamma_k} c_k h_0 t^{\delta_1} h_1 \cdots h_{m-1} t^{\delta_m} c_k^{-1} t^{-\gamma_k} c_{k-1}^{-1} t^{-\gamma_{k-1}} \cdots t^{-\gamma_1} c_0^{-1}.$$

Since u is cyclically reduced, some t-reduction must be applicable to the right hand side of the above equation. The only possibilities are $t^{\gamma_k} c_k h_0 t^{\delta_1}$ and $t^{\delta_m} c_k^{-1} t^{-\gamma_k}$. For definiteness, assume that $\gamma_k = -1$ and that $c_k h_0 \in A$. Then $\delta_1 = 1$ and

$$(**) \qquad t^{-1} c_k h_0 t = b \in B.$$

Using the above equation, the fact that $\gamma_k = -1$, and inserting a term bb^{-1}, equation $(*)$ becomes

$$(***) \quad u = c_0 t^{\gamma_1} \cdots t^{\gamma_{k-1}} c_{k-1} b h_1 t^{\delta_2} \cdots t^{\delta_m} c_k^{-1} \underline{tb} b^{-1} c_{k-1}^{-1} t^{-\gamma_{k-1}} \cdots t^{-\gamma_1} c_0^{-1}$$

From $(**)$, we have $tb = c_k h_0 t$, so replacing the underlined occurrence of tb in $(***)$, we have

$$u = c_0 t^{\gamma_1} \cdots t^{\gamma_{k-1}} c_{k-1} b (h_1 t^{\delta_2} \cdots h_{m-1} t^{\delta_m} h_0 t) b^{-1} c_{k-1}^{-1} t_{k-1}^{-\gamma_{k-1}} \cdots t^{-\gamma_1} c_0^{-1}.$$

Since the term in the middle is a cyclic permutation of v, the result follows by the induction hypothesis.

Finally, when $u = zv^*z^{-1}$ where z is in A or B, Lemma 2.3 shows that the sequence of $t^{\pm 1}$ in v^* is exactly the same as in u. □

We turn to free products with amalgamation. Let G and H be groups with subgroups $A \subseteq G$ and $B \subseteq H$, and with $\phi: A \to B$ an isomorphism. Form the group

$$P = \langle G * H;\, a = \phi(a),\, a \in A \rangle.$$

We can view P as the quotient of the free product $G * H$ by the normal subgroup generated by $\{a\,\phi(a)^{-1}: a \in A\}$. A sequence $c_1, \ldots, c_n$, $n \geqslant 0$, of elements of

$G * H$ will be called *reduced* if

(1) Each c_i is in one of the factors G or H.
(2) Successive c_i, c_{i+1} come from different factors.
(3) If $n > 1$, no c_i is in A or B.
(4) If $n = 1$, $c_1 \neq 1$.

It is clear that every element of P is equal to the product of the elements in a reduced sequence. On the other hand we have

Theorem 2.6. (Normal Form Theorem for Free Products with Amalgamation) *If $c_1, \ldots, c_n$ is a reduced sequence, $n \geqslant 1$, then the product $c_1 \cdots c_n \neq 1$ in P. In particular, G and H are embedded in P by the maps $g \to g$ and $h \to h$.*

□ The group $F^* = \langle G * H, t; t^{-1}at = \phi(a), a \in A\rangle$ is an HNN extension of the free product $G * H$. Define $\psi: P \to F^*$ by

$$\begin{cases} \psi(g) = t^{-1}g\,t & \text{if} \quad g \in G, \\ \psi(h) = h & \text{if} \quad h \in H. \end{cases}$$

Now ψ is a homomorphism since the defining relations of P go to 1. If $n = 1$ and $1 \neq c_1 = a \in A$, then $\psi(a) = t^{-1}at = \phi(a) \neq 1$. In all other cases, ψ sends a reduced sequence $c_1, \ldots, c_n$ of elements of P to a reduced sequence of elements in F^*. (For example, $\psi(h_1 g_1\, h_2 g_2) = h_1 t^{-1} g_1 t\, h_2 t^{-1} g_2 t$ and each $g_i \notin A$, $h_i \notin B$.) The theorem thus follows from the Normal Form Theorem for HNN Extensions. □

As with HNN extensions, there is an equivalent statement of the normal form theorem which involves choosing coset representatives for A and B, and obtaining a unique representation.

The above proof shows that ψ is, in fact, an embedding. Thus P is isomorphic to the subgroup of F^* generated by $t^{-1}Gt$ and H.

A sequence $c_1, \ldots, c_n$ of elements of P is called *cyclically reduced* if all cyclic permutations of $c_1, \ldots, c_n$ are reduced. As before, every element of P is conjugate to a cyclically reduced element. The torsion theorem for free products with amalgamation follows by the usual argument.

Theorem 2.7. (Torsion Theorem) *Every element of finite order in $P = \langle G * H; A = B, \phi\rangle$ is a conjugate of an element of finite order in G or H.* □

The Conjugacy Theorem for Free Products with Amalgamation (see Theorem 4.6 of Magnus, Karrass, and Solitar) is deducible from Collins' Lemma in the same way that the Normal Form Theorem for Free Products with Amalgamation is deducible from Theorem 2.1.

Theorem 2.8. (The Conjugacy Theorem for Free Products with Amalgamation) *Let $P = \langle G * H, A = B, \phi\rangle$ be a free product with amalgamation. Let $u = c_1 \cdots c_n$ be a cyclically reduced element of P where $n \geqslant 2$. Then every cyclically reduced conjugate of u can be obtained by cyclically permuting $c_1 \cdots c_n$ and then conjugating by an element of the amalgamated part A.* □

3. Some Embedding Theorems

Having discussed the basic properties of HNN extensions, we can prove some rather remarkable theorems. In their 1949 paper, Higman, Neumann, and Neumann proved the following famous result.

Theorem 3.1. *Every countable group C can be embedded in a group G generated by two elements of infinite order. The group G has an element of finite order n if and only if C does. If C is finitely presentable then so is G.*

☐ Assume that $C = \langle c_1, c_2, \ldots; s_1, \ldots \rangle$ is given with a countable set of generators. Let $F = C * \langle a, b \rangle$. The set

$$\{a, b^{-1} a\, b, b^{-2} a\, b^2, \ldots, b^{-n} a\, b^n, \ldots\}$$

freely generates a free subgroup of $\langle a, b \rangle$ since it is Nielsen-reduced. Similarly, the set

$$\{b, c_1 a^{-1} ba, \ldots, c_n a^{-n} ba^n, \ldots\}$$

freely generates a free subgroup of F. (To check this let π be the projection of F onto $\langle a, b \rangle$ defined by $a \mapsto a$, $b \mapsto b$, $c_i \mapsto 1$, for all i. Since the images b, $a^{-i}ba^i$, $i \geqslant 1$, are free generators, so also is the indicated set.)

Hence, the group

$$G = \langle F, t; t^{-1}at = b, t^{-1}b^{-i}ab^it = c_i a^{-i} ba^i, i \geqslant 1 \rangle$$

is an HNN extension of F. Thus C is embedded in G. That G is generated by t and a is immediate from the defining relations. That G has an element of order n if and only if C does follows from the Torsion Theorem for HNN Extensions. Finally, suppose that $C = \langle c_1, \ldots, c_m; s_1, \ldots, s_k \rangle$ is finitely presented. The HNN relations, $t^{-1}at = b$, $t^{-1}b^{-i}ab^it = c_i a^{-i}ba^i$, can all be eliminated by Tietze transformations since each relation contains a single occurrence of some generator (namely, b or c_i). ☐

The next theorem is due to B. H. Neumann (1937).

Theorem 3.2. *There are $2^{\aleph_0}$ non-isomorphic 2-generator groups.*

☐ Let S be any set of primes. Let $T_S = \sum_{p \in S} C_p$. where C_p is the cyclic group of order p, and embed each T_S in a 2-generator group G_S as in the previous theorem. Now T_S, and thus G_S, has an element of order p iff $p \in S$. Since there are $2^{\aleph_0}$ distinct sets of primes, the result follows. ☐

One of the embedding theorems proved by Higman, Neumann, and Neumann in their original paper is the following.

Theorem 3.3. *Any countable group C can be embedded in a countable group G in which all elements of the same order are conjugate.*

□ The first thing is to embed C in a group C^* in which any two elements of C which have the same order are conjugate. To do this, let $\{\langle a_i, b_i\rangle : i \in I\}$ be the set of all ordered pairs of elements of C which have the same order. The group

$$C^* = \langle c, t_i, i \in I; t_i a_i t_i^{-1} = b_i, i \in I\rangle$$

has the desired property. To prove the theorem, let $G_0 = C$. Suppose inductively that G_i has been defined. Embed G_i in a group G_{i+1} in which any two elements of G_i which have the same order are conjugate. The group

$$G^* = \bigcup_{i=1}^{\infty} G_i$$

is the desired group. □

Recall that a group G is said to be *divisible* if for every element $g \in G$ and every positive integer n, the equation $g = y^n$ has a solution in G. (In other words, every element has an n-th root for every n.)

Theorem 3.4. *Every countable group C can be embedded in a countable, simple, divisible group G.*

□ First, embed C in a countable group K which has elements of all orders. (For example, the direct sum of C, $\mathbb{Z}$, and cyclic groups of order n for all n.) Embed the group $K * \langle x\rangle$ in a two generator group U in which both generators have infinite order. Finally, embed U in a countable group G in which all elements of the same order are conjugate. In summary, we have embeddings

$$C \to K \to K * \langle x\rangle \to U \to G.$$

We claim that the group G is both simple and divisible. Let $1 \neq N \lhd G$. Since K contains elements of all orders and all elements of the same order are conjugate in G, N contains an element $1 \neq z \in K$. Now $x^{-1}z^{-1}x \in N$, and thus $x^{-1}z^{-1}xz$ is an element of N which has infinite order. Thus N contains the generators of U by the conjugacy property of G. Thus $K \subseteq U \subseteq N$. Since K contains elements of all orders and all elements of the same order are conjugate in G, $N = G$.

To check divisibility, let $g \in G$, and let n be any positive integer. Let g have order m (which may be infinite). Since G contains elements of all orders, G has an element z of order mn. Since z^n has order m, there is a $v \in G$ so that $g = v^{-1}z^n v$. Thus $g = (v^{-1}zv)^n$. □

In view of the last theorem and the fact that there are $2^{\aleph_0}$ two-generator groups (Theorem 3.2), there must be $2^{\aleph_0}$ non-isomorphic countable simple groups. (Any particular countable group has at most $\aleph_0$ two-generator subgroups.) Most techniques for constructing infinite simple groups yield groups which are not finitely generated. Indeed, the first proof of the existence of finitely generated infinite simple groups is the proof of G. Higman (1951). Ruth Camm (1953) constructed $2^{\aleph_0}$ non-isomorphic, torsion-free, two-generator simple groups. A remarkable theorem of P. Hall (1968) asserts that every countable group can be embedded in a finitely generated simple group. The number of generators required was subsequently reduced to two by Goryushkin (1974) and by Schupp (1976). We shall prove Hall's theorem by using a construction of M. O. Rabin (1958) which is well-known as a method for showing that certain group-theoretic decision problems are unsolvable. (We shall consider the decision problem aspect in the next section.) The version of Rabin's construction which we use follows C. F. Miller III (1971).

Theorem 3.5. *Every countable group C can be embedded in a six-generator simple group.*

□ First embed C in a countable simple group S. Embed the free product $S * \langle x \rangle$ in a two generator group U where the chosen generators u_1 and u_2 of U both have infinite order. Then the group

$$J = \langle U, y_1, y_2; y_1^{-1}u_1y_1 = u_1^2, y_2^{-1}u_2y_2 = u_2^2 \rangle$$

is an HNN extension of U with stable letters y_1 and y_2. The group

$$K = \langle J, z; z^{-1}y_1z = y_1^2, z^{-1}y_2z = y_2^2 \rangle$$

is an HNN extension of J.

We next consider the group

$$Q = \langle r, s, t; s^{-1}rs = r^2, t^{-1}st = s^2 \rangle.$$

Letting $P = \langle r, s; s^{-1}rs = r^2 \rangle$, P is an HNN extension of $\langle r \rangle$ and Q is an HNN extension of P with stable letter t. We claim that r and t freely generate a free subgroup of rank 2. For, let V be any non-trivial freely reduced word on r and t, and suppose that $V = 1$ in Q. If V does not contain t, then V is identically r^n for some $n \neq 0$. But r has infinite order in Q, so this is impossible. Hence, V contains t. By Britton's Lemma applied to Q over P, V contains a subword $t^{\varepsilon}Rt^{-\varepsilon}$ where R does not contain t and is in the subgroup $\langle s \rangle$ or $\langle s^2 \rangle$ depending on the sign of ε. Since V is freely reduced and contains only t's and r's, R must be r^n for some $n \neq 0$. Hence an equation $r^n = s^j$ with $n \neq 0$ holds in P. But this is impossible by Britton's Lemma applied to P. We thus have a contradiction and the claim is established.

Let w be an element of the group S with $w \neq 1$. The commutator $[w, x] = w^{-1}x^{-1}wx$ has infinite order in U. As in the proof of the previous claim, $[w, x]$ and z freely generate a free subgroup of K. Thus we can form the free product with amalgamation

$$D = \langle K * Q; r = z, t = [w, x] \rangle$$

We claim that D has the property that if $N \lhd D$, then $N \cap S = \{1\}$ or $N = D$. For suppose that $N \cap S \neq \{1\}$. Since S is simple, $w \in N$. Thus in the quotient D/N, $w = 1$. But we next see (and this is the main point of Rabin's construction) that $w = 1$ implies that $D/N = \{1\}$. For, if $w = 1$ then $[w, x] = 1$, and, using the defining relators, this successively implies that $t = 1, s = 1, r = 1, z = 1, y_1 = 1, y_2 = 1, u_1 = 1$, and $u_2 = 1$. Thus $N = D$.

There exists a normal subgroup M of D which is maximal with respect to $M \cap S = \{1\}$. Thus S is embedded in D/M and, by maximality and the property above, D/M is simple. Since the generators r and t can be eliminated, we see that D has six generators. □

It follows immediately from Theorem 3.2, that there exist $2^{\aleph_0}$ six-generator simple groups. An interesting aspect of Hall's theorem is that it is provably non-constructive. Recall that a group is said to be *recursively presented* if it is given by a presentation which is finitely generated and has a recursively enumerable set of defining relators. Kuznetsov (1958) observed the following.

Theorem 3.6. *A recursively presented simple group G has solvable word problem.*

□ Let $G = \langle x_1, \ldots, x_n; r_1, \ldots \rangle$. If $G = \{1\}$, the result certainly holds, so assume that $G \neq \{1\}$, and let $x \neq 1$ be a fixed element of G.

If w is any word of G, let G_w be the group obtained by adding w to the defining relators of G. Thus

$$G_w = \langle x_1, \ldots, x_n; w, r_1, r_2, \ldots \rangle.$$

If $w = 1$ in G, then, of course, G_w is isomorphic to G. If $w \neq 1$ in G, then, since G is simple, G_w is the trivial group. In particular, $x = 1$ in G_w if and only if $w \neq 1$ in G. Now G_w is also recursively presented.

By a familiar argument, in any recursively presented group, the set of words equal to 1 is recursively enumerable. Thus an algorithm for the word problem of G is the following. Given w, begin enumerating the words equal to 1 in G, and simultaneously begin enumerating the words equal to 1 in G_w. If $w = 1$ in G, w appears on the first list, and if $w \neq 1$ in G, x appears on the second list. Simply wait to see which occurs. □

We assume the existence of a finitely presented group H with unsolvable word problem. (This will be proved in Section 7.) By Hall's theorem, H can be embedded in a six-generator simple group G. The group G thus has unsolvable word problem. Since G is simple, we must conclude from Kuznetsov's theorem that G cannot be recursively presented.

We have not yet said anything about finitely presented infinite simple groups. The first example of a finitely presented infinite simple group is due to R. Thompson (1969). G. Higman (1973) exhibits $\aleph_0$ non-isomorphic finitely presented infinite simple groups. An interesting open question is whether every finitely presented group with solvable word problem is embeddable in a finitely presented simple group. Kuznetsov's theorem shows that solvability of the word problem is necessary for such an embedding to exist. In Section 7 we shall prove the following theorem of Boone and Higman (1973): A finitely generated group has solvable word problem if and only if it can be embedded in a simple subgroup of a finitely presented group.

4. Some Decision Problems

Throughout this section, we shall assume the existence of finitely presented groups with unsolvable word problem. (This will be proved in Section 7.) We first turn to the theorem of Adyan (1958) and Rabin (1958) showing that most group-theoretic properties are not recursively recognizable. The corresponding theorem for semigroups was proved earlier by Markov (1950) who introduced the concept of a Markov property which we now consider.

Let P be a property of finitely presented groups which is preserved under isomorphism. The property P is said to be a *Markov property* if:

(1) There is a finitely presented group G_1 with P.

(2) There is a finitely presented group G_2 which cannot be embedded in any finitely presented group which has P.

Familiar examples of Markov properties are being trivial (let G_2 be any finitely presented non-trivial group), finite, abelian, torsion-free, and free. A property P is called *hereditary* if whenever a group G has P, all subgroups of G must also have P. Any hereditary property of finitely presented groups is Markov as long as there are finitely presented groups with and without the property. To construct non-hereditary examples of Markov properties, we note that if P is any property such that all finitely presented groups with P have solvable word problem, then P is Markov. For, let H be a finitely presented group with unsolvable word problem. Any finitely presented group in which H can be embedded has unsolvable word problem and hence can not have P. Thus, for example, being simple is a Markov property by Theorem 3.6. Having rank 2 is not a Markov property since every finitely presented group can be embedded in a finitely presented group with rank 2 by the Higman-Neumann-Neumann embedding.

Theorem 4.1. *Let P be any Markov property of finitely presented groups. Then there is no algorithm which decides whether or not finitely presented groups have the property P.*

□ Let G_1 and G_2 be finitely presented groups as in the definition of P being a Markov property. Let H be a finitely presented group with unsolvable word problem. Let w be any word on the generators of H. We now regard Rabin's construction starting with the group $G_2 * H$ and the word w as directions for constructing a presentation. Recall that in the HNN embedding, given the presentation of $G_2 * H * \langle x \rangle$, one can effectively write down the finite presentation of the two generator group U in which $G_2 * H * \langle x \rangle$ is embedded. As before, we let

$$J = \langle U, y_1, y_2; y_1^{-1}u_1y_1 = u_1^2, y_2^{-1}u_2y_2 = u_2^2 \rangle,$$

$$K = \langle J, z; z^{-1}y_1z = y_1^2, z^{-1}y_2z = y_2^2 \rangle,$$

$$Q = \langle r, s, t; s^{-1}rs = r^2, t^{-1}st = s^2 \rangle,$$

$$D_w = \langle K * Q; r = z, t = [w, x] \rangle,$$

and, finally, let

$$E_w = D_w * G_1.$$

Let π_w be the indicated presentation for the group E_w. Given a word w on the generators of H, we have effectively described how to write down the finite presentation π_w. In our previous discussion of Rabin's construction, we have seen that if $w \neq 1$ in H, then G_2 is embedded in E_w. Thus E_w does not have P. If $w = 1$ in G, then $D_w = \{1\}$, and thus E_w is isomorphic to G_1 and does have P. Hence, the group E_w presented by π_w has P if and only if $w = 1$ in H. Thus an algorithm deciding whether or not groups given by finite presentations have P could be used to solve the word problem in H. Since H has unsolvable word problem, the existence of such an algorithm is impossible. □

Actually, the proof of the theorem shows that many properties other than Markov properties are not recursively recognizable. We say that a property P of finitely presented groups is *incompatible with free products* if:

(1) There exists a finitely presented group G_1 with P such that,

(2) if A is any non-trivial finitely presented group, then $A * G_1$ does not have P.

For example, let r be any positive integer. The property of having rank r is incompatible with free products for, by the Grushko-Neumann Theorem, if G_1 has rank r and $A \neq \{1\}$, then $G_1 * A$ has rank greater than r. Let G_1 be any finitely presented group. Again by the Grushko-Neumann Theorem, being isomorphic to G_1 is incompatible with free products.

In the last step of the construction in the theorem, if $w = 1$ in H, then E_w is isomorphic to G_1. If $w \neq 1$ in H, then E_w is the free product of G_1 and a non-trivial group. Thus the proof shows that if P is incompatible with free products there is no algorithm which determines if finite presentations present groups with P. In particular, given any particular finitely presented group G_1, one cannot tell what finite presentations are presentations of G_1.

We next turn to a construction of Mikhailova (1958) which shows that the direct product of two free groups may have unsolvable generalized word problem. Let

$$H = \langle x_1, \ldots, x_n; r_1, \ldots, r_m \rangle$$

be a finitely presented group. Let F_n be the free group on $x_1, \ldots, x_n$. We shall use ordered pair notation (u, v), for elements of the direct product $F_n \times F_n$. Let L_H be the subgroup of $F_n \times F_n$ generated by

$$(x_i, x_i),\ i = 1, \ldots, n,$$

$$(1, r_j),\ j = 1, \ldots, m.$$

Lemma 4.2. *$(u, v) \in L_H$ if and only if $u = v$ in H.*

□ It is clear that if $(u, v) \in L_H$ then $u = v$ in H since each of the generators has this property. Suppose that $u = v$ in H. Now $(u, u) \in L_H$ since all the diagonal pairs (x_i, x_i) are in L_H. Since $u = v$ in H, it follows that in F_n

$$v = u\prod_{i=1}^{t} (c_i r_{j_i}^{\varepsilon_i} c_i^{-1}).$$

Hence, in $F_n \times F_n$,

$$(u, v) = (u, u) \prod_{i=1}^{t} (c_i, c_i)(1, r_{j_i}^{\varepsilon_i})(c_i^{-1}, c_i^{-1})$$

and thus $(u, v) \in L_H$. □

In view of the lemma, the generalized word problem for L_H in $F_n \times F_n$ is equivalent to the word problem for H. Taking H to have unsolvable word problem, we have

Theorem 4.3. *Let $n \geqslant 2$. Then there is a finitely generated subgroup L_H of $F_n \times F_n$ such that the generalized word problem for L_H in $F_n \times F_n$ is unsolvable.* □

Let G be a finitely generated group. The *generating problem* for G is solvable if there exists an algorithm which, when given any finite subset of elements of G, decides whether or not the subgroup they generate is all of G.

Now consider Mikhailova's construction starting with a finitely presented group H. Note that $H = \{1\}$ if and only if $u = v$ for all pairs (u, v) of words on the generators of H. By Lemma 4.2, this happens if and only if $L_H = F_n \times F_n$.

Now Rabin's construction gives a class of presentations with six generators, so the triviality problem for presentations with six generators is unsolvable. Since a finitely presented group $H = \{1\}$ if and only if $L_H = F_n \times F_n$, the generating problem for $F_6 \times F_6$ is unsolvable. We can obtain the same result for any $n > 6$ by simply adding new generating symbols to the presentation and also adding the new generators as defining relators. Thus we have the following result of C. F. Miller (1971).

Theorem 4.4. *Let $n \geqslant 6$. Then the generating problem for $F_n \times F_n$ is unsolvable.* □

Problems concerning $F_n \times F_n$ are of considerable interest because of their close connections with problems about 3-manifolds. A compact connected orientable surface of genus g has fundamental group

$$S_g = \langle a_i, b_i, \ldots, a_g, b_g; \prod_{i=1}^{g} [a_i, b_i] = 1 \rangle$$

where $[a_i, b_i]$ is the commutator $a_i^{-1} b_i^{-1} a_i b_i$. The problem of deciding whether a given 3-manifold is simply connected is equivalent to deciding whether or not a homeomorphism from S_g to $F_g \times F_g$ is onto. This, in turn, is equivalent to the generating problem for $F_g \times F_g$ restricted to subsets $\{y_1, z_1, \ldots, y_g, z_g\}$ having $2g$ elements which satisfy the relation

$$\prod_{i=1}^{g} [y_i, z_i] = 1$$

in $F_n \times F_n$.

Let $\phi: S_g \to F_g \times F_g$ be onto. We say that ϕ *factors essentially through a free product* if there exists a non-trivial free product $A * B$, $A \neq \{1\}$, $B \neq \{1\}$, and homomorphisms ψ and α, with $\psi: S_g \to A * B$ onto, such that the diagram

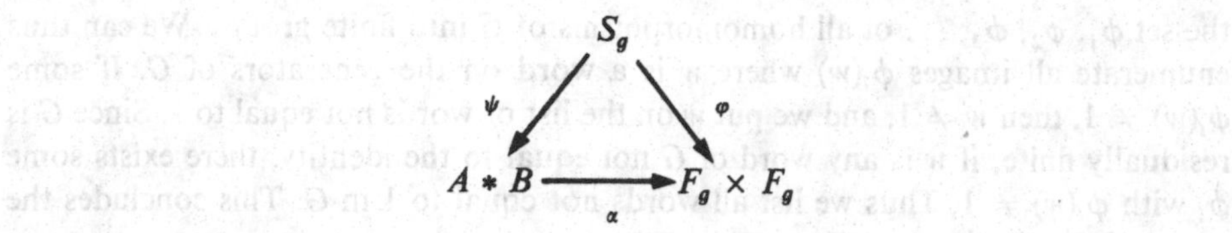

commutes.

The *Poincare Conjecture* surmises that every compact, connected, simply-connected 3-manifold is homeomorphic to the 3-sphere. We state a remarkable theorem of Stallings (1962) and Jaco (1969).

Theorem 4.5. *The Poincaré Conjecture is true if and only if, for every $g > 1$ and every homomorphism $\phi: S_g \to F_g \times F_g$ of S_g onto $F_g \times F_g$, ϕ factors essentially through a free product.* □

We next collect some useful theorems concerning groups being residually finite or hopfian. Recall that a group G is *residually finite* if for every non-trivial element $g \neq 1$ of G, there is a homomorphism ϕ from G into a finite group K such that $\phi(g) \neq 1$. The choice of K and ϕ depends, of course, on the element g. It is clear from the definition that if H is the direct product of a family of residually finite groups, then H is residually finite. Also, subgroups of residually finite groups are residually finite.

The fact that free groups are residually finite follows from the existence of a faithful representation of the free group of rank 2 by integer matrices. For example, (Sanov 1947), the matrices

$$\begin{pmatrix} 1 & 2 \\ 0 & 1 \end{pmatrix} \text{ and } \begin{pmatrix} 1 & 0 \\ 2 & 1 \end{pmatrix}$$

are free generators of a free subgroup of $\mathbb{GL}(2, \mathbb{Z})$.

The connection between finitely presented residually finite groups and decision problems is given by the next theorem. The argument really goes back to the "finite-reducibility" idea of J. C. C. McKinsey (1943) and was first applied to groups by V. Dyson (1964).

Theorem 4.6. *A finitely presented, residually finite group G has solvable word problem.*

□ Let $G = \langle x_1, \ldots, x_n; r_1, \ldots, r_m \rangle$. Since G is finitely presented, the set of words equal to 1 in G can be effectively enumerated. We show that the set of words not equal to 1 in G is also recursively enumerable. Fix an alphabet $y_1, y_2, \ldots$. We can effectively enumerate all multiplication table presentations of finite groups on this alphabet. Now a homomorphism from G into a finite group K is completely determined by its effect on the generators $x_1, \ldots, x_n$. Thus a "candidate" for a homomorphism of G into K is an n-tuple $(k_1, \ldots, k_n)$ of elements of K. The map $x_i \mapsto k_i$ is a homomorphism if and only if each r_i goes to 1. Since we can solve the word problem in K, we can check this condition. Thus we can effectively enumerate the set $\phi_1, \phi_2, \phi_3, \ldots$ of all homomorphisms of G into finite groups. We can thus enumerate all images $\phi_i(w)$ where w is a word on the generators of G. If some $\phi_i(w) \neq 1$, then $w \neq 1$, and we put w on the list of words not equal to 1. Since G is residually finite, if w is any word of G not equal to the identity, there exists some ϕ_i with $\phi_i(w) \neq 1$. Thus we list all words not equal to 1 in G. This concludes the proof of the theorem. □

V. Dyson (1974) and S. Meskin (1974) have exhibited finitely generated, recursively presented, residually finite groups with unsolvable word problem.

We next turn to a theorem of Marshall Hall (1949).

Theorem 4.7. *Let G be a finitely generated group. Then the number of subgroups of G having any fixed finite index n is finite. If H is a subgroup of finite index in G, then H contains a subgroup K characteristic in G with finite index in G.*

□ Let n be a positive integer. For each subgroup H of index n, choose a complete set $c_1, \ldots, c_n$ of representatives of the right cosets of H in G with $c_1 = 1$. Now G permutes the cosets Hc_i by multiplication on the right. This induces a homomorphism ψ_H from G into the symmetric group, S_n, of permutations of $\{1, \ldots, n\}$ as follows. For $g \in G$, $\psi_H(g)$ is the permutation which sends i to j if $Hc_ig = Hc_j$. Since $Hc_1 = H$, $\psi_H(g)$ fixes the number 1 if and only if $g \in H$. If H and L are distinct subgroups of index n, there is an element g in one subgroup but not the other. Thus $\psi_H(g) \neq \psi_L(g)$ and ψ_H and ψ_L are distinct. Since G is finitely generated, there are only finitely many homomorphisms from G into S_n, and the number of subgroups of index n is thus finite.

If H is a subgroup of finite index n in G, let $H_1, \ldots, H_m$ be all the distinct subgroups of index n. Let $K = \bigcap_{i=1}^m H_i$. Then K is of finite index since it is the intersection of finitely many subgroups of finite index. Let α be any automorphism of G. Since the image $\alpha(H_i)$ of each H_i is again a subgroup of index n, α permutes the H_i. Thus

$$\alpha(K) = \bigcap_{i=1}^m \alpha(H_i) = K$$

and K is characteristic in G. □

If G is any group, Aut(G) will denote the group of all automorphisms of G.

The next theorem is due to G. Baumslag (1963).

Theorem 4.8. *If G is a finitely generated residually finite group, then* Aut(G) *is also residually finite*

□ Let $A = \text{Aut}(G)$, and let $1 \neq \alpha \in A$. Then there is an element $c \in G$ such that $\alpha(c)c^{-1} = c^* \neq 1$. Since G is residually finite, there is a subgroup H of finite index in G with $c^* \notin H$. By the previous theorem, H contains a characteristic subgroup K of finite index in G. Since K is characteristic, we can define a homomorphism $\psi: A \to \text{Aut}(G/K)$ by

$$\psi(\beta)\,[Kg] = K\beta(g).$$

Now Aut(G/K) is finite and $\psi(\alpha) \neq 1$. □

Since free groups are residually finite, the theorem shows that the automorphism group of a free group of finite rank is again residually finite. Let

$$F_\omega = \langle x_1, x_2, x_3, \ldots \rangle$$

be the free group of rank $\aleph_0$ on the indicated generators. We can see that $\text{Aut}(F_\omega)$ is not residually finite as follows. Since $\text{Aut}(F_\omega)$ contains the symmetric group on $\{x_1, x_2, \ldots\}$, $\text{Aut}(F_\omega)$ contains an infinite simple group A. Certainly then, A is not residually finite, and thus $\text{Aut}(F_\omega)$ is not residually finite.

Recall that a group G is hopfian if every onto endomorphism $\theta: G \to G$ is also one-to-one. Equivalently, G is hopfian if G is not isomorphic to a proper quotient group of itself. The problem of whether finitely presented non-hopfian groups exist arose in a topological context (Hopf, 1931). Examples of non-hopfian groups were given by B. H. Neumann (1950) and G. Higman (1951). The simplest possible non-hopfian group is the following example of Baumslag and Solitar (1962).

Theorem 4.9. *The group $G = \langle b, t; t^{-1}b^2t = b^3\rangle$ is non-hopfian.*

□ Define $\theta: G \to G$ by $\theta(t) = t$ and $\theta(b) = b^2$. An application of θ squares both sides of the defining relation, so θ is well-defined. Since t and b^2 are in the image of θ and $t^{-1}b^2t = b^3$, θ is onto G. Applying θ to the commutator $[t^{-1}bt, b]$,

$$\theta([t^{-1}bt, b]) = [t^{-1}b^2t, b^2] = [b^3, b^2] = 1.$$

But

$$[t^{-1}bt, b] = t^{-1}btbt^{-1}b^{-1}tb^{-1} \neq 1 \quad \text{in} \quad G$$

by Britton's Lemma, and θ thus has non-trivial kernel. □

Remark. Let m and n be a pair of non-zero relatively prime integers, neither with absolute value 1. The proof above actually shows that $\langle b, t; t^{-1}b^mt = b^n\rangle$ is non-hopfian.

A theorem of Malcev (1940) shows that all finitely generated residually finite groups are hopfian.

Theorem 4.10. *A finitely generated residually finite group G is hopfian.*

□ Let $\theta: G \to G$ be onto, and let K be the kernel of θ. Let n be any positive integer. Since G is finitely generated, M. Hall's theorem states that there are only finitely many subgroups, say $M_1, \ldots, M_k$ of index n. Let $L_i = \theta^{-1}(M_i)$. It is easy to check that $[G: L_i] = n$. Since the preimages of the M_i are distinct and there are only finitely many M_i, the collection of the L_i is equal to the collection of the M_i. Thus K is contained in all the M_i. But since n is arbitrary, K is contained in the intersection of all subgroups of finite index. Since G is residually finite, this intersection is $\{1\}$. Thus $K = \{1\}$ and θ is an automorphism. □

Miller and Schupp (1971) have shown that every finitely presented group can be embedded in a finitely presented hopfian group. (See V.10.) It follows that there are finitely presented hopfian groups with unsolvable word problem. A construction of Miller (1971) exhibits finitely presented residually finite groups with unsolvable conjugacy problem. Using this construction, Miller is further able to deduce that if F_r is the free group of rank $r \geqslant 3$, then there is a finitely generated subgroup A of Aut(F_r) such that the generalized word problem for A in Aut(F_r) is unsolvable.

5. *One-Relator Groups*

The basic theorems about groups with one defining relator, the Freiheitssatz and the solvability of the word problem, were proved by Magnus in the early 1930's. There is now a well-developed theory of one-relator groups. (See section II.5 for a discussion of several aspects of this theory.) In this chapter we prove some of the main theorems about one-relator groups by using HNN extensions. Moldavanskii (1967), in his work on subgroups of one-relator groups, observed that if G is a one-relator group whose defining relator r is cyclically reduced and has exponent sum zero on some generator occurring in it, then G is an HNN extension of another one-relator group H. The proofs given here follow McCool and Schupp (1973). The basic strategy of using induction on the length of the defining relator and the method of dealing with the case of non-zero exponent sum are unchanged from the original papers of Magnus (1930, 1932).

Theorem 5.1. (The Freiheitssatz) *Let* $G = \langle t, b, c, \ldots; r\rangle$ *where r is cyclically reduced. If L is a subset of* $\{t, b, c, \ldots\}$ *which omits a generator occurring in r, then the subgroup M generated by L is freely generated by L.*

□ It suffices to consider sets L containing all the generators of G except one. The proof is by induction on the length of r. If r involves only one generator the theorem holds. We may thus assume that G has at least two generators, say t and b, occurring in r. There are two cases.

Case 1. Suppose that the exponent sum, $\sigma_t(r)$, of some generator t occurring in r is zero. We shall exhibit G as an HNN extension of a one-relator group H whose defining relator s has shorter length than r. We can assume, replacing r by a suitable cyclic permutation if necessary, that r begins with $b^{\pm 1}$. For i an integer, we put $b_i = t^i b t^{-i}$, $c_i = t^i c t^{-i}$, etc. As an element of the free group $F = \langle t, b, c, \ldots\rangle$, r belongs to the normal subgroup of F generated by $b, c, \ldots$ Thus r can be rewritten as a cyclically reduced word s on the $b_i, c_i, \ldots$, where the length of s is less than that of r. To rewrite r, simply replace each occurrence of a generator other than t by the generator subscripted by i, where i is the sum of the exponents on t's preceeding the given occurrence of the generator. (For example, if r is $b^2t^{-1}c^2b^2tc^2$, then s is $b_0^2c_{-1}^2b_{-1}^2c_0^2$.)

Let μ and m be respectively the minimum and maximum subscripts on b actually occurring in s. (Note that b_0 occurs in s since we are assuming that r starts with $b^{\pm 1}$). We claim that G has a presentation

$$\langle t, b_\mu, \ldots, b_m, c_i, d_i, \ldots, (i \in \mathbb{Z}); s = 1, tb_jt^{-1} = b_{j+1}; (j = \mu, \ldots, m-1),$$
$$tc_it^{-1} = c_{i+1}, \ldots, (i \in \mathbb{Z})\rangle.$$

To verify the claim, let G^* be the group defined by the new presentation. The map $\phi\colon G \to G^*$ defined by

$$t \mapsto t, b \mapsto b_0, c \mapsto c_0, \text{etc.}$$

is a homomorphism since $\phi(r) = s$. On the other hand, the map $\eta\colon G^* \to G$ defined by

$$t \mapsto t, b_i \mapsto t^i b t^{-i}, c_i \mapsto t^i c t^{-i}, \text{etc.}$$

is a homomorphism since all the relators of G^* are sent to 1. Since $\phi\eta$ and $\eta\phi$ are the identity maps on G and G^* respectively, ϕ is an isomorphism.

(Continuing our example, if

$$G = \langle t, b, c; b^2t^{-1}c^2b^2tc^2\rangle,$$

the new presentation of G is

$$\langle t, b_{-1}, b_0, c_i(i \in \mathbb{Z}); b_0^2c_{-1}^2b_{-1}^2c_0^2, tb_{-1}t^{-1} = b_0, tc_it^{-1} = c_{i+1}(i \in \mathbb{Z})\rangle.)$$

Now put $H = \langle b_\mu, \ldots, b_m, c_i, d_i, \ldots, (i \in \mathbb{Z}); s = 1\rangle$. It follows from the induction hypothesis that the subgroups X and Y of H generated respectively by $\{b_\mu, \ldots, b_{m-1}, c_i, d_i, \ldots, (i \in \mathbb{Z})\}$ and $\{b_{\mu+1}, \ldots, b_m, c_i, d_i, \ldots, (i \in \mathbb{Z})\}$ are freely generated by the indicated generators. In particular, the map $b_j \mapsto b_{j+1}, c_i \mapsto c_{i+1}, \ldots, (\mu \leqslant j < m, i \in \mathbb{Z})$ extends to an isomorphism $\theta\colon X \to Y$. Thus G is exhibited as HNN group with base H.

First suppose that our subset of the original generators for G is $L = \{b, c, \ldots\}$. Note that at least one generator of H with a non-zero subscript occurs in s (for otherwise t could not occur in r with zero exponent sum). By the induction hypothesis, L freely generates a free subgroup of H, and thus of G.

Suppose that $L = \{t, c, \ldots\}$. (The omitted generator is b.) Let w be a non-trivial freely reduced word on $\{t, c, \ldots\}$. If $\sigma_t(w) \neq 0$, then $w \neq 1$ in G since any word equal to 1 in G must be freely equal to a product of conjugates of $r^{\pm 1}$.

If $\sigma_t(w) = 0$, rewrite w as a word on the set $J = \{c_i, \ldots\}$, following the same procedure as in rewriting r. This yields a freely reduced non-trivial word w^*. By the induction hypothesis J freely generates a free subgroup of H. Hence, $w^* \neq 1$. Since $w^* = w$ in G, $w \neq 1$ in G.

Case 2. Up to a relabelling of generators, Case 1 covers all situations except that where all the generators occurring in r have non-zero exponent sum. Suppose $L = \{b, c, \ldots\}$. Let $\sigma_t(r) = \alpha$, and let $\sigma_b(r) = \beta$. The map Ψ defined by

$$t \mapsto yx^{-\beta}, b \mapsto x^\alpha, c \mapsto c, \ldots$$

is a homomorphism of G into the group

$$C = \langle y, x, c, \ldots; r(yx^\beta, x^\alpha, c, \ldots)\rangle$$

Let r_1 be the result of cyclically reducing $r(yx^{-\beta}, x^\alpha, c, \ldots)$. Then $\sigma_x(r_1) = 0$ and y occurs in r_1. We can rewrite C as an HNN group using x as a stable letter. If s is the rewritten form of $r_1(yx^{-\beta}, x^\alpha, c, \ldots)$, then the length of s will be less than the length of r since all x symbols will be eliminated. It follows that the subgroup of C generated by $\{x, c, \ldots\}$ is freely generated by this set, and thus the subgroup generated by $\{x^\alpha, c, \ldots\}$ is freely generated by these generators. Since Ψ sends $b \mapsto x^\alpha$, $c \mapsto c, \ldots$, L freely generates a free subgroup of G. This completes the proof of the theorem. □

We shall need one further observation about the group C and the map Ψ introduced in the case of non-zero exponent sum. By the Freiheitssatz, the element b has infinite order in G. Thus the group $C' = \langle t, b, c \ldots, x; r, b = x^\alpha \rangle$ is the free product of G and the infinite cyclic group $\langle x \rangle$, amalgamating $b = x^\alpha$. Now C is obtained from C' by the Tietze transformations of adding a new generator y and relation $t = yx^{-\beta}$, and then deleting the generators b and t and replacing them in r by x^α and $yx^{-\beta}$. Thus the map $\Psi\colon G \to C$ is an embedding.

We next turn to the theorem of Karrass, Magnus, and Solitar (1960) characterizing elements of finite order in one-relator groups.

Theorem 5.2. *Let $G = \langle t, b, c, \ldots; r \rangle$ where r is cyclically reduced. The group G is torsion-free if r is not a proper power in the free group $\langle t, b, c, \ldots \rangle$. If $r = u^n$, $n > 1$, where u itself is not a proper power, then u has order n in G and all elements of G of finite order are conjugates of powers of u.*

□ This theorem is almost immediate from the theorem characterizing elements of finite order in HNN groups. The proof is, of course, by induction on the length of r. If r involves only one generator, the theorem holds. We may thus assume that r involves at least two generators, say t and b. If r has exponent sum 0 on some generator, say t, then, as before, we consider G as an HNN extension with base

$$H = \langle b_\mu, \ldots, b_m, c_i, \ldots \; (i \in \mathbb{Z}); s = 1 \rangle$$

where s is the rewritten form of r. Note that s is an n-th power if and only if r is an n-th power. By the induction hypothesis, H, and thus G, is torsion-free unless r is a proper power. If $r = u^n$, $n > 1$, (where u is not a proper power), then $s = v^n$ where v is the rewritten form of u. The induction hypothesis guarantees that the only elements of finite order in H, and thus G, are conjugates of powers of v and that v has order n. Since $u = v$ in G we are done.

In the case where no generator in r has exponent sum 0, we must consider the group.

$$C = \langle y, x, c, \ldots; r(yx^{-\beta}, x^\alpha, c, \ldots) \rangle$$

as before. Now r_1, the cyclically reduced form of $r(yx^{-\beta}, x^\alpha, c, \ldots)$ is an n-th power if and only if r is an n-th power. Since the map $\Psi\colon G \to C$ is an embedding, it follows as in the previous case, that G is torsion-free unless r is a proper power. If $r = u^n$, $n > 1$, write $r_1 = u_1^n$. Since $\Psi(u)$ is conjugate to u_1, it follows that u has order n in G.

The only point remaining is to show that all elements of G which have finite order are conjugates of powers of u. We must check that if two elements of $\Psi(G)$ are conjugate in C, then they are already conjugate in G. To verify this, write, as in our discussion of the map Ψ,

$$C = \langle G * \langle x \rangle; b = x^{\alpha} \rangle$$

Suppose $cgc^{-1} = g'$ where $g, g' \in G$. Write $c = c_1 \cdots c_k$ in reduced form in the free product with amalgamation sense. We have

$$c_1 \cdots c_k g c_k^{-1} \cdots c_1^{-1} = g'$$

Without loss of generality, we may suppose that $c_k = x^j$. By the Normal Form Theorem for Free Products with Amalgamation, the only way that the above equality can hold is if g is in the amalgamated part. Then $x^j g x^{-j} = x^j x^m x^{-j} = g$. We have $c_{k-1} = g_1 \in G$, so

$$c_1 \cdots c_{k-2}(g_1 g g_1^{-1}) c_{k-2}^{-1} \cdots c_1^{-1} = g'$$

and the result follows by induction on the length of c. □

We next turn to the word problem. Recall that the generalized word problem with respect to a subgroup K of a recursively presented group $H = \langle S; D \rangle$ is solvable if there exists an algorithm which, when given any word w on S, determines whether or not $w \in K$. We shall simply say that K is *solvable in* H if the generalized word problem for K in H is solvable.

In our basic discussion of HNN extensions, we made the following observation. Let H be a group with solvable word problem. Let X and Y be subgroups of H which are solvable in H, and let $\theta: X \to Y$ be a recursive isomorphism. Then the HNN extension

$$G = \langle H, t; t^{-1} X t = Y, \theta \rangle$$

has solvable word problem. (This is because the process of performing t-reductions is effective under the assumptions made.)

In exhibiting a one-relator group G as an HNN extension of a group H with shorter defining relator, the associated subgroups are all generated by subsets of the generators of H. We must thus consider the generalized word problem for such subgroups.

Theorem 5.3. *Let $G = \langle t, b, c, \ldots; r \rangle$ be a countably generated one-relator group group where r is cyclically reduced. If M is the subgroup generated by a recursive subset L of the given generators of G, then the generalized word problem with respect to M in G is solvable.*

□ As usual, the proof is by induction on the length of r. If r contains only one generator, then G is the free product of a free group and a finite cyclic group. Using the Normal Form Theorem for Free Products, it is easy to see that the theorem holds. We first consider the situation where r has exponent sum zero on some generator, say t, which occurs in r. As before, we view G as an HNN extension.

$$G = \langle H, t; t^{-1}Xt = Y \rangle$$

where the one-relator group H has a shorter defining relator. Note that the induction hypothesis applies to the subgroups X and Y of H. Thus the process of performing t-reductions in G is effective. In particular, G has solvable word problem.

We consider three possibilities for the set L. First suppose that L contains all the generators which occur in r. Now G is the free product of the group G_1 on the set R of those generators which actually occur in r, and the free group G_2 on the set S of remaining generators. Using the solvability of the word problem for G, we can, given any element w, effectively calculate its free product normal form, say $w = w_1 \cdots w_n$. By the Normal Form Theorem for Free Products and the fact that G_2 is free, we have $w \in K = \text{Gp}\, L$ if and only $w_i \in \text{Gp}\,(L \cap S)$ for each normal form component w_i which is in G_2. Since $L \cap S$ is a recursive subset of the free generators for G_2, $\text{Gp}\,(L \cap S)$ is solvable in G_2.

The second possibility is that $L = \{b, c, \ldots\}$ omits the stable letter t. Thus, identifying b with b_0, etc., L is contained in the base H of G. Then $K = \text{Gp}\, L$ is solvable in H by the induction hypothesis. Given any word w of G, we can effectively calculate a t-reduced word w^* which is equal to w in G. By Britton's Lemma, we can have $w \in K$ only if w^* is t-free. But if w^* is t-free, we can decided if $w^* \in K$.

Finally, there is the possibility that $L = \{t, c, \ldots\}$ contains the stable letter t but omits some other generator, say b, which occurs in r. By choosing our notation in the rewriting process, we can assume that b is the generator with bounded subscript range. Let w be any word of G. Since $t \in L$, we have $w \in K = \text{Gp}\, L$ if and only if $w_1 = wt^{-\alpha} \in K$ where $\alpha = \sigma_t(w)$. Thus $\sigma_t(w_1) = 0$. If $w_1 \in K$ then w is equal to a word which does not contain any b. The crucial point is that since b is the generator with bounded subscript range, Britton's Lemma implies that if $w_1 \in K$ and $\sigma_t(w_1) = 0$, then performing all applicable t-reductions leads to a t-free word w_1^*. Let $L^* = \{c_i, \ldots (i \in \mathbb{Z})\} \subseteq H$, and let $K^* = \text{Gp}\, L^*$. Now K^* is solvable in H by the induction hypothesis. Putting together the above, we have $w \in K$ if and only if $w_1^* \in K^*$. This concludes the proof in the case that some generator r occurs with exponent sum zero.

Finally suppose that all generators occurring in r have non-zero exponent sum and that M is the subgroup generated by $L = \{b, c, \ldots\}$. We again consider the group C. Since the map $\Psi: G \to C$ is an embedding, a word $w(t, b, c, \ldots) \in M$ if and only if $w(yx^{-\beta}, x^{-\alpha}, c, \ldots) \in \Psi(M)$. As in the previous case, the subgroup K generated by $\{x, c, \ldots\}$ is solvable in C. Since K is freely generated by these generators, $\Psi(M)$, which is the subgroup generated by $\{x^\alpha, c, \ldots\}$, is solvable in K and thus C. Thus M is solvable in G. This concludes the proof of the theorem. ☐

The reader has undoubtedly noticed that in dealing with one-relator groups, one mainly considers subgroups generated by a subset of the generators which omits a generator occurring in the defining relator.

Definition. Let $G = \langle X; r \rangle$, where r is cyclically reduced. A subgroup M of G is called a *Magnus subgroup* if M is generated by a subset L of X where L omits at least one generator occurring in r.

In order to introduce our next topic, we first switch our attention to free products. Let $P = A * B$ be a non-trivial free product. Using the Normal Form Theorem for Free Products, it is easy to verify that if $c \in P - A$, then $cAc^{-1} \cap A = \{1\}$. In general, a subgroup K of a group G is said to be *malnormal in* G if $g \notin K$ implies that $gKg^{-1} \cap K = \{1\}$. It follows from the remark above that if $F = \langle X \rangle$ is the free group on the set X, and $Y \subseteq X$, then the subgroup K generated by Y is malnormal in F. B. B. Newman (1968) showed that if G is a one-relator group with torsion, then any Magnus subgroup of G is malnormal in G. We next turn to a surprising general result of G. H. Bagherzadeh (1973).

Theorem 5.4. *Let $G = \langle t, b, c, \ldots; r \rangle$ where r is cyclically reduced. If M is a Magnus subgroup of G and $g \notin M$, then $gMg^{-1} \cap M$ is cyclic.*

□ By the Freiheitssatz and the above remarks, it suffices to prove the theorem for subgroups M generated by sets containing all the generators of G except some one generator which occurs in r. Our notation will be as follows. We shall always assume that b occurs in r, and that M is the subgroup generated by all the generators except b.

The proof is, of course, by induction on the length of r. If r involves only one generator, then either $G = M$, or G is the free product of the free group M and a non-trivial finite cyclic group. The result then follows from the remarks on malnormality preceeding the statement of the theorem.

We now must consider the situation where r involves precisely two generators, say b and t. In this case, G is the free product with amalgamation of M and the group $K = \langle b, t; r \rangle$ amalgamating the cyclic subgroup $\langle t \rangle$. In brief,

$$G = \langle M * K; t = t \rangle$$

Suppose that $g \notin M$ and that $gmg^{-1} = m'$ where $m, m' \in M$. Write $g = g_1 g_2 \cdots g_n$ in reduced form in the free product with amalgamation sense. Without loss of generality, we may suppose that $g_n \in K$. First suppose that $n = 1$. We have

$$g_1 m g_1^{-1} = m'.$$

By the Normal Form Theorem for Free Products with Amalgamation, the only way that the above equation can hold is if m is in the amalgamated part. Hence, $m = t^k$ for some integer k. Thus $gMg^{-1} \subseteq \langle t \rangle$ and the result holds.

Now suppose that $n \geq 2$. We have

$$g_1 \cdots g_{n-1} g_n m g_n^{-1} g_{n-1}^{-1} \cdots g_1^{-1} = m'.$$

As before, we have $g_n m g_n^{-1} = t^k$ for some k. Again applying the Normal Form Theorem, we must have $g_{n-1} t^k g_{n-1}^{-1}$ equal to a power of t. Since M is a free group and $g_{n-1} \in M$, the only way that g_{n-1} can conjugate a power of t to a power of t is if $g_{n-1} = t^l$. But this contradicts g_{n-1} part of the reduced form of g.

Now suppose that r involves at least three generators, say t, b, and c. Suppose that one of the generators other than b, say t, has exponent sum 0 in r. As before, we write G as an HNN extension,

$$G = \langle H, t; tXt^{-1} = Y \rangle$$

Suppose that for some $g \in G - M$, we have $J = gMg^{-1} \cap M$ not cyclic. Since M is free, $J \subseteq M$, and J is not cyclic, it follows that J is free of rank at least two. Hence, J', the commutator subgroup of J, is free and non-cyclic. Now

$$J' \subseteq gM'g^{-1} \cap M' \tag{1}$$

where M' is the commutator subgroup of M. The crucial point is that since M omits the generator b, and all elements of M' have zero exponent sum on t, the group M' is contained in the base H. In fact, $M' \subseteq H^*$, where H^* is the Magnus subgroup of H generated by the set of generators which omits all the b_i. Note also that $H^* \subseteq X \cap Y$.

Conjugating both sides of (1) by g, we obtain

$$g^{-1}J'g \subseteq M' \cap g^{-1}M'g \tag{2}$$

Suppose that g has HNN length 0, i.e. $g \in H$. Since $g \notin M$, $g \notin M'$. Since H^* is a Magnus subgroup of H and $g^{-1}J'g$ is not cyclic, we have a contradiction to the induction hypothesis. Suppose next, that

$$g^{-1} = g_0 t^{\varepsilon_1} g_1 \cdots t^{\varepsilon_n} g_n$$

in HNN reduced form, $n \geq 1$. If $g_n \in M$, then $t^{\varepsilon_n} g_n M' g_n^{-1} t^{-\varepsilon_n} \subseteq M'$, and we could replace g^{-1} by the element $g, \ldots t^{\varepsilon_{n-1}} g_{n-1}$ of shorter length. Hence, we may assume that $g_n \notin M$. In particular, g is not in either of the associated subgroups X or Y. For definiteness, suppose that $\varepsilon_n = 1$.

For each $j \in J'$, we have

$$g_0 t^{\varepsilon_1} \cdots t g_n j g_n^{-1} t^{-1} \cdots g_0^{-1} \in M'.$$

By Britton's Lemma, the only way which this can happen is to have $g_n j g_n^{-1} \in X$. Since $J' \subseteq M' \subseteq X$, we have $J' \subseteq g_n^{-1} X g_n \cap X$, contradicting the induction hypothesis.

We have completed the proof in the case that some generator other than b, which occurs in r has exponent sum 0 in r. The proof used, in a crucial way, the fact that the generator b, omitted by M, became the generator with bounded subcript range in H. If r contains no generator other than b with 0 exponent sum, we use the fact that r involves at least two generators, t and c, other than b. We use the standard trick for creating a zero exponent sum, using the generators t and c. The map $\Psi: G \to C$ embeds the subgroup M of G in a Magnus subgroup M^* of C, where the omitted generator can again be taken to have bounded subscript range in rewriting C as an HNN extension. The result follows as in the previous case. □

In the case of a one-relator group with torsion, the "Spelling Theorem" of B. B. Newman (1968) gives a very sharp solution to the word problem.

Theorem 5.5. *Let $G = \langle t, b, c, \ldots; r^n = 1\rangle$ where r is cyclically reduced and $n > 1$. Suppose $w = v$ in G where w is a freely reduced word on $\{t, b, c, \ldots\}$ and v omits a generator occurring in w. Then w contains a subword S such that S is also a subword of $r^{\pm n}$ and the length of S is greater than $(n-1)/n$ times the length of r^n.*

□ Suppose that an equation $w = v$ holds in G where v omits some generator, say t, which occurs in w but not in the defining relator r. Let K be the subgroup of G generated by all the given generators except t. Then $G = K * \langle t\rangle$, and $v \in K$. Writing $w = w_1 \cdots w_n$ in free product syllables, some w_j is a non-trivial power of t. By the Normal Form Theorem for Free Products, the only way the equation $w = v$ can hold is if some $w_i = 1$ in K. But if the conclusion of the theorem holds for the equation $w_i = 1$ it holds for the equation $w = v$. Thus we need consider only equations in which the omitted generator occurs in the defining relator r^n. The proof, of course, is by induction on the length of r. If r involves only one generator the result holds, so we may assume that r involves at least two generators.

Case 1. We first consider the case where some generator t occurring in r has $\sigma_t(r) = 0$. As before, we consider G as an HNN group with base

$$H = \langle b_\mu, \ldots, b_m, c_i, \ldots (i \in \mathbb{Z}); P^n = 1\rangle.$$

The associated subgroups X and Y are freely generated by $\{b_\mu, \ldots, b_{m-1}, c_i, \ldots (i \in \mathbb{Z})\}$ and $\{b_{\mu+1}, \ldots, b_m, c_i, \ldots (i \in \mathbb{Z})\}$ respectively.

Suppose that w is a freely reduced word on $t, b, c, \ldots$, and that $w(t, b, \ldots) = v(b, \ldots)$ where t occurs in w but not in v. The equation $w(t, b_0, \ldots) = v(b_0, \ldots)$ implies that w can be reduced to a t-free word w^* by t-reductions. By a t-reduction which is simply a "*shifting of subscripts*" we mean replacing a subword $t^\varepsilon u(b_i, c_i, \ldots)t^{-\varepsilon}$, $\varepsilon = \pm 1$, by $u(b_{i+\varepsilon}, c_{i+\varepsilon}, \ldots)$ where all the generators occurring in u occur explicitely among the given generators of X(if $\varepsilon = 1$) or Y(if $\varepsilon = -1$). The point of considering such reductions is that if w' is obtained from w by t-reductions which simply shift subscripts, then w can be obtained from w' by replacing each $b_i, c_i, \ldots$ in w' by $t^i b_0 t^{-i}$, $t^i c_0 t^{-i}, \ldots$, and then freely reducing, and the only letters cancelled in the free reductions will be t-symbols.

Starting with the original word w perform, wherever possible, t-reductions which simply shift subscripts. Suppose we reach a word w' to which no such reductions can be applied but w' is not t-reduced. Then w' contains a subword $t^\varepsilon u t^{-\varepsilon}$ where u is t-free and u itself is not a word on the given generators for X or Y (depending on ε) but u is equal to a word z on the given generators. Thus z omits a generator of H occurring in u, and $u = z$ in H. By the induction hypothesis, u contains a subword Q of $P^{\pm n}$ of the required length. Since we have only shifted subscripts to obtain w', we can recover w from w' by replacing each $b_i, \ldots$, by $t^i b_0 t^{-i}, \ldots$, and freely reducing, cancelling only t-symbols. Note that the part S of u which is recovered from Q will contain a subword of $r^{\pm n}$ of the desired length even if we disregard any occurrences of $t^{\pm 1}$ at the beginning or end of S.

If w can be reduced to a t-free word w^* by shifting subscripts, then w^* must contain a generator with a non-zero subscript and $w^* = v$ in H. By the induction hypothesis, w^* must contain a subword Q of $P^{\pm n}$ of the desired length. As before, this implies that w contains a suitable subword S of $r^{\pm n}$ and, moreover, S can be chosen so that it does not begin or end with $t^{\pm 1}$. (We shall need later the fact that the subword S can be chosen not to begin or end with the stable letter t).

Next suppose that an equation $w(t, b_0, c_0, \ldots) = v(t, c_0, \ldots)$ holds in G where b_0 occurs in w but not in v. By Britton's Lemma, we have $\sigma_t(w) = \sigma_t(v) = \alpha$ say. Hence, $wt^{-\alpha} = vt^{-\alpha}$. Since $vt^{-\alpha}$ has exponent sum zero on t and does not contain any b_i-symbols, $vt^{-\alpha}$ can be rewritten as an t-free word v^* by shifting subscripts. The equation $wt^{-\alpha} = v^*$ holds in G. As in the previous argument, if $wt^{-\alpha}$ cannot be reduced to a t-free word by shifting subscripts we conclude that $wt^{-\alpha}$ must contain a subword S of $r^{\pm n}$ of the desired length where S does not begin or end with $t^{\pm 1}$. The latter condition ensures that S is a subword of w. If $wt^{-\alpha}$ can be reduced to a t-free word w^* by shifting subscripts, then some b_i occurs in w^*. Since $w^* = v^*$ in H, the induction hypothesis says that w^* contains a subword Q of $P^{\pm n}$ of the desired length. As in the first part of this paragraph, w must then contain a subword S of $r^{\pm n}$ of the desired length where S does not begin or end with $t^{\pm 1}$.

Case 2. Finally, suppose that all generators occurring in r have non-zero exponent sum. Suppose that an equation $w(t, b, \ldots) = v(b, \ldots)$ holds in G where t occurs in w but not v. Let $\alpha = \sigma_t(r)$ and let $\beta = \sigma_b(r)$. The map Ψ defined by $t \mapsto yx^{-\beta}$, $b \mapsto x^\alpha$, $c \mapsto c, \ldots$ is an embedding of G into the group $C = \langle y, x, c, \ldots; r_1(yx^{-\beta}, x^\alpha, c, \ldots)\rangle$. Let w' be the result of freely reducing $w(yx^{-\beta}, x^\alpha, c, \ldots)$ and let v' be $v(x^\alpha, c, \ldots)$. Now w' contains an occurrence of y and v' does not. As in Case 1, w' contains a subword Q' of $r^{\pm n}(yx^{-\beta}, x^\alpha, c, \ldots)$ of the desired length, and Q' does not begin or end with $x^{\pm 1}$. This implies that w contains a suitable subword of $r^{\pm n}$. $\square$

B. B. Newman (1968) used the above theorem to solve the conjugacy problem for one-relator groups with torsion. The conjugacy problem for one-relator groups which are the free product of two finitely generated free groups with cyclic amalgamation was solved by S. Lipschutz (1966). In conclusion, we point out that the conjugacy problem for one-relator groups in general is still unsolved and appears to be very difficult.

6. *Bipolar Structures*

In his work on the theory of ends, J. Stallings (1971) shows that if G is a finitely generated group with infinitely many ends, then G has a decomposition as a non-trivial free product with amalgamation or as an HNN extension where the amalgamated (respectively, associated) subgroups are finite. In his proof, Stallings introduces the concept of a bipolar structure. Bipolar structures provide a characterization for a group to be either a non-trivial free product with amalgamation or an HNN extension. We shall apply this characterization to obtain a theorem of Hanna Neumann (1948) on finitely generated subgroups of free products with amalgamation and HNN extensions.

We turn to the definition of a bipolar structure on a group. (The reader familiar with Stalling's work will notice two slight differences in our definition. In working with ends, it is crucial that the subgroup F mentioned below be finite. Here, of course, we must allow F to be infinite. Also, we shall not need Stallings' set S.)

Definition. A *bipolar structure* on a group G is a partition of G into five disjoint subsets F, EE, EE^*, E^*E, E^*E^* satisfying the following axioms. (The letters X, Y, Z will stand for the letters E or E^* with the convention that $(X^*)^* = X$, etc.)

1. F is a subgroup of G.
2. If $f \in F$ and $g \in XY$, then $gf \in XY$.
3. If $g \in XY$, then $g^{-1} \in YX$. (*Inverse axiom*)
4. If $g \in XY$ and $h \in Y^*Z$, then $gh \in XZ$. (*Product axiom*)
5. If $g \in G$, there is an integer $N(g)$ such that, if there exist $g_1, \ldots, g_n \in G$ and $X_0, \ldots, X_n$ with $g_i \in X_{i-1}^* X_i$ and $g = g_1 \cdots g_n$, then $n \leqslant N(g)$. (*Boundedness axiom*)
6. $EE^* \neq \varnothing$. (*Non-triviality axiom*)

We next show that every non-trivial free product with amalgamation and every HNN extension has a bipolar structure. Let $G = \langle A * B; F = \phi(F)\rangle$ be a free product with amalgamation where F and $\phi(F)$ are proper subgroups of A and B respectively. (It may be that $F = \{1\}$, so that G is an ordinary free product.) We can define a bipolar structure on G as follows. The subgroup F of G is the subgroup F in the bipolar structure. Every element $g \in G - F$ has a representation as

$$g = c_1 \cdots c_n$$

where no $c_i \in F$, each c_i is as one of the factors A or B, and successive c_i, c_{i+1} come from different factors. The Normal Form Theorem for Free Products with Amalgamation ensures that the number n and what factors the c_i come from are the same for any representation satisfying the stated restrictions. We define the sets EE, EE^*, E^*E, and E^*E^* as follows:

$$g \in EE \text{ iff } c_1 \in A \text{ and } c_n \in A,$$
$$g \in EE^* \text{ iff } c_1 \in A \text{ and } c_n \in B,$$
$$g \in E^*E \text{ iff } c_1 \in B \text{ and } c_n \in A,$$
$$g \in E^*E^* \text{ iff } c_1 \in B \text{ and } c_n \in B.$$

Verification of the axioms is immediate. For example, if $g \in XY$ and $h \in Y^*Z$, then g and h have representations

$$g = c_1 \cdots c_n \quad \text{and} \quad h = d_1 \cdots d_m$$

where c_n and d_1 are in different factors. Thus a representation of gh is

$$c_1 \cdots c_n d_1 \cdots d_m,$$

and axiom 4 holds. The number $N(g)$ in axiom 5 is simply the length of g, in the free product with amalgamation length sense. Since F and $\phi(F)$ are proper subgroups of A and B respectively, there are elements $c \in A - F$ and $d \in B - \phi(F)$. Thus $cd \in EE^*$, verifying the non-triviality axiom.

We now consider the HNN case. Let

$$G = \langle H, t; tFt^{-1} = \phi(F)\rangle$$

be an HNN extension. We can define a bipolar structure on G as follows. The subgroup F of G is the subgroup F of the bipolar structure. Each element $g \in G - F$ has a representation as a product of elements in a reduced sequence; say

$$g = h_0 t^{\varepsilon_1} h_1 \cdots t^{\varepsilon_n} h_n,$$

where each $h_i \in H$.

We put

$$g \in EE \text{ iff } \quad h_0 \in H - F, \text{ or } h_0 \in F \text{ and } \varepsilon_1 = +1,$$
$$\text{and } h_n \in H - F, \text{ or } h_n \in F \text{ and } \varepsilon_n = -1,$$

$$g \in EE^* \text{ iff } \quad h_0 \in H - F, \text{ or } h_0 \in F \text{ and } \varepsilon_1 = +1,$$
$$\text{and } h_n \in F \text{ and } \varepsilon_n = +1,$$

$$g \in E^*E \text{ iff } \quad h_0 \in F \text{ and } \varepsilon_1 = -1,$$
$$\text{and } h_n \in H - F, \text{ or } h_n \in F \text{ and } \varepsilon_n = -1,$$

$$g \in E^*E^* \text{ iff } \quad h_0 \in F \text{ and } \varepsilon_1 = -1,$$
$$\text{and } h_n \in F \text{ and } \varepsilon_n = +1.$$

In particular, all elements of $H - F$ are in EE. It follows from Britton's Lemma that the above definition is independent of the choice of the reduced sequence for g.

We verify the product axiom (axiom 4.) As with free products with amalgamation, the point is that if $g \in XY$ and $k \in Y^*Z$, then we can obtain a reduced sequence for gk by putting together the sequences for g and k. Let $g = h_0 t^{\varepsilon_1} \cdots t^{\varepsilon_n} h_n$, and let $k = k_0\, t^{\delta_1} \cdots t^{\delta_m} k_m$. Suppose $g \in XE$ and $k \in E^*Z$. Then $h_n \in H - F$, or $g_n \in F$ and $\varepsilon_n = -1$, while $k_0 \in F$ and $\delta_1 = -1$. Thus the sequence

$$h_0 t^{\varepsilon_1} \cdots t^{\varepsilon_n} (h_n k_0) t^{\delta_1} \cdots t^{\delta_n} k_m$$

is reduced and $gk \in XZ$. A similar verification works for $g \in XE^*$ and $k \in EZ$.

To verify the boundedness axiom, consider a product $g = g_1 \cdots g_n$ where $g_i \in X_{i-1}^* X_i$. The condition $g_i \in X_{i-1}^* X_i$, implies that at most half the g_i can be in EE. Each $g_i \notin EE$ must have a t-symbol in its reduced form. Since we have seen that we can obtain a reduced sequence for g by putting together the reduced sequences for the g_i, merely consolidating elements of H at the beginning and end of the sequences for the g_i, we see that n is less than or equal to twice the number of t-symbols in the reduced form of g.

Finally, $t \in EE^*$, verifying non-triviality.

We note that a group may possess many different bipolar structures. Consider, for example, the fundamental group of the surface of genus 3. The bipolar structure arising from viewing G as a free product with amalgamation, say

$$G = \langle a, b, c, d, d, f; [a, b][c, d] = [f, e]\rangle,$$

and that arising from viewing G as an HNN extension, say

$$G = \langle a, b, c, d, e, f; f^{-1}ef = e[d, c][b, a]\rangle,$$

are rather different.

We next investigate some of the consequences of the axioms for a bipolar structure. The following sequence of four lemmas follows Stallings (1972). Let G be a group with a bipolar structure. An element $g \in G$ is said to be *irreducible* if $g \in F$, or $g \in XY$ and g is not equal to a product $g = hk$ with $h \in XZ$ and $k \in Z^*Y$.

The boundedness axiom, axiom 5, immediately implies that G is generated by irreducible elements. It follows from the inverse axiom (axiom 3) and the fact that F is a subgroup, that g is irreducible if and only if g^{-1} is irreducible.

Lemma 6.1. *If $g \in XY$, $h \in YZ$, and h is irreducible, then $gh \in F$ or $gh \in XW$ for some W.*

☐ If $gh \in F$, we are done. Suppose $gh \in X^*W$. Now $g^{-1} \in YX$ by the inverse axiom. But then $h = g^{-1}(gh)$, which contradicts h being irreducible. ☐

Lemma 6.2. *If $h \in ZX$, $g \in XY$, and h is irreducible, then $hg \in F$ or $hg \in WY$ for some W.*

☐ Similar to Lemma 6.1. ☐

Lemma 6.3. *If $g \in XY$ and $h \in YZ$ are both irreducible, then gh is an irreducible element of $F \cup XZ$.*

☐ By Lemmas 6.1 and 6.2, $gh \in F \cup XZ$. If gh is not irreducible, then $gh \in XZ$ and $gh = pq$ where $p \in XW$ and $q \in W^*Z$. Now $g = p(qh^{-1})$. Since $h^{-1} \in ZY$ and is irreducible, we have $qh^{-1} \in F$ or $qh^{-1} \in W^*V$ by Lemma 6.1. We cannot have $qh^{-1} \in W^*V$, since this would contradict g being irreducible. Hence, $qh^{-1} \in F$. Thus $g = p(qh^{-1}) \in XW$ by axiom 2. Also, $h^{-1} = q^{-1}(qh^{-1})$, so $h^{-1} \in ZW^*$ by the inverse axiom and axiom 2. Hence, $h \in W^*Z$. This contradicts $g \in XY$ and $h \in YZ$. ☐

Lemma 6.4. *If $g \in XY$, $f \in F$, and g is irreducible, then gf is an irreducible element of XY. Similarly, fg is an irreducible element of XY.*

☐ We have $gf \in XY$ by axiom 2. If gf is not irreducible, then $gf = pq$ where $p \in XW$ and $q \in W^*Y$ for some W. But then $g = p(qf^{-1})$. Since $p \in XW$ and $(qf^{-1}) \in W^*Y$ by axiom 2, this contradicts g being irreducible. Note that $g^{-1}f^{-1}$

is an irreducible element of YX by the inverse axiom and the first part of the proof. Thus fg is an irreducible element of XY. □

We can now prove Stallings' characterization theorem.

Theorem 6.5. *A group G has a bipolar structure if and only if G is either a non-trivial free product with amalgamation (possibly an ordinary free product) or an HNN extension.*

□ Let G have a bipolar structure. Define

$$G_1 = F \cup \{x: x \text{ is an irreducible element of } EE\}, \text{ and}$$

$$G_2 = F \cup \{x: x \text{ is an irreducible element of } E^*E^*\}.$$

We claim that G_1 and G_2 are subgroups of G. The inverse of an element of G_1 is in G_1 by axiom 1 and the inverse axiom. Consider a product hk of two elements of G_1. If both h and k are in F, then $hk \in F$ since F is a subgroup. If both h and k are irreducible elements of EE, then $hk \in F$ or hk is an irreducible element of EE by Lemma 6.3. If exactly one of h, k is in F, then hk is an irreducible element of EE by Lemma 6.4. Similarly, G_2 is a subgroup of G.

Case 1. If there are no irreducible elements of EE^*, then $G = \langle G_1 * G_2; F = F \rangle$.

Since the elements of E^*E are inverses of elements of EE^*, there are no irreducible elements in E^*E. Thus $G_1 \cup G_2$ contains all the irreducible elements of G. Since G is generated by irreducible elements, $G_1 \cup G_2$ generates G.

Take disjoint copies $\bar{G}_1$ and $\bar{G}_2$ of G_1 and G_2. For any element $g_i \in G_i$, $i = 1, 2$, $\bar{g}_i$ will denote the corresponding element of $\bar{G}_i$. Let

$$\bar{G} = \langle \bar{G}_1 * \bar{G}_2; \bar{F} = \bar{F} \rangle$$

Define $\psi: \bar{G} \to G$ by $\psi(\bar{g}_1) = g_1$ if $\bar{g}_1 \in \bar{G}_1$, and $\psi(\bar{g}_2) = g_2$, $\bar{g}_2 \in \bar{G}_2$. We claim that ψ is an isomorphism. First, ψ is onto G by the remark of the preceeding paragraph. Now ψ is certainly one-to-one on $\bar{G}_1$ and $\bar{G}_2$. If $\bar{g}$ is an element not in a factor of $\bar{G}$, write $\bar{g} = \bar{c}_1 \cdots \bar{c}_n$ where each $\bar{c}_i$ is in a factor, no $\bar{c}_i \in \bar{F}$, and successive $\bar{c}_i$, $\bar{c}_{i+1}$ come from different factors. The images $c_i = \psi(\bar{c}_i)$ thus come alternately from EE and E^*E^*. Thus, by the product axiom,

$$\psi(\bar{g}) = c_1 \cdots c_n$$

is in one of the sets XY and is not equal to 1. Hence, ψ is an isomorphism.

If F were not a proper subgroup of both G_1 and G_2, say $F = G_1$, then $G_1 \cup G_2 = G_2$. Since G_2 then generates G, we have $G = G_2 \subseteq F \cup EE$, which contradicts the non-triviality axiom, $EE^* \neq \emptyset$.

Case 2. If there is an irreducible element $t \in EE^*$, then

$$G = \langle G_1, t; tFt^{-1} = \phi(F) \rangle.$$

We first show that $G_1 \cup \{t\}$ generates G. If g is an irreducible element of E^*E, then tg is an irreducible element of $F \cup EE$ by Lemma 6.3, and $g = t^{-1}(tg)$. The irreducible elements of EE^* are inverses of irreducible elements of E^*E. If g is an irreducible element of E^*E^*, then gt^{-1} is an irreducible element of $E^*E \cup F$ by Lemma 6.3.

Certainly, conjugation by t induces an isomorphism ϕ between F and a subgroup $\phi(F)$ of G. We check that $tFt^{-1} \subseteq G_1$. If $f \in F$, then tf is an irreducible element of EE^* by Lemma 6.4, and $(tf)t^{-1}$ is thus an irreducible element of $F \cup EE$ by Lemma 6.3.

Recall that G_1 is a subgroup of G and that $G_1 \subseteq F \cup EE$. Now $t \in EE^*$ which is disjoint from $F \cup EE$. Hence, for any choice of elements g_1 and g_2 of G_1 and $\varepsilon = \pm 1$, we have $g_1 t^{\varepsilon} g_2 \notin F$. We shall often implicitely use this observation.

Let $\bar{G}_1$ be an isomorphic copy of G_1, and let

$$\bar{G} = \langle \bar{G}_1, \bar{t}; \bar{t}\bar{F}\bar{t}^{-1} = \overline{\phi(F)} \rangle.$$

Define $\psi: \bar{G} \to G$ by $\psi(\bar{g}_1) = g_1$ if $\bar{g}_1 \in G_1$, and $\psi(\bar{t}) = t$. We know that ψ is onto G since $G_1 \cup \{t\}$ generates G. If $\bar{g} \in \bar{G} - \bar{G}_1$, write $\bar{g}$ as the product of elements in a reduced sequence, say

$$g = \bar{g}_0 \bar{t}^{\varepsilon_1} \cdots \bar{t}^{\varepsilon_n} \bar{g}_n, \; n \geqslant 1,$$

where each $\bar{g}_i \in \bar{G}_1$. We must show that

$$\psi(\bar{g}) = g_0 t^{\varepsilon_1} \cdots t^{\varepsilon_n} g_n \neq 1.$$

In exhibiting a bipolar structure for an arbitrary HNN extension, we gave a scheme for putting elements into the sets XY. We claim that $\psi(\bar{g})$ is in XY according to the same scheme. (In the present context, G_1 plays the role of H.) The proof is by induction on n. We will first analyze the case where $n > 1$. The case $n = 1$ is easily seen to follow from the same analysis.

We consider the sign of ε_{n-1}. Suppose $\varepsilon_{n-1} = 1$. Then $g = w g_{n-1} t^{\varepsilon_n} g_n$ where $w = g_0 \cdots g_{n-2} t$. Now $w \in XE^*$ by the induction hypothesis. We cannot have both $g_{n-1} \in F$ and $\varepsilon_n = -1$ since the sequence for $\bar{g}$ is reduced. Suppose $\varepsilon_n = -1$. Then $g_{n-1} \in EE$. Regardless of whether $g_n \in EE$ or $g_n \in F$, we have $t^{-1} g_n \in E^*E$ by applying either Lemma 6.3 or axiom 2. Thus $w g_{n-1}(t^{-1} g_n) \in XE$ by the product axiom. Suppose $\varepsilon_n = 1$. Regardless of whether $g_{n-1} \in EE$ or $g_{n-1} \in F$, we have $g_{n-1} t \in EE^*$. If $g_n \in EE$, we have $w(g_{n-1} t) g_n \in XE$. If $g_{n-1} \in F$, we have $w(g_{n-1} t) g_n \in XE^*$.

Suppose $\varepsilon_{n-1} = -1$. Write $g = v t^{-1} g_{n-1} t^{\varepsilon_n} g_n$ where $v = g_0 \cdots g_{n-2}$. Suppose that v does not consist solely of $g_0 \in F$. Then we claim that $v \in XE$, for, otherwise, v would have to end in $t g_{n-2}$ with $g_{n-2} \in F$. This contradicts the original sequence for $\bar{g}$ being reduced. Now $t^{-1} g_{n-1}$ is an irreducible element of E^*E regardless of whether $g_{n-1} \in EE$ or $g_{n-1} \in F$. (Apply either Lemma 6.3 or 6.4.) Suppose $\varepsilon_n = 1$. Then $t^{-1} g_{n-1} t \in F \cup E^*E^*$ by Lemma 6.3. Now $t^{-1} g_{n-1} t \in F$ is impossible since this implies $g_{n-1} \in \phi(F)$ which contradicts the original sequence for $\bar{g}$ for being reduced. Thus $t^{-1}g_{n-1}t \in E^*E^*$. If $g_n \in EE$, $v(t^{-1}g_{n-1}t)g_n \in XE$, while, if $g_n \in F$, $v(t^{-1}g_{n-1}tg_n) \in XE^*$. Finally, suppose that $\varepsilon_n = -1$. Then $t^{-1}g_n \in E^*E$ and $v(t^{-1}g_{n-1})(t^{-1}g_n) \in XE$. The result for the case $v \in F$ follows easily from the above analysis.

The case where $n = 1$ follows easily by analyzing the product $g_0 t^{\varepsilon_1} g_1$ along the lines above. Thus we see that $g = \psi(\bar{g})$ is in one of the sets XY and cannot be equal to 1. Hence, ψ is one-to-one and is thus an isomorphism. This concludes the proof of the theorem. □

We have seen that a group G has a bipolar structure if and only if G is a non-trivial free product with amalgamation or an HNN extension. We shall now use the bipolar structure characterization to prove a theorem of H. Neumann (1948) on finitely generated subgroups of free products with amalgamation or HNN extensions.

Theorem 6.6. *Let $G = \langle A * B;\ F = \phi(F)\rangle$ be a non-trivial free product with amalgamation. (Respectively, let $G = \langle A, t;\ t^{-1}Ft = \phi(F)\rangle$ be an HNN extension.) Let H be a finitely generated subgroup of G such that all conjugates of H intersect F trivially. Then*

$$H = K * (*_\alpha H_\alpha)$$

where K is a free group and each H_α is the intersection of a subgroup of H with a conjugate of a factor (respectively, the base) of G.

The theorem remains true without the assumption that G is finitely generated. For a complete discussion of subgroup theorems for free products with amalgamation and HNN extensions see Serre (1969) or Karrass and Solitar (1970, 1971). An immediate corollary of the theorem is the following.

Corollary 6.7. *Let $G = \langle A * B;\ F = \phi(F)\rangle$ be a non-trivial free product with amalgamation. (Respectively, let $G = \langle A, t;\ tFt^{-1} = \phi(F)\rangle$ be an HNN extension.) If H is a finitely generated subgroup of G which has trivial intersection with all conjugates of the factors, A and B, (respectively, the base A) of G, then H is free.* □

Before proving the theorem, we need a short lemma.

Lemma 6.8. *Let $G = \langle A * B;\ F = \phi(F)\rangle$ be a non-trivial free product with amalgamation. Let H be a finitely generated subgroup of G. Then either H is contained in a conjugate of a factor of G, or some conjugate of H contains a cyclically reduced element of length at least two. Similarly, let $G = \langle A, t;\ tFt^{-1} = \phi(F)\rangle$ be an HNN extension. If H is a finitely generated subgroup of G, then H is contained in a conjugate of the base, A, or some conjugate of H contains a cyclically reduced element of length at least two.*

□ We prove the lemma for free products with amalgamation. The proof for HNN extensions is similar. The proof is by induction on s, the sum of the lengths of the elements in a finite set of generators for H. If $s = 1$, H is contained in a factor. Let $H = \langle h_1, \ldots, h_n\rangle$. If any of the h_i are cyclically reduced of length at least two we are done. Assuming that this is not the case, if we write any $h_i = c_1 \cdots c_k$ in reduced form (possibly $k = 1$), then c_1 and c_k are in the same factor. If two generators for H, say h_i and h_j, begin and end with elements from different factors, the product $h_i h_j$ is cyclically reduced of length at least two. So suppose that reduced forms of all the h_i begin and end with elements from the same factor, say A. If all the h_i have length one, $H \subset A$. So assume that some $h_i = c_1 \cdots c_k$, $k > 1$, $c_1, c_k \in A$. We can then replace H by $c_1^{-1} H c_1 = \langle h_1^*, \ldots, h_n^* \rangle$, where $h_j^* = c_1^{-1} h_j c_1^{-1}$. The sum of the lengths of the h_j^* is less than the sum of the lengths of the h_j, and the result follows. □

We now turn to the theorem. The reader familiar with Stallings' proof of Serre's conjecture in the finitely generated case, will note that the overall strategy of our proof, while not involving ends, is the same.

Proof of the theorem. We use the notation in the statement of the theorem. If H is contained in a conjugate of a factor (respectively, the base) of G, the result holds trivially, so we assume that this is not the case. The proof is by induction on n, the minimum number of generators of H. If $n = 1$ and $H = \langle h_1 \rangle$ is not in a conjugate of a factor, then h_1 has infinite order, so H is free.

Assume the result true for $1 \leqslant n \leqslant k$, and prove it for $n = k + 1$. Note that a subgroup H of G has a decomposition of the desired type stated in the theorem if and only if all conjugates of H have a decomposition of the desired type. By Lemma 6.8, some conjugate H^* of H contains a cyclically reduced element of length greater than one. We replace H by H^*.

Give G the bipolar structure associated with viewing G as the given free product with amalgamation or HNN extension. We put a bipolar structure on H^* by simply taking the set-theoretic intersection of H^* with the sets F, EE, etc. Thus $F_{H^*} = H^* \cap F$, $EE_{H^*}^* = H^* \cap EE^*$, etc. Note that axioms 1–5 for a bipolar structure are hereditary, and thus hold in the proposed bipolar structure for H^*. We must check the non-triviality axiom. But H^* contains a cyclically reduced element h^* of length at least two, whence one of h^* or $(h^*)^{-1}$ is in EE^*. Thus $EE_{H^*}^* \neq \varnothing$.

By the hypothesis on H, $H^* \cap F = \{1\}$. But $F_{H^*} = \{1\}$ means that H^* is a non-trivial free product, say $H^* = H_1 * H_2$. By the Grushko-Neumann Theorem, H_1 and H_2 have fewer generators than H^*. Thus H_1 and H_2 have decompositions of the desired type by the induction hypothesis. But it is immediate that the free product of two groups having a decomposition of the desired type again has a decomposition of the desired type. This concludes the proof of the theorem. □

We conclude this section by pointing out that bipolar structures may be useful in showing that various groups have nice decompositions as free products with amalgamations or HNN extensions. The following theorem is due to Nagao (1959). (See section III.12.)

Theorem 6.9. *Let $K[x]$ be the polynomial ring in one variable over a field K. Then*

$$\mathbb{GL}_2(K[x]) = \langle \mathbb{GL}_2(K) * T; U = U \rangle$$

where U is the group of upper triangular matrices with entries from K, and T is the *group of matrices of the form* $\begin{bmatrix} k_1 & f(x) \\ 0 & k_2 \end{bmatrix}$ *where* k_2 *and* k_2 *are non-zero elements of* K *and* $f(x) \in K[x]$.

For generalizations of Nagao's result, see Serre (1969). The easiest way to prove Nagao's result is a direct proof. It turns out, however, that $\mathbb{GL}_2(K[x])$ has a rather natural bipolar structure, which we now describe.

□ Let $F = U$, and put all matrices in $\mathbb{GL}_2(K) - U$ into EE. If $f \in K[x]$, $\delta(f)$ will denote the degree of f. Now consider any matrix $M = \begin{bmatrix} f_{11} & f_{12} \\ f_{21} & f_{22} \end{bmatrix}$ where at least one entry has degree greater than zero. Put

$$M \in EE \text{ iff } \delta(f_{12}) \leqslant \delta(f_{11}) \text{ and } \delta(f_{12}) \leqslant \delta(f_{22}),$$
$$M \in EE^* \text{ iff } \delta(f_{12}) \leqslant \delta(f_{11}) \text{ and } \delta(f_{12}) > \delta(f_{22}),$$
$$M \in E^*E \text{ iff } \delta(f_{12}) > \delta(f_{11}) \text{ and } \delta(f_{12}) \leqslant \delta(f_{22}),$$
$$M \in E^*E^* \text{ iff } \delta(f_{12}) > \delta(f_{11}) \text{ and } \delta(f_{12}) > \delta(f_{22}).$$

In short, one compares the degree of f_{12} with the degrees of the entries on the main diagonal. The inverse axiom is an immediate consequence of the formula for inverting 2×2 matrices; $M^{-1} = \frac{1}{\det M}\begin{bmatrix} f_{22} & -f_{12} \\ -f_{21} & f_{11} \end{bmatrix}$. To verify the product axiom and the axiom for the amalgamated part, it seems that one must multiply out the several cases. The boundedness axiom holds because these multiplications show that if $M \in XY$ and $N \in Y^*Z$, then the maximum of the degrees of the entries in MN is strictly greater the degree of any entry in either M or N. □

7. The Higman Embedding Theorem

Long before the notion of an "algorithm" was made precise, algorithms had, of course, been given for solving many problems. In cases of positive solutions of decision problems, as, for example, the word problem for one-relator groups, the algorithm was actually produced and everyone agreed that an effective decision procedure had been supplied. Note, however, that negative unsolvability results could not be proved before a precise definition of "algorithm" had been given. For a nonexistence proof requires a survey of all possible algorithms. In the 1930's, a precise definition of an algorithm was given. One could then replace the intuitive ideas of "effectively decidable" and "effectively enumerable" by the precise concepts "recursive" and "recursively enumerable."

In the 1950's, Novikov (1955) and Boone (1959) independently proved that there exist finitely presented groups with unsolvable word problem. In 1961, G. Higman proved a remarkable theorem, firmly establishing that the connection between the logical notion of recursiveness and questions about finitely presented groups is not accidental but very deep. Recall that a recursive presentation is a presentation on a finite number of generators such that the set of defining relators is recursively enumerable.

Theorem 7.1. (The Higman Embedding Theorem). *A finitely generated group G can be embedded in some finitely presented group if and only if G can be recursively presented.*

Our goal in this section is to prove the Higman Embedding Theorem and some of its consequences.

Before proving the Higman Embedding Theorem, we shall discuss some of its consequences, retaining the use of an intuitive concept of "recursive." When we discuss a precise definition of "recursive," we shall prove that there exists a recursively enumerable non-recursive set S of positive integers. Given this fact, the existence of a finitely presented group with unsolvable word problem follows easily from the Higman Embedding Theorem. We give such a proof now. Actually, all the facts needed to exhibit a finitely presented group with unsolvable word problem will be established halfway through the proof of the embedding theorem. At that point we will again consider the unsolvability of the word problem.

Theorem 7.2. *There exists a finitely presented group H with unsolvable word problem.*

□ Let S be a recursively enumerable non-recursive set of positive integers. Let

$$G = \langle a, b, c, d; a^{-i}ba^i = c^{-i}dc^i, i \in S \rangle.$$

It is clear that G has unsolvable word problem, for, in G,

$$a^{-n}ba^n = c^{-n}dc^n \quad \text{iff} \quad n \in S.$$

Since the set of defining relations of G is recursively enumerable, G can be embedded in a finitely presented group H. Since G is finitely generated with unsolvable word problem, H must have unsolvable word problem. □

The next theorem is due to Higman (1961).

Theorem 7.3. *There exists a finitely presented group H such that every recursively presented group is embeddable in H.*

□ The set of all finite presentations $G_i = \langle X_i; R_i \rangle$ is clearly countably infinite and recursively enumerable. Clearly we can choose an enumeration such that the X_i are successive disjoint segments of a set $X = \{x_1, x_2, \ldots\}$. Now $\langle X; \bigcup R_i \rangle$ is clearly a recursive presentation for a group G isomorphic to the free product of the G_i, and hence containing a subgroup isomorphic to every finitely presented group. Therefore the Higman-Neumann-Neumann embedding puts G in a recursively presented two-generator group G^*. Then G^* can be embedded in a finitely presented group H. Clearly, H contains a copy of every finitely presented group. Again applying the Higman Embedding Theorem, H contains a copy of every recursively presented group. □

We now turn to a theorem of Boone and Higman (1973) giving a succinct algebraic characterization of finitely generated groups with solvable word problem.

Theorem 7.4. *A finitely generated group G has solvable word problem if and only if G can be embedded in a simple subgroup of a finitely presented group.*

☐ Suppose that G can be embedded in a simple subgroup S of a finitely presented group H. The fact that G then has solvable word problem is really contained in Kuznetsov's Theorem (Theorem 3.6.). Since G is finitely generated and embeddable in a finitely presented group, the set of words equal to 1 in G is recursively enumerable. It thus suffices to show that the set of words not equal to 1 in G is also recursively enumerable. Let $\psi: G \to H$ be an embedding with $\psi(G) \subseteq S$ where S is a simple subgroup of H. Pick a fixed element $1 \neq s \in S$. For $w \in G$, let H_w be the group obtained from H by adding $\psi(w)$ as a defining relator. Since S is simple, if $\psi(w) \neq 1$ in H, then all elements of S, in particular s, are equal to 1 in H_w. Thus $w \neq 1$ in G if and only if $s = 1$ in H_w. Since G is finitely generated and H is finitely presented, the set of w such that $s = 1$ in H_w is recursively enumerable.

We must now show that if G is a finitely generated group with solvable word problem, then G can be embedded in a simple subgroup of a finitely presented group. The first step is to embed G in a simple group S with a recursive set of defining relators. The construction of S is reminiscent of the construction of a group in which any two elements of the same order are conjugate, but we must be careful to ensure a solvable word problem.

Since G has solvable word problem, the set

$$\{\langle u_1, v_1\rangle, \langle u_2, v_2\rangle, \ldots\}$$

of pairs of elements of G, neither of which is equal to 1, is recursive. Let

$$G_1 = \langle G, x_1, t_i (i \geq 1); t_i^{-1} u_i x_1^{-1} u_i x_1 t = v_i x_1^{-1} u_i x_1, i \geq 1\rangle.$$

The elements $u_i x^{-1} u_i x_1$ and $v_i x^{-1} u_i x_1$ are cyclically reduced with free product length four. Thus they all have infinite order and, furthermore, the generalized word problem with respect to the cyclic subgroups generated by these elements is uniformly solvable. Thus G_1 is an HNN extension of $G * \langle x_1\rangle$, and the indicated presentation of G_1 has solvable word problem.

Suppose, inductively, that G_k has been defined, and obtain G_{k+1} from G_k as in the preceding paragraph. Let

$$S = \bigcup_{k=1}^{\infty} G_k.$$

Since our construction process is uniform, S has solvable word problem. We next check that S is simple. Let u and v be any non-identity elements of S. Pick an index $k - 1$ such that both u and v are in G_{k-1}. Then there is a stable letter p such that the equation

$$p^{-1} u x_k^{-1} u x_k p = v x_k^{-1} u x_k$$

holds in G_k. Solving this equation for v, we see that v is in the normal closure of u. Since u and v are arbitrary, this shows that S is simple.

The set of defining relations of S is recursive. Thus the Higman-Neumann-Neumann embedding puts S into a recursively presented two-generator group K. By the Higman Embedding Theorem, K can be embedded in a finitely presented group H. Since we have embeddings

$$G \to S \to K \to H$$

the theorem is proved. □

In order to prove the Higman embedding theorem, we must have precise definitions of "recursive" and "recursively enumerable." Many definitions have been given: Turing machines, formal systems, λ-computability, etc. All the definitions proposed have been shown to be equivalent. The equivalence of all these notions, which are formally quite different, has led logicians to the belief that the precisely defined concept of being recursive is an adequate formalization of the intuitive notion of "effective." This philosophical position is called the Church-Turing thesis. In practice this means that if someone proves that a certain function f is not recursive, people do not waste time trying to find a procedure (necessarily non-recursive) for computing f which is in some sense "effective."

In what may initially seem to the reader to be an abrupt change of thought, let us turn to some concepts involving polynomials with integer coefficients. Let $P(X_1, \ldots X_k)$ be a polynomial (in several variables) with integer coefficients. A k-tuple $(z_1, \ldots z_k)$ of integers such that

$$P(z_1, \ldots, z_k) = 0$$

is said to be a *root* of P.

Definition. A subset S of $\mathbb{Z}^n$ is said to be *Diophantine* if there exists a polynomial $P(X_1, \ldots, X_n; Y_1, \ldots, Y_m)$ such that

$(s_1, \ldots, s_n) \in S$ if and only if $P(s_1, \ldots s_n; Y_1, \ldots, Y_m)$ has an integer root.

We say that P *enumerates* S.

As a non-trivial example, the set $\mathbb{N}$ of natural numbers is Diophantine. For, by the famous theorem of Lagrange, an integer is non-negative if and only if it is a sum of four squares. Thus $s \in \mathbb{N}$ if and only if the polynomial $P(s; Y_1, \ldots, Y_4) = Y_1^2 + \cdots + Y_4^2 - s$ has a root.

Note that a Diophantine set S is certainly intuitively effectively enumerable. For, let $P(X_1, \ldots, X_n, Y_1, \ldots Y_m)$ be the polynomial which enumerates S. We can effectively enumerate all $(n + m)$-tuples $(s_1, \ldots, s_n, d_1, \ldots, d_m)$ of integers. As each is enumerated, compute $P(s_1, \ldots, s_n, d_1, \ldots, d_m)$ and see if the value is 0. If so, put $(s_1, \ldots, s_n)$ on the list of elements of S. If not, go on to the next $(n + m)$-tuple.

One of the most famous decision problems is Hilbert's Tenth Problem. Hilbert asked for an algorithm which, when given a polynomial $P(X_1, \ldots X_m)$ with integer coefficients, decides whether or not P has an integer root. Matiyasevich (1970)

showed that no such algorithm exists. In settling Hilbert's Tenth Problem, Matiyasevich actually established much more. Namely, all recursively enumerable sets are Diophantine! This is now a basic result of recursive function theory. For our purposes, it will be convenient to take being Diophantine as the definition of recursively enumerable. There are two reasons for our adopting this approach. First, it will allow us to explain some basic facts about recursively enumerable sets with a minimum of logical formalism. Secondly, our proof of the Higman Embedding Theorem will follow Valiev (1968) who makes ingenious use of the Diophantine character of recursively enumerable sets.

The reader who favors a standard definition of "recursive" may view the theorem of Matiyasevich as establishing the equivalence of that definition and the one which we offer below. Also, in what follows we shall not prove that various sets which are obviously intuitively "effectively enumerable" are actually Diophantine. Suffice it to say that this can be done. For an excellent exposition of the work of Matiyasevich, we urge the reader to consult M. Davis (1973). Within the understanding above, our development will be self-contained.

Definition. A set $S \subseteq \mathbb{Z}^n$ is *recursively enumerable* if S is Diophantine. The set S is said to be *recursive* if both S and its complement, $\mathbb{Z}^n - S$, are recursively enumerable.

The first thing we shall do is to exhibit a recursively enumerable set which is not recursive. The way to do this is to "arithmetize" one's formalism by assigning numbers to everything in sight. Since this was first done by Gödel, the numbers assigned are called "Gödel numbers." We shall assign positive integers to polynomials as follows. The function $\alpha: \mathbb{Z} \to \mathbb{N}$ defined by

$$\alpha(z) = \begin{cases} 2|z| + 1 & \text{if } z \leqslant 0 \\ 2|z| & \text{if } z > 0 \end{cases}$$

is clearly one-to-one.

Fix $X_0, X_1, \ldots, X_n, \ldots$ as our infinite list of variables. Assign to each monomial term

$$T = cX_{i_1}^{e_1} \cdots X_{i_n}^{e_n}$$

where $0 \neq c \in \mathbb{Z}$, each $e_i \geqslant 1$, and $i_1 < i_2 < i_2 < \cdots < i_n$, the number

$$\beta(T) = 2^{\alpha(c)} p_{(i_1+2)}^{e_1} \cdots p_{(i_n+2)}^{e_n}$$

where p_j is the j-th prime. (Thus $\beta(5X_0^3 X_4^2) = 2^{10}3^3 13^2$.)

Each non-zero polynomial P in the X_i can be uniquely written as a sum of monomial terms

$$P = T_1 + \cdots + T_k$$

where the T_i do not differ only in their coefficients from $\mathbb{Z}$, and $\beta(T_1) < \cdots <$

$\beta(T_k)$. To the polynomial P written as above, assign the number

$$\gamma(P) = 2^{\beta(T_1)} \ldots p_k^{\beta(T_k)}$$

Certainly, given any non-zero polynomial P we can effectively calculate its Gödel number $\gamma(P)$.

Theorem 7.5. *There exists a recursively enumerable non-recursive set of positive integers.*

☐ Let

$$S = \{\gamma(P(X_{i_1}, \ldots, X_{i_n})) : P(e, X_{i_2}, \ldots, X_{i_n}) \text{ has a root where } e = \gamma(P).\}$$

In words, S is the set of Gödel numbers of polynomials such that, when their own number is substituted for the first variable occurring, the resulting polynomial has a root. The set S is clearly intuitively effectively enumerable. On the other hand, $S^* = \mathbb{Z} - S = \{z : z$ is not in the range of γ or $z = \gamma(P(X_{i_2}, \ldots X_{i_n}))$ but $P(\gamma(P), X_{i_2}, \ldots, X_{i_n})$ does not have a root.$\}$

If S^* is recursively enumerable, let Q be a polynomial enumerating S^*. That is $z \in S^*$ if and only if $Q(z, X_{i_2}, \ldots, X_{i_m})$ has a root.

We can now apply the classic diagonal argument. Let $e^* = \gamma(Q)$. The embarrassing question to ask is "In which of the sets S or S^* is e^*?" By the definition of Q we have

$$e^* \in S^* \text{ iff } Q(e^*, X_{i_2}, \ldots, X_{i_n}) \text{ has a root.}$$

But then $e^* = \gamma(Q) \in S$ by definition. This contradiction completes the proof. ☐

We begin the proof of the Higman Embedding Theorem by introducing one of Higman's key concepts.

Definition. A subgroup H of a finitely generated group G is called *benign in G* if the group

$$G_H = \langle G, t; t^{-1}ht = h, h \in H \rangle$$

is embeddable in a finitely presented group.

Note that if we have

$$H \subseteq G \subseteq K$$

where G and K are finitely generated, and H is benign in K, then H is benign in G. We shall often implicitely use this remark.

The relation of the concept of being benign to our goal is given by the following lemma.

Lemma 7.6. (The Higman Rope Trick) *If R is a benign normal subgroup of the finitely generated group F, the F/R is embeddable in a finitely presented group.*

☐ By hypothesis the group

$$F_R = \langle F, t; t^{-1}rt = r, r \in R \rangle$$

is embeddable in a finitely presented group H. Suppose the given generators of F are $x_1, \ldots, x_n$. Without altering the fact that we have a finite presentation, we may assume that $x_1, \ldots, x_n$ are included among the generating symbols of the given finite presentation of H. Let $\bar{F}$ be an isomorphic copy of F with generators $\bar{x}_1, \ldots, \bar{x}_n$. If w is a word in the generators of F, let $\bar{w}$ denote the word of $\bar{F}$ obtained by replacing each x_i by $\bar{x}_i$.

In F_R, the subgroup L generated by F and $t^{-1}Ft$ is the free product of F and $t^{-1}Ft$ with R amalgamated. Define a homomorphism $\phi: L \to \bar{F}/\bar{R}$ by $\phi(w) = \bar{w}$ and $\phi(t^{-1}wt) = 1$. Since the two definitions of ϕ agree on the amalgamated part, ϕ is well-defined.

Consider the group $H \times \bar{F}/\bar{R}$. We shall use ordered pair notation to denote elements of this group. Viewing L as a subgroup of H, the map $\psi: L \to L \times \bar{F}/\bar{R}$ defined by $\psi(l) = (l, \phi(l))$ is one-to-one. Hence, we can form the HNN extension

$$K = \langle H \times \bar{F}/\bar{R}, s; s^{-1}(l, 1)s = (l, \phi(l)), l \in L \rangle.$$

A set of defining relations for K can be obtained by taking the union of the defining relations for $\bar{F}/\bar{R}$, the defining relations for H, the relations saying that the generators of H commute with the generators of $\bar{F}/\bar{R}$, and the relations $s^{-1}(l, 1)s = (l, \phi(l))$ for a set of generators of L. Since all the groups involved are finitely generated and H is finitely presented, if we can show that the defining relations of $\bar{F}/\bar{R}$ follow from the other relations, we shall have established that K can be finitely presented. Suppose that $\bar{w}$ is a word on the generators of $\bar{F}/\bar{R}$ such that $\bar{w} = 1$ in $\bar{F}/\bar{R}$. Then the corresponding word w on the generators of F is in R. Now

$$s(w, 1)s^{-1} = (w, \bar{w}).$$

Since $w \in R$, $t^{-1}wt = w$ so

$$(w, 1) = (t^{-1}wt, 1).$$

But, by the definition of ϕ,

$$s(t^{-1}wt, 1)s = (w, 1).$$

Hence $\bar{w} = 1$ follows. Thus K is a finitely presented group in which F/R is embedded. ☐

Since any recursively presented group has the form F/R where F is a finitely generated free group and R is a recursively enumerable normal subgroup of F, the lemma shows that in order to prove the Higman embedding theorem, it suffices to show that recursively enumerable subgroups of finitely generated free groups are benign. This is the overall strategy of the proof.

Having embarked on the study of benign subgroups, we need some initial examples and ways of constructing benign subgroups from subgroups already known to be benign. If H and K are subgroups of G, then $Gp\{H, K\}$ will denote the subgroup generated by H and K. For this section, the notation $\langle G, t; t^{-1}Ht = H\rangle$ will denote the HNN extension of G with $t^{-1}ht = h$ for $h \in H$.

Lemma 7.7. *Let G be a finitely generated group which is embeddable in a finitely presented group.*

(i) *Every finitely generated subgroup of G is benign in G.*

(ii) *If H and K are benign subgroups of G, then $H \cap K$ and $Gp\{H, K\}$ are benign in G.*

☐ Statement (i) is clear, so we turn to the proof of (ii). By assumption, $G_H = \langle G, t; t^{-1}Ht = H\rangle$ embeds in a finitely presented group M, and $G_K = \langle G, s; s^{-1}Ks = K\rangle$ embeds in a finitely presented group N. The free product with amalgamation

$$P = \langle M * N; G = G\rangle$$

is finitely presented since G is finitely generated. It is easily verified that the subgroup $Gp\{G, ts\}$ of P is isomorphic to

$$\langle G, u; u^{-1}(H \cap K)u = H \cap K\rangle$$

by the map $g \to g$, $u \to ts$. Hence, $H \cap K$ is benign.

By Britton's Lemma, we have in P,

$$Gp\{H, K\} = Gp\{s^{-1}Gs, t^{-1}Gt\} \cap G.$$

Since the groups on the right hand side are finitely generated and we have checked intersections, $Gp\{H, K\}$ is benign. ☐

We now follow Valiev's (1968) proof. The version given here incorporates several later simplifications (unpublished) which Valiev made after his original argument, and which he very kindly made available to us. The major step is

Lemma 7.8. (The principal lemma). *Let S be a recursively enumerable set of integers. Then the subgroup*

$$Gp\{a_0^z b_0 c_0^z; z \in S\}$$

is a benign subgroup of the free group $\langle a_0, b_0, c_0\rangle$.

☐ *Step* 1. We shall heavily use the Diophantine character of the set S. There is a polynomial $P(X_0, \ldots, X_t)$ with integer coefficients such that

$$z_0 \in S \text{ iff } \exists z_1 \cdots z_t[P(z_0, \ldots, z_t) = 0] \tag{1}$$

Even this characterization is too complicated for us to use directly. We can convert (1) to a characterization

(2) $$z_0 \in S \text{ iff } \exists z_1 \cdots z_m \mathcal{M}(z_0, \ldots, z_m)$$

where $w_{(z_0,\ldots,z_m)} = c_m^{-z_m} b_m^{-1} a_m^{-z_m}$ is a conjunction of elementary formulas of one of the forms

$$\begin{aligned}
&X_i = c \quad (c \text{ an integer}),\\
&X_i = X_j,\\
&X_i + X_j = X_k \quad (i, j, k \text{ distinct}), \text{ or}\\
&X_l = X_i \cdot X_j \quad (0 < l < i < j \leqslant m).
\end{aligned}$$

(The restriction on the subscripts in the last type of formula is a technicality which will be used later.)

For the reader unfamiliar with this sort of trick, we do an example. Let P be $6X_1 - X_2^2 + X_0$, and suppose that

$$z_0 \in S \text{ iff } P(z_0, X_1, X_2) \text{ has a root.}$$

Introducing auxillary variables, we write

$$\begin{aligned}
&X_4 = 6, \quad X_5 = X_1, \quad X_4 \cdot X_5 = X_3\\
&X_7 = X_2, \quad X_8 = X_2, \quad X_7 \cdot X_8 = X_6\\
&X_{11} = -1, \quad X_{12} = X_6, \quad X_{11} \cdot X_{12} = X_{10}\\
&X_{13} = X_3 + X_{10}, \quad X_{14} = X_{13} + X_0, \quad X_{14} = 0.
\end{aligned}$$

Letting $\mathcal{M}(X_0, \ldots, X_{14})$ be the conjunction of the above formulas, we have

$$z_0 \in S \text{ iff } \exists z_1 \cdots z_{14} \mathcal{M}(z_0, \ldots, z_{14}).$$

Step 2. Using the representation (2), we next reduce the problem of proving the lemma to establishing that some particular subgroups of the free group

$$F = \langle a_0, b_0, c_0, \ldots, a_m, b_m, c_m \rangle$$

are benign.

With each tuple $(z_0, \ldots, z_m)$ we will associate a code word $w_{(z_0,\ldots,z_m)}$ in the free group F. Namely, let

$$w_{(z_0,\ldots,z_m)} = c_m^{-z_m} b_m^{-1} a_m^{-z_m} \cdots c_1^{-z_1} b_1^{-1} a_1^{-z_1} a_0^{z_0} b_0 c_0^{z_0} a_1^{z_1} b_1 c_1^{z_1} \cdots a_m^{z_m} b_m c_m^{z_m}.$$

Let

$$A = Gp\{w_{(z_0,\ldots,z_m)} : (z_0, \ldots, z_m) \in \mathbb{Z}^{m+1}\}.$$

Note that the set of $w_{(z_0,\ldots,z_m)}$ is a free set of generators for A since it is Nielsen reduced.

We shall use the letter Γ as a variable for either the formula $\mathcal{M}$ or one of the elementary formulas involved in $\mathcal{M}$. If $\Gamma(X_0, \ldots, X_m)$ is a formula, let

$$A_\Gamma = Gp\{w_{(z_0,\ldots,z_m)}: \Gamma(z_0, \ldots, z_m) \text{ is true}\}.$$

For the elementary formulas

$$X_i = c,\ X_i = X_j,\ X_i + X_j = X_l,\ X_i \cdot X_j = X_l$$

we shall also use the notations

$$A_i^c,\ A_{i,j}^=,\ A_{i,j,l}^+,\ A_{i,j,l}^\cdot$$

respectively. Thus

$$A_{i,j}^= = Gp\{w_{(z_0,\ldots,z_m)}: z_i = z_j\},$$

etc..

We next show that if the subgroups A_i^c, $A_{i,j,k}^=$, $A_{i,j,l}^+$, and $A_{i,j,l}^\cdot$ are benign subgroups of F, then the subgroup

$$Gp\{a_0^{z_0} b_0 c_0^{z_0}: z_0 \in S\}$$

is benign in F, and consequently, benign in $\langle a_0, b_0, c_0 \rangle$.

For, let $\Gamma_1, \ldots, \Gamma_p$ be the elementary formulas of which $\mathcal{M}$ is the conjunction. Note that

$$A_\mathcal{M} = \bigcap_{q=1}^p A_{\Gamma_q}.$$

The inclusion $\subseteq$ is clear, and the reverse inclusion follows since the set of all $w_{(z_0,\ldots,z_m)}$ is free. Note that

$$Gp\{a_0^{z_0} b_0 c_0^{z_0}: z \in S\} = Gp\{A_\mathcal{M}, a_1, b_1, c_1, \ldots, a_m, b_m, c_m\} \cap Gp\{a_0, b_0, c_0\}.$$

The desired conclusion follows from Lemma 7.7.

Step 3. In order to show that the subgroup A_Γ is benign (where Γ is an elementary formula), we shall construct a finitely presented group M containing F such that for each Γ there is a finitely generated subgroup L_Γ of M with

$$L_\Gamma \cap F = A_\Gamma.$$

Another application of Lemma 7.7 will then complete the proof.

We construct M in two stages, each an HNN extension with several stable letters.

(I) The group F^* is obtained from F by adding the generators $t_0, \ldots, t_m$ and, for each i with $0 \leqslant i \leqslant m$, the defining relations

$$t_i^{-1} b_i t_i = a_i b_i c_i,$$

$$t_i \text{ commutes with all the other generators of } F.$$

It is clear that F^* is an HNN extension of F since conjugation by each t_i sends a free set of generators of F to a free set of generators.

(II) The group M is obtained from F^* by adding the generators $p_{j,l}$ where the subscripts range over ordered pairs (j, l) with $0 < l < j \leqslant m$. We also add, for each pair (j, l) the defining relations

$$p_{j,l}^{-1} c_j p_{j,l} = t_l c_j,$$

$$p_{j,l} \text{ commutes with all the other generators of } F \text{ and with } t_l.$$

The subgroup of F^* associated with $p_{j,l}^{-1}$ is $Gp\{F_j, t_l\}$. Let E_l be the free group $F * \langle t_l \rangle$. It is clear that the map $\phi_{j,l}$ defined by sending $c_j \mapsto t_l c_j$ and all other generators to themselves is an automorphism of E_l. Let $\phi_{j,l}^{-1}$ be the inverse of $\phi_{j,l}$. In order to verify that $\phi_{j,l}$ defines an automorphism of $Gp\{F, t_l\}$ in F^*, it is sufficient to check that both $\phi_{j,l}$ and $\phi_{j,l}^{-1}$ send all the defining relators of $Gp\{F, t_l\}$ to 1. For relations not containing the generator c_j this is clear. For the defining relation $t_l^{-1} c_j t_l = c_j$, we have

$$\phi_{j,l}(t_l^{-1} c_j t_l) = t_l^{-1} t_l c_j t_l = c_j t_l = t_l c_j = \phi_{j,l}(c_j),$$

$$\phi_{j,l}^{-1}(t_l^{-1} c_j t_l) = t_l^{-1} t_l^{-1} c_j t_l = t_l^{-1} c_j = \phi_{j,l}^{-1}(c_j).$$

This proves the claim.

Step 4. We claim that for each elementary formula Γ, there is a finitely generated subgroup L_Γ of M with $L_\Gamma \cap F = A_\Gamma$. Namely,

$$L_i^c = Gp\{w_{(0,\ldots,0,c,0,\ldots 0)}, t_s, s \neq i\}$$

$$L_{i,j}^{=} = Gp\{w_{(0,\ldots,0)}, t_s (s \neq i, j), t_i t_j\},$$

$$L_{i,j,l}^{+} = Gp\{w_{(0,\ldots,0)}, t_s (s \neq i, j, l), t_i t_l, t_j t_l\},$$

$$L_{i,j,l}^{\bullet} = Gp\{w_{(0,\ldots,0)}, t_s (s \neq i, j, l), t_i p_{j,l}, t_j p_{i,l}\}.$$

To prove the claim, first note that a simple verification reveals that

$$t_i^{-\varepsilon} w_{(z_0,\ldots,z_m)} t_i^{\varepsilon} = w_{(z_0,\ldots,z_{i-1},z_i+\varepsilon,z_{i+1},\ldots,z_m)} \tag{1}$$

$$p_{j,l}^{-\varepsilon} w_{(z_0,\ldots,z_m)} p_{j,l}^{\varepsilon} = w_{(z'_0,\ldots,z'_m)} \tag{2}$$

where $z'_l = z_l + \varepsilon z_j$, and $z'_s = z_s$, for $s \neq l$.

(In verifying (2), recall that $0 < l < j$.)

The purpose of the generators t_i and $p_{j,l}$ is now clear. If Γ is an elementary formula, it follows from the definition of L_Γ and equations (1) and (2) above, that $L_\Gamma \cap F \supseteq A_\Gamma$. But the reverse inclusion follows easily from Britton's Lemma, since, if an element u of L_Γ is contained in F, it must be reducible to a word w of F by successive stable letter reductions. But this ensures that $w \in A_\Gamma$, concluding the proof of the lemma. □

The principal lemma, 7.8, is sufficient to establish the existence of a finitely presented group with unsolvable word problem. (Note that only Lemma 7.7 was necessary in the proof of the previous lemma. Lemma 7.6 was not used.)

Theorem 7.2. *There exists a finitely presented group H with unsolvable word problem.*

□ Let S be a recursively enumerable non-recursive set of positive integers. By Lemma 7.8, the subgroup

$$B = Gp\{a^s bc^s; s \in S\}$$

is a benign subgroup of the free group $K = \langle a, b, c\rangle$. Since the subgroup $Gp\{a^z bc^z: z \in \mathbb{Z}\}$ is freely generated by the indicated generators, we have

$$z \in S \quad \text{iff} \quad a^z bc^z \in B.$$

Since B is benign, there is an embedding ϕ of the group $K_B = \langle K, t; t^{-1}Bt = B\rangle$ into a finitely presented group H. Because K_B is an HNN extension, we have, for every element y of K,

$$y \in B \quad \text{iff} \quad t^{-1}yt = y.$$

Thus

$$z \in S \quad \text{iff} \quad \phi(a^z bc^z) = \phi(t^{-1}a^z bc^z t).$$

Hence, a solution of the word problem for H would allow one to decide membership in S. Since S is not recursive, H must have unsolvable word problem. □

We now turn to completing the proof of the Higman Embedding Theorem. First, we note that since the standard Higman-Neumann-Neumann embedding into a two-generator group preserves the recursiveness of presentations, it suffices to show that any recursively enumerable subgroup N of the free group $L = \langle a, b\rangle$ is benign in L.

We must define precisely what we mean in saying that a set W of words on the generators a and b is recursively enumerable. To do this, we effectively assign a Gödel number, $\gamma(w)$, to each word w of L. A set W of words is then defined to be recursively enumerable if and only if the set

$$\gamma(W) = \{\gamma(w): w \in W\}$$

is recursively enumerable.

Let the empty word have Gödel number 0. If w is any non-empty word, not necessarily reduced, on the letters a, b, a^{-1}, b^{-1}, then $\gamma(w)$ is the number obtained by regarding w as representing a number to the base 10, where the letters a, b, a^{-1}, b^{-1} correspond respectively to 1, 2, 3, and 4. Thus $\gamma(ba) = 21$, while $\gamma(a^{-1}b^2) = 322$.

To each word w we assign a code word g_w in the free group $F = \langle a, b, c, d, e, h\rangle$ defined by

$$g_w = whc^{\gamma(w)}de^{\gamma(w)}$$

Let

$$G = Gp\{g_w : w \text{ a word on } a, b, a^{-1}, b^{-1}\}$$

be the subgroup of F generated by all the code words. Note that G is freely generated by the indicated generators.

Let $N \subseteq L$ be a subgroup generated by a subset X of L. Since the group

$$Y = Gp\{h, a, b, c^i de^i, i \in \gamma(X)\}$$

is freely generated by the indicated generators, we have, in F,

$$N = Gp\{G \cap Y, h, c, d, e\} \cap Gp\{a, b\}.$$

Suppose that X is recursively enumerable. This means that $\gamma(X)$ is recursively enumerable, and thus, by Lemma 7.8, that Y is benign. If we can establish that G is benign, then it follows from Lemma 7.7 that N is benign, and the proof of the theorem is complete.

To prove that G is benign, consider the HNN extension F^* of F obtained by adding the stable letters t_λ, for $\lambda = a^{\pm 1}, b^{\pm 1}$, and the defining relations

$$t_\lambda^{-1} h\, t_\mu = \lambda h$$

$$t_\lambda a = at_\lambda,\ t_\lambda b = bt_\lambda$$

$$t_\lambda^{-1} ct_\lambda = c^{10},\ t_\lambda^{-1} et_\lambda = e^{10},$$

$$t_\lambda^{-1} dt_\lambda = c^{\gamma(\lambda)} de^{\gamma(\lambda)}$$

From these relations it is easy to verify that if $w = \lambda_1 \cdots \lambda_n$ is a word on a, b, a^{-1}, b^{-1}, then

$$(*) \qquad t_{\lambda_n}^{-1} \cdots t_{\lambda_1}^{-1} hdt_{\lambda_1} \cdots t_{\lambda_n} = whc^{\gamma(w)}de^{\gamma(w)} = g_w.$$

It also follows from the defining relators that if w is a word ending in the letter λ, say $w = u\lambda$, then

$$(**) \quad t_\lambda g_w t_\lambda^{-1} = t_\lambda u\lambda hc^{\gamma(u\lambda)}de^{\gamma(u\lambda)}t_\lambda^{-1} = u\lambda\lambda^{-1}hc^{\gamma(u)}t_\lambda c^{\gamma(\lambda)}de^{\gamma(\lambda)}t_\lambda^{-1}e^{\gamma(u)} = g_u.$$

We claim that in F^*,

$$G = Gp\{hd, t_a, t_{a^{-1}}, t_b, t_{b^{-1}}\} \cap F.$$

It is immediate from (*) that G is contained in the right hand side. We shall use Britton's Lemma to establish the reverse inclusion. Let T be a freely reduced word on hd and the t_λ. If $T \in F$, then there is a sequence of words $T = T_0, T_1, \ldots, T_m$, where each T_{i+1} is obtained from T_i by a single stable letter reduction, and T_m contains no stable letters. We claim that in each T_i, if z is a subword between successive occurrences of stable letters, that is, $T_i \equiv S_1 t_\lambda^\varepsilon z t_\beta^\delta S_2$ where z does not contain any t_λ, then $z \in G$. Since $hd \in G$, this is true for T. It is immediate from (*) that if $z \in G$, then $t_\lambda^{-1} z t_\lambda \in G$.

We thus need to worry only about stable letter reductions of the form $t_\lambda z t_\lambda^{-1}$ where $z \in G$. Write

$$z = g_{w_1}^{\varepsilon_1} \cdots g_{w_n}^{\varepsilon_n}$$

where each $\varepsilon_i = \pm 1$ and there are no successive inverse pairs g_w, g_w^{-1} in the product. Note that in freely reducing this product, the occurrence of $(c^{\gamma(w_i)}d)^{\varepsilon_i}$ in $g_{w_i}^{\varepsilon_i}$ is not cancelled. Also, from the definition of the function γ, if $w = u\lambda$, then

$$\gamma(w) \equiv \gamma(\lambda) \text{ (modulo 10)}.$$

Now the subgroup C_λ associated with t_λ is freely generated by h, a, b, c^{10}, e^{10}, and $c^{\gamma(\lambda)} d e^{\gamma(\lambda)}$. If $z \in C_\lambda$, we can write z as

$$z = y_1 c^{n_2} y_2 \cdots y_k c^{n_k} y_{k+1}$$

where the y_i are words on h, a, b, and d, and each y_i is non-empty if $1 < i < k + 1$. From the form of the generators of C_λ, it is clear that each n_i is congruent modulo 10 to one of

$$0, \pm\gamma(\lambda)$$

Note that if β is a letter different from λ, then $\pm\gamma(\beta)$ is not congruent modulo 10 to any of the above numbers. Also, an element of C_λ does not contain an occurrence of hd. Hence, z cannot be in C_λ unless for each code word g_{w_i} in the product for z, w_i ends in the letter λ. But then, from (**), $t_\lambda z t_\lambda^{-1}$ is again a product of code words. This concludes the proof of the theorem. □

8. Algebraically Closed Groups

We conclude this chapter with a topic which has recently yielded some remarkable theorems. Let G be a group. The notation $W(x_j, g_k)$ will denote a word in variables x_j and elements $g_k \in G$.

A finite set of equations and inequations:

$$W_i(x_j, g_k) = 1 \quad (i = 1, \ldots, m)$$
$$V_l(x_j, g_k) \neq 1 \quad (l = 1, \ldots, n)$$

is said to be *consistent with G* if there is a group H and an embedding $\phi: G \to H$ such that the system

$$W_i(x_j, \phi(g_k)) = 1 \quad (i = 1, \ldots, m)$$
$$V_l(x_j, \phi(g_k)) \neq 1 \quad (l = 1, \ldots, n)$$

has a solution in H.

A group A is said to be *algebraically closed* if every finite set of equations and inequations which is consistent with A already has a solution in A. The concept of an algebraically closed group was introduced by W. R. Scott (1951) who proved

Theorem 8.1. *Every countable group C can be embedded in a countable algebraically closed group A.*

□ The first step is to embed C in a group C^* in which every finite set of equations and inequations with coefficients in C which is consistent with C^* has a solution in C^*.

There are only countably many finite systems of equations and inequations with coefficients in C. Fix an enumeration $S_1, S_2, \ldots$ of such systems. Let $C_0 = C$. Suppose inductively that C_{i-1} is already defined and contains C. Then C_i is defined as follows. If S_i is not consistent with C_{i-1}, then $C_i = C_{i-1}$. If S_i has a solution in an extension H of C_{i-1}, let C_i be the subgroup of H generated by the embedded copy $\phi_i(C_{i-1})$ and the elements $h_1, \ldots, h_t$ of H substituted for the variables x_i in solving the system S_i. Identify C_{i-1} with its image in C_i. Note that C_i is countable.

Let

$$C^* = \bigcup_{i=1}^{\infty} C_i.$$

Now define a new ascending chain of groups as follows. Let $A_0 = C^*$. Suppose inductively that A_i has already been defined. As in the previous paragraph, construct a countable group A_{i+1} containing A_i and in which every finite system of equations and inequations with coefficients from A_i which is consistent with A_{i+1} has a solution in A_{i+1}. Then the group

$$A = \bigcup_{i=1}^{\infty} A_i$$

is algebraically closed. It is easy to see that "countable" can be replaced by "having cardinality less then or equal to $\aleph_\lambda$," and the proof is essentially the same. □

Shortly after Scott's paper, B. H. Neumann (1952) showed that algebraically closed groups are simple. He later observed (1973) that an algebraically closed group cannot be finitely generated.

Theorem 8.2. *Every algebraically closed group is simple. An algebraically closed group cannot be finitely generated.*

□ Let A be any algebraically closed group. Let $w \neq 1$ and $a \neq 1$ be any pair of non-trivial elements of A. In the free product $A * \langle x \rangle$, the elements $wxw^{-1}x^{-1}$ and $axw^{-1}x^{-1}$ both have infinite order. Hence, we can form the HNN extension

$$\langle A * \langle x \rangle, t; twxw^{-1}x^{-1}t^{-1} = axw^{-1}x^{-1} \rangle.$$

Now regard t and x as variables. Since the equation

$$twxw^{-1}x^{-1}t^{-1} = axw^{-1}x^{-1}$$

has a solution in an extension of A, and A is algebraically closed, there is a solution in A. Solving the above equation for a, we have a in the normal closure of w. Since a and w are arbitrary non-trivial elements, A is simple.

Let $1 \neq a \in A$. Since the inequation $ax \neq xa$ has a solution in an extension of A (say $A * \langle x \rangle$), A has trivial center. On the other hand, we shall show that every finitely generated subgroup of A has non-trivial centralizer. Let $\{a_1, \ldots, a_n\}$ be a finite subset of A. The set of equations and inequations

$$a_1 y = y a_1, \ldots, a_n y = y a_n, y \neq 1$$

has a solution in $A \times \langle y \rangle$. Since A is algebraically closed, there is a solution in A. Thus the centralizer of the subgroup H generated by $\{a_1, \ldots, a_n\}$ is non-trivial. Hence, $H \neq A$. □

It is immediate from the definition of an algebraically closed group that every finite group is embedded in every algebraically closed group A. For, if G is a finite group with distinct elements $g_0 = 1, g_1, \ldots, g_n$ and multiplication table $g_i g_j = g_k$; the finite system

$$x_t \neq 1 \quad t = 1, \ldots, n$$

$$x_i x_j = x_k \quad 1 \leqslant i, j \leqslant n$$

has a solution in $A \times G$, and hence in A.

Next, we observe that every finitely presented group

$$G = \langle x_1, \ldots, x_n; r_1 = 1, \ldots, r_m = 1 \rangle$$

is *residually embeddable* in every algebraically closed group A. By this we mean that if $1 \neq w \in G$, there is a homomorphism $\phi \colon G \to A$ with $\phi(w) \neq 1$. The proof is simply to note that the system

$$r_i(x_j) = 1, \quad i = 1, \ldots, m$$

$$w(x_j) \neq 1$$

has a solution in $A \times G$ and thus a solution

$$r_i(a_j) = 1 \quad i = 1, \ldots, m$$
$$w(a_j) \neq 1$$

in A. The map $\phi: G \to A$ defined by $x_j \to a_j$ is a homomorphism since each defining relator goes to the identity. Clearly $\phi(w) \neq 1$.

Before proving the next theorem we need one more definition. We shall say that a group G can be *infinitely recursively presented* if G has a presentation of the form

$$G = \langle x_i, i \in \mathbb{N}; r_1, r_2, \ldots \rangle$$

where the set of r_i is recursively enumerable.

The reader has noticed that we have not given any explicit examples of algebraic closed groups and that the existence proof was highly non-constructive. We see that this is necessarily the case from the next theorem, which is due to C. F. Miller, III.

Theorem 8.3. *No algebraically closed group can be infinitely recursively presented.*

☐ Suppose that an algebraically closed group A has an infinite recursive presentation

$$A = \langle x_i, i \in \mathbb{N}; r_1, r_2, \ldots \rangle.$$

Since A is simple, the given presentation of A has solvable word problem by Kuznetsov's Theorem (Theorem 3.6). Let

$$G = \langle z_1, \ldots, z_n; s_1, \ldots, s_m \rangle$$

be a finitely presented group with unsolvable word problem. We shall show, by an argument exactly analogous to the one showing that finitely presented residually finite groups have solvable word problems, that the solution of the word problem for the given presentation of A can be used to solve the word problem for G. Since G has unsolvable word problem, this contradiction forces us to conclude that no infinite recursive presentation of A exists.

Since G is finitely presented, the set of words equal to 1 in G is recursively enumerable. To solve the word problem for G, it thus suffices to show that the set of words not equal to 1 in G is also recursively enumerable. Enumerate all n-tuples $(w_1, \ldots, w_n)$ of words on the generating symbols x_i of A. The function $z_i \mapsto w_i$ defines a homomorphism of G into A if and only if each defining relator s_j of G goes to 1, that is, $s_j(w_i) = 1$ in A. Using the solution of the word problem in A, we can effectively check this condition. Thus, we can effectively enumerate all homomorphisms $\phi_1, \phi_2, \ldots$ from G into A. Let $v_1, v_2, \ldots$ be an enumeration of all words of G. By a diagonal procedure, we can effectively enumerate all images $\phi_i(v_j)$.

Using the solution of the word problem in A, we can check if $\phi_i(v_j) \neq 1$ in A.

If so, $v_j \neq 1$ in G, and we put v_j on the list of words not equal to 1 in G. But we have noted that G is residually embeddable in A. Thus every word $v_j \neq 1$ in G appears on the above list. We have shown that the word problem for G is solvable relative to the word problem for any presentation of A. As noted above, this implies that A cannot have an infinite recursive presentation. □

The subject of algebraically closed groups remained dormant until B. H. Neumann (1973) proved the following remarkable theorem.

Theorem 8.4. *Every finitely generated group G with solvable word problem is embedded in every algebraically closed group A.*

□ By the theorem of Boone and Higman (Theorem 7.4), G is embeddable in a simple subgroup S of a finitely presented group

$$H = \langle z_1, \ldots, z_n; r_1, \ldots, r_m \rangle.$$

Pick an element $1 \neq w \in S$. The system of equations and inequations

$$r_i(z_j) = 1, \quad i = 1, \ldots, m$$
$$w(z_j) \neq 1$$

has a solution in $A \times H$ and thus a solution in A since A is algebraically closed. Let $a_1, \ldots, a_n$ be elements of A satisfying the above equations. The map $z_0 \mapsto a_i$ defines a homomorphism $\phi: H \to A$ since each defining relator r_i of H goes to 1. Since S is simple, if $\phi(v) = 1$ for any $1 \neq v \in S$, then $\phi(w) = 1$. But $\phi(w) \neq 1$. Hence, ϕ restricted to S is an embedding. In particular ϕ embeds G in A. (Neumann proved his theorem before the theorem of Boone and Higman, which we have used to point out the connection between embeddings into algebraically closed groups and the existence of sufficiently many simple subgroups of finitely presented groups.) □

In 1972, A. Macintyre proved another remarkable theorem, namely, the converse of Neumann's theorem. That is, if a finitely generated group G is embeddable in all algebraically closed groups, then G has solvable word problem. Putting the two theorems together, we have the following algebraic characterization of having solvable word problem: A finitely generated group G has solvable word problem if and only if G is embeddable in every algebraically closed group. A remarkable feature of this characterization is that it characterizes an effectiveness notion, having solvable word problem, in terms of a class of groups so wild that no member has any effective presentation!

We now turn to a proof of Macintyre's theorem.

Theorem 8.5. *If a finitely generated group G is embeddable in all algebraically closed groups, then G has solvable word problem.*

□ Given any finitely generated group

$$H = \langle h_1, \ldots, h_n; r_1, r_2, \ldots \rangle$$

with unsolvable word problem, we must construct an algebraically closed group A in which H is not embedded.

In order to construct the group A, we will need the following enumerations. Let $x_1, x_2, \ldots$ be an enumeration of a countably infinite set of generating symbols. (These will eventually be the generators of A.) Let $v_1, v_2, \ldots$ be a countably infinite set of *variables*. Let $S_0, S_1, \ldots$ be an enumeration of all finite sets of equations and inequations involving the x's and v's. Let $\tau_1, \tau_2, \ldots$ be an enumeration of all n-tuples of words on the x_i. Finally, let $z_1, \ldots, z_n$ be n distinct variables disjoint from the x_i and v_i.

A finite set of equations and inequations:

$$W_i(x_j, v_j) = 1, \quad (i = 1, \ldots, m)$$
$$Y_l(x_j, v_j) \neq 1, \quad (l = 1, \ldots, n)$$

is *consistent* if there is a group G and elements a_j, b_k of G with

$$W_i(a_j, b_j) = 1, \quad (i = 1, \ldots, m)$$
$$Y_l(a_j, b_j) \neq 1, \quad (j = 1, \ldots, n)$$

in G.

We shall construct the group A in successive stages. The overall strategy used to construct A is quite simple. At odd numbered stages, $2i + 1$, if the system S_i of equations and inequations is consistent with what we have already constructed, we shall ensure a solution. At even numbered stages, $2i$, we shall ensure that the subgroup generated by the elements in the i-th tuple, τ_i, is not isomorphic to H.

At each stage, k, we shall have a finite set X_k of generating symbols *already used*, and a finite set Σ_k of equations and inequations *already assumed*. Put $X_0 = \varnothing = \Sigma_0$. Suppose that X_{k-1} and Σ_{k-1} are already defined. We construct X_k and Σ_k as follows.

First suppose that k is odd, $k = 2i + 1$. Then the set X_k' consists of X_{k-1} together with all generating symbols x_j which appear in the system S_i.

Consider the system S_i; say

$$W_h(x_j, v_j) = 1, \quad h = 1, \ldots, m$$
$$U_l(x_j, v_j) \neq 1, \quad l = 1, \ldots, d.$$

Suppose that $\Sigma_{k-1} \cup S_i$ is consistent.

Let the variables which occur in S_i be $v_{j_1}, \ldots, v_{j_q}$. Select generating symbols $x_{k_1}, \ldots, x_{k_q}$ which do *not* occur in X_k'. (This is certainly possible since X_k' is finite.) Let X_k be X_k' together with $x_{k_1}, \ldots, x_{k_q}$. Let Σ_k be Σ_{k-1} together with

$$W_h(x_j, x_{k_j}) = 1, \quad h = 1, \ldots, m$$
$$U_l(x_j, x_{k_j}) \neq 1, \quad l = 1, \ldots, d.$$

Clearly, Σ_k is consistent.

If $\Sigma_{k-1} \cup S_i$ is not consistent, let $X_k = X'_k$ and $\Sigma_k = \Sigma_{k-1}$.

Next suppose that $k = 2i$. We shall now use Macintyre's ingenious argument. Let $\tau_i = \langle t_1, \ldots, t_n \rangle$ be the i-th n-tuple in the enumeration of all words on the generating symbols x_j. Let X_k consist of X_{k-1} together with all generators occurring in members of τ_i.

We next define four sets of words on the variables $z_1, \ldots, z_n$. Let

$$\Delta^+ = \{w(z_1, \ldots, z_n): w(h_1, \ldots, h_n) = 1 \text{ in } H\},$$

and let

$$\Delta^- = \{u(z_1, \ldots, z_n): u(h_1, \ldots, h_n) \neq 1 \text{ in } H\}.$$

Note that since H has unsolvable word problem, not both Δ^+ and Δ^- can be recursively enumerable.

Let A_k be the group whose set of generators is X_k and whose defining relations are the equations $w = 1$ in Σ_{k-1}. Let

$$D^+ = \{w(z_1, \ldots, z_n); w(t_1, \ldots, t_n) = 1 \text{ in } A_k\}.$$

Since A_k is finitely presented, D^+ is recursively enumerable.

For each word $u(z_1, \ldots, z_n)$, let $A_{k,u}$ be the group obtained from A_k by adding $u(t_1, \ldots, t_n)$ as a defining relator. Since each $A_{k,u}$ is finitely presented, the set of words on the generators X_k which are equal to 1 in $A_{k,u}$ is recursively enumerable. By a diagonal enumeration, the set

$$D^- = \{u(z_1, \ldots, z_n); \text{ there is an inequation } w \neq 1 \text{ in } \Sigma_{k-1} \text{ such that } w = 1 \text{ in } A_{k,u}\}$$

is recursively enumerable. (In short, a word u is in D^- if adding $u(t_1, \ldots, t_n)$ as a defining relator contradicts an inequation in Σ_{k-1}.)

Since D^+ and D^- are both recursively enumerable but at least one of Δ^+ and Δ^- is not, either $D^+ \neq \Delta^+$ or $D^- \neq \Delta^-$. We consider the four possibilities. Suppose $\Delta^+ - D^+ \neq \varnothing$. Choose $v \in \Delta^+ - D^+$. Then $v(t_1, \ldots, t_n) \neq 1$ in A_k. Form Σ_k by adding the inequation $v(t_1, \ldots, t_n) \neq 1$ to Σ_{k-1}. (Clearly, Σ_k is consistent.)

If $D^+ - \Delta^+ \neq \varnothing$. Choose $v \in D^+ - \Delta^+$. Then $v(t_1, \ldots, t_n) = 1$ in A_k. Form Σ_k by adding the equation $v(t_1, \ldots, t_n) = 1$ to Σ_{k-1}. If $D^+ = \Delta^+$ and $\Delta^- - D^- \neq \varnothing$, choose $v \in \Delta^- - D^-$. Form Σ_k by adding the equation $v(t_1, \ldots, t_n) = 1$ to Σ_{k-1}. Since $v \notin D^-$, all the inequations of Σ_{k-1} still hold in $A_{k,u}$ and Σ_k is consistent. If $D^+ = \Delta^+$ and $D^- - \Delta^- \neq \varnothing$, choose $v \in D^- - \Delta^-$. Since $v \in D^-$, $v(t_1, \ldots, t_n) \neq 1$ in A_k. Form Σ_k by adding $v(t_1, \ldots, t_n) \neq 1$ to Σ_{k-1}.

Let B be any group with a set of generators $X \supseteq X_k$, and in which all the equations and inequations of Σ_k hold. A proposed correspondence $h_j \to t_j$ cannot define an isomorphism from H into B since it is not correct on the element $v(h_1, \ldots, h_n)$, where v is chosen as above.

By induction, the sets Σ_k are specified for all $k \geqslant 0$. Let

$$\Sigma = \bigcup_{k=1}^{\infty} \Sigma_k.$$

Let A be the group with generators the set $X = \{x_1, x_2, \ldots\}$ and defining relations all equations $w = 1$ which belong to Σ. We claim that all the equations and inequations of Σ are simultaneously satisfied in A. This is clear for equations since they are defining relations. Suppose that there is an inequation $u \neq 1$ in Σ but $u = 1$ is deducible from the defining relations of A. Then $u = 1$ is derivable from a finite number of relations, say $w_1 = 1, \ldots, w_m = 1$. Choose a subscript k large enough so that the equations $w_j = 1, j = 1, \ldots, m$, and $u \neq 1$ are all in Σ_k. This contradicts Σ_k being consistent.

Since all the equations and inequations of Σ hold in A, it follows from the construction that A is algebraically closed and that no subgroup is isomorphic to H. This completes the proof. □

Macintyre's original proof used concepts of mathematical logic and applies in a very general setting. Indeed, the reader has probably noticed that many of the proofs given are of a universal algebra nature and have little to do with the fact that we are working with groups. In particular, we call attention to the case of semigroups with 1. There, a finite system of equations and inequations looks like

$$U_i(s_j, y_j) = U_i(s_j, y_j) \quad i = 1, \ldots, n$$

$$W_k(s_j, y_j) \neq Z_k(s_j, y_j) \quad k = 1, \ldots, m$$

since we cannot transpose everything to one side. Since we are working in the variety of semigroups with 1, we assume that homomorphisms send 1 to 1. We have written this section so that not only all the statements of the theorems but also, with only one exception, the proofs given remain valid upon replacing the word *group* by *semigroup with* 1. The exception is the proof that an algebraically closed semigroup (with 1) is simple. This has been proved by B. H. Neumann (1971) but here we adopt a trick from Boone and Higman (1974).

□ Let A be an algebraically closed semigroup with 1. Let u and v be any pair of unequal elements and let w be any element of A. Enlarge A by adding the new generators c, d, and b, and defining relations

$$cvd = b, \; cud = 1, \; bw = b.$$

It is not difficult to verify that A is embedded in the new semigroup. Hence, regarding b, c, d as variables, there is a solution of the above set of equation in A. But setting $u = v$ then forces $w = 1$. Since u, v, w are arbitrary, A must be simple. □

For further results on algebraically closed groups see Macintyre (1970). In general, investigation of algebraically closed structures is currently an active area of research.

Chapter V. Small Cancellation Theory

1. Diagrams

In 1911 M. Dehn posed the word and conjugacy problems for groups in general and provided algorithms which solved these problems for the fundamental groups of closed orientable two-dimensional manifolds. A crucial feature of these groups is that (with trivial exceptions) they are defined by a single relator r with the property that if s is a cyclic conjugate of r or r^{-1}, with $s \neq r^{-1}$, there is very little cancellation in forming the product rs. Dehn's algorithms have been extended to large classes of groups possessing presentations in which the defining relations have a similar *small cancellation* property. At first, investigations were concerned with the solution of the word problem for groups G presented as *small cancellation* quotients of a free group F. The theory was subsequently extended to the case where F is a free product, a free product with amalgamation, or an HNN extension. Moreover, strong results were obtained about algebraic properties; for example, one can classify torsion elements and commuting elements in small cancellation quotients.

Dehn's methods were geometric, making use of regular tessellations of the hyperbolic plane. The first extensions of Dehn's results to larger classes of groups were obtained using cancellation arguments of combinatorial group theory, independent of any geometric considerations. More recently, the geometric character of Dehn's argument has been restored in the form of elementary combinatorial geometry. Small cancellation theory is now emerging as a unified and powerful theory. In this chapter we shall develop the central ideas of the theory and present some important and typical results.

The basic idea of our geometric approach is the following. Suppose a group G has a presentation $G = \langle X; R\rangle$. Let F be the free group on X, and let N be the normal closure of R in F. Then, of course, $G = F/N$. An element w of F represents the identity in the quotient group G if and only if $w \in N$. Now $w \in N$ if and only if, in the free group F, w is a product of conjugates of elements of $R^{\pm 1}$; say $w = c_1 \ldots c_n$ where $c_i = u_i r_i u_i^{-1}$ with r_i or r_i^{-1} in R. With each such product $c_1 \ldots c_n$ we shall associate a diagram in the Euclidean plane which contains all the essential information about the product $c_1 \ldots c_n$. It then turns out that diagrams are an adequate tool for studying membership in the normal subgroup N of F, and hence, for studying equality in the quotient group G. Diagrams were discovered by E. R. van Kampen (1933) but van Kampen did not make much use of diagrams, and, as far as we know, the idea was totally neglected for thirty years. R. C. Lyndon (1966) independently arrived at the idea of cancellation diagrams and used them to initiate a geometric study of small cancellation theory. At the same time, C. M. Weinbaum (1966) rediscovered van Kampen's paper and also used diagrams to prove results in small cancellation theory.

Let $\mathbb{E}^2$ denote the Euclidean plane. If $S \subseteq \mathbb{E}^2$, then ∂S will denote the boundary of S, the topological closure of S will be denoted by $\bar{S}$, and $-S$ will denote $\mathbb{E}^2 - S$. A *vertex* is a point of $\mathbb{E}^2$. An *edge* is a bounded subset of $\mathbb{E}^2$ homeomorphic to the open unit interval. A *region* is a bounded set homeomorphic to the open unit disk. A *map* M is a finite collection of vertices, edges, and regions which are pairwise disjoint and satisfy:

(i) If e is an edge of M, there are vertices a and b (not necessarily distinct) in M such that $\bar{e} = e \cup \{a\} \cup \{b\}$.

(ii) The boundary, ∂D, of each region D of M is connected and there is a set of edges $e_1, \ldots, e_n$ in M such that $\partial D = \bar{e}_1 \cup \cdots \cup \bar{e}_n$.

We shall also use M to denote the set-theoretic union of its vertices, edges, and regions. The boundary of M will be denoted by ∂M. If e is an edge with $\bar{e} = e \cup \{a\} \cup \{b\}$, the vertices a and b are called the *endpoints* of e. A *closed edge* is an edge e together with its endpoints.

We shall consider maps as being oriented. An edge may be traversed in either of two directions. If e is an oriented edge running from endpoint v_1 to endpoint v_2, the vertex v_1 is the *initial vertex* of e and v_2 is the *terminal vertex* of e. The oppositely oriented edge, or *inverse* of e, is denoted by e^{-1} and runs from v_2 to v_1.

A *path* is a sequence of oriented closed edges $e_1, \ldots, e_n$ such that the initial vertex of e_{i+1} is the terminal vertex of e_i, $1 \leqslant i \leqslant n-1$. We also allow the empty path. The endpoints of a path are the initial vertex of e_1 and the terminal vertex of e_n. A *closed path* or a *cycle* is a path such that the initial vertex of e_1 is the terminal vertex of e_n. A path is *reduced* if it does not contain a successive pair of edges of the form ee^{-1}. A reduced path $e_1 \cdots e_n$ is *simple* if, for $i \neq j$, e_i and e_j have different initial points.

Since M is planar, it is possible to orient the regions of M and the components of $-M$ so that in traversing the boundaries of the regions of M and the components of $-M$, each edge of M is traversed twice, once in each of its possible orientations. If D is a region of M with the given orientation, any cycle of minimal length which includes all the edges of ∂D, and in which the edges are oriented in accordance with the orientation of D, is a *boundary cycle* of D. If M is connected and simply connected, a *boundary cycle* of M is a cycle α of minimal length which contains all the edges in the boundary of M which does not cross itself, in the sense that, if e_i and e_{i+1} are consecutive edges of α with e_i ending at a vertex v, then e_i^{-1} and e_{i+1} are adjacent in the cyclically ordered set of all edges of M beginning at v.

A *diagram* over a group F is an oriented map M and a function ϕ assigning to each oriented edge e of M as a *label*, an element $\phi(e)$ of F such that if e is an oriented edge of M and e^{-1} is the oppositely oriented edge, then $\phi(e^{-1}) = \phi(e)^{-1}$.

If α is a path in M, $\alpha = e_1 \cdots e_k$, we define $\phi(\alpha) = \phi(e_1) \cdots \phi(e_k)$. If D is a region of M, a *label of D* is an element $\phi(\alpha)$ for α a boundary cycle of D.

Let F be a free group with a given basis. With each finite sequence $(c_1, \ldots, c_n)$ of non-trivial elements of the free group F we shall associate a diagram $M(c_1, \ldots, c_n)$ which will be an oriented map labeled by a function ϕ into F and satisfying the following conditions:

(i) If e is an edge of M, $\phi(e) \neq 1$.
(ii) M is connected and simply connected, with a distinguished vertex O on ∂M. There is a boundary cycle $e_1 \ldots e_t$ of M beginning at O such that the product $\phi(e_1) \cdots \phi(e_t)$ is reduced without cancellation and $\phi(e_1) \cdots \phi(e_t) = c_1 \cdots c_n$.
(iii) If D is any region of M and $e_1 \cdots e_j$ is any boundary cycle of D, then $\phi(e_1) \cdots \phi(e_j)$ is reduced without cancellation and is a cyclically reduced conjugate of some c_i.

Theorem 1.1. *If F is a free group and $c_1, \ldots, c_n$, $n \geqslant 0$, is a sequence of non-trivial elements of F, there is a diagram $M(c_1, \ldots, c_n)$ which satisfies* (i)–(iii).

□ Each element c of a free group can be written uniquely as uru^{-1} where uru^{-1} is reduced without cancellation and r is cyclically reduced. We thus write each c_i as $u_i r_i u_i^{-1}$. The proof is by induction on n. If $n = 0$, we take M to consist of a single vertex O.

If $n = 1$, $c_1 = uru^{-1}$, take a vertex v_1 and a loop e at v_1 with label r. If $u = 1$, take $O = v_1$ and M is constructed. If $u \neq 1$, take a vertex O external to the loop e and an arc from O to v_1 with label u.

For $n > 1$, we proceed as follows. Form M' by taking diagrams $M_1, \ldots, M_n$ for each of the single factors $c_1, \ldots, c_n$ and arrange these in order around a common base point O.

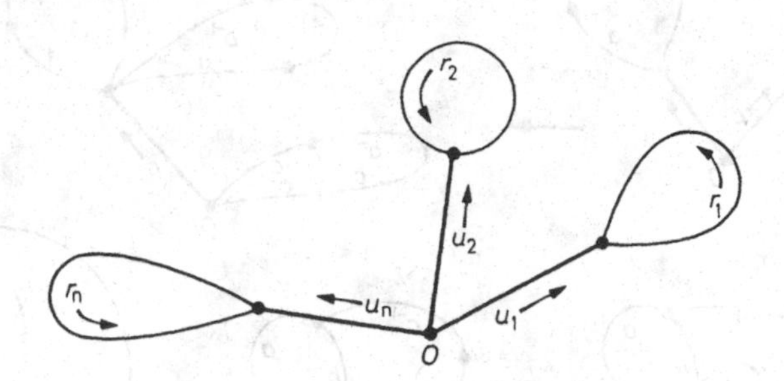

Fig. 1.1. The first stage of construction for $n > 1$

If the product $(u_1 r_1 u_1^{-1}) \cdots (u_n r_n u_n^{-1})$ is reduced without cancellation, then M' satisfies (i)–(iii) and is the desired diagram. Suppose that M' does not satisfy (ii), i.e., the product is not reduced without cancellation. If an edge e has label $s = x_1 \cdots x_j$ (each x_i a generator or its inverse), we can subdivide e into $e_1, \ldots, e_j$ so that each e_i has label x_i. We may thus suppose that each edge has a label which is a generator or the inverse of a generator.

The idea is to identify successive edges whose labels are inverses. Let α be the boundary cycle of M' which begins at O. Then $\phi(\alpha) = c_1 \cdots c_n$. By assumption,

α contains two successive edges e and f such that $\phi(e)$ and $\phi(f)$ are inverses. Let e and f respectively have initial and terminal vertices v_1 and v_2, and v_2 and v_3. Suppose that v_1 is not the same as either v_2 or v_3. We can then fold the edge e over onto the edge f (whether or not $v_2 = v_3$) without otherwise altering the structure of M' (See Figure 1.2.)

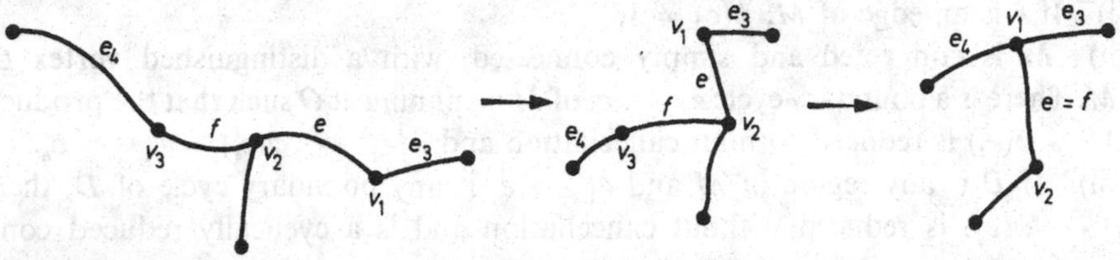

Fig. 1.2

In the resulting M'', $(\partial M'')$ contains fewer edges than α. If v_3 is distinct from v_1 and v_2 we can proceed in the same way.

It is possible that $v_1 = v_3$. In this case the closed edges e and f form a loop δ at the vertex v_1. We form M'' by deleting $\delta - v_1$ and all of M' interior to δ. Again, $\partial M''$ contains fewer edges than α. In both cases M'' satisfies (i) and (iii). Iteration of the process yields an M which satisfies (i)–(iii). M is the desired diagram. ☐

We illustrate the construction of Theorem 1.1 for the sequence ca^2bc^{-1}, $cb^{-1}c^{-1}ac^{-1}$, $ca^{-1}c^2$.

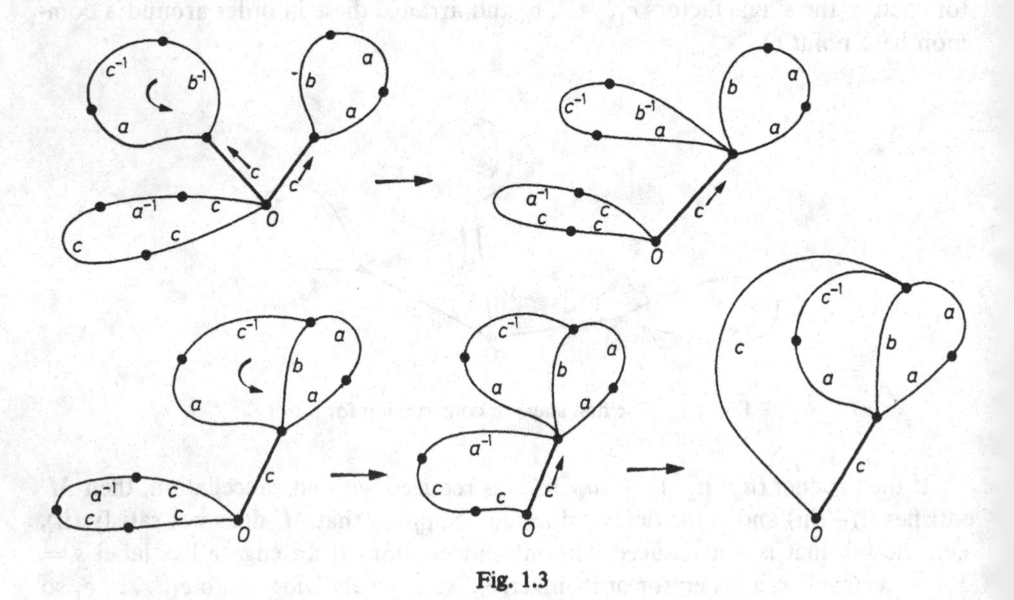

Fig. 1.3

Even this simple example illustrates that cancellation is a two-dimensional process. The region corresponding to $(b^{-1}ca)$ has no edges on the boundary of the final diagram.

The next lemma provides a converse of Theorem 1.1.

Lemma 1.2. (Normal Subgroup Lemma) *Let M be a connected, simply connected diagram with regions $D_1, \ldots, D_m$. Let α be a boundary cycle of M beginning at a vertex $v_0 \in \partial M$, and let $w = \phi(\alpha)$. Then there exist labels r_i of D_i and elements u_i of F, $1 \leqslant i \leqslant m$, such that*

$$w = (u_1 r_1 u_1^{-1}) \cdots (u_m r_m u_m^{-1}).$$

(Also, the u_i will satisfy the length restriction in the remark following the proof of the lemma.)

□ The proof is by induction on m. If $m = 0$ there is nothing to prove, but note that then M is a tree and thus $\phi(\alpha) = 1$. Now assume the theorem true for maps with k regions, and let M be a map with $k + 1$ regions.

There must exist a region D of M such that $\partial D \cap \partial M$ contains an edge. Form the map M' from M by deleting a single edge e in $\partial D \cap \partial M$. Now M' is still connected and simply connected. (See Fig. 1.4.)

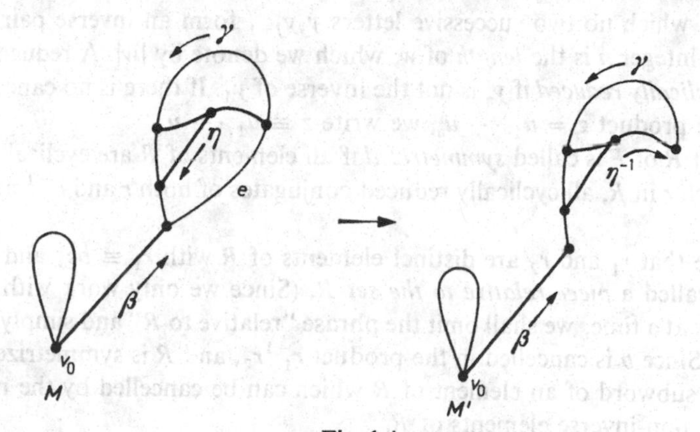

Fig. 1.4

Write $\alpha = \beta e \gamma$. There is a boundary cycle $e\eta$ of D which begins with the edge e. Let $\phi(\beta) = b$, $\phi(e) = z$, $\phi(\gamma) = c$, and $\phi(\eta) = d$. Then $w = \phi(\alpha) = bzc$. The boundary cycle μ of M' beginning at v_0 is $\beta\eta^{-1}\gamma$, so $\phi(\mu) = bd^{-1}c$.

By the induction hypothesis, the regions of M' (i.e., the regions of M other than D) can be numbered $D_1, \ldots, D_k$ so that $bd^{-1}c = (u_1 r_1 u_1^{-1}) \cdots (u_k r_k u_k^{-1})$, where r_i is a label of D_i. Now $w = bzc = (bd^{-1}c)(c^{-1}dzc)$ and dz is a label of D. Take D as D_{k+1}, dz as r_{k+1}, and c^{-1} as u_{k+1}. □

Remark. Let $K_M = \sum_{i=1}^{n} |\phi(e_i)|$, where the sum is over all the oriented edges of M. Note that we conjugated only by elements which are labels of parts of M'. Also, $K_{M'} < K_M$. Hence $|u_i| \leqslant mK_M$, $i = 1, \ldots, m$.

A subset R of a free group F is *symmetrized* if all elements of R are cyclically reduced and $r \in R$ implies that all cyclically reduced conjugates of $r^{\pm 1}$ are also in R.

Definition. Let R be a symmetrized subset of F. An *R-diagram* is a diagram M such that if δ is any boundary cycle of any region D of M, then $\phi(\delta) \in R$.

Let R be a symmetrized subset of the free group F, and let N be the normal subgroup of F generated by R. As a consequence of Theorem 1.1 and Lemma 1.2, we have the following fact. For any element w of F, $w \in N$ if and only if there is a connected, simply connected R-diagram M such that the label on the boundary of M is w. Connected, simply connected diagrams are therefore an adequate tool for studying membership in normal subgroups.

2. The Small Cancellation Hypotheses

We now turn to the formulation of the small cancellation hypotheses. In order to fix our notation and terminology, let F be a free group on a set X of generators. A *letter* is an element of the set Y of generators and inverses of generators. A *word* w is finite string of letters, $w = y_1 \cdots y_m$. We shall not distinguish between w and the element of F that it denotes. We denote the identity of F by 1. Each element of F other than the identity has a unique representation as a *reduced word* $w = y_1 \cdots y_n$ in which no two successive letters $y_j y_{j+1}$ form an inverse pair $x_i x_i^{-1}$ or $x_i^{-1} x_i$. The integer n is the *length* of w, which we denote by $|w|$. A reduced word w is called *cyclically reduced* if y_n is not the inverse of y_1. If there is no cancellation in forming the product $z = u_1 \cdots u_n$, we write $z \equiv u_1 \cdots u_n$.

A subset R of F is called *symmetrized* if all elements of R are cyclically reduced and, for each r in R, all cyclically reduced conjugates of both r and r^{-1} also belong to R.

Suppose that r_1 and r_2 are distinct elements of R with $r_1 \equiv bc_1$ and $r_2 \equiv bc_2$. Then b is called a *piece relative to the set* R. (Since we only work with one symmetrized set at a time, we shall omit the phrase "relative to R" and simply say that b is a *piece*.) Since b is cancelled in the product $r_1^{-1} r_2$, and R is symmetrized, a piece is simply a subword of an element of R which can be cancelled by the multiplication of two non-inverse elements of R.

The hypotheses of *small cancellation* assert that pieces are relatively small parts of elements of R. The most usual condition takes a metric form, $C'(\lambda)$, where λ is a positive real number.

Condition $C'(\lambda)$: If $r \in R$, $r \equiv bc$ where b is a piece, then $|b| < \lambda |r|$.

A closely related, non-metric, condition is $C(p)$, where p is a natural number.

Condition $C(p)$: No element of R is a product of fewer than p pieces.

Observe that $C'(\lambda)$ implies $C(p)$ for $\lambda \leqslant 1/(p-1)$. As illustration, the fundamental group of a closed, orientable 2-manifold of genus g has a presentation

$$G = \langle a_1, b_1, \ldots, a_g, b_g; a_1^{-1} b_1^{-1} a_1 b_1 \cdots a_g^{-1} b_g^{-1} a_g b_g \rangle.$$

In this case R consists of all cyclic permutations of r and r^{-1} where r is $a_1^{-1} b_1^{-1} a_1 b_1 \cdots a_g^{-1} b_g^{-1} a_g b_g$. Clearly, non-trivial pieces are single letters, and R satisfies $C'(1/(4g-1))$ and $C(4g)$. Groups which have a presentation $G = \langle X, R \rangle$ where

R satisfies $C'(\frac{1}{6})$ are sometimes called sixth-groups. Analogously, we have eighth-groups, etc..

We shall sometimes need a condition $T(q)$, for q a natural number, whose intuitive meaning will be clarified shortly.

Condition $T(q)$: Let $3 \leqslant h < q$. Suppose $r_1, \ldots, r_h$ are elements of R with no successive elements r_i, r_{i+1} an inverse pair. Then at least one of the products $r_1 r_2, \ldots, r_{h-1} r_h, r_h r_1$ is reduced without cancellation.

The cancellation conditions just introduced can be extended naturally to the case where F is a free product or a free product with amalgamation by using the appropriate normal forms and associated length functions. We defer precise definitions of the cancellation conditions in the more general cases until later.

We shall consistently use the notation introduced above. F will denote a free group on generators X, and R will denote a symmetrized subset of F with N the normal closure of R in F. G will be the quotient group F/N.

We now turn to investigating the geometric consequences of the small cancellation hypotheses.

Let R be a symmetrized subset of the free group F. A sequence $c_1, \ldots, c_n$ of conjugates of elements of R will be called a *minimal R-sequence* if the product $w = c_1 \cdots c_n$ cannot be written as a product of fewer than n conjugates of elements of R.

Let M be an arbitrary diagram over F. Let D_1 and D_2 be regions (not necessarily distinct) of M with an edge $e \subseteq \partial D_1 \cap \partial D_2$. Let $e\delta_1$ and $\delta_2 e^{-1}$ be boundary cycles of D_1 and D_2 respectively. Let $\phi(\delta_1) = f_1$, and $\phi(\delta_2) = f_2$. M will be called *reduced* if one never has $f_2 = f_1^{-1}$.

Lemma 2.1. *If M is the diagram of a minimal R-sequence, then M is reduced.*

□ Suppose that $w = c_1 \cdots c_n$ where $c_1, \ldots, c_n$ is a minimal R-sequence, and let M be the diagram for $c_1, \ldots, c_n$. Suppose that M is not reduced. Using the notation in the definition above, first assume that there are distinct regions D_1 and D_2 which make M not reduced. Delete the edge e, combining D_1 and D_2 into a single region D with boundary label 1. Call the resulting diagram M'. Since D_1 and D_2 were distinct, M' is still connected and simply connected. Now M' has the same boundary label, w, as M, but has one fewer region. By the Normal Subgroup Lemma (Lemma 1.2), w is the product of conjugates of the labels of the regions of M'. All regions of M' except D are labelled by elements of R. The label on D is 1 and can be deleted from the product. Hence, w is a product $q_1 \cdots q_{(n-2)}$ of conjugates of elements of R, which contradicts the original sequence $c_1, \ldots, c_n$ being minimal.

We are left with the possibility that two boundary cycles, δ_1 and δ_2, of a single region D make M not reduced. This means that two cyclic conjugates of a nontrivial element of a free group are inverses. But this is impossible in a free group. □

Let M be a map. A *boundary vertex* or a *boundary edge* of M is a vertex or edge in ∂M. A *boundary region* of M is a region D of M such that $\partial D \cap \partial M \neq \emptyset$. Thus if D is a boundary region of M, $\partial D \cap \partial M$ need not contain an edge, but may consist only of one or more vertices. A vertex, edge, or region of M which is not a boundary vertex, edge or region is called *interior*.

If v is a vertex of a map M, $d(v)$, the *degree* of v, will denote the number of oriented edges having v as initial vertex. Thus, if an edge has both endpoints at v we count it twice. If D is a region of M, $d(D)$, the *degree of D*, is the number of edges in a boundary cycle of D. The symbol $i(D)$ will denote the number of *interior* edges of ∂D, again with an edge counted twice if it appears twice in a boundary cycle of D.

It follows from their construction that most R-diagrams which we consider have no interior vertices of degree one. Suppose that in an R-diagram we have two interior edges e_1 and e_2 meeting in a vertex v of degree two. Then we can delete the vertex v and unite e_1 and e_2 into a single edge e with label $\phi(e) = \phi(e_1)\phi(e_2)$. Thus we may assume, if desired, that if M is an R-diagram, all interior vertices of M have degree at least three.

Lemma 2.2. *Let R be a symmetrized set of elements of a free group F, and let M be a reduced R-diagram.*

(1) *If R satisfies $C(k)$, then each region D of M such that $\partial D \cap \partial M$ does not contain an edge has $d(D) \geqslant k$.*

(2) *If R satisfies $T(m)$, then each interior vertex v of M has $d(v) \geqslant m$.*

□ We first show that if e is an interior edge of M, then the label $c = \phi(e)$ is a piece. Since e is an interior edge, e is on the common boundary of regions D_1 and D_2 of M. Then D_1 and D_2 have labels r_1 and r_2 in R with $r_1 = ca$ and $r_2 = c^{-1}b$. Since R is symmetrized, $cb^{-1} \in R$. Since M is reduced, $a \neq b^{-1}$. Thus c is a piece by definition. If D is a region of M and all edges of ∂D are interior edges, say $\partial D = e_1 \cdots e_{d(D)}$ with $\phi(e_i) = c_i$, then D has label $r = c_1 \cdots c_{d(D)} \in R$, and r is a product of $d(D)$ pieces. Hence, $C(k)$ implies that $d(D) \geqslant k$ for all regions D of M such that $\partial D \cap \partial M$ does not contain an edge. This shows, in particular, that each interior region of M has degree at least k.

Let v be an interior vertex of degree h and let $e_1, \ldots, e_h$ be, in order, the oriented edges incident at v. Then, for each i (modulo h), e_{i+1} and e_i^{-1} are consecutive edges on the boundary of a region D_i of M. There are paths α_i such that the boundary of D_i is described by a cycle at v of the form $e_i^{-1}\alpha_i e_{i+1}$. If f_i is the label on e_i and a_i the label on α_i, then D_i has label $r_i = f_i^{-1}a_i f_{i+1}$.

Since M is reduced, no $r_i = r_{i+1}^{-1}$, and since each $f_i \neq 1$, there is cancellation in each of the products $r_1 r_2, \ldots, r_{h-1}r_h, r_h r_1$ and $T(m)$ fails if $m > h$. Thus the condition $T(m)$ implies that $d(v) \geqslant m$ for each interior vertex v of M. □

The geometric interpretation of the small cancellation hypotheses shows that we must turn to a study of maps where the degrees of the vertices and regions satisfy certain inequalities.

3. The Basic Formulas

The results on maps obtained in this section are combinatorial generalizations of properties of the regular tessellations of the plane and are due in this context to

Lyndon (1966); similar results had been used in a different context by Blanc (1940, 1941) and Fiala (1946). There are only three regular tessellations of the plane: by triangles, squares, and hexagons. The types of more general maps which we will consider fall into three corresponding types.

Let p and q be positive real numbers such that $1/p + 1/q = 1/2$. As is well-known, the only positive integral solutions are (3, 6), (4, 4), and (6, 3). Two types of maps will arise in our considerations. If M is a non-empty map such that each interior vertex of M has degree at least p and *all* regions of M have degree at least q, then M will be called a *$[p, q]$ map*. If M is a non-empty map such that each interior vertex of M has degree at least p and each *interior* region of M has degree at least q, M will be called a *(p, q) map*.

Summation signs $\sum$ will denote summations over vertices or regions of M. Thus $\sum d(v)$ is the sum of the degrees of all the vertices of M and $\sum d(D)$ is the sum of the degrees of all the regions of M. The notation $\sum^{\bullet}$ denotes summation restricted to boundary vertices or regions, and $\sum^{\circ}$ summation over interior vertices or regions. Thus $\sum^{\bullet} d(v)$ is the sum of the degrees of the boundary vertices of M, and $\sum^{\circ} d(D)$ is the sum of the degrees of the interior regions. When necessary, a subscript naming the map will be added.

Let M be an arbitrary map. Then V will denote the number of vertices of M. (We will avoid using subscripts to name the map unless more than one map is under consideration.) The number of unoriented edges of M will be denoted by E, and F will denote the number of regions of M. $V^{\bullet}$ is the number of boundary vertices of M, $F^{\bullet}$ is the number of boundary regions of M, and $E^{\bullet}$ is the number of boundary edges of M, *counted with multiplicity*. If M is connected and simply connected, then $E^{\bullet}$ is the number of edges in a boundary cycle of M. To obtain $E^{\bullet}$ in general, we must add the number of edges in the cycles necessary to describe the boundary of M. Note that it is possible that $E^{\bullet} > E$. Let Q be the number of components of M, and let h be the number of holes (that is, the number of bounded components of $-M$) of M. Let p and q be positive real numbers such that $1/p + 1/q = 1/2$.

The following formulas will be basic to our considerations.

Theorem 3.1. *Let M be an arbitrary map. Then*

$$p(Q - h) = \sum^{\bullet}[p - d(v)] + \sum^{\circ}[p - d(v)] + \frac{p}{q}\sum[q - d(D)] - \frac{p}{q}E^{\bullet}. \tag{3.1}$$

$$p(Q - h) = \sum^{\bullet}\left[\frac{p}{q} + 2 - d(v)\right] + \sum^{\circ}[p - d(v)] + \frac{p}{q}\sum[q - d(D)] + \frac{p}{q}(V^{\bullet} - E^{\bullet}). \tag{3.2}$$

□ Euler's formula for a connected graph Γ is $1 = V - E + F$ if we do not count the unbounded region of the division of the plane into regions by Γ. Now let Γ be the 1-skeleton of M. Adding over each component of a possibly disconnected graph we have $Q = V - E + F$. Since we allow holes in a map, we subtract one for each hole (each region bounded by Γ which is not a region of M). Thus $(Q - h) = V - E + F$.

We have the following equations.

$$(1) \qquad (Q - h) = V - E + F.$$

(2) $2E = \sum d(v)$. (The sum of the degrees of the vertices counts each edge twice.)

$$(3) \qquad 2E = \sum d(D) + E^{\bullet}.$$

Let n be a positive real number. We eliminate E from the above equations.

$$(1)' \qquad 2(n+1)(Q-h) = 2(n+1)V - 2(n+1)E + 2(n+1)F.$$

$$(2)' \qquad 2E = \sum d(v).$$

$$(3)' \qquad 2nE = n\sum d(D) + nE^{\bullet}.$$

Using (2)′ and (3)′ in (1)′ we have

$$(4) \quad 2(n+1)(Q-h) = 2(n+1)V - \sum d(v) + 2(n+1)F - n\sum d(D) - nE^{\bullet}.$$

Since V is the number of vertices and F is the number of regions,

$$(5) \quad 2(n+1)(Q-h) = \sum [2(n+1) - d(v)] + n\sum\left[\frac{2(n+1)}{n} - d(D)\right] - nE^{\bullet}.$$

Splitting the first sum over boundary and interior vertices,

$$(6) \qquad 2(n+1)(Q-h) = \sum{}^{\bullet} [2(n+1) - d(v)] + \sum{}^{\circ} [2(n+1) - d(v)] + n\sum\left[\frac{2(n+1)}{n} - d(D)\right] - nE^{\bullet}.$$

Let $p = 2(n+1)$ and $q = 2(n+1)/n$. Then $n = p/q$, $1/p + 1/q = 1/2$, and $(p+2)/2 = p/q + 2$.

So we can rewrite (6) as

$$(7) \qquad p(Q-h) = \sum{}^{\bullet} [p - d(v)] + \sum{}^{\circ} [p - d(v)] + \frac{p}{q}\sum [q - d(D)] - \frac{p}{q}E^{\bullet}.$$

This is formula (3.1). We want to split the first sum in (6). If we sum n over the boundary vertices, $\sum^{\bullet} n = nV^{\bullet} = (p/q)V^{\bullet}$. Hence

$$(8) \quad p(Q-h) = \sum{}^{\bullet}[n + 2 - d(v)] + \sum{}^{\bullet} n + \sum{}^{\circ}[p - d(v)] + \frac{p}{q}\sum [q - d(D)] - \frac{p}{q}E^{\bullet}.$$

$$(9) \qquad p(Q-h) = \sum{}^{\bullet}\left[\frac{p}{q} + 2 - d(v)\right] + \sum{}^{\circ}[p - d(v)] + \frac{p}{q}\sum [q - d(D)] + \frac{p}{q}(V^{\bullet} - E^{\bullet}).$$

This is formula (3.2). □

Before looking at some corollaries of Theorem 3.1, we consider dual maps.

Given a map M, we form a *dual map* M^* as follows. Pick a point v_i^* in each region D_i of M. The collection of the v_i^* are the vertices of M^*. If D_1 and D_2 are regions of M, $D_1 \neq D_2$, but having an edge e in common, an edge e^* is drawn from v_1^* to v_2^* crossing e but no other edges of M or edges of M^* already constructed. Since $e \subseteq \partial D_1 \cap \partial D_2$, e is an interior edge of M. Also, if a region D of M has an edge e such that D lies on both sides of e, a loop is drawn at v_i^* crossing e but no other edges. The edges and vertices of M^* form a graph Γ^*. The regions of M^* are the regions bounded by Γ^* which contain an interior vertex of M.

This construction is the same as the usual construction of the dual of a plane graph except that boundary edges of M are ignored. The process could also be given in the following fashion. The 1-skeleton of M is a graph Γ, which divides the plane into various regions (counting the unbounded region). Form a dual graph Γ^*. Now delete the vertices and any incident edges which correspond to regions which are not regions of M.

We see that M^* has the following properties.

(1) The vertices v^* of M^* are in one-to-one correspondence with the regions D of M with $v^* \in D$. If v^* corresponds to D, then, since one edge is drawn from v^* across each interior edge of ∂D, $d(v^*) = i(D)$.

(2) The edges e^* of M^* are in one-to-one correspondence with the interior edges e of M.

(3) The regions D^* of M^* are in one-to-one correspondence with the interior vertices v of M, with $v \in D^*$. If v is an interior vertex of M there are $d(v)$ edges at v. Each of these edges is crossed by an edge of M^*, forming a region D^* of M^* with $d(D^*) = d(v)$.

(4) The boundary vertices v^* of M^* are in one-to-one correspondence with the boundary regions D of M. For, suppose v^* arises from a region D of M. If $\partial D \cap \partial M \neq \varnothing$, then there is a vertex $v_2 \in \partial D \cap \partial M$, and it is possible to construct a curve λ lying entirely in D from v^* to v_2 which does not cross any edges of M or M^*. Then λ can be extended into $-M$ which is contained in $-M^*$. Hence, v^* is a boundary vertex of M^*. If $\partial D \cap \partial M = \varnothing$, then every vertex of ∂D is an interior vertex of M. There are edges from v^* across each edge of ∂D, and these are connected by a sequence of edges through the regions which have a boundary edge emanating from a vertex on ∂D. Thus v^* is an interior vertex of M^*.

(5) If M has h holes, then M^* has h or fewer holes.

(6) If M is (p, q), then M^* is $[q, p]$.

Lemma 3.2. *If M is a map without isolated vertices, then $V^{\bullet} \leqslant E^{\bullet}$.*

□ $V^{\bullet}$ is the number of boundary vertices of M and $E^{\bullet}$ is the number of boundary edges of M counted with appropriate multiplicity. □

Corollary 3.3. (The Curvature Formula) *Let M be a simply-connected $[p, q]$ map which contains more than one vertex. Then*

$$\Sigma_M^{\bullet}\left[\frac{p}{q} + 2 - d(v)\right] \geqslant p. \tag{3.3}$$

□ Suppose first that M does not consist entirely of isolated vertices. Let M_1 be the submap of M obtained by deleting all isolated vertices. Let Q_1 be the number of components of M_1. By Lemma 3.2, $V_{M_1}^{\bullet} \leqslant E_{M_1}^{\bullet}$. Since M is a $[p, q]$ map and is without holes, $pQ_1 \leqslant \sum_{M_1}^{\bullet}[p/q + 2 - d(v)]$ from formula (3.2) since the first term is the only one which can be positive.

If there are Q_0 isolated vertices and M_0 consists of these vertices, $\sum_{M_0}^{\bullet}[p/q + 2 - d(v)] = Q_0[p/q + 2]$. If M consists entirely of isolated vertices, $Q_0 \geqslant 2$. In either case, $\sum_{M}^{\bullet}[p/q + 2 - d(v)] \geqslant p$. □

Corollary 3.4. (The Curvature Formula) *Let M be a simply-connected* (q, p) *map which contains more than one region. Then*

$$\sum_{M}^{\bullet}\left[\frac{p}{q} + 2 - i(D)\right] \geqslant p. \tag{3.4}$$

□ Let M^* be a dual map of M. Then M^* is a $[p, q]$ map satisfying the hypothesis of Corollary 3.3. If v^* is a vertex of M^* arising from a region D of M, then $d(v^*) = i(D)$, and the conclusion follows from Corollary 3.3. □

Corollaries 3.3 and 3.4 are basic to the study of small cancellation theory. We call these results "The Curvature Formula." To illustrate the reason for the name, let T be a regular tessellation of the plane by triangles, and let S be a finite submap of T whose boundary is a simple closed curve. Then the total curvature around the boundary of S is equal to 2π. For S, we can easily calculate the curvature. Let v be a boundary vertex of S. The interior angle at v is $[d(v) - 1]2\pi/6$. The curvature at v is then $\pi - [d(v) - 1]2\pi/6 = [4 - d(v)]2\pi/6$. The total curvature is then $2\pi = \sum_{S}^{\bullet}[4 - d(v)]2\pi/6$, which implies $\sum_{S}^{\bullet}[4 - d(v)] = 6$. All interior vertices of S have degree 6 and all regions of S have degree 3. For a general $[6, 3]$ map M which is simply-connected and has more than one vertex we have shown that $\sum_{M}^{\bullet}[4 - d(v)] \geqslant 6$. A similar interpretation applies to the regular tessellations of the plane by squares and by hexagons.

4. Dehn's Algorithm and Greendlinger's Lemma

In his study of the word problem for fundamental groups of orientable 2-manifolds, Dehn concluded that if a freely reduced non-trivial word w is equal to 1 in the fundamental group, then w contains more than half of some cyclic permutation of the defining relator or its inverse.

This conclusion gives *Dehn's algorithm* for the word problem. Suppose a group G has a presentation $G \doteq \langle x_1, \ldots, x_n; R\rangle$ where R is a recursive symmetrized set of defining relators, and that it has been established that freely reduced non-trivial words which are equal to 1 in G contain more than half of some element of R. Let w be a non-trivial word of G. If $w = 1$ in G, then w has some factorization $w \equiv bcd$ where, for some r in R, $r \equiv ct$ with $|t| < |c|$. Now such an r has $|r| < 2|w|$. The set S of all words on $x_1, \ldots, x_n$ which have length less than $2|w|$ is finite. Since R is recursive we can effectively list all elements of $R' = R \cap S$. If we find a suitable r then $w = bt^{-1}d$ in G, and $bt^{-1}d$ is a word of shorter length. A finite number of such reductions either leads to 1, giving a "proof" that $w = 1$ in G, or to a word w^* which cannot be so shortened, establishing $w \neq 1$ in G.

The most fundamental result of small cancellation theory is that Dehn's algorithm is valid for R satisfying either of the metric hypotheses $C'(\frac{1}{6})$, or $C(\frac{1}{4})$ and $T(4)$. Actually, as discovered by Greendlinger (1960) a considerably stronger result, now known as Greendlinger's Lemma, is true. Our approach here is to prove a strengthened version of the Curvature Formula (Theorem 4.3) and then deduce Greendlinger's Lemma as a corollary.

Lemma 4.1. *Let M be a simply-connected (q, p) map with (q, p) one of* (3, 6), (4, 4), *or* (6, 3). *Assume that if D is a region of M such that ∂D does not contain an edge of ∂M, then $d(D) \geqslant p$. Then the boundary of any region of M is a simple closed path.*

□ Let D be a region of M and suppose that there is a loop η in ∂D with η not all of ∂D. Then η and all of M interior to η form a simply connected submap K of M. Among all such loops η in ∂D, pick one so that K has a minimal number of regions

Because of the choice of η enclosing a minimal number of regions, there is at most one vertex, say v_0, contained in $\eta \cap \partial M$. With the exception of v_0, all vertices of K are interior vertices of M and so have degree at least q. Because η does not contain any boundary edges of M, no region of K can contain any boundary edges of M. By the hypothesis on M, it follows that all regions of K have degree at least p. Hence, K is a $[q, p]$ map. If K had only one vertex, then K would consist of one or more regions bounded by loops at v_0, contradicting the hypothesis that M is a (q, p) map. Thus we may now assume that K has more than one vertex.

Then by Corollary 3.3, $\sum_K^{\bullet}[q/p + 2 - d(v)] \geqslant q$. But since only v_0 can make a positive contribution to this sum, $\sum_K^{\bullet}[q/p + 2 - d(v)] < q/p + 2 < q$, which is a contradiction. □

Let M be a map. An *extremal disk* of M is a submap K of M which is topologically a disk and which has a boundary cycle $e_1, \ldots, e_n$ such that the edges $e_1, \ldots, e_n$ occur in order in some boundary cycle of the whole map M.

Lemma 4.2. *Let M be a connected, simply connected map with no vertices of degree one. If the boundary of M is not a simple closed path, then M has at least two extremal disks.*

□ We argue by induction on the number m of regions of M. If $m = 1$, then M is a simple closed path. Now assume that $m > 1$ and let $\delta = e_1 \ldots e_n$ be any boundary cycle of M. Let $\alpha = e_{i_1} \ldots e_{i_k}$ be the shortest closed subpath of δ. Since M does not contain any vertices of degree one, α has no consecutive edges of the form e, e^{-1}. Thus α is a simple closed path which bounds an extremal disk of M. Let J' be the submap of M which is bounded by $\delta - \alpha$. Since J' may have vertices of degree one, remove, one at a time, any vertices of degree one and the edges incident to such vertices. This process yields a submap J of M to which the induction hypothesis applies. If ∂J is a simple closed curve, then J is an extremal disk of M.

If ∂J is not a simple closed path, then J contains two extremal disks and at least one of these is extremal in M. □

Let D be a region of a map M. We say that $\partial D \cap \partial M$ is a *consecutive part* of M if $\partial D \cap \partial M$ is the union of a sequence $e_1, \ldots, e_n$ of closed edges, and the edges $e_1, \ldots, e_n$ occur consecutively in a boundary cycle of D and in some boundary cycle of M.

If M is a map, we will use the notation $\sum_M^*[p/q + 2 - i(D)]$ to denote summation only over those boundary regions D of M such that $\partial D \cap \partial M$ is a consecutive part of ∂M. If $1/p + 1/q = 1/2$, then $p/q + 2 = p/2 + 1$. We will use both these forms in our computations.

Theorem 4.3. *Let M be a connected, simply-connected (q, p) map. Suppose that M contains no vertices of degree one, and that M has more than one region. Suppose further that if D is a region of M, $d(D) \geq p$ unless $\partial D \cap \partial M$ contains an edge. Then*

$$\sum\nolimits_M^*\left[\frac{p}{q} + 2 - i(D)\right] \geq p.$$

□ We first prove the theorem for maps M such that ∂M is a simple closed path. The proof is by induction on the number, m, of regions of M.

Suppose $m = 2$. The only possibility is that M consists of two regions, D_1 and D_2, having a single edge in common. Hence $i(D_j) = 1$, $j = 1, 2$, and the theorem holds.

Now suppose the theorem is true for all maps satisfying the hypothesis and having t regions, $2 \leq t$.

Since the only regions of M with $d(D) < p$ are the regions D such that $\partial D \cap \partial M$ contains an edge, these regions are the only ones which can make a positive contribution to the sum $\sum_M^*[p/2 + 1 - i(D)]$. Corollary 3.4 says that

$$\sum\nolimits_M^{\cdot}[p/2 + 1 - i(D)] \geq p.$$

Hence, if all regions D of M such that $\partial D \cap \partial M$ contains an edge have $\partial D \cap \partial M$ a consecutive part of ∂M, then

$$p \leq \sum\nolimits_M^{\cdot}\left[\frac{p}{2} + 1 - i(D)\right] = \sum\nolimits_M^*\left[\frac{p}{2} + 1 - i(D)\right]$$

and we are done.

Now suppose that M contains a region E such that $\partial E \cap \partial M$ contains an edge, but $\partial E \cap \partial M$ is not a consecutive part of M. Then $M - \bar{E}$ has at least two components, say C_1 and C_2, each containing a region. Let $M_1 = C_1 \cup \bar{E}$, and let $M_2 = C_2 \cup \bar{E}$.

If D is a region of M_j, $j = 1, 2$, then $\partial D \cap \partial M_j = \partial D \cap \partial M$ unless $D = E$. The only region common to M_1 and M_2 is E, and $i(E)$ is at least 1 in both M_1 and M_2.

Applying the induction hypothesis to M_1 and M_2 gives

$$(4.1) \qquad \textstyle\sum_{M_1}^{*}\left[\frac{p}{2} + 1 - i(D)\right] + \sum_{M_2}^{*}\left[\frac{p}{2} + 1 - i(D)\right] \geqslant 2p.$$

At worst, E appears in both sums and has $i(E) = 1$ in each. Then

$$(4.2) \qquad \sum_{\substack{M_1 \\ D \neq E}}^{*}\left[\frac{p}{2} + 1 - i(D)\right] + \sum_{\substack{M_2 \\ D \neq E}}^{*}\left[\frac{p}{2} + 1 - i(D)\right] \geqslant p.$$

This concludes the proof in the case that ∂M is a simple closed path.

If the boundary of M is not a simple closed path then, by Lemma 4.2, M has at least two extremal disks, say K_1 and K_2. If a K_i consists of a single region D_0 then $\partial D_0 \cap \partial M$ is a consecutive part of ∂M and $\sum_{K_i}^{*}[p/2 + 1 - i(D)] = p/2 + 1$. If a K_i contains more than one region then $\sum_{K_i}^{*}[p/2 + 1 - i(D)] \geqslant p$ by the first part of the proof. Since an extremal disk is connected to the rest of M by a single vertex, there can be at most one region E in K_i such that $\partial E \cap \partial K_i$ is a consecutive part of ∂K_i but $\partial E \cap \partial M$ is not a consecutive part of ∂M. Putting together the contributions from K_1 and K_2 we have $\sum_{M}^{*}[p/q + 2 - i(D)] \geqslant p$. □

Definition. A word s is called a *j-remnant* (with respect to R) if some $r \in R$ has the form $r \equiv sb_1 \cdots b_j$ where $b_1, \ldots, b_j$ are pieces.

The point of all this is the following.

Theorem 4.4. *Let F be a free group. Let R be a symmetrized subset of F with N the normal closure of R. Assume that R satisfies the hypothesis $C(p)$ and $T(q)$ where (q, p) is one of the pairs* (6, 3), (4, 4), *or* (3, 6).

If $w \in N$, $w \neq 1$, then for some cyclically reduced conjugate w^* of w, $w^* \in R$ or has the form $w^* \equiv u_1 s_1 \cdots u_n s_n$ where each s_k is an $i(s_k)$-remnant. The number n of the s_k and the numbers $i(s_k)$ satisfy the relation

$$\sum_{k=1}^{n}\left[\frac{p}{q} + 2 - i(s_k)\right] \geqslant p.$$

In particular, if R satisfies

(i) *$C'(\lambda)$ for $\lambda \leqslant \frac{1}{6}$, or*
(ii) *$C'(\lambda)$ and $T(4)$ for $\lambda \leqslant \frac{1}{4}$,*

then every non-trivial element $w \in N$ contains a subword s of some $r \in R$ with

(i) *$|s| > (1 - 3\lambda)|r| > \frac{1}{2}|r|$, or*
(ii) *$|s| > (1 - 2\lambda)|r| > \frac{1}{2}|r|$.*

□ Let w be a non-trivial element of N with w' a cyclically reduced conjugate of w. Let M be the diagram of a minimal R-sequence for w'. Either M consists of a single region, in which case $w' \in R$ or M satisfies the hypothesis of Theorem 4.3.

Let D be a region of M with $\sigma = \partial D \cap \partial M$ a consecutive part of ∂M. Suppose that σ begins at vertex v_1 and ends at v_2. Since ∂D is a simple closed path by Lemma 4.1, there is a boundary cycle $\sigma\tau$ of D. Write $s = \phi(\sigma)$ and $t = \phi(\tau)$. Now $st \in R$ since it is a label of D. Thus s is a subword of an element of R.

If α is any boundary cycle of M, then $\phi(\alpha)$ is a cyclically reduced conjugate w^* of w'. Suppose α begins at a vertex v_0 not interior to the arc σ. Since σ is a consecutive part of ∂M we can write $\alpha = \alpha_1\sigma\alpha_2$. Thus s is also a subword of w^*.

Now we ask how "large" the subword s is. We know that the label on an interior edge is a piece. If $i(D) = j$, then t is a product of j pieces and s is a j-remnant.

Pick a boundary cycle α which does not begin at a vertex interior to an arc of the form $\partial D \cap \partial M$. Then for all D such that $\partial D \cap \partial M$ is a consecutive part of M, $\phi(\partial D \cap \partial M)$ is a subword of $w^* = \phi(\alpha)$ and is a j-remnant where $j = i(D)$. The formula $\sum_M[p/q + 2 - i(D)] \geqslant p$ gives the first part of the theorem.

In the $C'(\lambda)$, $\lambda \leqslant \frac{1}{6}$, case we have $(q, p) = (6, 3)$ and the formula is

$$\textstyle\sum_M^*[4 - i(D)] \geqslant 6.$$

For the inequality to hold there must be at least two regions D_k with $i(D_k) \leqslant 3$. The corresponding subwords s_k have length greater than $(1 - 3\lambda)|r_k|$. In the $C'(\lambda)$, $\lambda \leqslant \frac{1}{4}$, and $T(4)$ case we have $\sum_M^*[3 - i(D)] \geqslant 4$. This yields at least two regions with $i(D) \leqslant 2$.

In either case, if $w \in N$ write $w = uw'u^{-1}$ where w' is cyclically reduced. Since an appropriate cyclic permutation of w' contains at least two occurrences of more than half of an element of R, it follows that w' contains at least one such occurrence. □

If s is a word of F, we introduce the notation $s > cR$, c a rational number, to mean that there is an $r \in R$ with $r \equiv st$ in reduced form, and $|s| > c|r|$.

A more detailed analysis of the number of regions and the numbers $i(D)$ needed to make $\sum_M^*[4 - i(D)] \geqslant 6$ yields

Theorem 4.5. (Greendlinger's Lemma for Sixth-Groups) *Let R satisfy $C'(\frac{1}{6})$. Let w be a non-trivial, cyclically reduced word with $w \in N$. Then either*

(1) $w \in R$,

or some cyclically reduced conjugate w^* of w contains one of the following:

(2) *two disjoint subwords, each $> \frac{5}{6}R$,*

(3) *three disjoint subwords, each $> \frac{4}{6}R$,*

(4) *four disjoint subwords, two $> \frac{4}{6}R$ and two $> \frac{3}{6}R$,*

(5) *five disjoint subwords, four $> \frac{3}{6}R$ and one $> \frac{4}{6}R$, or*

(6) *six disjoint subwords, each $> \frac{3}{6}R$.*

□ We sketch the proof. From our geometric point of view, the present theorem is a slight strengthening of the previous theorem in the special case that R satisfies $C'(\frac{1}{6})$. Let w' be a cyclically reduced conjugate of w, and let M be the diagram of a minimal R-sequence for w'. Now a subword s of w' with $s > (j/6)R$ comes from a region D with $i(D) = 6 - j$. The crucial point is that if M does not contain any regions of interior degree 0 or 1, the result follows from Theorem 4.4 by counting. For example, if all regions D which make a positive contribution to the sum $\sum_M^*[4 - i(D)]$ have interior degree 3, there must be at least six such regions.

Although the conclusion of the present theorem is stated in terms of subwords, we think of each of the possibilities (1)–(6) as being a condition on the regions making a positive contribution to the sum $\sum_M^*[4 - i(D)]$. Thus for example, (3) asserts that M contains at least three regions which have interior degree at most 2, and which are such that the intersection of each of their boundaries with ∂M is a consecutive part of ∂M.

With this understanding, we prove by induction on the number, m, of regions of M, that M contains regions such that the conclusion of the theorem holds. If $m = 1$, then $w' \in R$. If $m = 2$, then M has two regions, both of interior degree either 0 or 1, and case (2) of the conclusion holds. Now suppose that $m \geqslant 3$. As noted above, if M does not contain any regions of interior degree 0 or 1, the conclusion follows from Theorem 4.4. Suppose that M contains a region D_1 with $i(D_1) = 1$. Obtain the map M' by removing D_1 and $\partial D_1 \cap \partial M$ from M. The theorem holds for M' by the induction hypothesis. But it is easy to see that a map which is obtained by attaching a region to one edge of a map satisfying one of the conclusions (1)–(6) also satisfies one of these conclusions.

Finally, suppose that M contains a region with interior degree 0. Then ∂M is not a simple close path, so M has at least two extremal disks. By the induction hypothesis, each of these disks satisfies one of the conclusions (1)–(6). Since an extremal disk is attached to the rest of M at a single vertex, it is easy to verify that M must satisfy one of the desired conclusions. □

A similar analysis yields the corresponding theorem for the $C'(\frac{1}{4})$ and $T(4)$ case. Compare Greendlinger (1965).

Theorem 4.6. *Let R satisfy $C'(\frac{1}{4})$ and $T(4)$. Let w be a non-trivial, cyclically reduced word with $w \in N$. Then either*

(1) *$w \in R$,*

or some cyclically reduced conjugate w^* of w contains one of the following:

(2) *two disjoint subwords, each $> \frac{3}{4}R$, or*

(4) *four disjoint subwords, each $> \frac{1}{2}R$.* □

For groups $G = \langle X; R \rangle$ in which Dehn's algorithm is valid, there is a rather natural definition of "reduced."

Definition. A word w on the generators X is called *R-reduced* if w is freely reduced and there is no subword s of w with $s > \frac{1}{2}R$. We call w *cyclically R-reduced* if w is cyclically reduced in the free group sense and all cyclic permutations of w are R-reduced.

Note that Dehn's algorithm says that the only R-reduced word equal to 1 in G is 1 itself. Also as long as X is finite and R is recursive we can effectively go from a word w to an R-reduced word equal to w in G. Namely, keep replacing subwords which are $> \frac{1}{2}R$ by shorter words equal in the group. In general, different R-reduced words may represent the same group element. For example, if

$$G = \langle a_1, b_1, a_2, b_2; a_1^{-1}b_1^{-1}a_2b_2a_2^{-1}b_2^{-1}a_2b_2 \rangle,$$

then $a_1^{-1}b_1^{-1}a_1b_1 = b_2^{-1}a_2^{-1}b_2a_2$.

We give an indication of the historical development of the ideas in this section.

Dehn's methods (1911, 1912) were geometric. He used the fact that with the fundamental group G of an orientable closed 2-manifold there is an associated regular tessellation of the hyperbolic plane which is composed of transforms of a fundamental region for G. Using the hyperbolic metric, Dehn inferred that a non-trivial word w equal to 1 in G contained more than half of an element of R. Reidemeister (1932) pointed out that Dehn's conclusion followed from the combinatorial properties of the tessellation, without metric considerations.

V. A. Tartakovskii (1949) initiated the algebraic study of small cancellation theory. Tartakovskii solved the word problem for finitely presented quotients of free products of cyclic groups by symmetrized R satisfying $C(7)$. Britton (1957) independently investigated quotient groups of arbitrary free products by R satisfying $C'(\frac{1}{6})$. The triangle condition, Condition $T(4)$, was introduced in by Schiek (1956) who solved the word problem for R satisfying $C'(\frac{1}{4})$ and $T(4)$. Greendlinger (1960) proved Greendlinger's Lemma and obtained several other important results. Greendlinger (1964, 1965) subsequently also investigated the $C'(\frac{1}{4})$ and $T(4)$ hypothesis.

The general "geometrization" of small cancellation theory is due to Lyndon (1966). As we have remarked earlier, the existence of the type of diagrams we are using was observed by van Kampen (1933). Lyndon independently discovered such diagrams and the geometric significance of the small cancellation hypotheses. Also, Weinbaum (1966) came across van Kampen's work and used diagrams to give a geometric proof of Greendlinger's Lemma in the $C'(\frac{1}{6})$ case. The curvature formula $\sum [(p/q) + 2 - i(D)] \geqslant p$ is due to Lyndon (1966).

5. The Conjugacy Problem

Our study of conjugacy begins with a discussion of the algorithm which Dehn (1912) found for solving the conjugacy problem for the fundamental groups of closed 2-manifolds. Let $G = \langle X; R\rangle$, where X is finite and R is recursive, be a group in which Dehn's algorithm for the word problem is valid. Let u' and z' be any two elements of G. We can effectively replace u' and z' respectively by conjugates u and z which are cyclically R-reduced. Two trivial cases arise. If both u and z are 1, they are certainly conjugate in G, while if one of u or z is 1 and the other is not, they are not conjugate in G. The conjugacy problem is thus reduced to considering pairs of non-trivial cyclically R-reduced words. We say that *Dehn's algorithm solves the conjugacy problem for G* if there is a fixed integer k such that the following condition is satisfied:

Two non-trivial cyclically R-reduced words u and z are conjugate in G if and only if there are cyclic permutations u^* and z^* of u and z respectively such that $u^* = cz^*c^{-1}$ in G where c is a subword of some $r \in R$ which satisfies the length inequality $|r| < k \max(|u|, |z|)$.

The above condition implies that the conjugacy problem is solvable as follows. Since X is finite, there are only finitely many $r \in R$ satisfying the given length restriction, and since R is recursive, all such r can be effectively found. In view of the solvability of the word problem for G, one can then decide if the above equation holds for any permutations u^* and z^*, and any of the finitely many conjugating elements c that must be tried.

Greendlinger (1960) showed that Dehn's algorithm solves the conjugacy problem if F is a free group and R satisfies $C'(\frac{1}{8})$. Greendlinger (1965, 1966) subsequently showed that slight generalizations of Dehn's algorithm solve the conjugacy problem for R satisfying $C'(\frac{1}{6})$, and $C'(\frac{1}{4})$ and $T(4)$. A geometric proof of these results is given by Schupp (1970).

We turn to interpreting conjugacy in terms of diagrams. An *annular map* M is a connected map such that $-M$ has exactly two components. Let M be an annular map. Let K be the unbounded component of $-M$, and let H be the bounded component of $-M$. We call $\partial M \cap \partial K$ the *outer boundary* of M, while $\partial M \cap \partial H$ is the *inner boundary* of M. A cycle of minimal length (that does not cross itself) which contains all the edges in the outer (inner) boundary of M is an *outer* (*inner*) *boundary cycle* of M. (A note on orientation is called for. We read boundary cycles in the orientation of M. Thus outer boundary cycles are read counterclockwise while inner boundary cycles are read clockwise.)

Let F be a free group, and let R be a symmetrized subset of F. As usual, N will denote the normal closure of R in F, and G will denote the quotient group F/N. We shall see that annular diagrams are an adequate tool for studying conjugacy in G.

Lemma 5.1. *Let M be an annular R-diagram. If u is a label of an outer boundary cycle of M, and z^{-1} is a label of an inner boundary cycle of M, then u and z are conjugate in G.*

□ Since M is connected, there is a simple path β from the outer boundary of M to the inner boundary of M. Suppose that β begins at the vertex v_1 and ends at the vertex v_2. Let σ be the outer boundary cycle of M beginning at v_1, and let τ be the inner boundary cycle of M beginning at v_2. Let $\phi(\sigma) = u_1$, $\phi(\tau) = z_1$, and $\phi(\beta) = b$.

Cut open the map M along the path β to obtain a connected simply connected map M'. (See Figure 5.1.) A boundary cycle of M' is $\sigma\beta\tau\beta^{-1}$, and thus $u_1 b z_1^{-1} b^{-1} \in N$ by Lemma 1.2. Since u_1 and z_1 are conjugates of u and z respectively, the result follows. □

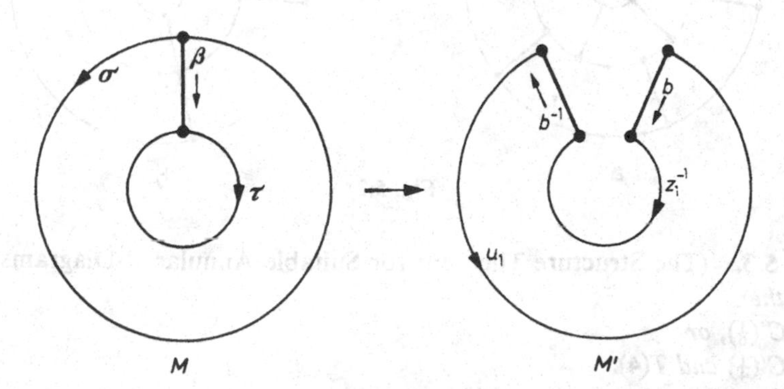

Fig. 5.1

Lemma 5.2. *Let u and z be two cyclically reduced words of F which are not in N and which are not conjugate in F. If u and z represent conjugate elements of G, then there is a reduced annular R-diagram M containing at least one region such that:*

If $\sigma = e_1 \cdots e_s$ and $\tau = f_1 \cdots f_k$ are respectively outer and inner boundary cycles of M, then the product $\phi(e_1) \cdots \phi(e_s)$ is reduced without cancellation and is a conjugate of u, while the product $\phi(f_1) \cdots \phi(f_k)$ is reduced without cancellation and is a conjugate of z^{-1}.

□ Since u and z represent conjugate elements of G, u is equal to some product $pp_1 \cdots p_n$, with $p = czc^{-1}$, each $p_i = c_i r_i c_i^{-1}$ with $r_i \in R$. Among all such products equal to u pick one $p'p'_1 \cdots p'_m$ with m minimal. Let M' be the diagram for the sequence $p'p'_1 \cdots p'_m$. Since u is not conjugate to z in F, there must be at least one p_i. It is clear that since $u \notin N$, the region with label z was not deleted in the construction of M'. If $\sigma = e_1 \cdots e_s$ is the boundary cycle of M' beginning at the base point v_0, then $\phi(e_1) \cdots \phi(e_s)$ is reduced without cancellation and is equal to u.

Form M from M' by deleting the region with label z. M is the desired diagram. Finally, since m is minimal, M is reduced (as in the proof of Lemma 2.1). □

We call M a *conjugacy diagram* for u and z. The construction of the conjugacy diagram did not require any hypothesis on R. If R satisfies the cancellation conditions $C(p)$ and $T(q)$, then M is an annular (q, p) map by Lemma 2.2.

We now turn to the case where R satisfies one of the cancellation conditions $C'(1/6)$, or $C'(1/4)$ and $T(4)$. Let u and z be non-trivial cyclically R-reduced words which are conjugate in G, but which are not conjugate in F. Our goal is to describe the geometry of the conjugacy diagram, M, for u and z. We shall obtain a very strong structure theorem. We shall prove that either all regions of M have edges on both boundaries, or M has a "thickness" of two regions as indicated in Figure 5.2. (The $C'(1/6)$ case is illustrated in Fig. (a), while Fig. (b) illustrates the $C'(1/4)$ and $T(4)$ case. The number of regions per layer is variable.)

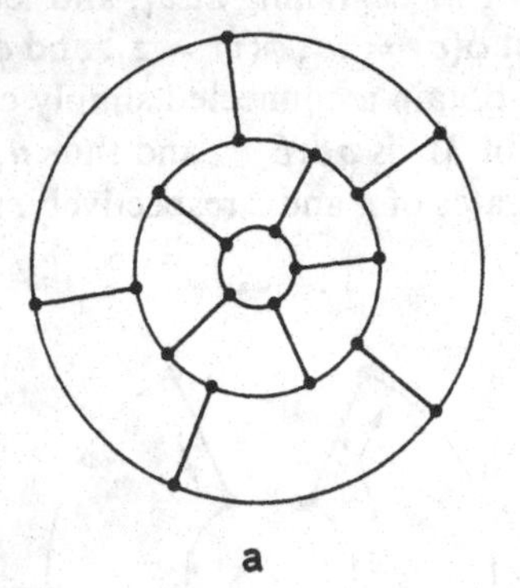

Fig. 5.2

Theorem 5.3. (The Structure Theorem for Suitable Annular R-Diagrams) *Let R satisfy either*

(1) $C'(\frac{1}{6})$, *or*

(2) $C'(\frac{1}{4})$ *and* $T(4)$.

Assume the following three hypotheses.

(A) *M is a reduced annular R-diagram.*

(B) *Let σ and τ be respectively the outer and inner boundaries of M. If D is a region of M with $\sigma_1 = \partial D \cap \sigma$ connected, then $\phi(\sigma_1)$ is not $> \frac{1}{2}R$. Assume the same hypothesis replacing σ by τ.*

(C) *M does not contain a region D such that ∂D contains an edge of both σ and τ.*

Let (q, p) be (3, 6) or (4, 4) in cases (1) and (2) respectively. Then M satisfies all of the following conditions:

(i) *For each region D, ∂D contains a boundary edge of M.*

(ii) *$i(D) = p/q + 2$ for all regions D of M.*

(iii) *$d(v) = q$ for all interior vertices v of M.*

☐ We shall prove the theorem in Case (1). The proof in Case (2) differs only in the numbers used.

As usual, we may assume that M has no vertices of degree two. First of all, σ and τ are simple closed paths. For suppose there is a loop $\eta \subseteq \sigma$, $\eta \neq \sigma$. Then η together with its interior is a simply-connected R-diagram M_1. But then by Theorem 4.3, M_1 must contain a region D which contradicts (B) of the hypothesis. The same remarks apply to τ.

Suppose D is a region of M such that $\eta = \partial D \cap \sigma$ is a consecutive part of σ. We show that ∂D has at least four interior edges. Since R satisfies $C'(\frac{1}{6})$ and the label on an interior edge is a piece, if D had three or fewer interior edges, then we would have $|\phi(\eta)| > \frac{3}{6}|r|$, where r is a label of D. Then D would contradict hypothesis (B). The same argument applies to regions D such that $\partial D \cap \partial M$ is a consecutive part of τ.

We now show that there are no regions D such that $\partial D \cap \sigma$ is disconnected. Suppose there is such a region D. Then $M—D$ has a component which is a non-empty simply connected submap K of M. Let D be chosen among regions with $\partial D \cap \partial M$ disconnected such that K has a minimal number of regions. It follows from the minimal choice of D that if D_j is any region of K with $\partial D_j \cap \sigma \neq \emptyset$, then $\partial D_j \cap \sigma$ is connected. Let $K' = K \cup D$. Then every $\partial K \cap \partial D_j$ is connected and every such region D_j of K' except D has at least four interior edges in K'. But by Theorem 4.3, K' contains at least two boundary regions each with at most three interior edges. Hence, some region of K' other than D has at most three interior edges, which is a contradiction. Again, the same argument applies to a region D with $\partial D \cap \tau$ disconnected.

Since there are no vertices of degree two, it follows that if D is any region of M, then $\partial D \cap \partial M$ contains at most one boundary edge. If ∂D contains a boundary edge, then $i(D) \geqslant 4$. If ∂D has no edge in ∂M, then $d(D) \geqslant 7$.

We apply Theorem 3.1 to a dual map, M^*, of M. We have

$$(5.1) \quad 6(Q_{M^*} - h_{M^*}) \leqslant \textstyle\sum^{\bullet}_{M^*}[4 - d(v)] + \sum^{\circ}_{M^*}[6 - d(v)] + 2\sum_{M^*}[3 - d(D)] + 2(V^{\bullet}_{M^*} - E^{\bullet}_{M^*})$$

Since M^* has at most one hole, $6(Q_{M^*} - h_{M^*}) \geqslant 0$. Since each region of M has interior edges, M^* has no isolated vertices and $V^{\bullet}_{M^*} \leqslant E^{\bullet}_{M^*}$. Hence,

$$(5.2) \quad 0 \leqslant \textstyle\sum^{\bullet}_{M^*}[4 - d(v)] + \sum^{\circ}_{M^*}[6 - d(v)] + 2\sum_{M^*}[3 - d(D)].$$

Using the correspondence between a map and a dual map, we have

$$0 \leqslant \sum\nolimits_M^{\bullet}[4 - i(D)] + \sum\nolimits_M^{\circ}[6 - d(D)] + 2\sum\nolimits_M[3 - d(v)]. \tag{5.3}$$

We have shown that each term in the first sum is non-positive. Also, each term in the last sum is non-positive. Now a term in the middle sum would be negative. Hence, we conclude that there are no interior regions in M. If some boundary region D had $i(D) > 4$, the first sum would be negative. Hence $i(D) = 4$ for all regions D of M. Similarly, from the last term we conclude that $d(v) = 3$ for all vertices v of M. □

Theorem 5.4. *Let R satisfy either*

(1) $C'(\frac{1}{6})$, *or*

(2) $C'(\frac{1}{4})$ *and* $T(4)$.

Let u and z be non-trivial elements of F which are cyclically R-reduced and which are not conjugate in F.

Then u and z are conjugate in G if and only if there exists an h in F such that $u^* = h^{-1}z^*h^{-1}$ in G, where u^* and z^* are cyclically reduced conjugates of u and z respectively, and h satisfies the following conditions:

(i) $h = b_1$ *or* $h = b_1b_2$, *where each* b_j, $j = 1, 2$, *is a subword of an element of* r_j *of* R. (*If R satisfies $C'(\frac{1}{8})$, then $h = b_1$*)

(ii) $|r_j| < 2q \max(|u|, |z|)$, where q is 3 or 4 in cases (1) or (2) respectively.

Thus if F is finitely generated and R is recursive, then $G = F/N$ has solvable conjugacy problem.

□ Sufficiency is trivial. Suppose that u and z are conjugate in G. The hypotheses allow us to construct the conjugacy diagram, M, for u and z. Let σ and τ be respectively the outer and inner boundaries of M. There are two cases.

Case 1. Suppose there is a region of M whose boundary contains an edge of both σ and τ. The proof of Theorem 5.3 shows that if E is a region of M such that ∂E does not contain an edge of both σ and τ, then $i(E) \geqslant p/q + 2$. Hence,

$$0 \leqslant \sum\nolimits_M^{\bullet}\left[\frac{p}{q} + 2 - i(D)\right] \leqslant \sum\nolimits_M'\left[\frac{p}{q} + 2 - i(D)\right]$$

where the latter sum is only over those regions whose boundary contains an edge of both σ and τ. Hence, there is at least one such region D with $i(D) \leqslant p/q + 2$.

In the $C'(\frac{1}{6})$ case, $i(D) \leqslant 4$. Thus more than 2/6 of the label r of ∂D appears on the boundary of M. Therefore more than 1/6 of r must appear in either $\phi(\sigma)$ or $\phi(\tau)$. Hence, either $|r| < 6|u|$ or $|r| < 6|z|$. In the $C'(\frac{1}{4})$ case, we obtain $|r| < 8|u|$ or $|r| < 8|z|$. This proves assertion (ii).

There is a simple path β from σ to τ with $\beta \subseteq \partial D$. Cut the map M open along the path β to obtain the simply connected map M'. We then have $u^*b(z^*)^{-1}b^{-1} \in N$ where u^* and z^* are cyclically reduced conjugates of u and z respectively, and b is the label on β.

Case 2. Suppose no region of M is such that its boundary contains an edge of both σ and τ. In this case, Theorem 5.3 applies. Let M_1 be the union of σ and the closures of all regions whose boundaries contain an edge of σ. Define M_2 similarly, replacing σ by τ. Then $M_1 \cup M_2 = M$ and M_1 and M_2 are both annular maps. Take any region D_1 with a boundary edge e on the inner boundary of M_1. Now e is an edge in the common boundary of D_1 and a region D_2 of M_2. Then we can construct a simple path β from σ to τ by going first along the boundary of D_1 and then along the boundary of D_2. Cutting M open along the path β, we obtain $u^*b(z^*)^{-1}b^{-1} \in N$. The label on b is b_1b_2 where b_i is the label on the part of β in D_i.

Let D_1 have label r_1. Since $d(D_1) = p/q + 2$, more that 2/6 of r_1 occurs in u in the one-sixth case. In the $C'(\frac{1}{4})$ and $T(4)$ case, more than 1/4 of r_1 occurs in u. The same remarks apply to the amount of the label on D_2 which occurs in z^{-1}.

If R is assumed to satisfy a cancellation condition $C'(\frac{1}{8})$, a diagram satisfying the hypothesis of Theorem 5.3 cannot exist. Because of the condition $C'(\frac{1}{8})$ and hypothesis (B), a region D which did not contain edges of both σ and τ would have at least five interior edges. This would force the sum in (5.3) to be negative, a contradiction. Thus a conjugacy diagram M for u and z must contain a region with edges on both boundaries of M and Case 1 must apply. □

Although the previous theorem solves the conjugacy problem, we have not pinned down the detailed structure of the conjugacy diagram when some region contains an edge of both boundaries. We do this in the following theorem.

Theorem 5.5. *Let R satisfy either $C'(\frac{1}{6})$, or $C'(\frac{1}{4})$ and $T(4)$. Assume that*

(A) *M is a reduced annular R-diagram.*

(B) *Let σ and τ be respectively the outer and inner boundaries of M. If D is a region of M with $\sigma_1 = \partial D \cap \sigma$ connected, then $\phi(\sigma_1)$ is not $> \frac{1}{2}R$. Assume the same hypothesis with σ replaced by τ.*

(C) *There is a region E of M such that ∂E intersects both boundaries of M.*

Then every region D of M has edges on both σ and τ and $i(D) \leqslant 2$.

□ We begin with a definition. An *island* of M is a submap of M bounded by a simple closed path of the form $\sigma_1\tau_1$ where $\sigma_1 \subseteq \sigma$ and $\tau_1 \subseteq \tau$. A *bridge* is an edge in $\sigma \cap \tau$. We shall show that M "looks like" Fig. 5.3. If M has no islands, then each region will have interior degree two. Otherwise, M will consist of various islands connected by bridges or joined at common vertices. A region with interior degree zero is itself an island, while a region with interior degree one is at the end of an island.

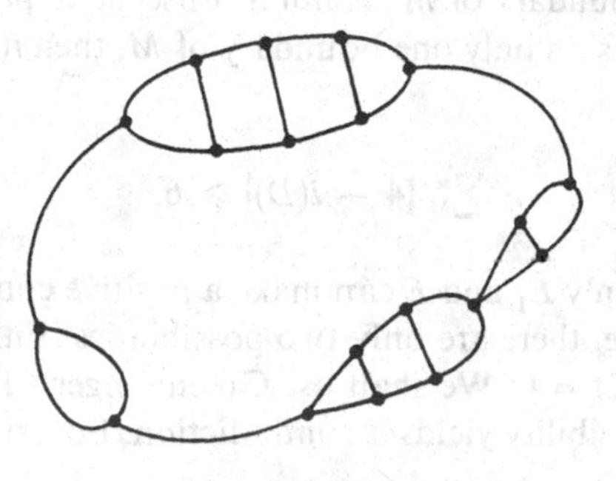

Fig. 5.3

As before, we shall prove the theorem in the $C'(\frac{1}{6})$ case. The proof for $C'(\frac{1}{4})$ and $T(4)$ differs only in the numbers used. As usual, we may assume that M has no vertices of degree two. In view of hypotheses (A) and (B) it follows, exactly as in the proof of Theorem 5.3, that if D is a region such that D intersects at most one of the boundaries of M, then $i(D) \geqslant 4$. Furthermore, there is no region whose boundary has disconnected intersection with one of the boundaries of M.

The overall proof is by induction on the number, m, of regions of M. If $m = 1$, the theorem holds. We now make the special assumption that if β is a simple path from σ to τ which is contained in the boundary of a region D, then D does not lie on both sides of β. We shall show later that if this assumption is violated, then M has exactly one region.

Suppose that M contains a region E with $i(E) = 0$. Then E is an island. Write $\partial E = \sigma_1\tau_1$, and let σ_1 begin at the vertex v_1 and end at v_2. Form the map M' by by deleting the region E and its boundary (excluding v_1 and v_2), and identifying v_1 and v_2. The map M' has fewer regions than M and satisfies all the hypotheses of the theorem. The result follows by induction for M', and thus also for M.

We are left with the situation where M contains a region E such that $i(E) \geqslant 1$ and ∂E intersects both boundaries of M. Since $i(E) \geqslant 1$, there is a region J on one side of E and a simple path β from σ to τ such that $\beta \subseteq \partial E$ and β contains an edge of ∂J. Form the map M' as follows. Cut M open along the path and adjoin a copy E_1 of the region E along the side of β which borders J. (See Fig. 5.4.)

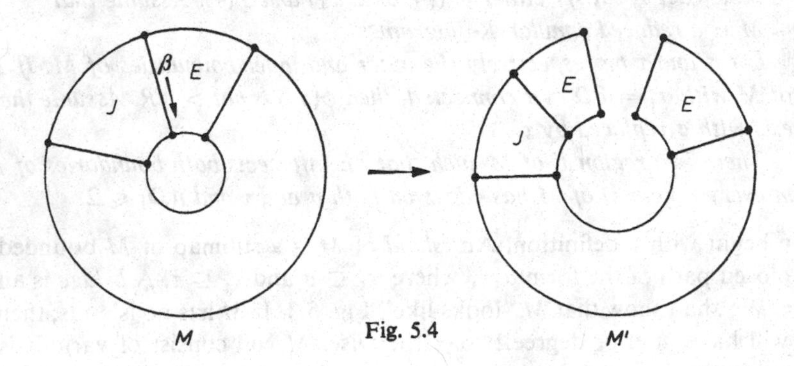

Fig. 5.4

Note that if a region D of M, $D \neq E$, has edges on both σ and τ, then the intersection of ∂D and the boundary of M' is not a consecutive part of the boundary of M'. Again, if D has edges on only one boundary of M, then $i(D)$ is still at least four in M'. By Theorem 4.3,

$$\Sigma^*_{M'}[4 - i(D)] \geqslant 6. \tag{5.4}$$

By the above remarks, only E_1 and E can make a positive contribution to this sum. Since $i(E_1)$ is at least one, there are only two possibilities. Either $i(E_1) = i(E) = 1$, or $i(E_1) = 2$, forcing $i(E) = 0$. We shall use Greendlinger's Lemma (Theorem 4.5) to show that the last possibility yields a contradiction. For, since M' contains more than one region, and only E_1 and E make positive contributions to the sum (5.4), if $i(E_1) = 2$, M' does not contain two regions both of interior degree less than or equal to one. This contradicts Greendlinger's Lemma. (In the $C'(\frac{1}{4})$ and $T(4)$ case, one uses Theorem 4.6 at this point.)

Hence, in M', $i(E_1) = 1$, and $i(E)$ is either 1 or 0. Thus in M, the region E has exactly one boundary edge in common with J. Further, if there is a region K on the other side of E, then E has exactly one boundary edge in common with K. We can now apply the same argument to J and K. Thus, working outward from E, we can prove that all regions in the same island as E have interior degree at most two. This process of working outward from E covers all of M if M does not contain any islands, so we suppose that M does contain islands. Form the map M_1 from M by deleting the island in which E occurs, and identifying its end vertices. The theorem holds for M_1 by induction, and thus the theorem holds for M.

We are left with justifying our special assumption. Suppose that some region E of M contains a simple path β from σ to τ in its boundary, and that E lies on both sides of β. In this situation, form the simply connected map M' by cutting M open along β. (Do not add an extra region.) If M' contains more than one region, the inequality (5.3) holds. Since E is the only region which can make a positive contribution to this sum, the inequality is impossible. Thus M has only one region. □

There are now two equally interesting but independent directions to pursue. The next three sections are devoted to a more detailed examination of the geometry of (q, p) maps, the solution of the word and conjugacy problems for free F and finite R satisfying the non-metric conditions $C(p)$ and $T(q)$, and applications to knot groups.

The second possibility is to proceed to examine the algebraic applications of small cancellation theory. These applications use the theory over free products, free products with amalgamation, and HNN extensions. The reader interested in algebraic applications may turn to Section 9.

6. The Word Problem

In this section we shall investigate further properties of simply connected $[p, q]$ maps and the solvability of the word problem under the non-metric hypotheses $C(p)$ and $T(q)$. The results obtained are due to Lyndon (1966). Our main result will be an "area theorem." Combinatorially, it is reasonable to define the "area" of a map M as either the total number, V_M, of vertices of M, or the total number, F_M, of regions of M. If the reader draws several $[p, q]$ maps he will find that they "grow toward the boundary," that is, an increase in the size of the map is reflected in the boundary. We shall show that the area of a simply connected $[p, q]$ map is bounded by a function of the boundary alone. This fact quickly yields a solution of the word problem.

Lemma 6.1. *If M is a $[p, q]$ map such that each component of M is either simply-connected or annular, then*

$$E_M^{\bullet} \leqslant \frac{q}{p}\sum_M^{\bullet}[p - d(v)], \quad \textit{and} \tag{6.1}$$

$$V_M^{\bullet} \leqslant \frac{q}{p}\sum_M^{\bullet}[p - d(v)]. \tag{6.2}$$

□ We can rewrite formula (3.1) as

$$E_M^{\bullet} = \frac{q}{p}\sum{}^{\bullet}[p - d(v)] + \frac{q}{p}\sum{}^{\circ}[p - d(v)] + \sum[q - d(D)] - q(Q - h). \tag{6.3}$$

Since M is a $[p, q]$ map and $Q \geqslant h$, the first term is the only one which can be positive. Hence,

$$E_M^{\bullet} \leqslant \frac{q}{p}\sum_M^{\bullet}[p - d(v)].$$

Let M_1 be the submap of M obtained by deleting all the isolated vertices. Since $V_{M_1}^{\bullet} \leqslant E_{M_1}^{\bullet}$ by Lemma 3.2, we have $V_{M_1}^{\bullet} \leqslant q/p\sum_{M_1}^{\bullet}[p - d(v)]$.

If there are no isolated vertices the conclusion holds. If there are isolated vertices, let Q_0 be the number of isolated vertices, and let M_0 be the submap of M consisting of the isolated vertices. Then

$$\frac{q}{p}\sum_{M_0}^{\bullet}[p - d(v)] = qQ_0 > Q_0 = V_{M_0}.$$

Since $V_M^{\bullet} = V_{M_1}^{\bullet} + V_{M_0}$, the conclusion follows. □

Definition. Let M be an arbitrary map. The *boundary layer* of M consists of all boundary vertices of M, all edges of M incident with boundary vertices, and all boundary regions of M.

If M is a $[p, q]$ map, we introduce the notation

$$\sigma(M) = \sum_M^{\bullet}[p - d(v)].$$

Theorem 6.2. (The Area Theorem) *Let M be a simply connected* $[p, q]$ *map. Then*

$$V_M \leqslant \frac{q}{p^2}\sigma(M)^2.$$

Dually, if M is a simply connected (q, p) map, then

$$F_M \leqslant \frac{q}{p^2}(\sum_M[p - i(D)])^2.$$

□ We prove first that if M is a $[p, q]$ map which contains an interior vertex, and if M_1 is obtained from M by removing the boundary layer of M, then

$$\sigma(M) - \sigma(M_1) \geqslant 2p.$$

We first modify M to M' by removing, one at a time, boundary vertices of degree one and isolated vertices. If there are any boundary vertices of degree one, let v be one such. Let M''' be obtained from M by removing v and the edge e incident to v. The vertex v contributes $(p - 1)$ to $\sigma(M)$. Since $p > 2$, $(p - 1) > 1$. Let v_2 be the other endpoint of e. In M''', $d(v_2)$ is decreased by one so $\sigma(M) - \sigma(M''') = [(p - 1) - 1] > 0$ and $\sigma(M) \geqslant \sigma(M''')$. Continue removing boundary vertices of degree one, one at a time, until there are no boundary vertices of degree one remaining. Let M'' be the final result of this process. Then $\sigma(M) \geqslant \sigma(M'')$. The effect of this removal process is to remove any components of M which are trees, and any spines which are attached to M.

Let M' be obtained from M'' by deleting any isolated vertices. If there are Q_0 isolated vertices they contribute $Q_0 p$ to $\sigma(M'')$. Hence $\sigma(M'') \geqslant \sigma(M')$.

We can now show that $\sigma(M') - \sigma(M_1') \geqslant 2p$. So we assume that M contains no isolated vertices or boundary vertices of degree one, and drop the prime notation.

(1) Let $n = \sum^{\bullet}_M [p - d(v)]$.

(2) Let $n_1 = \sum^{\bullet}_{M_1} [p - d_1(v)]$ where d_1 is the degree function for M_1.

Let ξ be the set of edges with an endpoint on ∂M.

(3) Let ε_1 be the number of edges with exactly one endpoint on ∂M.

(4) Let ε_2 be the number of edges with two endpoints on ∂M.

(5) Let $s = \sum^{\bullet}_M d(v)$. Then

(6) $s = \varepsilon_1 + 2\varepsilon_2$.

(7) Let $f(v) = d(v) - d_1(v)$. Then $f(v)$ is the number of edges incident at v which are in ξ.

If $v \in \partial M_1$, then v is an interior vertex of M and $d(v) \geqslant p$. Hence, using (7),

(8) $n_1 = \sum^{\bullet}_{M_1} [p - d_1(v)] \leqslant \sum^{\bullet}_{M_1} [d(v) - d_1(v)] = \sum^{\bullet}_{M_1} f(v)$.

(9) $\sum_{M_1} f(v) = \varepsilon_1$.

(10) We can write $n = \sum^{\bullet}_M p - \sum^{\bullet}_M d(v) = pV^{\bullet}_M - s$.

Hence, using (6), (8), and (9),

(11) $n - n_1 = pV^{\bullet}_M - s - n_1 \geqslant pV^{\bullet}_M - s - \varepsilon_1 = pV^{\bullet}_M - 2s + 2\varepsilon_2$.

Since M has no isolated vertices or boundary vertices of degree one,

(12) $V^{\bullet}_M \leqslant \varepsilon_2$. Therefore

(13) $n - n_1 \geqslant pV^{\bullet}_M - 2s + 2V^{\bullet}_M = 2[(p/2 + 1)V^{\bullet}_M - s]$, or, using (5) and rewriting,

(14) $n - n_1 \geqslant 2\sum^{\bullet}_M [(p/2 + 1) - d(v)] = 2\sum^{\bullet}_M [(p/q) + 2 - d(v)]$.

By Corollary 3.3, the last sum is greater than or equal to $2p$. Hence,

(15) $\sigma(M) - \sigma(M_1) \geqslant 2p$.

We now want to prove that $V_M \leqslant (q/p^2)\, \sigma(M)^2 = (q/p^2)n^2$.

Note that this holds by Lemma 6.1 if the boundary layer of M contains all of M. For, in that case, $V_M = V^{\bullet}_M \leqslant (q/p)\sum^{\bullet}_M [p - d(v)]$ and $\sum^{\bullet}_M [p - d(v)] \geqslant p$ for all non-empty $[p, q]$ maps. The proof is by induction on the number of vertices in M. The above remark allows us to assume that M contains an interior vertex.

Now V_M is equal to V_{M_1} plus the number of vertices in the boundary layer, that is, $V_M = V_{M_1} + V_M^{\bullet}$. By the induction hypothesis and Lemma 6.1,

$$V_M \leqslant \frac{q}{p^2}(n - 2p)^2 + \frac{q}{p}n = \frac{q}{p^2}[n^2 - 4pn + 4p^2 + np] < \frac{q}{p^2}[n^2 - 2np + 4p^2].$$

We note that if $n < 2p$ the boundary layer must contain all the vertices of M, for otherwise we would obtain a contradiction from (15). So we can assume $n \geqslant 2p$, $2pn \geqslant 4p^2$. Hence,

$$V_M \leqslant \frac{q}{p^2}n^2 = \frac{q}{p^2}\sigma(M)^2.$$

The second part of the theorem follows immediately from the first part by considering dual maps. □

We can now quickly obtain the solvability of the word problem for finite R satisfying one of our hypotheses.

Theorem 6.3. *Let F be a finitely generated free group, let R be a finite symmetrized set of elements of F, and let N be the normal closure of R. If R satisfies $C(6)$, or $C(4)$ and $T(4)$, or $C(3)$ and $T(6)$, then the word problem for F/N is solvable.*

□ Let w be any word of F. If $w \in N$, let M be diagram of a minimal R-sequence for w. Then M is a (q, p) map where (q, p) is (3, 6), (4, 4), or (6, 3) depending on the case.

By the Area Theorem, the number of regions in M is less than or equal to $(q/p^2)(\sum_M^{\bullet}[p - i(D)])^2$. A region of M can have $[p - i(D)] > 0$ only if ∂D contains a boundary edge. Since there can be no more than $|w|$ regions of M which contain a boundary edge, we have

$$0 \leqslant \textstyle\sum_M^{\bullet}[p - i(D)] \leqslant p|w|.$$

If $d = (q/p^2)(p^2|w|^2) = q|w|^2$, then the number of regions of M is less than or equal to d. Set $L = \max_{r_i \in R}|r_i|$.

By Lemma 1.2, $w = (u_1' r_1' u_1'^{-1}) \cdots (u_m' r_m' u_m'^{-1})$ where $m \leqslant d$, each $|u_i'| \leqslant d(L + |w|)$, and each $r_i' \in R$. Since any such product *is* in N, we have $w \in N$ if and only if $w = (u_1' r_1' u_1'^{-1}) \cdots (u_m' r_m' u_m'^{-1})$ where $m \leqslant d$ and $|u_i| \leqslant d(L + |w|)$.

There are only a finite number of such products, which can all be tested to see whether or not any of them is equal to w. Thus the word problem is solvable. □

7. The Conjugacy Problem

In this section we develop the necessary results to deal with annular (q, p) maps and the conjugacy problem. To illustrate the falsity of the area theorem for annular maps, take, for example, a rectangle divided into mn squares and bend the rectangle around to form an annulus, identifying along the side with n subdivisions We have a tessellation of an annulus by a [4, 4] map. The *length* of the boundary is $2m$ and the number of regions is mn, with n arbitrary. Thus there is no function of the number of boundary vertices which bounds the number of regions of an annular (q, p) map.

However, if the reader tries to construct annular (q, p) maps with several layers, he will see that the number of regions in a layer must remain constant or increase toward one or both of the boundaries. Let M be an annular (q, p) map and consider the sequence of maps $M = M_0, M_1, \ldots, M_k$ where M_{i+1} is obtained from M_i by removing the boundary layer of M_i. We shall prove that there is a function of the boundary of M which bounds the number of boundary regions in any of the M_i. It is this property which will allow us to solve the conjugacy problem. Results in this section are taken from Schupp (1968).

Lemma 7.1. *Let M be a $[p, q]$ map such that each component of M is either simply-connected or annular. Then*

$$\sum\nolimits_M^{\cdot}\left[\frac{p}{q} + 2 - d(v)\right] \geqslant 0. \tag{7.1}$$

□ The proof is like the proof of Corollary 3.3 from the basic formulas of Theorem 3.1. □

We connect dual maps and the operation of removing the boundary layer.

Lemma 7.2. *If M is a map, M^* a dual of M, and M_1 is obtained by removing the boundary layer of M, then M_1 is a dual of M^*.*

□ Since M^* is a dual of M, the interior vertices v of M are in one-to-one correspondence with the regions D^* of M^*, with $v \in D^*$. Furthermore, each interior edge e of M crosses exactly one edge e^* of M^*. It is thus necessary only to show that the edges of M_1 are exactly the edges of M which cross interior edges of M^*. This is equivalent to saying that an edge of M^* is a boundary edge of M^* if and only if it crosses an edge of M which is incident to a boundary vertex of M.

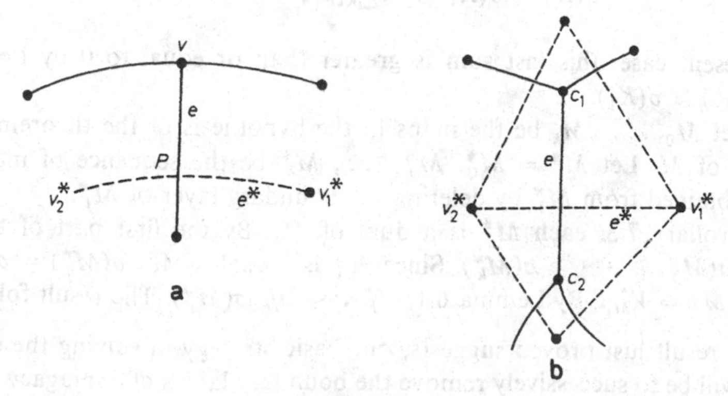

Fig. 7.1

Let e be an interior edge of M incident with a boundary vertex v in ∂M (Fig. 7.1(a)). The edge e is crossed by an edge e^* of M^*, say at a point P (not a vertex). The arc composed of e from P to v runs to $-M$ and hence $-M^*$. Since e cannot be crossed by any other edges of M^*, e^* is a boundary edge of M^*.

Let e be an edge of M both of whose endpoints, c_1 and c_2, are interior vertices of M. (Fig. 7.1(b)). The edge e is crossed by edge e^* of M^*. The sequence of edges other than e which connect the vertices arising from regions D of M which have either c_1 or c_2 on their boundaries must completely enclose e^*, so e^* is an interior edge of M^*. □

Corollary 7.3. *If M is a map, M^* a dual of M, and M_1 and M_1^* are obtained by removing the boundary layers of M and M^* respectively, then M_1^* is a dual of M_1.* □

If M is a map, let $\sigma'(M) = \sum_M^{\bullet}[p - i(D)]$, and let $\beta(M)$ denote the number of regions in the boundary layer of M.

Theorem 7.4. (Layer Theorem) *Let M be a (q, p) map such that each component of M is either simply-connected or annular. Consider the sequence of maps $M = M_0$, $M_1, \ldots, M_k$ where M_i is obtained by deleting the boundary layer of M_{i-1}, and the process is continued until the boundary layer of M_k is equal to M_k. Then*

$$\text{(7.2)} \qquad \frac{q}{p}\sigma'(M) \geqslant \max\{\beta(M_i) | i = 0, \ldots, k\}.$$

□ Let K be any $[p, q]$ map such that each component of K is either annular or simply-connected. We claim that if K_1 is the submap of K obtained by removing the boundary layer of K then

$$\text{(7.3)} \qquad \sigma(K) \geqslant \sigma(K_1).$$

To see this look back at the proof of the Area Theorem. From the beginning of the proof through step (14), the assumption that the map was simply-connected was not used. What we actually proved was that for an arbitrary $[p, q]$ map having an interior vertex,

$$\sigma(K) - \sigma(K_1) \geqslant 2\sum_K^{\bullet}[p/q + 2 - d(v)].$$

In the present case, this last sum is greater than or equal to 0 by Lemma 7.1. Hence, $\sigma(K) \geqslant \sigma(K_1)$.

Now let $M_0, \ldots, M_k$ be the maps in the hypothesis of the theorem. Let M^* be a dual of M. Let $M^* = M_0^*, M_1^*, \ldots, M_k^*$ be the sequence of maps where M_{i+1}^* is obtained from M_i^* by deleting the boundary layer of M_i^*.

By Corollary 7.3, each M_i^* is a dual of M_i. By the first part of the proof, $\sigma(M^*) \geqslant \sigma(M_1^*) \geqslant \cdots \geqslant \sigma(M_k^*)$. Since M_i^* is a dual of M_i, $\sigma(M_i^*) = \sigma'(M_i)$. By duality, $\beta(M_i) = V_{M_i^*}^{\bullet}$. By Lemma 6.1, $V_{M_i^*}^{\bullet} \leqslant (q/p)\sigma(M_i^*)$. The result follows. □

As the result just proved suggests, our basic strategy in solving the conjugacy problem will be to successively remove the boundary layers of conjugacy diagrams, obtaining new conjugacy diagrams. We shall use Theorem 7.4 to bound the length of the labels on the boundaries of the new conjugacy diagrams. We must be a bit careful, however, since, in general, if we remove the boundary layer of an annular map, the resulting map need not be annular.

Let A be an annular map, and let B be the boundary layer of A. The map $C = A - B$ may have several components. However, C has at most one annular component. We call a simply connected component of C a *gap* of B. Thus, a gap is a connected, simply connected submap of A which does not contain any boundary regions but which is entirely surrounded by boundary regions.

Let $K_1, \ldots, K_n$ be the gaps of B, and let $B' = B \cup K_1 \cup \cdots \cup K_n$. Then $H = A - B'$ is the annular component of $A - B$ if there is an annular component. Otherwise, H is empty. We say that H is *obtained from A by removing the boundary layer and its gaps.* We next formulate a condition which will ensure that H is annular.

Let A be an annular map, and let σ and τ be respectively the outer and inner boundaries of M. A pair (D_1, D_2) of regions (not necessarily distinct) of A is called a *boundary linking pair* if $\sigma \cap \partial D_1 \neq \emptyset$, $\partial D_1 \cap \partial D_2 \neq \emptyset$, and $\partial D_2 \cap \tau \neq \emptyset$.

Lemma 7.5. *Let A be an annular map having at least one region. Let H be obtained from A by removing the boundary layer and its gaps. If there are no boundary linking pairs in A, then H is an annular map having at least one region.*

☐ Let σ and τ be respectively the outer and inner boundaries of A. If D is a region of A with $\partial D \cap \sigma \neq \emptyset$, we call D an *outer* boundary region. If D is a region of A with $\partial D \cap \tau \neq \emptyset$, we call D an *inner* boundary region. We similarly distinguish inner and outer boundary vertices and edges. No region D of A is both an inner and an outer boundary region, for then (D, D) would be a boundary linking pair.

If K is a gap, it is surrounded by boundary regions D_i. Since there are no boundary linking pairs in A, successive D_i must both be inner or both be outer. Thus K is surrounded entirely by inner boundary regions or is surrounded entirely by outer boundary regions. We call K an *inner gap* or an *outer gap*, according to the case.

Let C_1 be the union of all the inner boundary vertices, the edges incident to inner boundary vertices, the inner boundary regions, and the inner gaps. Define C_2 similarly, replacing "inner" by "outer." Then $B' = C_1 \cup C_2$. Let τ_1 be the boundary of the unbounded component of $-C_1$, and let σ_1 be the boundary of the bounded component of $-C_2$. Then τ_1 is interior to σ_1, and σ_1 and τ_1 are the boundaries of H. Any vertex in either σ_1 or τ_1 is on the boundary of a boundary region of A. Since there are no boundary linking pairs in A, $\sigma_1 \cap \tau_1 = \emptyset$. Since H contains all of A which lies between σ_1 and τ_1, H must contain at least one region. ☐

We can now proceed with the solution of the conjugacy problem.

Theorem 7.6. *Let F be a finitely generated free group. Let R be a finite non-empty symmetrized subset of F, and let N be the normal subgroup of F generated by R. If R satisfies one of the conditions C(6), C(4) and T(4), or C(3) and T(6), then the conjugacy problem is solvable for $G = F/N$.*

☐ Before proceeding with the proof of the theorem, we state the algorithm which we shall obtain. Assume the hypothesis of the theorem. Let w_1 and w_2 be elements of F. Let L be the length of the longest relator in R. (We assume that $L \geqslant 2$.) Define $w_1 \sim w_2$ if and only if there exists b in F such that $|b| \leqslant L/2$ and $bw_1b^{-1}w_2^{-1} \in N$. Since F is finitely generated and the word problem for G is solvable, the relation $w_1 \sim w_2$ is decidable.

Let u and z be cyclically reduced. Let $d = q(|u| + |z|)$ (where q is 3, 4, or 6 depending upon the case). Let $W = \{w: w \in F, |w| \leqslant dL\}$. Define the relation $u \sim\sim z$ to hold if there exist $w_1, \ldots, w_k$ in W such that

$$u \sim w_1 \sim \cdots \sim w_k \sim z.$$

Since F is finitely generated, W is a finite set. It is easy to see that all w such that $w \in W$ and $u \sim\sim w$ can be effectively enumerated. We prove that u and z are conjugate in G if and only if $u \sim\sim z$. The sufficiency part of this claim is trivial.

Suppose that $w \in W$ and that w^* is a cyclic permutation of w. Certainly then, $w \sim\sim w^*$, for we can successively conjugate by generators of F until w is transformed into w^*. We shall often use this property of the relation $\sim\sim$ without comment.

Let u and z be cyclically reduced words which represent conjugate elements of G. If u and z are conjugate in the free group F, then z is a cyclic permutation of u, and $u \sim\sim z$ by the remark above. Now assume that u and z are not conjugate in F, and let M be the conjugacy diagram for u and z. Then M is an annular (q, p) map with $(q, p) = (3, 6), (4, 4)$, or $(6, 3)$, according to the case. Since M has boundary labels u and z^{-1}, there can be no more than $(|u| + |z|)$ regions having edges on ∂M. If D is a region of M with $\partial D \cap \partial M$ not containing an edge then $i(D) \geqslant p$. Certainly then,

$$\frac{q}{p} \sum\nolimits_M^{\bullet} [p - i(D)] \leqslant q(|u| + |z|).$$

Let $d = q(|u| + |z|)$.

Now consider the sequence of maps $M = H_0, H_1, \ldots, H_k$ where H_i is obtained from H_{i-1} by removing the boundary layer and gaps of H_{i-1}, and H_k is the first map obtained by this process which has a boundary linking pair. Let $M = M_0, M_1, \ldots, M_k$ be the sequence of maps where M_i is obtained from M_{i-1} by removing the boundary layer of M_{i-1}. By construction, the number, $\beta(M_i)$, of boundary regions of each M_i is greater than or equal to the number, $\beta(H_i)$, of boundary regions of the corresponding H_i. By Theorem 7.4, each $\beta(M_i) \leqslant d$. Thus $\beta(H_i) \leqslant d$, $0 \leqslant i \leqslant k$.

If $i > 0$, then every boundary edge of H_i is an edge on the boundary of a region in the boundary of H_{i-1}. Thus, if w is the label on any boundary cycle of any of the H_i, $i = 0, \ldots, k$, then $|w| \leqslant dL$ and $w \in W$.

Let σ_i be the outer boundary of H_i, and let τ_i be the inner boundary of H_i. Let S_i, $i = 0, \ldots, k-1$, be the submap of M consisting of σ_i, σ_{i+1}, and all of M between σ_i and σ_{i+1}. Let T_i, $i = 0, \ldots, k-1$, be the submap of M consisting of τ_i, τ_{i+1}, and all of M between τ_i and τ_{i+1}. (See Fig. 7.2.)

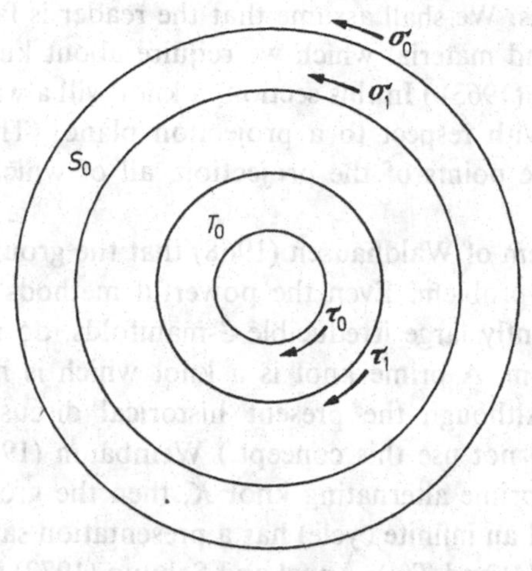

Fig. 7.2

Because of the nature of the maps S_i, $i \geqslant 0$, every boundary region D of S_i intersects both the inner and outer boundaries of S_i. There is a simple path γ_i from σ_i to σ_{i+1} with $|\phi(\gamma)| \leqslant L/2$. Cutting S_i open along the path γ_i, we have $s_i \sim s_{i+1}$ where s_i and s_{i+1}^{-1} are respectively labels of outer and inner boundary cycles of S. Now s_{i+1} will be a label of an outer boundary cycle of S_{i+1}. Similarly, we have $t_i \sim t_{i+1}$ where t_i^{-1} and t_{i+1} are respectively labels of inner and outer boundary cycles of T_i.

There is a boundary linking pair (D_1, D_2) in H_k. Then there are vertices $v_0 \in \sigma_k \cap \partial D_1$, $v_1 \in \partial D_1 \cap \partial D_2$, and $v_2 \in \partial D_2 \cap \tau_k$. Thus there is a simple path $\beta_1 \subseteq \partial D_1$ from v_0 to v_1 with label b_1 where $|b_1| \leqslant L/2$, and a simple path β_2 from v_1 to v_2 with label b_2 where $|b_2| \leqslant L/2$. Let $\beta = \beta_1\beta_2$. Let s be the label of the outer boundary cycle of H_k starting at v_0, and let t^{-1} be the label of the inner boundary cycle of M beginning at v_2. Cutting H open along the path β, we have $sb_1b_2t^{-1}b_2^{-1}b_1^{-1} \in N$. Thus

$$s \sim b_1^{-1}\, s\, b_1 \sim b_2 t b_2 \sim t.$$

Since s_0 and t_0 are cyclic permutations of u and z respectively, we have

$$u \sim\sim s_0 \sim s_1 \sim \cdots \sim s_k \sim\sim s \sim\sim t \sim\sim t_k \sim \cdots \sim t_0 \sim\sim z.$$

Since all the s_i and t_i are in W, we have established that $u \sim\sim z$. □

8. Applications to Knot Groups

One of the interesting developments in small cancellation theory is the application of the theory to solve the word and conjugacy problems for the groups of tame alternating knots. We shall assume that the reader is familiar with the small amount of background material which we require about knots and their groups. (See Crowell and Fox (1963).) In this section, a knot will always mean a tame knot in general position with respect to a projection plane. (That is, there are only finitely many multiple points of the projection, all of which are isolated double points.)

It is a deep theorem of Waldhausen (1968) that the group G of any tame knot has a solvable word problem. Even the powerful methods of Waldhausen's approach, using sufficiently large irreducible 3-manifolds, do not shed any light on the conjugacy problem. A prime knot is a knot which is not the "join" of two non-trivial knots. (Although the present historical discussion mentions prime knots, our proof will not use this concept.) Weinbaum (1971) discovered that if G is the group of a prime alternating knot K, then the group $H = G * \langle x \rangle$ (the free product of G and an infinite cycle) has a presentation satisfying the small cancellation condition $C(4)$ and $T(4)$. Appel and Schupp (1972) subsequently extended the solution of the conjugacy problem to the group of any alternating knot.

In discussing knot projections, we shall assume that all projections lie within some fixed plane, and we work within that plane. If Π is a knot projection, then the complement of Π in the plane of projection consists of some finite number of domains (connected components) which we shall always number as $X_0, X_1, \ldots, X_{m+1}$ where X_0 is the unbounded domain. We shall need to work with projections having certain properties. First of all, given any projection of a knot K, we can effectively obtain a projection Π of K which satisfies condition (1) below:

(1) Any vertex of Π is on the boundary of four distinct domains.

Suppose that we are given a projection Π^* containing a vertex v such that only three distinct domains meet at v. There is a simple closed curve δ in the plane of Π^* which intersects Π^* only in v, and which separates Π^* into two parts. By turning over that part of the projection which is interior to δ, the crossing v may be eliminated. (See Figure 8.1. This "untwisting operation" is operation $\Omega.4$ of Reidemeister (1932b) and is discussed fully there.)

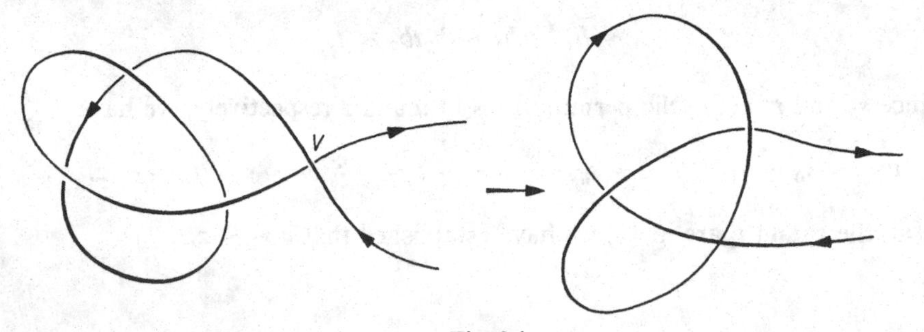

Fig. 8.1

If Π^* is alternating, then so is the new projection. The untwisting operation is effective and reduces the number of crossings in the projection. We can thus obtain a projection satisfying (1) in a finite number of steps. From now on, we shall assume that projections satisfy (1).

Given a knot projection Π one can read off a presentation for the group G of the knot. The most commonly used presentation is the Wirtinger presentation. In order to use small cancellation theory, however, it is necessary to use the *Dehn presentation* for G, which is obtained as follows. Let F be the free group on generators $X_0, \ldots, X_{m+1}$. (We intentionally use the same notation for the generators of F and the domains of the complement of Π. The generator X_j corresponds to a path which starts at a distant basepoint above the plane E of Π, pierces E through the domain X_j, passes below E, and returns to the basepoint through the domain X_0.)

Each vertex v_i of Π determines a defining relator r_i as follows. There are exactly four domains meeting at the vertex v_i. Let these domains be, in clockwise order, X_a, X_b, X_c, X_d, where X_a meets X_b along the overcrossing coming into v_i. Put $r_i = X_a X_b^{-1} X_c X_d^{-1}$.

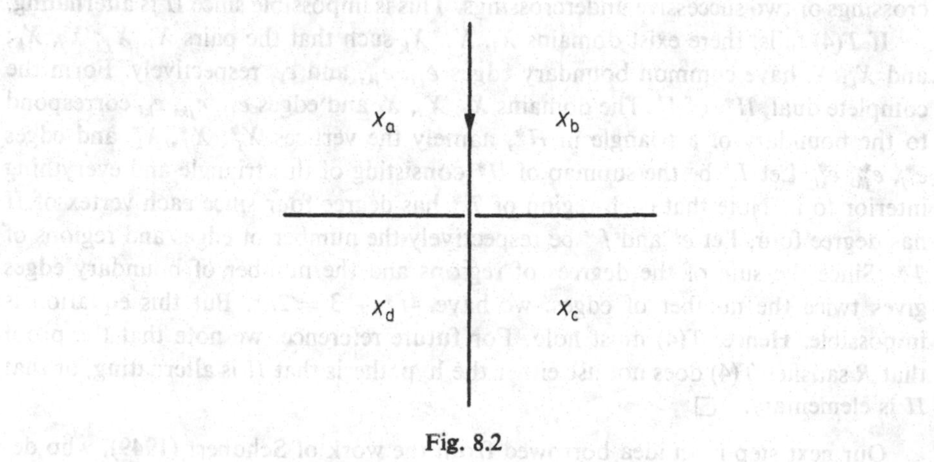

Fig. 8.2

The group of the knot is the group $G = \langle X_0, \ldots, X_{m+1}; r_1, \ldots, r_m, X_0 \rangle$.

The presence of the defining relator X_0 makes it unsuitable to work directly with the group G. In fact, we shall work with the group H obtained by deleting the relator X_0 from the presentation for G.

Lemma 8.1. *The group $H = \langle X_0, \ldots, X_{m+1}; r_1, \ldots, r_m \rangle$ is the free product of G and an infinite cyclic group.*

□ Let η be the endomorphism of F defined by $\eta(X_0) = 1$, and $\eta(X_j) = X_j$ for $1 \leqslant j \leqslant m+1$. Then $G \simeq \langle X_1, \ldots, X_{m+1}; \eta(r_1), \ldots, \eta(r_m) \rangle$. Let α be the automorphism of F defined by $\alpha(X_0) = X_0$, and $\alpha(X_j) = X_j X_0$ for $1 \leqslant j \leqslant m+1$. From the form of the defining relators, it is easy to check that $\alpha(r_i) = \eta(r_i)$ for $1 \leqslant i \leqslant m$.

Since α is an automorphism of F, $H \simeq \langle X_0, \ldots, X_{m+1}; \alpha(r_1), \ldots, \alpha(r_m) \rangle$. By the above remark, $G \simeq \langle X_1, \ldots, X_{m+1}; \alpha(r_1), \ldots, \alpha(r_m) \rangle$. □

From the theory of free products, it follows that the word or conjugacy problem for G is solvable if and only if the corresponding problem for H is solvable.

A knot projection Π is called *elementary* if it satisfies both condition (1) and condition (2) below:

(2) Any two domains have at most one boundary edge in common.

If K is a prime knot, then any projection of K which has a minimal number of crossings is elementary. Note, however, that being elementary is simply a property of projections. We turn to Weinbaum's basic discovery.

Theorem 8.2. *Let Π be an alternating elementary projection. Then the presentation of the group H satisfies $C(4)$ and $T(4)$.*

□ We mean, of course, that if R is the symmetrized subset generated by the relators $r_1, \ldots, r_m$, then R satisfies $C(4)$ and $T(4)$. If $C(4)$ fails, there is a piece $X_j X_k^{-1}$ or $X_j^{-1} X_k$ arising from distinct elements r, s in R. The corresponding domains X_j, X_k have exactly one boundary edge e in common. The relators r and s must thus arise from the vertices on the endpoints of this edge. But then, from the way the defining relators are read from Π, there must be two successive over-crossings or two successive undercrossings. This is impossible since Π is alternating.

If $T(4)$ fails, there exist domains X_i, X_j, X_k such that the pairs X_i, X_j; X_j, X_k; and X_k, X_i have common boundary edges e_{ij}, e_{jk}, and e_{ki} respectively. Form the complete dual, Π^*, of Π. The domains X_i, X_j, X_k and edges e_{ij}, e_{jk}, e_{ki} correspond to the boundary of a triangle in Π^*, namely the vertices X_i^*, X_j^*, X_k^* and edges e_{ij}^*, e_{jk}^*, e_{ki}^*. Let T^* be the submap of Π^* consisting of this triangle and everything interior to it. Note that each region of T^* has degree four since each vertex of Π has degree four. Let e^* and f^* be respectively the number of edges and regions of T^*. Since the sum of the degrees of regions and the number of boundary edges gives twice the number of edges, we have $4f^* + 3 = 2e^*$. But this equation is impossible. Hence, $T(4)$ must hold. For future reference, we note that the proof that R satisfies $T(4)$ does not use either the hypothesis that Π is alternating, or that Π is elementary. □

Our next step is an idea borrowed from the work of Schubert (1949), who described a method for decomposing knots into prime parts. Fortunately, we shall need to work only with properties of projections. A projection Π will be called *standard* if it satisfies condition (1) and condition (3) below:

(3) There is a fixed domain X_1 such that no pair of distinct domains have more than one boundary edge in common except X_1 and X_0 (the unbounded domain).

In a standard projection, only the domains X_0 and X_1 violate condition (2) in the definition of an elementary projection.

Lemma 8.3. *Every knot K has a standard projection. If K is an alternating knot, then K has an alternating standard projection.*

□ Let Π be a projection of K. Fix a domain X_1 having a boundary edge in common with X_0. Call a pair (X_a, X_b) of domains, where $a < b$, a *bad pair* if (X_a, X_b) is not the pair (X_0, X_1) and X_a and X_b have more than one boundary edge in common. A *bad vertex* is a vertex lying on the boundaries of both domains in a bad pair. If Π is not standard, pick a bad pair (X_a, X_b). Since X_a and X_b have more than one boundary edge in common, there is a simple closed curve Γ lying entirely in X_a and X_b such that there are vertices of Π on both sides of Γ. Further, Γ can be chosen so that X_1 is not in the interior of Γ.

The following is an intuitive description of what is essentially Schubert's argument. Let S be a sphere which encloses that part of the knot whose projection is enclosed by Γ. The knot pierces S exactly twice. Regard the point at which the knot enters S as being fixed. Shrink S and its interior to a "suitably small" size. By stretching the knot, pull S along the knot until an "unused" portion of an edge e on the common boundary of X_0 and X_1 is reached. (See Fig. 8.3.)

In view of this discussion, we define a *transfer* operation on the projection Π as follows. Let Π' be the part of Π interior to Γ, and let Π'' be the part of Π exterior to Γ. Obtain Π^* from Π as follows.

(i) Delete Π' and replace it by a simple arc interior to Γ which joins the ends of Π''.

(ii) Delete a small arc δ from the edge e. Replace δ by a curve Σ geometrically similar to δ, but small enough so that Σ does not intersect Π except at the joining points. Perform this replacement so that the orientation in going around the knot is preserved.

(iii) Suppose that the projection Π is alternating. Since the projection enters Γ once and leaves Γ once, each vertex interior to Γ is traversed twice, once as an undercrossing and once as an overcrossing. Hence, if Π is alternating, both Π' and Π'' are also alternating. When Σ is moved to the edge e, there may be a pair of consecutive undercrossings (or overcrossings) consisting of the last vertex traversed in Σ and the next vertex traversed. If this happens, turn Σ over. This reverses overcrossings and undercrossings in Σ, and the projection Π^* is now alternating.

Now a transfer operation reduces the number of bad vertices. Hence, after a finite number of transfers, we obtain a standard projection. The knot type is not changed since we have performed allowable deformations on the knot. □

Let Π be a projection which is standard but not elementary. Remove a single point (not a crossing) from each edge e_i common to the boundaries of X_0 and X_1. This separates Π into parts J_i which, if their loose ends are joined, are elementary projections. We call the J_i the *elementary parts* of Π.

If the reader calculates the Dehn presentation for the group H from an alternating standard projection which is not elementary, that of Figure 8.3 for example, he will see that $C(4)$ fails. The presentation is "nice enough" however, in the following sense. Let F be a free group, and let R be a finite symmetrized subset of F, all elements of which have length four. We say that *R satisfies $C(4)$ and $T(4)$ for minimal sequences* if the following two conditions hold.

(1) If two elements r_1, r_2 of R cancel two or more letters, then either $r_2 = r_1^{-1}$ or r_1r_2 is already an element of R.

(2) If r_1, r_2, r_3, are elements of R and there is cancellation in all the products r_1r_2, r_2r_3, and r_3r_1, then $r_1r_2r_3$ is a product of two or fewer elements of R.

Lemma 8.4. *Let F be a free group, and let $R \subseteq F$ be a finite symmetrized set of elements of length four. Let N be the normal closure of R in F. If R satisfies $C(4)$ and $T(4)$ for minimal sequences, then $G = F/R$ has solvable word and conjugacy problems.*

□ In constructing diagrams to study the word and conjugacy problems, we needed to consider only diagrams of minimal sequences. The hypotheses on R ensure that if M is the diagram of a minimal sequence, then M is a (4, 4) map.

Thus the proofs of Theorems 6.3 and 7.6 solve the word and conjugacy problems for G. □

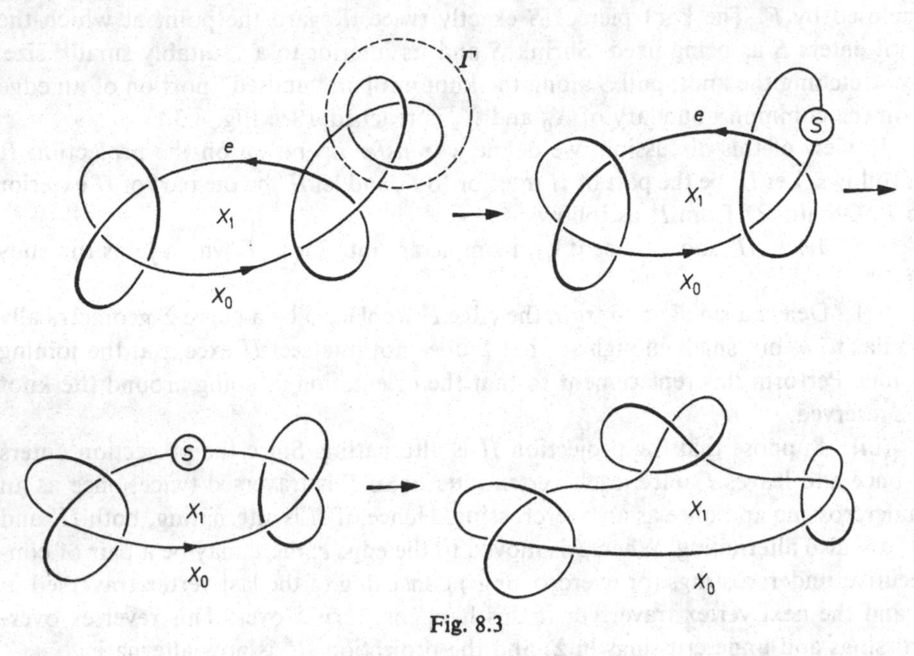

Fig. 8.3

Let K be an alternating knot, and let Π be an alternating standard projection of K. We assume that Π is not elementary, for otherwise Theorem 8.2 is directly applicable. The rest of this section is devoted to proving that the group H can be presented so that $C(4)$ and $T(4)$ are satisfied for minimal sequences.

Choose an orientation of K. In each elementary part J_i consider the first and last crossings traversed. Since Π is alternating, we may assume without loss of generality that the first crossing is an overcrossing. This crossing is called the overcrossing of J_i. Similarly, the last crossing encountered is called the undercrossing of J_i. We define domains U_i, V_i, P_i, Q_i as follows. U_i and V_i are the domains other than X_0 and X_1 at the undercrossing of J_i, with U_i adjacent to X_0 and V_i adjacent to X_1. The domains P_i and Q_i are the domains other than X_0 and X_1 on the overcrossing of J, with P_i adjacent to X_0 and Q_i adjacent to X_1. (See Fig. 8.4.) It is possible that $P_i = U_i$ or that $Q_i = V_i$, but both of these equations cannot hold, for then P_i and Q_i would be adjacent along two distinct boundary edges, contradicting J_i being elementary.

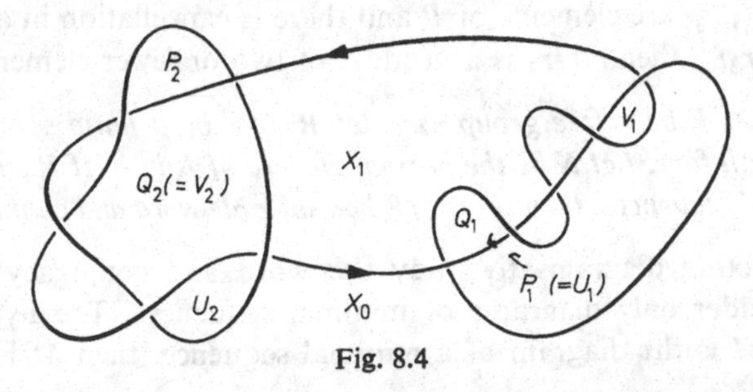

Fig. 8.4

Note that in the Dehn presentation, the symmetrized set generated by the relator corresponding to the overcrossing on J_i is generated by $X_1X_0^{-1}P_iQ_i^{-1}$, while the symmetrized set corresponding to the undercrossing is generated by $X_0^{-1}X_1V_i^{-1}U_i$. The presentation we consider is the Dehn presentation augmented by the symmetrized set generated by the relators $P_iQ_i^{-1}Q_jP_j$ (which we call *derived overcrossing relators*) and $V_i^{-1}U_iU_j^{-1}V_j$ (which we call *derived undercrossing rerators*) where i, j range over all pairs of distinct indices of elementary parts of K. Any of these additional relators is called a *derived relator*.

If two relators from distinct elementary parts have any generators in common, these generators must be among X_0 and X_1. The following observation is crucial to our proof. In any derived overcrossing relator, in reading two successive occurrences of generators from the same elementary part, the exponents are positive followed by negative. In reading successive occurrences of generators from different elementary parts, the exponents are negative then positive. For derived undercrossing relators the exponent patterns are opposite.

We recall the following two facts from the proof of Theorem 8.2. The relators arising from each elementary part satisfy $C(4)$ among themselves. The symmetrized collection of non-derived relators satisfies $T(4)$.

To verify $C(4)$ for minimal sequences, we must show that if r_1 and r_2 are relators such that r_1r_2 has length four or less, then r_1r_2 is either trivial or is another relator. Theorem 8.2 shows that two non-inverse relators from the same elementary part cannot cancel more than one letter. If neither r_1 nor r_2 is a derived relator and they come from different elementary parts, then the cancelled generators must be X_0 and X_1. Since the relators from each elementary part satisfy $C(4)$, r_1 is a relator arising from the undercrossing or the overcrossing of its elementary part. Since two letters of r_2 are cancelled, r_2 is a relator arising from the corresponding crossing of its elementary part, and r_1r_2 is a derived relator. We may now assume that at least one of the relators, without loss generality r_1, is a derived relator. The argument is symmetric for overcrossings and undercrossings, so we shall assume that r_1 is a derived overcrossing relator.

Case 1. Suppose that r_1 is $P_iQ_i^{-1}Q_jP_j^{-1}$. If r_2 is a relator corresponding to a crossing on J_j, then it must be $P_jQ_j^{-1}X_1X_0^{-1}$ by $C(4)$ on relators from elementary parts. Hence, $r_1r_2 = P_iQ_i^{-1}X_1X_0^{-1}$. If r_2 is a derived overcrossing relator, it must be $P_jQ_j^{-1}Q_kP_k^{-1}$, and r_1r_2 is $P_iQ_i^{-1}Q_kP_k^{-1}$. Now suppose that r_2 is a derived undercrossing relator. Then r_2 must begin with $U_jV_j^{-1}$ (where $U_j = P_j$ and $V_j = Q_j$). But this is impossible.

Case 2. Suppose that r_1 is $Q_i^{-1}Q_jP_j^{-1}P_i$. Clearly, r_2 must be a derived relator. If it is a derived overcrossing relator, it must be r_1^{-1}. If r_2 is a derived undercrossing relator, it must begin with $U_i^{-1}U_j$ (where $U_i = P_i$ and $U_j = P_j$). But such an exponent pattern is impossible for an undercrossing relator.

To verify $T(4)$ for minimal sequences, we may assume that r_1 is a derived relator, and that precisely one letter from each factor is cancelled in the products r_1r_2, r_2r_3, and r_3r_1.

Case 1. Suppose that r_1 is $P_iQ_i^{-1}Q_jP_j^{-1}$. If r_2 is a derived overcrossing relator, then the product r_1r_2 is not minimal. Thus this possibility can be discarded.

Subcase (i). Suppose that $P_j = U_j$ and $r_2 = U_j U_k^{-1} V_k V_j^{-1}$. Then r_3 has the form $V_j A^{-1} B P_i^{-1}$. Since $P_j = U_j$, we must have $V_j \neq Q_j$. Hence, r_3 is the derived undercrossing relator $V_j V_i^{-1} U_i U_j^{-1}$. But then $P_i = U_j$, contradicting the uniqueness of the elementary part in which P_i lies.

Subcase (ii). The situation where r_3 is a derived relator is the same as that where r_1 and r_2 are derived relators. (Consider the sequence r_3, r_1, r_2.) We may thus suppose that neither r_2 nor r_3 are derived relators. Then r_2 comes from the elementary part J_j and r_3 comes from the elementary part J_i. The generator cancelled in the product $r_2 r_3$ must be either X_0 or X_1. Now r_2 begins with P_j, which is adjacent to X_0. The domain P_j cannot also be adjacent to X_1, for then P_j, X_0, and X_1 are three domains, each pair of which has a boundary edge in common. The proof of Theorem 8.2 showed that this is impossible. We conclude that the last letter in r_2 is X_0^{-1}. By $C(4)$ on relators from the elementary part J_j, $r_2 = P_j Q_j^{-1} X_1 X_0^{-1}$. Hence, $r_3 = X_0 A^{-1} B P^{-1}$. By $C(4)$ on J_i, $r_3 = X_0 X_1^{-1} Q_i P_i^{-1}$. Thus $r_2 r_3$ is not minimal.

Case 2. Suppose that r_1 is $Q_i^{-1} Q_j P_j^{-1} P_i$. As before, if r_2 is a derived overcrossing relator, then the product $r_1 r_2$ is not minimal.

Subcase (i). If r_2 is a derived undercrossing relator, then $P_i = U_i$ and $r_2 = U_i^{-1} V_i V_k^{-1} U_k$. Then r_3 has the form $U_k^{-1} A B^{-1} Q_i$. Since $Q_i \neq V_i$, $r_3 = P_i^{-1} P_l Q_l^{-1} Q_i$, yielding the contradiction $P_i = U_k$ where $i \neq k$.

Subcase (ii). Suppose that neither r_2 nor r_3 is derived. Then both come from the elementary part J_i. Since r_1, r_2, r_3 all have cancellation in their products, so do r_1', r_2, r_3 where $r_1' = Q_i^{-1} X_1 X_0^{-1} P_i$. This violates $T(4)$ on the relators from J_i unless one of r_2 or r_3 is $(r_1')^{-1}$. This assumption yields a contradiction, since it implies that either r_2 or r_3 is not cyclically reduced. If, for example, $r_2 = (r_1')^{-1}$, then r_3 must begin with Q_i^{-1} and end with Q_i for cancellation to occur in $r_2 r_3$ and $r_3 r_1$. This completes the proof that the augmented presentation for H satisfies $C(4)$ and $T(4)$ for minimal sequences. We have thus established.

Theorem 8.5. *If K is an alternating knot, then the group G of K has solvable conjugacy problem.* □

9. The Theory over Free Products

In this section we develop small cancellation theory over free products. Our basic approach follows Lyndon (1966). If F is the free product of non-trivial groups X_j, then each non-identity element w of F has a unique representation in *normal form* as $w = y_1 \cdots y_n$ where each of the *letters* y_i is a non-trivial element of one of the factors X_j, and where no adjacent y_i, y_{i+1} come from the same factor. The integer n is the *length* of w, written $|w|$.

If $u = y_1 \cdots y_k c_1 \cdots c_t$ and $v = c_t^{-1} \cdots c_1^{-1} d_1 \cdots d_s$ in normal form where $d_1 \neq y_k^{-1}$, we say that the letters $c_1, \ldots, c_t$ are *cancelled* in forming the product

uv. If y_k and d_1 are in different factors of F, then $w = uv$ has normal form $y_1 \cdots y_k d_1 \cdots d_s$. It is possible that d_1 and y_k are in the same factor of F with $d_1 \neq y_k^{-1}$. Let $a = y_k d_1$. Then $w = uv$ has normal form $y_1 \cdots y_{k-1} a d_2 \cdots d_t$. We say that y_k and d_1 have been *consolidated* to give the single letter a in the normal form of uv.

We say that a word w has *reduced form uv* if the normal form for w is obtained by concatenating the normal forms for u and v. Thus there is neither cancellation nor consolidation between u and v. We say that w has *semi-reduced form uv* if $w = uv$ and there is no cancellation between u and v. Consolidation is expressly allowed.

Recall that element w of F with normal form $w = y_1 \cdots y_n$ is said to be *cyclically reduced* if $|w| \leqslant 1$ or y_1 and y_n are in different factors of F. We say that w is *weakly cyclically reduced* if $|w| \leqslant 1$ or $y_n \neq y_1^{-1}$. Thus there is no cancellation between y_n and y_1 although consolidation is allowed.

A subset R of F is called *symmetrized* if every $r \in R$ is weakly cyclically reduced and every weakly cyclically reduced conjugate of r and r^{-1} is also in R.

A word b is called a *piece* if R contains distinct elements r_1 and r_2 with semi-reduced forms $r_1 = bc_1$ and $r_2 = bc_2$. Note that the last letter of b does not have to be a letter of the normal form of r_1 or r_2.

Condition $C'(\lambda)$: If $r \in R$, $r = bc$ in semi-reduced form where b is a piece, then $|b| < \lambda|r|$. To avoid pathological cases, we further require that if $r \in R$ then $|r| > 1/\lambda$.

There are obvious analogues for free products of the conditions $C(p)$ and $T(q)$, but we shall not formulate them explicitly. We shall work only with the metric hypothesis $C'(\lambda)$ for $\lambda \leqslant 1/6$. As an illustration of the hypothesis, and the importance of the theory over free products, note that the $C'(\frac{1}{6})$ hypothesis applies to "most" Fuchsian groups

$$G = \langle a_1, b_1, \ldots, a_g, b_g, x_1, \ldots, x_n, f_1, \ldots, f_k; x_1^{m_1} = 1, \ldots, x_n^{m_n} = 1,$$
$$f_1 \cdots f_k x_1 \cdots x_n \textstyle\prod_{i=1}^{g} [a_i, b_i] = 1\rangle.$$

Regard G as a quotient group of the free product $F = \langle a_1, \ldots, b_g, x_1, \ldots, x_m, f_1, \ldots, f_k; x_1^{m_1}, \ldots, x_n^{m_n}\rangle$ by the normal closure of $f_1 \cdots f_k x_1 \cdots x_m \prod_{i=1}^{g} [a_i, b_i]$.

Since in the definition of a piece the r_i need be only weakly cyclically reduced and the factorizations $r_i = bc_i$ are semi-reduced, the $C'(\lambda)$ hypothesis is stronger than it appears. Suppose that $b = x_1 \cdots x_n$ in normal form and that

$$r_1 = (x_1 \cdots x_n)(y_1 \cdots y_t)$$

and $r_2 = (x_1 \cdots x_n)(z_1 \cdots z_s)$ are semi-reduced factorizations demonstrating that b is a piece. Suppose that y_1 is in the same factor as x_n. If $z_1 = y_1$ then $x_1 \cdots (x_n y_1)$ is certainly a piece. However, if $z_1 \neq y_1$ then $(x_1 \cdots (x_n y_1))(y_1^{-1} z_1 \cdots z_s)$ is a semi-reduced factorization of r_2 and $x_1 \cdots (x_n y_1)$ is a piece. If y_t is in the same factor of F as x_1, then $r_1' = ((y_t x_1) \cdots x_n)(y_1 \cdots y_{t-1})$ and $r_2' = ((y_t x_1) \cdots x_n)(z_1 \cdots z_s y_t^{-1})$ are semi-reduced factorizations of elements of R and r_1 is cyclically reduced. From these considerations we have

Lemma 9.1. *Let R satisfy $C'(\lambda)$ and suppose an $r \in R$ has a semi-reduced factorization $r = b_1 \cdots b_j c$ where $b_1, \ldots, b_j$ are pieces. If c' is the maximal subword of c consisting of the letters of c which appear consecutively in the normal form of a cyclically reduced conjugate r' of r, then $|c'| > (1 - j\lambda)|r'|$.* □

This lemma will allow us to make exactly the same length deductions in the free product situation as we made in the free group case.

We now turn to the construction of diagrams over free products. Let $F = *X_i$ be the free product of groups X_i. Let R be a symmetrized subset of F. With each sequence $p_1, \ldots, p_n$ of conjugates of elements of R we shall associate a diagram $M(p_1, \ldots, p_n)$ which will be a connected, simply-connected, oriented planar map with a distinguished vertex $O \in \partial M$. M will be labelled by a function ϕ into F satisfying the following conditions:

(1) There is a boundary cycle $s_1 \ldots s_t$ of M beginning at O such that $\phi(s_1) \ldots \phi(s_t)$ is a semi-reduced form of $w = p_1 \ldots p_n$.

(2) If D is any region of M and $e_1, \ldots, e_j$ are the edges in a boundary cycle δ of D, then $\phi(e_1) \cdots \phi(e_j)$ is in semi-reduced form and is a weakly cyclically reduced conjugate of one of the p_i.

If p is a conjugate of an element of R, we can write $p = uru^{-1}$ where $r \in R$, and $u = 1$, or u has a normal form $u = z_1 \cdots z_k$, where r is weakly cyclically reduced with normal form $r = x_1 \cdots x_m$, and where z_k is not in the same factor of F as either x_1 or x_m. Then $z_1 \cdots z_k x_1 \cdots x_m z_k^{-1} \cdots z_1^{-1}$ is the normal form of p_i.

We first describe the initial construction of the diagram M for a single p_i. Vertices are divided into two types, *primary* and *secondary*. The label on every edge of M will belong to a factor X_i of F, with the labels on successive edges meeting at primary vertices belonging to different factors X_j, while the labels on the edges at a secondary vertex all belong to the same factor of F. We call two successive edges e_i, e_i', each with label from the same factor, a *segment*, and call the individual edges *half-segments*.

For a single $p = z_1 \cdots z_k x_1 \cdots x_m z_k^{-1} \cdots z_1^{-1}$ in normal form the initial diagram is as follows. If x_1 and x_m are in different factors of F, the initial diagram for p is a loop at a vertex v joined to the base point O by a path. The path Ov consists of $2k$ edges $e_1, e_1', \ldots, e_k, e_k'$ where each $\phi(e_i e_i') = z_i$. The loop at v consists of $2m$ edges $d_1, d_1', \ldots, d_m, d_m'$ with $\phi(d_i d_i') = x_i$. If x_1 and x_n lie in the same factor of F, take Ov to end with an additional edge e, and the loop at v to consist of edges $b, d_2, \ldots, d_{m-1}, d_{m-1}, c$ with $\phi(d_i d_i) = x_i$ for $2 \leqslant i \leqslant m - 1$. The three edges e, b, c which meet at the secondary vertex v are labelled to satisfy the necessary (and compatible) conditions $\phi(eb) = x_1$, $\phi(ce^{-1}) = x_m$, and $\phi(cb) = x_m x_1$. Note that the label on an individual edge may be 1, but if e and e' are the two edges in a segment, the product $\phi(e)\phi(e') \neq 1$. The vertex O is considered a primary vertex.

Example. Let $F = \langle a, b; a^6 \rangle * \langle c; c^5 \rangle$. Possible initial diagrams for $b^2a^2c^3b^{-2}$ and $b^2a^2c^3ab^{-2}$ are illustrated below. Primary vertices are marked with on asterisk. (See Fig. 9.1)

Note that among the half-segments with a common secondary vertex v, there is an arbitrary choice of label on one edge. This arbitrary choice is used in adjusting labels later.

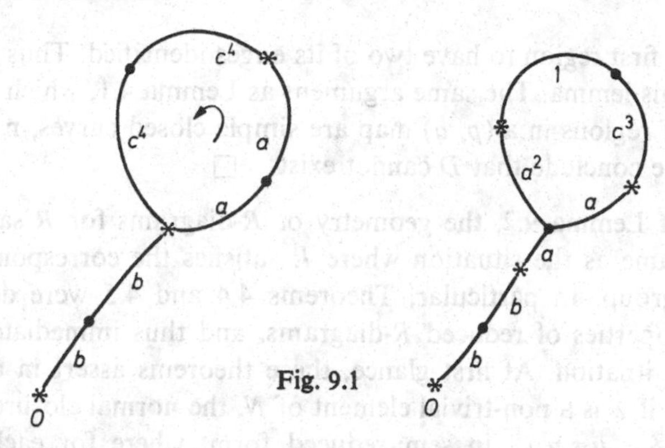

Fig. 9.1

The initial diagram for the sequence $p_1, \ldots, p_n$ consists of the initial diagrams for each p_i arranged, in order, around the base point O. The initial diagram has the desired properties except possibly condition (1).

In making identifications, we shall always identify primary vertices with primary vertices and secondary vertices with secondary vertices, preserving this distinction. The construction proceeds as follows. There may be successive segments e, e' and f, f' in ∂M where e' and f are separated by a primary vertex v, but the labels $\phi(ee')$ and $\phi(ff')$ are in the same factor of F. If so, change the label on the edge f to $\phi(e')^{-1}$, readjusting the labels on the other edges at the secondary vertex separating f and f'. Identify the edges e' and f, which now have inverse labels. Either $\phi(e) \neq \phi(f)^{-1}$, in which case one goes on to consider other edges; or $\phi(e) = \phi(f')^{-1}$, in which case e and f' can be identified, or, if ef' forms a closed loop α with $\phi(\alpha) = 1$, the loop α together with its interior can be deleted from the diagram M.

A finite number of interations of the above process yields a diagram satisfying (1) and (2). When the process is completed we can, as usual, delete vertices of degree two, combining edges and labels.

Lemma 9.2. *Let F be a free product, and let R be a symmetrized subset of F which satisfies $C'(1/p)$ for $p \geqslant 6$. Then the following statements hold*:

(1) *If M is a reduced R-diagram, then the label on an interior edge is a piece. Thus $d(D) > p$ for all regions D of M such that $\partial D \cap \partial M$ does not contain an edge.*

(2) *The diagram of a minimal R-sequence is reduced.*

□ The proof of statement (1) is exactly the same as in Lemma 2.2. Statement (2) however, does require a slight amount of argument. In a free group, no non-trivial element is conjugate to its own inverse. Thus in constructing diagrams over free groups it is impossible for two edges of a single region to be identified in such a way that the diagram becomes not reduced. We must, however, consider this possibility over free products.

It follows, exactly as in Lemma 2.1, that in the diagram M of a minimal R-sequence, there cannot be two distinct regions which make the diagram not reduced. If, in the construction of M, two edges of the same region are ever identified, let D be the first region to have two of its edges identified.

There must be a loop η interior to the rest of ∂D. Now η cannot have a vertex of degree one, since this would contradict the fact that the label on ∂D is in normal form. Hence, η bounds a simply connected submap K of M. Now K is reduced since D is the first region to have two of its edges identified. Thus K satisfies statement (1) of this lemma. The same argument as Lemma 4.1, which showed that the boundaries of regions in a (p, q) map are simple closed curves, now yields a contradiction. We conclude that D cannot exist. □

In view of Lemma 9.2, the geometry of R-diagrams for R satisfying $C'(\frac{1}{6})$ is exactly the same as the situation where R satisfies the corresponding hypothesis over a free group. In particular, Theorems 4.4 and 4.5 were derived from the geometric properties of reduced R-diagrams, and thus immediately apply to the free product situation. At first glance, these theorems assert in the free product situation that if w is a non-trivial element of N, the normal closure of R in F, then $w = u_1 s_1 u_2 s_2 \cdots u_j s_j u_{j+1}$ in semi-reduced form, where for each s_i there is an $r_i \in R$ with $r_i = s_i t_i$ in semi-reduced form, and the number j of the s and their lengths, $|s_i|$, satisfy one of the conclusions of the theorems. Using Lemma 9.1, however, we can conclude that $w = u'_1 s'_1 u'_2 s'_2 \cdots u'_j s'_j u'_{j+1}$ in reduced form, where, for each s_i there is a cyclically reduced $r_i \in R$ with $r_i = s_i t_i$ in reduced form, and the number j of the s_i and the lengths of the s_i satisfy one of the conclusions of Theorem 4.5. We have thus established

Theorem 9.3. *Let F be a free product. Let R be a symmetrized subset of F which satisfies $C'(\lambda)$ for $\lambda \leqslant 1/6$. Let N be the normal closure of R in F. If w is a non-trivial element of N, then w has a reduced factorization*

$$w = usv$$

in reduced form, where there is a cyclically reduced $r \in R$ with $r = st$ in reduced form and $|s| > (1 - 3\lambda)|r|$.

Indeed, for some cyclically reduced conjugate w^* of w,

$$w^* = u_1 s_1 u_2 s_2 \cdots u_j s_j u_{j+1}$$

in reduced form, where, for each s_i there is a cyclically reduced $r_i \in R$ with $r_i = s_i t_i$ in reduced form, and the number j of the s_i and their lengths satisfy one of the conclusions of Greendlinger's Lemma. □

In particular, N does not contain any elements of length one. We single out this important property of small cancellation quotients.

Corollary 9.4. *Let $F = * X_i$ be a free product, and let R be a symmetrized subset of F which satisfies $C'(\frac{1}{6})$. Let N be the normal closure of R in F. Then the natural map $\gamma: F \to F/N$ embeds each factor X_i of F.* □

Our discussion so far is independent of any finiteness or effectiveness assumptions on either R or F. The conclusion that a non-trivial element of N contains more than half of an element of R allows one to use Dehn's algorithm to solve the word problem in many cases where F is a free product and R is infinite. The hypotheses in the next theorem allow us to effectively use Dehn's algorithm to attempt to shorten any word w. In the free product situation, we are led to a word w which represents 1 in F, or to a non-trivial element of F which cannot be shortened.

Theorem 9.5. *Let $F = X_1 * \cdots * X_n$ be a finitely generated free product with solvable word problem. Let R be a symmetrized subset of F which satisfies $C'(\frac{1}{6})$. Assume that there is an algorithm which, when given a word $c \in F$, decides if there is a cyclically reduced $r \in R$ where $|r| < 2|c|$ and $r = cd$ in reduced form, and which produces the r if it exists. (The cancellation condition implies that r is unique if it exists.)*

Let N be the normal closure of R in F. Then $G = F/N$ has solvable word problem. □

If s is a word of F, by the notation $s > kR$ we mean that there is an $r \in R$ with $r = st$ in reduced form and $|s| > k|r|$. We call a word w *R-reduced* if it is not the case that $w = bsc$ in reduced form and $s > \frac{1}{2}R$. Call w *cyclically R-reduced* if w is cyclically reduced and all cyclically reduced conjugates of w are R-reduced.

We turn to a study of conjugacy. The argument of Lemma 9.1 showing that the diagram M of a minimal R-sequence is reduced used the fact that M is simply connected. In our investigation of conjugacy we shall therefore assume

Condition J: If $r \in R$, then r is not conjugate to r^{-1} in F.

By assuming Condition J, we do not need to worry about identifications of edges of a single region making conjugacy diagrams not reduced. Our analysis of the structure of conjugacy diagrams is then exactly the same as for F a free group.

Theorem 9.6. *Let F be a free product, let R be a symmetrized subset of F, let N be the normal closure of R in F, and let $G = F/N$. Assume that R satisfies $C'(\frac{1}{6})$ and condition J.*

Let u and z be non-trivial cyclically R-reduced words which are conjugate in G but not in F. Then there is an $h \in F$ such that $u^* = hz^*h^{-1}$ in G, where u^* and z^* are cyclically reduced conjugates of u and z respectively, and h satisfies the following condition:

(1) $h = b_1$ or $h = b_1b_2$, where each b_j, $j = 1, 2$, is a block of successive letters occurring in a cyclically reduced element r_j of R such that $|r| < 6\max(|u|, |z|)$.

Furthermore, at least one of u or z has length greater than one.

If F is finitely generated with solvable conjugacy problem, and there is an algorithm which, when given $c \in F$ decides if there is a cyclically reduced $r \in R$ such that $|r| < 6|c|$ and $r = cd$ in reduced form, and which produces the r if it exists, then G also has solvable conjugacy problem.

□ The geometry of the conjugacy diagram M for u and z is exactly the same as in the proof of Theorem 5.4. We use the notation of that theorem. In Case 1, there is a region D having more that 1/6 of its label on one of the boundaries of M and there is a simple path β from σ to τ with $\beta \subseteq \partial D$. Cut the map M open along the path β to obtain a simply connected map M'. We then have $u'b(z')^{-1}b^{-1} \in N$ where u' and z' are weakly cyclically reduced conjugates of u and z respectively, and b is the label on β.

Some slight adjustment may be necessary to obtain the situation in the conclusion of the theorem. Note that u' is cyclically reduced if and only if β does not begin at a secondary vertex. Also, $(z')^{-1}$ is cyclically reduced if and only if β does not end at a secondary vertex.

Consider, for example, the case that β begins and ends at secondary vertices. This is illustrated in Fig 9.2. Primary vertices are marked with an asterisk.

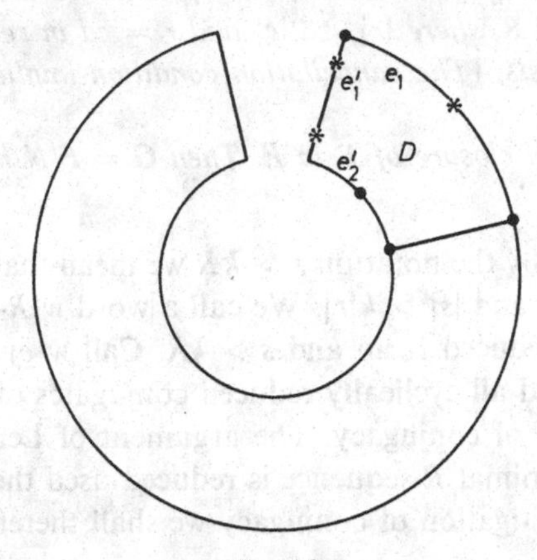

Fig. 9.2

Now the half segments e_1 and e_2 both belong to ∂D. Let $\phi(e_1) = u_1$, and let $\phi(e_2') = z_2^{-1}$. Write $u' = u_2u_1$, and $(z')^{-1} = z_2^{-1}z_1^{-1}$. We have

$$u'b(z')^{-1}b^{-1} \in N.$$

Inserting $z_2^{-1}z_2$ after $(z')^{-1}$ and conjugating by u_1 we have

$$(u_1u_2)(u_1bz_2^{-1})(z_1^{-1}z_2^{-1})(z_2b^{-1}u_1^{-1}) \in N.$$

Now $u^* = u_1u_2$ and $z^* = z_2z_1$ are cyclically reduced, and $b_1 = u_1bz_2^{-1}$ is exactly a subsequence of the letters appearing in a cyclically reduced label of ∂D. The other possibilities for β beginning and ending at a half segment are handled as easily. In case (2), where the conjugacy diagram has a thickness of two regions, we can also adjust for secondary vertices if necessary.

The fact that at least one of u or z has length greater than one follows immediately from the fact that some region has more than 1/6 of its label on one of the boundaries of M. Actually, using the proof of Theorem 4.6, one can conclude that both u and z have length greater than one. The important thing here is that taking the small cancellation quotient G does not introduce any new conjugacy between elements of the factors X_i of F. □

10. Small Cancellation Products

In this section we discuss some of the algebraic applications of small cancellation theory.

A group G will be called a *product* of groups X_i if there are isomorphisms ν_i

of the X_i into G such that G is generated by the images $v_i(X_i)$. In this case, if F is the free product $F = *X_i$, then the v_i have a common extension to an epimorphism v from F onto G, with kernel N. If N is the normal closure in F of a set R satisfying the small cancellation hypothesis $C'(1/6)$, we call G a *small cancellation product.* Note that if $F = *X_i$ and $v: F \to G$ has kernel N, the normal closure of R where R satisfies $C'(1/6)$, then, by Corollary 9.4, each v_i is an monomorphism, whence G is a small cancellation product.

We shall see that these products have several nice properties and are powerful tools in dealing with embedding problems and with adjunction of solutions to equations over groups.

Our next theorem shows that small cancellation products are well behaved with respect to torsion.

Theorem 10.1. (The Torsion Theorem) *Let F be a free group or a free product, and let R be a symmetrized subset of F satisfying $C'(\frac{1}{8})$. Let $v: F \to F/N$ be the natural map.*

If w has finite order in $G = F/N$ then either

(i) *$w = v(w')$ where w' is an element of finite order in F, or*

(ii) *some $r \in R$ has the form $r = v^n$ with w conjugate to a power of v in G.*

Theorem 10.1 says that the only elements of finite order in G are the "obvious" ones. If R contains no proper powers and F is torsion free (certainly the case if F is free), then F/N is torsion free. In general, if R contains no proper powers, then small cancellation products introduce no new finite orders.

A basic idea of the proof is a lemma due to Lipschutz (1960).

Lemma 10.2. *Let F be a free group or a free product. Let R be a symmetrized subset of F which does not contain any elements of length one. If $r \in R$, $r = x^m a$ in semi-reduced form, $m > 1$, and r is not a proper power in F, then x and x^{m-1} are pieces.*

□ Write $r = x^{m-1}(xa)$ and $r^* = x^{m-1}(ax)$. Then x^{m-1} (and thus x) is a piece by definition unless $xa = ax$. Suppose that $xa = ax$. Now, not both x and a are in the same conjugate of a factor of F since r is cyclically reduced and has length greater than one. Hence $xa = ax$ implies that a and x are powers of a common element. Therefore, r is a proper power in F. □

□ We now proceed with the proof of Theorem 10.1. Let w be any element of F. Let C be the set of all elements of F which are conjugate to w in G. Certainly, all elements of C have the same order in G as w. Let z be an element of least length in C. If $|z| = 1$, we are done. For, since the factors of F are embedded in G by the natural map, $z^n = 1$ in G if and only if $z^n = 1$ in F. Note that, by minimality of length, z is cyclically R-reduced. Suppose that $|z| > 1$, $z^n \in N$ for some $n > 1$. If $z^n \in R$, we are done.

By Theorem 9.3 we can write $z^n = z_1 u z_2$ in reduced form where some cyclically reduced $r \in R$ has reduced form $r = uv$ and $|u| > \frac{5}{8}|r|$. Now $u z_2 z_1 = (z^*)^n$ where z^* is a cyclically reduced conjugate of z.

We want to argue about $(z^*)^n$. For simplicity of notation we drop the superscript and write $z^n = ub$ in reduced form. Now u cannot be a subword of z since z is cyclically R-reduced. Hence, $u = z^m t$ in reduced form where $m \geqslant 1$ and t does not begin with a power of z. Write $z = ts$ in reduced form. (Possibly $t = 1$). We have $r = uv = (ts)^m tv$ in semi-reduced form.

First consider the possibility that $m > 1$. Then $(ts)^{m-1}$, (ts), and t are all pieces by the lemma unless ts and t are powers of a common element. If the latter holds, then z and r are powers of a common element in F, and we are done. If $(ts)^{m-1}$, (ts), and t are all pieces, then $u = (ts)^m t$ is a product of three pieces, and would have length less than $\frac{3}{8}|r|$. But $|u| > \frac{5}{8}|r|$. Hence, $m > 1$ is impossible unless z and r are powers of a common element, and r is a proper power.

Now suppose that $m = 1$. Then $r = tstv$. If $tstv = tvts$ in F, then ts and tv commute, again yielding r and z powers of a common element. If $ts \neq tv$, then t is a piece and $|t| < \frac{1}{8}|r|$. Now in G, $z = ts = (tv)^{-1}$. But since $|u| = |tst| > \frac{5}{8}|r|$, we have $|tv| \leqslant |t| + |v| < \frac{1}{8}|r| + \frac{3}{8}|r| < \frac{4}{8}|r|$. This contradicts the choice of z of minimal length and concludes the proof. □

The torsion theorem can be strengthened to the case where R satisfies $C'(\frac{1}{6})$, but the proof is slightly more complicated. In the $C'(\frac{1}{6})$ case, the torsion theorem was proved for F free by Greendlinger (1960), and for F a free product by McCool (1968).

We mention some other investigations of algebraic properties of small cancellation groups. Let F be a free group. Greendlinger (1962, 1966) showed, first for R satisfying $C'(\frac{1}{8})$ and then for $C'(\frac{1}{6})$, that if two elements of $G = F/N$ commute, then they are powers of a common element. Truffault (1973) and Seymour (1974) independently strengthed the conclusion and showed that non-trivial elements have cyclic centralizers.

Let F be either a free group of a free product, and let R satisfy either $C'(\frac{1}{6})$, or $C'(\frac{1}{4})$ and $T(4)$. Assume further that R contains no even powers and satisfies condition J. Comerford (1973) gives a geometric proof that, under these conditions, no non-trivial element of G is conjugate to its own inverse. Where F is free and R satisfies $C'(\frac{1}{8})$, this result had been obtained earlier by Gowdy (1972). Using the same hypothesis, Lipschutz (1971) had showen that if a is a non-trivial element of G and $|m| \neq |n|$, then a^m is not conjugate to a^n in G.

The theorem of Higman-Neumann-Neumann (1949) that a countable group can be embedded in a two-generator group is well-known. As an illustration of the use of small cancellation products we will prove a stronger result. The idea of using small cancellation theory to prove embedding theorems is originally due to J. L. Britton and to F. Levin (1968).

A countable group K is called *SQ-universal* if every countable group can be embedded in a quotient group of K.

Theorem 10.3. *Let P be any non-trivial free product $P = X * Y$, with the single exception of the free product of two copies of C_2, the cyclic group of order two. Then P is SQ-universal.*

□ Since we have excluded the case of $C_2 * C_2$, we can pick distinct elements x_1, x_2, neither the identity, in one group, X say, and an element $y \neq 1$ in Y. Let H be a countable group with presentation $H = \langle h_1, \ldots ; S\rangle$.

Let $F = H * X * Y$. Let

$$r_1 = h_1(x_1y)x_2y(x_1y)^2x_2y(x_1y)^3x_2y \cdots (x_1y)^{80}x_2y$$

and, in general, let

$$r_i = h_i(x_1y)^{80(i-1)+1}x_2y \cdots (x_1y)^{80i}x_2y.$$

Let R be the symmetrized set generated by the r_i. It is not difficult to see that R satisfies the cancellation condition $C'(\frac{1}{10})$. This follows from the fact that no piece can contain a subword of the form

$$(x_2y(x_1y)^kx_2y(x_1y)^{k+1}x_2y)^{\pm 1}.$$

Let N be the normal closure of R in F. Then $G = F/N$ is a small cancellation product, and thus embeds all the factors of F, in particular, H.

Now G is certainly generated by the images of X and Y, since each $r_i = 1$ in G and each h_i is thus equal to a word on x_1, x_2, and y. Indeed, since each r_i contains precisely one h_i, we can eliminate the relations R by Tietze transformations, rewriting the relations S in terms of x_1, x_2, and y. Hence, G is actually a quotient group of $X * Y$ which embeds H. □

It turns out that endomorphisms of certain small cancellation products may be severely limited. We need to recall some definitions. A group K is *hopfian* if every endomorphism of K onto K is an automorphism. Dually, K is *co-hopfian* if all one-to-one endomorphisms of K are onto. K is *complete* if all automorphisms of K are inner and K has trivial center.

Let $F = H * C_m * C_n$ where H is an arbitrary countable group, and C_m and C_n are cyclic of orders $m \geqslant 3$ and $n \geqslant 2$. Miller and Schupp (1971) investigated the endomorphisms of $G = F/N$ where N is the normal closure of a set R similar to that defined in the proof of Theorem 10.3. They proved that G is always complete and hopfian. In addition, if H has no elements of order m, or no elements or order n, then G is co-hopfian. In particular, we have

Theorem 10.4. *Any countable group H can be embedded in a two generator, complete hopfian group G. If H is finitely presentable, then so is G. If H has no elements of some finite order p, then G can be chosen to be co-hopfian.*

□ Let $H = \langle h_1, \ldots, S\rangle$ be any countable group. Let $F = H * C_5 * C_7$, and let x, y be generators of C_5 and C_7 respectively. Let

$$r_0 = xy\, xy^2(xy)^2xy^2 \cdots (xy)^{80}xy^2,$$

and, for $i = 1, 2, \ldots$, let

$$r_i = h_i^{-1}\textstyle\prod_{j=80i+1}^{80(i+2)}((xy)^jxy^2)$$

The symmetrized set R generated by the $r_i (i \geqslant 0)$ satisfies $C'(\frac{1}{10})$. Let $G = F/N$ where N is the normal closure of R in F. As in Theorem 10.3, G is a quotient group of $C_5 * C_7$ and can be finitely presented if H is finitely presented. Further, H, C_5, and C_7 are embedded in G.

We now show that G is complete and hopfian. Let $\psi: G \to G$ be a epimorphism. Now ψ is determined by its values on x and y, and $\psi(x)$ and $\psi(y)$ must generate G.

Since R contains no proper powers of elements of F and satisfies $C'(\frac{1}{10})$, any element of finite order in H must lie in a conjugate of a factor of F by Theorem 10.1. Thus $\psi(x)$ and $\psi(y)$ are in conjugates of factors of F. Note that neither $\psi(x)$ nor $\psi(y)$ can be 1, for then G would be cyclic of order dividing 5 or 7. But G embeds both C_5 and C_7. Thus $\psi(x)$ and $\psi(y)$ have orders 5 and 7 respectively.

Our plan is to show that ψ differs from the identity map by an inner automorphism. This will prove that G is hopfian and all automorphisms of G are inner. For ease of notation we retain the letter ψ even when we replace ψ by its composition with an inner automorphism of G.

To begin with, since $\psi(x)$ is in a conjugate of H or a conjugate of C_5, following ψ by an inner automorphism we may assume that either $\psi(x) \in H$ or $\psi(x) \in C_5$ and that $\psi(y) = uvu^{-1}$ where $v \in H$ or $v \in C_7$. Moreover, we can assume that, as an element of F, u has the following properties: (i) u does not contain more than $\frac{1}{2}$ of an element of R; (ii) u does not end in a letter lying in the same factor as v: and (iii) u does not begin with a letter lying in the same factor of F as $\psi(x)$.

To see that we may assume (iii), observe that otherwise we could follow ψ by an inner automorphism which would shorten u and leave $\psi(x)$ in the same factor.

First we show that $u = 1$ in F. Since $\psi(x)$ and $\psi(y)$ generate G, x and y differ in F from words on $\psi(x)$ and $\psi(y)$ by elements of N. We have some word

$$W_y = y^{-1}\psi(x)^{m_1}uv^{m_2}u^{-1}\psi(x)^{m_3} \cdots uv^{m_k}u^{-1} \in N.$$

By the assumptions on u, the word W_y is in normal form except possibly for an initial cancellation of length 1 (m_1 may be zero). Since $\psi(x) \notin C_7$, W_y cannot equal 1 in F unless $u = 1$ and $\psi(y) \in C_7$.

If W_y is not identically 1, then W_y must contain a subword which is $> \frac{7}{10}R$. Observe that each element of R has length greater than 1000. On the other hand, from the form of the elements of R, it follows that no element $r \in R$ contains subwords of form ztz^{-1} where $|t| = 1$ and $z \neq 1$. Hence we must again have $u = 1$ and $\psi(y) \in C_7$. A similar argument yields $\psi(x) \in C_5$.

We have $\psi(x) = x^\delta$ and $\psi(y) = y^\gamma$ with neither equal to 1. Now calculate

$$\psi(r_0) = (x^\delta y^\gamma)x^\delta y^{2\gamma} \cdots (x^\delta y^\gamma)^{80}x^\delta y^{2\gamma}.$$

Since ψ sends relators to relators, we have $\psi(r_0) \in N$. The above word is in normal form in F.

Thus $\psi(r_0)$ must contain more than $\frac{7}{10}$ of an element of R. This is clearly impossible unless $\delta = \pm 1 \pmod 5$ and $\gamma = \pm 1 \pmod 7$. We claim it is also impossible for ψ to send x or y to their inverses. Note that blocks of the form $[(x^{-1}y^{-1})^j x^{-1}y^{-1}]$ which are present in r_0^{-1} occur in order of decreasing j (reading from left to right.) Even if $\delta = \gamma = -1$, blocks of the above form in $\psi(r_0)$ would occur in order of increasing j. Thus $\psi(x) = x$ and $\psi(y) = y$ and the original epimorphism was an inner automorphism.

To see that G has trivial center, consider $wxw^{-1}x^{-1}$ where w does not contain more that $\frac{1}{2}$ of an element of R. If this word is non-trivial and belongs to N, then it contains $\frac{7}{10}$ of an element of R, which is again impossible, so $wxw^{-1}x^{-1} = 1$ in F.

Hence $w = x^\delta$ or 1. Thus any element of the center of G is a power of x. But clearly x^δ is not in the center of G because $xyx^{-1}y^{-1} \neq 1$ in G. This concludes the proof that G is complete and hopfian.

We now turn to the proof that if H has no elements of order 5, then G is co-hopfian. (In general, if H omitted elements of order p, we would carry out the proof using the free product $H * C_p * C_q$ where q is a prime greater than p.) Let $\theta: G \to G$ be a monomorphism. Since $\theta(x)$ must have order 5, $\theta(x)$ is in a conjugate of C_5. Then, following θ by an inner automorphism, we may assume that $\theta(x) = x^\delta$. Since $\theta(y)$ must be in a conjugate of H or a conjugate of C_7, $\theta(y) = uvu^{-1}$ where $v \in H$ or $v \in V_7$. We can assume that, as an element of F, u has properties (i), (ii), (iii) exactly as before.

We have

$$\theta(r_0) = x^\delta uvu^{-1}x^\delta uv^2u^{-1} \cdots uv^2v^{-1} \in N$$

The above word is in normal form as written and so is not 1 in F. Thus $\theta(r_0)$ must contain at least 7/10 of an element of R. As before, this is impossible unless θ is the identity. □

The universal finitely presented group H of Higman (Theorem IV.7.3) properly contains a copy of every recursively presented group. No recursively presented group C in which H is embedded can be co-hopfian, since C is isomorphic to a proper subgroup of H. However, the construction of the theorem applied to Higman's group does yield a finitely presented complete hopfian group which contains a copy of every recursively presented group. In general, the construction applied to any finitely presented group with unsolvable word problem yields a finitely presented complete hopfian group with unsolvable word problem.

11. Small Cancellation Theory Over Free Products with Amalgamation and HNN Extensions

In this section we will discuss small cancellation theory over free products with amalgamation and HNN extensions. The cancellation conditions will be natural generalizations of the usual hypotheses over free groups or free products. We begin with free products with amalgamation, where our development follows Schupp (1972). We work in the following context. Let $X_1, \ldots, X_m$ be groups with proper subgroups $A_i \subseteq X_i$. Let $A = A_1$. Let $\psi_i: A \to A_i$ be isomorphisms, $i = 2, \ldots, m$. We use the notation $F = \langle *X_i: A = \psi_i(A_i)\rangle$ to denote the free product of the X_i, amalgamating the subgroups A_i under the mappings ψ_i.

In discussing normal forms for elements of F, it is usual to choose coset representatives for each A_i in X. We specifically do *not* want to choose coset representatives. Since we already are using the word "reduced" in several meanings, we will depart from the usual usage of "normal form." From now on, if w is an element of F, $w \neq 1$, a *normal form* of w is any sequence $y_1 \cdots y_n$ such that each y_i is in a factor of F, successive y_i come from different factors of F, and no y_i is in the amalgamated part unless $n = 1$. Under this definition, an element has many normal forms. However, the length, n, of every normal form of w is the same.

A word $w = y_1 \cdots y_n$ in normal form is *cyclically reduced* if $n \leqslant 1$ or if y_n and y_1 are in different factors of F. We say that w is *weakly cyclically reduced* if $n \leqslant 1$ or if the product $y_n y_1 \notin A$.

Suppose u and v are elements of F with normal forms $y = y_1 \cdots y_n$ and $v = x_1 \cdots x_m$. If $y_n x_1 \in A$, the amalgamated part, we say that there is *cancellation* between u and v in forming the product $w = uv$. If y_n and x_1 are in the same factor of F but $y_n x_1 \notin A$, we say that y_n and x_1 are *consolidated* in forming a normal form of uv. A word w is said to have semi-reduced form $u_1 \cdots u_k$ if there is no cancellation in the product $u_1 \cdots u_k$. Consolidation is expressly allowed.

A subset R of F is *symmetrized* if $r \in R$ implies r is weakly cyclically reduced and every weakly cyclically reduced conjugate of $r^{\pm 1}$ is also in R. A word b is said to be a *piece* (relative to R) if there exist distinct elements r_1, r_2 of R such that $r_1 = bc_1$ and $r_2 = bc_2$ in semi-reduced form.

For a positive real number λ we define:

Condition $C'(\lambda)$: If $r \in R$ has semi-reduced form $r = bc$ where b is a piece, then $|b| < \lambda |r|$. Further, $|r| > 1/\lambda$ for all $r \in R$.

The condition $C'(\lambda)$ is quite strong in the case of free products with amalgamation since *all* normal forms of elements of R must be used to determine pieces. A great deal thus depends on the amalgamated part.

To see what can happen, consider the following example. Let $F = (\langle x \rangle * \langle y \rangle; x^2 = y^2)$, the free product of two infinite cyclic groups, amalgamating the squares of the generators. Let n be a positive integer $n \geqslant 3$, and let R be the smallest symmetrized set containing $(xy)^n$. Since R is symmetrized, $(yx)^{-n} \in R$. Now $(xy)^n \neq (yx)^{-n}$ in F, but, letting $c = x^2 = y^2$ which is in the center of F, we have

$$(yx)^{-n} = (x^{-1}y^{-1})^n = (x^{-1}cy^{-1}c^{-1})^n = (xyc^{-2})^n = (xy)^n c^{-2n} = (xy)^{n-1}xy^{-(4n-1)}$$

Thus $(xy)^{n-1}x$ is a piece relative to R and any cancellation condition $C'(\lambda)$, $\lambda \leqslant 1/2$, fails badly.

We now turn to the construction of diagrams over free products with amalgamation. The construction is essentially the same as that for diagrams over ordinary free products.

Let $F = (*X_i; A = \psi_i(A_i))$ be the free product of the groups X_i, amalgamating the subgroups A_i. Let R be a symmetrized subset of F which satisfies $C'(\frac{1}{6})$. With each sequence $p_1, \ldots, p_n$ of conjugates of elements of R we shall associate a diagram $M(p_1, \ldots, p_n)$ which will be a connected, simply-connected, oriented planar map with a distinguished vertex $O \in \partial M$. M will be labelled by a function ϕ into F satisfying:

(1) There is a boundary cycle $s_1 \ldots s_t$ of M beginning at O such that $\phi(s_1) \ldots \phi(s_t)$ is a semi-reduced form of $w = p_1 \ldots p_n$.

(2) If D is any region of M and $e_1, \ldots, e_j$ are the edges in a boundary cycle δ of D, then $\phi(e_1) \cdots \phi(e_j)$ is in semi-reduced form and is a weakly cyclically reduced conjugate of one of the p_i.

Suppose for the moment that a diagram satisfying (1) and (2) exists. We may, as usual, suppose that M has no vertices of degree two. Then exactly as in the proof of Lemma 9.2 for diagrams over free products we have:

(i) If M is reduced diagram, then the label on an interior edge of M is a piece. Thus if R satisfies $C'(\frac{1}{6})$ and M is a reduced R-diagram, then M is a (3, 6) map.

(ii) The diagram of a minimal sequence is reduced.

We shall need these observations in our proof of

Theorem 11.1. *Let R be a symmetrized subset of F which satisfies $C'(\frac{1}{6})$. For each sequence $p_1, \ldots, p_n$ of conjugates of elements of R there exists a diagram which satisfies* (1) *and* (2).

☐ If p_i is a conjugate of an element of R, we can write $p_i = u_i r_i u_i^{-1}$ where $r_i \in R$, and $u_i = 1$, or u_i has a normal form $u_i = z_1 \cdots z_k$, where r_i is weakly cyclically reduced and has a normal form $r_i = x_1 \cdots x_m$, and where z_k is not in the same factor of F as either x_1 or x_m. Then $z_1 \cdots z_k x_1 \cdots x_m z_k^{-1} \cdots z_1^{-1}$ is a normal form of p_i under our extended definition of normal form.

Recall the initial construction of the diagram over a free product. We follow exactly the same construction of the initial diagrams for each p_i. Then the initial diagram for the sequence $p_1, \ldots, p_n$ consists of the initial diagrams for each p_i, arranged, in order, around the base point O. The initial diagram has all the desired properties except possibly condition (1). The product of the labels in the edges in M need not be reduced with cancellation.

The construction then proceeds as follows. There may be successive segments e, e' and f, f' in M' where e' and f are separated by a primary vertex v, but the labels $\phi(ee')$ and $\phi(ff')$ are in the same factor of F. If so, change the label on the edge f to $\phi(e')^{-1}$, readjusting the labels on the other edges at the secondary vertex separating f and f'. Identify the edges e' and f, which now have inverse labels.

In the case of diagrams over free products there are two possibilities. If $\phi(e) \neq \phi(f')^{-1}$, then one can go on to consider other edges. If $\phi(e) = \phi(f')^{-1}$, then e and f' can be identified, or, if ef' forms a closed loop α with $\phi(\alpha) = 1$, the loop α together with its interior can be deleted from the diagram M.

Over free products with amalgamation the possibilities are enlarged. It may be that the two successive edges e and f' in ∂M have labels x and y respectively such that $xy \in A$, the amalgamated part, although xy is not 1. If this happens, then $y = x^{-1}a$ for some $a \in A$.

Let e begin at vertex v_1 and end at vertex v_2, while f' begins at v_2 and ends at vertex v_3. There are two cases to consider. First, assume that the vertices v_1, v_2, v_3 are all distinct. Suppose that f' is not the last edge in ∂M (in the boundary cycle beginning at O). Let the edges outgoing from v_3, other than $(f')^{-1}$, be in order, $f_1, \ldots, f_j$. Let $\phi(f_i) = y_i$, $i = 1, \ldots, j$. (See Fig. 11.1)

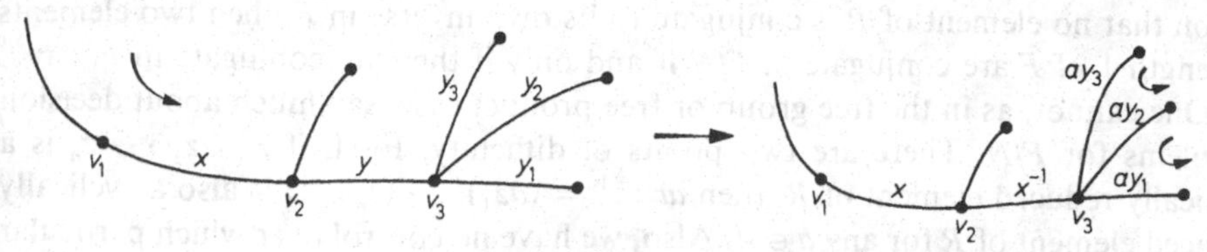

Fig. 11.1

Change the label on f' to x^{-1}. Change the label on each edge f_i to ay_i. (Since a is in the amalgamated part, ay_i is in the same factor of F as y_i.) It is immediate that this process preserves the label on ∂M (up to equality in F, of course) and property (2). The edges e and f' now have inverse labels and can be identified. (If f' is the last edge in ∂M, then e cannot be the first edge of ∂M since we are assuming that v_1 and v_3 are distinct vertices. In this situation change the label on e to y^{-1}, adjust the labels on the edges outgoing from v_1, and then identify e and f'.)

We next show that the case where the successive edges e and f' have labels x and y with $xy \in A$, but the vertices v_1, v_2, v_3 are not all distinct cannot arise. If two of the vertices coincide there is a loop β in ∂M with $|\phi(\beta)| = 1$.

There are no loops whose labels have length 1 in the initial stage of the diagram M. Consider the first time such a loop β exists. Since we are considering the first time such a loop exists, all previous identifications were made by identifying edges with distinct vertices v_1, v_2, v_3. Let K be the subdiagram of M consisting of β and its interior. By the first part of our argument, K satisfies (1) and (2) and thus properties (i) and (ii), cited before the theorem, apply to K. It then follows that the label on ∂K contains more than half of a normal form of some element in R. Hence, $|\phi(\beta)| > 1$, and we have a contradiction.

We conclude that if we are required to identify successive edges e and f' in the construction of M, then the vertices v_1, v_2, v_3 are all distinct. Hence, we eventually arrive at a diagram satisfying both (1) and (2). □

Note one contrast with the free group and free product situations. Over free groups or free products one is able to construct a diagram satisfying (1) and (2) for an arbitrary sequence of elements. Here, we used the assumption that R satisfies a small cancellation condition to rule out the possibility of some of the vertices v_1, v_2, v_3 coinciding. If the edges e and f' formed a closed loop with $v_1 = v_3$, the described adjustment of labels would not work since e itself would need its labe changed

The geometry of R-diagrams for R satisfying $C'(\frac{1}{6})$ is exactly the same as for R satisfying the corresponding hypothesis over a free group or an ordinary free product. We can thus draw the usual conclusion.

Theorem 11.2. *Let F be a free product with amalgamation, let R be a symmetrized subset of F, and let N be the normal closure of R in F with $G = F/N$. Suppose that R satisfies $C'(\lambda)$ with $\lambda \leqslant 1/6$. If w is a non-trivial element of N, then $w = usv$ in reduced form, where there is a cyclically reduced $r \in R$ with $r = st$ in reduced form and $|s| > (1 - 3\lambda)|r|$.*

In particular, the natural map $\nu: F \to F/N$ embeds each factor X_i of F. □

Our analysis of the geometry of possible conjugacy diagrams for R satisfying $C'(\frac{1}{6})$ goes through without change. In particular, if R satisfies the additional condition that no element of R is conjugate to its own inverse in F, then two elements of length 1 of F are conjugate in F/N if and only if they are conjugate in F.

One cannot, as in the free group or free product case, say much about decision problems for F/N. There are two points of difficulty. First, if $r = z_1 \cdots z_n$ is a cyclically reduced element of R, then $ara^{-1} = (az_1) \cdots (z_n a^{-1})$ is also a cyclically reduced element of R for any $a \in A$. Also, we have no control over which particular normal forms of elements are used. In considering the word problem, for example, all we know is that if w is a non-trivial element of N then some normal form of w contains more than half of a normal form of some cyclically reduced element of R. To attempt to apply Dehn's algorithm to solve the word problem we would need to be able to decide the following question. Given a string $s_1 \cdots s_t$ of elements, each in a factor of F and none in the amalgamated part A, does there exist a cyclically reduced element of R with a normal form $s_1 \cdots s_t s_{t+1} \cdots s_n$ such that $t > \frac{1}{2}n$?

Using Theorem 11.2, we can establish that "many" free products with amalgamation are *SQ*-universal.

Let A be a subgroup of the group H. Let $\{x_1, x_2\}$ be a pair of distinct elements of H, neither of which is in A. We say that $\{x_1, x_2\}$ is a *blocking pair for A in H* if the following condition is satisfied:

(1) If $a \in A$, $a \neq 1$, then $x_i^\varepsilon a x_j^\delta \notin A$, $1 \leqslant i, j \leqslant 2$, $\varepsilon = \pm 1$, $\delta = \pm 1$.

Note that (1) implies that $x_i^\varepsilon x_j^\delta \notin A$, $1 \leqslant i, j \leqslant 2$, $\varepsilon = \pm 1$, $\delta = \pm 1$, unless $x_i^\varepsilon x_j^\delta = 1$.

We shall prove

Theorem 11.3. *Let $P = \langle H * K, A = B\rangle$ be a free product amalgamating the proper subgroups A and B of H and K. If there is a blocking pair for A in H, then P is SQ-universal.*

The existence of blocking pairs is not an unreasonable condition in groups in which there is a lot of "freeness." For example, consider the following situation. Let A be a subgroup of H. Suppose there is a subgroup B of H which has a non-trivial decomposition as a free product, $B = B_1 * B_2$, and $A \subseteq B_1$. Then any pair of distinct non-identity elements of B_2 is a blocking pair for A in H.

M. Hall (1949; see I.3.7) has shown that if H is a free group and A is a finitely generated subgroup of H, then there exists a subgroup B of finite index in H which contains A as a free factor. If A is of infinite index in H it follows that B has a free product decomposition $B = A * B_2$, where B_2 is a non-trivial free group. By the remarks of the preceding paragraph, there exists a blocking pair for A in H. We thus have the following corollary.

Corollary 11.4. *Let H be a free group. Let A be a finitely generated subgroup with infinite index in H. Let K be any group containing, as a proper subgroup, an isomorphic copy, A′, of A. Then the free product with amalgamation $P = (H * K; A = A')$ is SQ-universal.* □

□ We turn to the proof of Theorem 11.3. Let $P = \langle H * K; A = B\rangle$ be a free product with amalgamation where A and B are proper subgroups of H and K respectively, and such that there exists a blocking pair, $\{x_1, x_2\}$, for A in H. The idea is to imitate the proof that ordinary free products are *SQ*-universal.

Let C be an arbitrary countable group, $C = \langle c_1, \ldots; S\rangle$, S a set of defining relators among the c_i. Let A' be an isomorphic copy of A. Let $C' = C * A'$ be the ordinary free product of C and A'. Finally, let $F = \langle C' * H * K; A' = A = B\rangle$. Let $y \in K - B$. Define

$$r_1 = c_1 x_1 y x_2 y (x_1 y)^2 x_2 y \cdots (x_1 y)^{80} x_2 y,$$

and, in general, let

$$r_i = c_i(x_1y)^{80(i-1)+1}x_2y \cdots (x_1y)^{80i}x_2y.$$

Let R be the symmetrized set generated by the r_i.

Let r and r' be two strictly cyclically reduced elements of R. By Theorem IV.2.8, r and r' are each conjugate, by elements of the amalgamated part A, to cyclic permutations of the $r_i^{\pm 1}$ listed above. Hence, we can write $r_1 = a_1z_1 \cdots a_na_1^{-1}$, and $r' = a_2z_m \cdots z_1'a_2^{-1}$, where $z_1 \cdots z_n$ and $z_m' \cdots z_1'$ are cyclic permutations of two of the $r^{\pm 1}$, and $a_1, a_2 \in A$.

Now consider how there can be cancellation in the product $r'r = a_2z_m' \cdots z_1'a_2^{-1}a_1z_1 \cdots z_na_2^{-1}$. The fact that $\{x_1, x_2\}$ is a blocking pair for A in H excludes the possibility of much cancellation unless $r' = r^{-1}$. We illustrate the situation.

Assume that "several" of the z_i' and z_i cancel each other. For z_1' and z_1 to cancel, they must be in the same factor of F. In each r_i, alternate letters, except for the single c_i, are $x_1^{\pm 1}$ or $x_2^{\pm 1}$, and then $y^{\pm 1}$. Thus, one of z_1 or z_2 must be an x. Suppose, for example, that z_1 is $y^{\pm 1}$, and that the single c_i is not among the cancelled z's.

Then $r'r = a_2^{-1}z_m' \cdots z_3'(x_j^{\varepsilon}ax_k^{\delta})z_3 \cdots z_na_1^{-1}$ where $a \in A$ is the result of previous cancellation; that is, $a = z_1'a_2^{-1}a_1z_1$. Since z_2' and z_2 cancel, we must have $x_j^{\varepsilon}ax_k^{\delta} \in A$. But since $\{x_1, x_2\}$ is a blocking pair for A, this is impossible unless $a = 1$ and $x_j^{\varepsilon}x_k^{\delta} = 1$. Hence, $z_2' = z_2^{-1}$.

Now z_3' and z_3' are y's. Thus $z_3z_3 = y^{\pm 2}$ or $z_3z_3' = 1$. *A priori*, it is possible that $1 \neq y^{\pm 2} = a^* \in A$. But then it would be impossible for z_3 and z_4 to cancel since z_4' and z_4 are x's and we could not have $x_s^{\varepsilon}a^*x_t^{\delta} \in A$. Hence, $z_3' = z_3^{-1}$. Thus either $y = y^{-1}$, or, since all the y's occurring in an element of R are of the same exponent, ± 1, all y's in r have opposite exponent to those in r'. Returning to the original cancellation in $r'r$, we have $1 = a = z_1'a_2^{-1}a_1z_1 = y^{\varepsilon}a_2^{-1}a_1y^{-\varepsilon}$. Thus $a_2^{-1}a_1 = 1$ and $a_1 = a_2$.

Continuing in the above fashion, we see that if z_j' and z_j cancel, then $z_j' = z_j^{-1}$. Indeed, in the general case suppose $z_1 \cdots z_s$ and $z_s' \cdots z_1'$ cancel, where $s \geqslant 6$. Then we can deduce that for each z_j, $1 \leqslant j \leqslant s$, $z_j' = z^{-1}$. Also, we have $a_1 = a_2$.

It is not difficult to see that if $z_1 \cdots z_s$ contains a sequence of letters of the form $[x_2y(x_1y)^kx_2y(x_1y)^{k+1}x_2y]^{\pm 1}$, then a particular permutation of one of the $r_i^{\pm 1}$ is uniquely determined, and we have $r' = r^{-1}$. It is also not difficult to see that if s is as much as one tenth of the length of either r or r', then $z_1 \cdots z_s$ contains a sequence of letters of the above form. Hence R satisfies $C'(\frac{1}{10})$.

By Theorem 11.2, the group C is embedded in $G = F/N$. Since each r_i contains exactly one c symbol we can eliminate the relators r_i by by Tietze transformations rewriting the relators S in terms of x_1, x_i and y. Thus G is actually a quotient group of $P = \langle H * K; A = B \rangle$. $\square$

We mention that Theorem 11.3 can be used to show that the four-generator, four-relator group

$$H = \langle a, b, c, d; b^{-1}ab = a^2, c^{-1}bc = b^2, d^{-1}cd = c^2, a^{-1}da = d^2 \rangle$$

used by Higman (1951) to establish the existence of a finitely generated infinite simple group, is itself *SQ*-universal. (See Schupp, 1972.)

Our discussion of small cancellation theory over HNN extensions follows Sacerdote and Schupp (1973). Let $F = \langle H, t; t^{-1}At = B, \psi \rangle$ be an HNN extension of the group H. If w is an element of F, a *normal form* of w is any sequence

$$h_0 t^{\varepsilon_1} h_1 \cdots h_n t^{\varepsilon_n} h_{n+1} = w$$

to which no t-reductions are applicable. Any two normal forms of w contain the same number of t-symbols. If u and v have normal forms $u = h_0 t^{\varepsilon_1} \cdots h_n t^{\varepsilon_n} h_{n+2}$ and $v = h'_0 t^{\delta_1} \cdots t^{\delta_m} h'_{m+1}$, we say that there is *cancellation* in forming the product uv if either $\varepsilon_n = -1$, $h_{n+1} h'_0 \in A$, and $\delta_1 = 1$, or if $\varepsilon_n = 1$, $h_{n+1} h'_0 \in B$, and $\delta_1 = -1$ We say that $w = uv$ in reduced form if there is no cancellation in forming the product uv.

A subset R of F is called *symmetrized* if $r \in R$ implies that r is cyclically reduced and all cyclically reduced conjugates of $r^{\pm 1}$ are also in R. A word b is said to be a *piece* (relative to R) if there exist distinct elements r_1, r_2 of R such that $r_1 = bc_1$ and $r_2 = bc_2$ in reduced form.

For λ a positive real number, the condition $C'(\lambda)$ is defined as follows:

Condition $C'(\lambda)$. If $r \in R$ has reduced form $r = bc$ where b is a piece then $|b| < \lambda |r|$. Also, $|r| > 1/\lambda$ for all $r \in R$.

The condition $C'(\lambda)$ is quite strong since all normal forms of elements of R must be used to determine pieces.

Let R be a symmetrized subset of F. With each sequence $p_1, \ldots, p_n$ of conjugates of elements of R we shall associate a diagram $M(p_1, \ldots, p_n)$ which will be a connected, simply connected, oriented planar map with a distinguished vertex $O \in \partial M$, the boundary of M. The edges of M will be labelled by a function ϕ into F satisfying the following two conditions:

(1) If $e_1, \ldots, e_s$ are, in order, the edges in the boundary cycle of M beginning at O, then $\phi(e_1) \cdots \phi(e_s)$ is a reduced form of $w = p_1 \cdots p_n$.

(2) If D is any region of M and $e_1, \ldots, e_j$ are the edges in a boundary cycle of D, then $\phi(e_1) \cdots \phi(e_j)$ is a reduced form of a cyclically reduced conjugate of one of the p_i.

Now if p is a cyclically reduced conjugate of an element of R we can write $p = uru^{-1}$ where u has normal form $u = h_1 t^{\varepsilon_1} \cdots h_n t^{\varepsilon_n} h_{n+1}$, $\varepsilon_i = \pm 1$, and $r \in R$ with normal form

$$r = t_{n+1}^{\varepsilon_{n+1}} h_{n+2} \cdots t_{n+m}^{\varepsilon_{n+m}} h_{n+m+1}, \; \varepsilon_j = \pm 1,$$

where some of the h_i may be 1.

The initial diagram for a single p consists of a loop at a vertex v joined to the basepoint O by a path. The path Ov consists of $2n + 1$ edges, $e_1, f_1, \ldots e_n, f_n, e_{n+1}$ where $\phi(e_i) = h_i$ and $\phi(f_i) = t^{\varepsilon_i}$. Edges labelled by H will be called *H-edges* and edges labelled by $t^{\pm 1}$ will be called *t-edges*. The loop at v consists of $2m$ edges,

$$f_{n+1}, e_{n+1}, \ldots, f_{n+m}, e_{n+m+1}, \text{ where } \phi(e_{n+j}) = h_{n+j}$$

and $\phi(f_{n+j}) = t^{\varepsilon_{n+j}}$.

The initial diagram for the sequence $p_1, \ldots p_n$ consists of the initial diagrams for each p_i arranged around the basepoint O. The initial diagram has all the usual properties except possibly condition (1); the product of the labels on the edges in ∂M need not be reduced.

Suppose that there is an arc $f_1, e_1, \ldots, e_k, f_2$ in ∂M where $\phi(f_1) = t^{-1}$, $\phi(f_2) = t$, the e_i are H-edges, and the product $a = \phi(e_1) \cdots \phi(e_k)$ is in the subgroup A. Subdivide the edge f_2 into successive edges $e'_k, \ldots, e'_1, f_3, e_{k+1}$ with labels $\phi(e'_i) = \phi(e_i)^{-1}$, $i = 1, \ldots, k$, $\phi(f_3) = t$, and $\phi(e_{k+1}) = \psi(a)$. (See Fig. 11.2.)

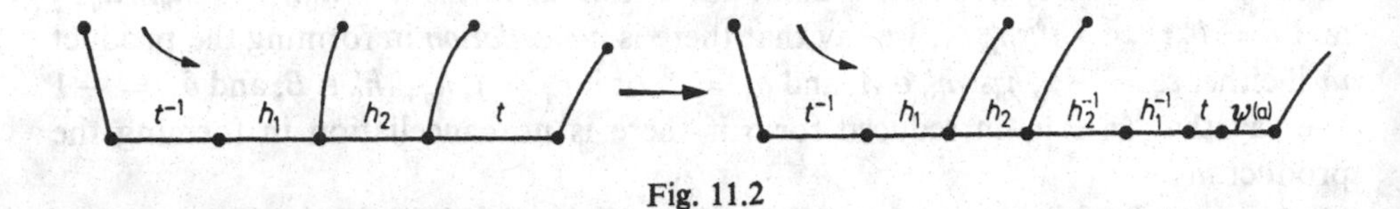

Fig. 11.2

Since the relation $t^{-1}at = \psi(a)$ holds in F, we have $t = a^{-1}t\psi(a)$. Thus the product of the labels on the edges of ∂M remains unchanged. Similarly, if the original edge f_2 is in the boundary of a region D, the product of the labels on the edges of a boundary cycle of D remains unchanged. Now successively identify the edges e'_i and e_i, $i = k, \ldots, 1$, and the edges f_1 and f_3. Note that this procedure reduces the number of t-edges in ∂M.

The procedure for an arc $f_1, e_1, \ldots, e_k, f_2$ in ∂M where $\phi(f_1) = t$, $\phi(f_2) = t^{-1}$, and the e_i are H-edges with $\phi(e_1) \cdots \phi(e_k) = b \in B$ is similar. Subdivide f_2 into edges $e'_k, \ldots, e'_1, f_3, e_{k+1}$, with labels $\phi(e'_i) = \phi(e_i)^{-1}$, $i = k, \ldots, 1$, $\phi(f_3) = t^{-1}$, and $\phi(e_{k+1}) = \psi^{-1}(b)$. Then successively identify e_i with e'_i, $i = k, \ldots, 1$, and then identify f_3 with f_1. After a finite number of applications of these procedures we arrive at a diagram satisfying both (1) and (2). Hence, we have the following.

Theorem 11.5. *Let R be a symmetrized subset of G. For each sequence $p_1, \ldots, p_n$ of conjugates of elements of R there exists a diagram which satisfies* (1) *and* (2). □

In the usual way, we deduce

Theorem 11.6. *Let $F = \langle H, t; t^{-1}At = B, \psi\rangle$ be an HNN extension of the group H. Let R be a symmetrized subset of F which satisfies $C'(\lambda)$, $\lambda \leqslant \frac{1}{6}$ and let N be the normal closure of R in F. If w is a non-trivial element of N, then $w = w_1 s w_2$ in reduced form, where there is a cyclically reduced $r \in R$ with $r = sv$ in reduced form, and $|s| > (1 - \lambda)|r|$.*

In particular, the natural map $v\colon F \to F/N$ embeds H in F/N. □

As the reader has surmised, we can now show that many HNN extensions are SQ-universal.

Theorem 11.7. *Let $H^* = \langle H, t; t^{-1}At = B, \psi\rangle$ be an HNN extension. If H has an element $z \neq 1$ such that*

$$z^{-1}Az \cap A = \{1\} = zBz^{-1} \cap B,$$

then H^* is SQ-universal.

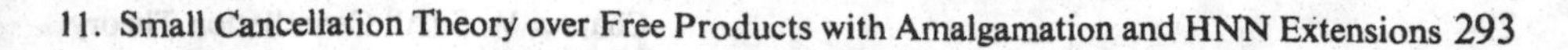

☐ Let $C = \langle c_1, \ldots ; S \rangle$ be a countable group. Let $F = \langle C * H, t; t^{-1}At = B, \psi \rangle$. Let z be an element of H satisfying the hypothesis of the theorem. Let

$$r_i = c_i z t^{80(i-1)+1} z t^{80(i-1)+2} \cdots z t^{80i}.$$

Let R be the symmetrized set generated by the r_i.

We now show that R satisfies $C'(\frac{1}{6})$. Let r and r' be elements of R. In order to study cancellation in the product rr', we may assume that r ends with t^{ε}, $\varepsilon = \pm 1$, and r' begins with $t^{-\varepsilon}$. For definiteness, assume that r ends with t. (The other case is similar.) By Collins' Lemma (Theorem IV.2.5), we have $r = b_1 s_1 b_1^{-1}$ and $r' = b_2 s_2 b_2^{-1}$ where s_1 and s_2 are cyclic permutations of the $r_i^{\pm 1}$ as written above, and b_1 and b_2 are in B. From the form of the r_i, note that an initial string of the form $t^j z^{\delta} t^m z^{\delta} t^n z^{\delta}$, $\delta = \pm 1$, uniquely determines a permutation of one of the r_i. Thus if as much as three blocks of powers of t cancel in the product rr', we have $s_2 = s_1^{-1}$. Three consecutive blocks of powers of t have length much less than 1/6 of the length of any element of R in which it occurs. Therefore, if cancellation of 1/6 of the length of r or r' occurs in the product rr', we have $s_2 = s^{-1}$.

In order to show that $r' = r^{-1}$, it remains only to show that $b_1 = b_2$. Cancelling the first t-symbols, we have $tb_1^{-1}b_2t^{-1} = \psi^{-1}(b_1^{-1}b_2)$. Cancelling the first block of t-symbols we arrive at

$$rr' = \cdots tzb^*z^{-1}t^{-1} \cdots$$

where $b^* = \psi^{-j}(b_3) \in B$ for some j. Since further cancellation occurs, we must have $zb^*z^{-1} \in B$. By the hypothesis on z, this implies that $b^* = 1$, and thus that $b_1 = b_2$. ☐

The theorem just proved has an interesting application to one-relator groups. Recall that a one-relator group $G = \langle t, b, c, \ldots ; r \rangle$, where r is cyclically reduced and some generator occurring in r has exponent sum zero, say $\sigma_t(r) = 0$, is an HNN extension of another one-relator group; see (IV.5). We shall need the following lemma.

Lemma 11.8. *Let $G = \langle a, b, \ldots ; r \rangle$ be a one-relator group with at least two generators. Then G has a presentation $\langle t, \ldots ; r' \rangle$ where $\sigma_t(r') = 0$.*

☐ If either a or b has zero exponent sum in r, then let t be whichever of a or b is appropriate. If neither a nor b has zero exponent sum we proceed by induction on $(|\sigma_a(r)| + |\sigma_b(r)|)$. Suppose $0 < |\sigma_a(r)| \leqslant |\sigma_b(r)|$. Then G has presentation $G = \langle a, b, \ldots ; r' \rangle$ where $r' = r(ab^{-\varepsilon}, b, \ldots)$. For suitable choice of $\varepsilon = \pm 1$, $|\sigma_b(r')| < |\sigma_b(r)|$. Consequently, G has a presentation of the desired type. ☐

Theorem 11.9. *Let $G = \langle t, b, c, \ldots ; r \rangle$ be a group presented with one relator and at least three generators. Then G is SQ-universal.*

☐ As usual, we assume that r is cyclically reduced, and, by the preceeding lemma, we may suppose that $\sigma_t(r) = 0$. We view G as an HNN extension of a one relator group H. It is usually most convenient, as we did in section IV.5, to allow the subscripts on the generators of H other than the b's to range over all the integers. We do not want to follow this procedure here. Let s be the rewritten form of r. For each generator x of G, let $\mu(x)$ be the minimum subscript on an occurrence of an x in s, and let $m(x)$ be the maximum subscript on an occurrence of an x in s. Let

$$H = \langle b_i, c_j, \ldots, \mu(b) \leqslant i \leqslant m(b), \mu(c) \leqslant j \leqslant m(c), \ldots ; s\rangle$$

Let U and V be the subgroups of H defined by

$$U = \langle b_i, c_j, \ldots, \mu(b) \leqslant i < m(b), \mu(c) \leqslant j < m(c), \ldots\rangle,$$

and

$$V = \langle b_i, c_j, \ldots, \mu(b) < i \leqslant m(b), \mu(c) < j \leqslant m(c), \ldots\rangle.$$

Then

$$G = \langle H, t; tUt^{-1} = V\rangle.$$

Suppose first that $\mu(b) < m(b)$ and $\mu(c) < m(c)$. Let $z = b_{\mu(b)}c_{m(c)}$. Suppose that u_1 and u_2 are non-identity elements of U. Applying the Freiheitssatz, an equation of the form $zu_1z^{-1} = u_2$ cannot hold in H since neither side contains $b_{m(b)}$ (which occurs in s). Similarly, if v_1 and v_2 are non-identity elements of V, the equation $z^{-1}v_1z = v_2$ cannot hold in H since neither side contains $c_{\mu(c)}$. Thus

$$zUz^{-1} \cap U = \{1\} = z^{-1}Vz \cap V$$

and G is SQ-universal by Theorem 11.7.

If the inequalities assumed above do not hold, suppose for definiteness that $\mu(b) = m(b)$. This means that no b_i occurs among the generators of either U or V. Let $z = c_{\mu(c)}c_{m(c)}$ (whether or not $\mu(c) = m(c)$), and apply an argument similar to the one above. □

One direction upon which we have not even touched is small cancellation theory for semigroups. For an excellent geometric development of this subject see Remmers (1971).

We have focused on small cancellation theory in this chapter. The use of diagrams in proving theorems is, however, by no means limited to small cancellation theory. Lyndon's (1973) proof by diagrams of the Freiheitssatz (Theorem II.5.1) was given earlier. We also mention the geometric proof by Miller and Schupp (1974) of Britton's and Collins' Lemmas. Also, diagrams are used in the work of Hurwitz (1976) showing that if G is the free product of two free groups with finitely generated commuting subgroups, then G has solvable conjugacy problem.

Bibliography

Accola, R. D. M.: On the number of automorphisms of a closed Riemann surface. Trans. Amer. Math. Soc. **131**, 398–408 (1968).

Ackca, J.: Untergruppen speziell präsentierter Gruppen. Boun: Gesellsch. für Math. und Datenverarbeitung. 1974.

Adelsberger, H.: Über unendliche diskrete Gruppen. J. Reine Angew. Math. **163**, 103–124 (1930).

Adyan, S. I.: Algorithmic unsolvability of problems of recognition of certain properties of groups. Dokl. Akad. Nauk SSSR **103**, 533–535 (1955).

Adyan, S. I.: The unsolvability of certain algorithmic problems in the theory of groups. Trudy Moskov. Mat. Obsc. **6**, 231–298 (1957).

Adyan, S. I.: On algorithmic problems in effectively complete classes of groups. Dokl. Akad. Nauk SSSR **123**, 13–16 (1958).

Adyan, S. I.: Defining relations and algorithmic problems for groups and semigroups. Proc. Steklov Inst. **85** (1966). Amer. Math. Soc. Transl. 152 (1967).

Adyan, S. I.: *See also* Novikov, P. S.

Ahlfors, L. V.: Finitely generated Kleinian groups. Amer. J. Math. **86**, 413–429 (1964).

Akagawa, Y.: On the number of fundamental relations with respect to minimal generators of a *p*-group. J. Math. Soc. Japan **20**, 1–12 (1968).

Albert, A. A., Thompson, J.: Two-element generation of the projective unimodular group. Illinois J. Math. **3**, 421–439 (1959).

Allenby, R. B. J. T., Gregorac, R. J.: Generalised free products which are free products of locally extended residually finite groups. Math. Z. **120**, 323–325 (1971).

Allenby, R. B. J. T., Tang, C. Y.: On the Frattini subgroup of a residually finite generalized free product. Proc. Amer. Math. Soc. **47**, 300–304 (1975).

Allenby, R. B. J. T., Tang, C. Y.: On the Frattini subgroups of generalized free products and the embedding of amalgams. Trans. Amer. Math. Soc. **203**, 319–330 (1975).

Althoen, S. C.: A Seifert-van Kampen theorem for the second homotopy group. Thesis, New York: City Univ. of New York 1973.

Althoen, S. C.: A geometric realization of a construction of Bass and Serre. J. Pure Appl. Algebra **5**, 233–237 (1974).

Althoen, S. C.: A van Kampen theorem. J. Pure Appl. Math. **6**, 41–47 (1975).

Andreadakis, S.: On some series of groups of automorphisms of groups. Bull. Soc. Math. Grèce **4**, 111–120 (1963).

Andreadakis, S.: On the automorphisms of free groups and free nilpotent groups. Proc. London Math. Soc. **15**, 239–268 (1965).

Andreadakis, S.: On the embedding of a free product of cyclic groups. Bull. Soc. Math. Grèce **10**, 19–34 (1969).

Andreadakis, S.: On semicomplete groups. J. London Math. Soc. **44**, 361–364 (1969).

Andreadakis, S.: Semicomplete one-relator groups. Bull. Soc. Math. Grèce **12**, 1–6, (1971).

Andrews, J. J., Curtis, M. L.: Free groups and handlebodies. Proc. Amer. Math. Soc. **16**, 192–195 (1965).

Andrews, J. J., Curtis, M. L.: Extended Nielsen operations in free groups. Amer. Math. Monthly

73, 21–28 (1966).

Anshel, M.: The endomorphisms of certain one-relator groups and the generalized Hopfian problem. Bull. Amer. Math. Soc. **77**, 348–350 (1971).

Anshel, M.: Non-Hopfian groups with fully invariant kernel, I, II. Trans. Amer. Math. Soc. **170**, 231–237 (1972), J. Algebra **24**, 473–485 (1973).

Anshel, M.: Conjugate powers in HNN groups. Proc. Amer. Math. Soc. **54**, 19–23 (1976).

Anshel, M.: Decision problems for HNN groups and vector addition systems. Math. Comput. **30**, 154–156 (1976).

Anshel, M., Prener, R.: On free products of finite abelian groups. To appear.

Anshel, M., Stebe, P.: The solvability of the conjugacy problem for certain HNN groups. Bull. Amer. Math. Soc. **80**. 266–270 (1974).

Anshel, M., Stebe, P.: Conjugate powers in free products with amalgamation. Houston J. Math. **2**, 139–147 (1976).

Appel, K. I.: One-variable equations in free groups. Proc. Amer. Math. Soc. **19**, 912–918 (1968).

Appel, K. I.: On two-variable equations in free groups. Proc. Amer. Math. Soc. **21**, 179–181 (1969).

Appel, K. I.: The conjugacy problem for tame alternating knot groups is solvable. Notices Amer. Math. Soc. **18**, 42 (1971).

Appel, K. I.: On the conjugacy problem for knot groups. Math. Z. **138**, 273–294 (1974).

Appel, K. I., Djorup, F. M.: On the equation $z_1^n \cdots z_k^n = y^n$ in a free semigroup. Trans. Amer. Math. Soc. **134**, 461–470 (1968).

Appel, K. I., Schupp, P. E.: The conjugacy problem for the group of any tame alternating knot is solvable. Proc. Amer. Math. Soc. **33**, 329–336 (1972).

Artin, E.: The free product of groups. Amer. J. Math. **69**, 1–4 (1947).

Artin, R.: Theory of braids. Ann. of Math. **48**, 101–126 (1947).

Artin, E.: Braids and permutations. Ann. of Math. **48**, 643–649 (1947).

Artin, E.: The theory of braids. Amer. Scientist **38**, 112–119 (1950).

Aselderov, Z. M.: On equations with one unknown in a free group. Akad. Nauk Ukrain. SSR, Kiev, 3–16 (1969).

Aumann, R. J.: Asphericity of alternating knots. Ann. of Math. **64**, 374–392 (1956).

Aust, C.: Primitive elements and one relation algebras. Trans. Amer. Math. Soc. **193**, 375–387 (1974).

Bachmann, F., Grünenfelder, L.: Homological methods and the third dimension subgroup. Comment. Math. Helv. **47**, 526–531 (1972).

Bachmuth, S.: Automorphisms of free metabelian groups. Trans. Amer. Math. Soc. **118**, 93–104 (1965).

Bachmuth, S.: Induced automorphisms of free groups and free metabelian groups. Trans. Amer. Math. Soc. **122**, 1–17 (1966).

Bachmuth, S.: Automorphisms of a class of metabelian groups. Trans. Amer. Math. Soc. **127**, 284–293 (1967).

Bachmuth, S., Hughes, I.: Applications of a theorem of Magnus. Arch. Math. **17**, 380–382 (1966).

Bachmuth, S., Mochizuki, H. Y.: Automorphisms of a class of metabelian groups, II. Trans. Amer. Math. Soc. **127**, 294–301 (1967).

Bachmuth, S., Mochizuki, H. Y.: Automorphisms of solvable groups. Bull. Amer. Math. Soc. **81**, 420–422 (1975).

Bachmuth, S., Mochizuki, H. Y.: Triples of 2 × 2 matrices which generate free groups. Proc. Amer. Math. Soc. **59**, 25–28 (1976).

Bachmuth, S., Formanek, E., Mochizuki, H. Y.: IA-automorphisms of certain two-generator torsion-free groups. J. Alg. **40**, 19–30 (1976).

Baer, R., Levi, F.: Freie Produkte und ihre Untergruppen. Compositio Math. **3**, 391–398 (1930).

Bagherzadeh, G. H.: Commutativity in one-relator groups. J. London Math. Soc. **13**, 459–471 (1975).

Bagherzadeh, G. H.: Commutativity in groups with bipolar structure. J. London Math. Soc. **13**, 443–453 (1976).

Baker, R. P.: Cayley diagrams on the anchor ring. Amer. J. Math. **53**, 645–669 (1931).

Balcerzyk, S., Mycielski, J.: On free subgroups of topological groups. Bull. Akad. Polon. Sci. Cl. III. **4**, 415 (1956).

Balcerzyk, S., Mycielski, J.: On the existence of free subgroups in topological groups. Fund. Math. **44**, 303–308 (1957).

Balcerzyk, S., Mycielski, J.: Some theorems on the representations of free products. Bull. Acad. Polon. Sci. Cl. III. **5**, 1029–1030 (1957).

Balcerzyk, S., Mycielski, J.: On faithful representations of free products of groups. Fund. Math. **50**, 63–74 (1961/62).

Bass. H.: The degree of polynomial growth of finitely generated nilpotent groups. Proc. London Math. Soc. **25**, 603–614 (1972).

Bass, H.: Growth of groups. SL_2 of local fields. Groups acting on trees. Queen's Papers in Pure and Applied Math. (Kingston) **36**, 11–12; 13–15; 16–17 (1973).

Bass, H.: Some remarks on group actions on trees. Comm. Algebra **4**, 1091–1126 (1976).

Bass, H., Lazard, M., Serre, J.-P.: Sousgroupes d'indice fini dans $\mathbb{SL}(n, \mathbb{Z})$. Bull. Amer. Math. Soc. **70**, 385–392 (1964).

Baumslag, B.: Intersections of finitely generated subgroups in free products. J. London Math. Soc. **41**, 673–679 (1966).

Baumslag, B.: Residually free groups. Proc. London Math. Soc. **17**, 402–418 (1967).

Baumslag, B.: Generalised free products whose two-generator subgroups are free. J. London Math. Soc. **43**, 601–606 (1968).

Baumslag, G.: Wreath products and p-groups. Proc. Cambridge Philos. Soc. **55**, 224–231 (1959).

Baumslag, G.: On a problem of Lyndon, J. London Math. Soc. **35**, 30–32 (1960).

Baumslag, G.: On generalized free products. Math. Z. **78**, 423–438 (1962).

Baumslag, G.: A remark on generalised free products. Proc. Amer. Math. Soc. **13**, 53–54 (1962).

Baumslag, G.: A non-Hopfian group. Bull. Amer. Math. Soc. **68**, 196–198 (1962).

Baumslag, G.: Automorphism groups of residually finite groups. J. London Math. Soc. **38**, 117–118 (1963).

Baumslag, G.: Groups with one defining relator. J. Austral. Math. Soc. **4**, 385–392 (1964).

Baumslag, G.: Residual nilpotence and relations in free groups. J. Algebra **2**, 271–282 (1965).

Baumslag, G.: Finitely presented groups. Proc. Conf. Canberra 1965, pp. 37–50 New York: Gordon and Breach, 1967.

Baumslag, G.: Residually finite one-relator groups. Bull. Amer. Math. Soc. **73**, 618–620 (1967).

Baumslag, G.: On the residual nilpotence of certain one-relator groups. Comm. Pure Appl. Math. **21**, 322–326 (1968).

Baumslag, G.: A non-cyclic one-relator group all of whose finite quotients are cyclic. J. Austral. Math. Soc. **10**, 497–498 (1969).

Baumslag, G.: A finitely generated, infinitely related group with trivial multiplicator. Bull. Austral. Math. Soc. **5**, 131–136 (1971).

Baumslag, G.: Positive one-relator groups. Trans. Amer. Math. Soc. **156**, 165–183 (1971).

Baumslag, G.: Lecture notes on nilpotent groups. In: Regional Conf. Ser. in Math. Amer. Math. Soc. **2**, (1971).

Baumslag, G.: On finitely generated subgroups of free products. J. Austral. Math. Soc. **12**, 358–364 (1971).

Baumslag, G.: Residually finite groups with the same finite images. Compositio Math. **29**, 249–252 (1974).

Baumslag, G.: Some problems on one-relator groups. In: Proc. Conf. Canberra 1973 (Lecture Notes in Math., Vol. 372, pp. 75–81). Berlin-Heidelberg-New York: Springer 1974.

Baumslag, G. (Editor): Reviews on Infinite Groups, Parts I, II. Amer. Math. Soc. (1974).

Baumslag, G.: A remark on groups with trivial multiplicator. Amer. J. Math. **97**, 863–864 (1976).

Baumslag, G., Boone, W. W., Neumann, B. H.: Some unsolvable problems about elements and subgroups of groups. Math. Scand. **7**, 191–201 (1959).

Baumslag, G., Gruenberg, K. W.: Some reflections on cohomological dimension and freeness. J. Algebra, **6**, 394–409 (1967).

Baumslag, G., Karrass, A., Solitar, D.: Torsion-free groups and amalgamated products. Proc. Amer. Math. Soc. **24**, 688–690 (1970).

Baumslag, G., Mahler, K.: Equations in free metabelian groups. Michigan Math. J. **12**, 375–379 (1965).

Baumslag, G., Solitar, D.: Some two-generator one-relator non-Hopfian groups. Bull. Amer.

Math. Soc. **68,** 199–201 (1962).

Baumslag, G., Steinberg, A.: Residual nilpotence and relations in free groups. Bull. Amer. Math. Soc. **70,** 283–284 (1964).

Baumslag, G., Taylor, T. (= Lewin, T.): The centre of groups with one defining relator. Math. Ann. **175,** 315–319 (1968).

Baumslag, G., Strebel, R.: Some finitely generated, infinitely related metabelian groups with trivial multiplicator. J. Alg. **40,** 46–62 (1976).

Baur, W.: Eine rekursiv präsentierte Gruppe mit unentscheidbaren Wortproblem. Math. Z. **131,** 219–222 (1973).

Beaumont, R. A.: Groups with isomorphic proper subgroups. Bull. Amer. Math. Soc. **51,** 381–387 (1945).

Beetham, N. J.: A set of generators and relations for the group $\mathbb{PSL}(2, q)$, q odd. J. London Math. Soc. **3,** 554–557 (1971).

Beetham, M. J., Campbell, C. M.: A note on the Todd-Coxeter coset enumeration algorithm. Proc. Edinburgh Math. Soc. **20,** 73–78 (1976).

Behr, H.: Über die endliche Definierbarkeit verallgemeinerter Einheitengruppen. J. Reine Angew. Math. **211,** 123–135 (1962).

Behr, H.: Über die endliche Definierbarkeit von Gruppen. J. Reine Angew. Math. **211,** 116–122 (1962).

Behr, H.: Endliche Erzeugbarkeit arithmetischer Gruppen über Funktionenkörpern. Invent. Math. **7,** 1–32 (1969).

Behr, H.: Eine endliche Präsentation der symplektischen Gruppe $Sp_4(\mathbb{Z})$. Math. Z. **141,** 47–56 (1975).

Behr, H., Mennicke, J.: A presentation of the groups $\mathbb{PSL}(2, q)$. Canad. J. Math. **20,** 1432–1438 (1968).

Benson, C. T., Grove, L. C.: Generators and relations for Coxeter groups. Proc. Amer. Math. Soc. **24,** 545–554 (1970).

Benson, C. T., Grove, L. C.: Finite reflection groups. Bogden and Quigley 1971.

Bergman, G. M.: On groups acting on locally finite graphs. Ann. of Math. **88,** 335–340 (1968).

Best, L. A.: Subgroups of one-relator Fuchsian groups. Canad. J. Math. **25,** 888–891 (1973).

Bezverkhnii, V. N.: Solution of the occurrence problem for a certain class of groups. Questions in the Theory of Groups and Semigroups, pp. 3–86. Tulsk Gos. Ped. Inst. Tula 1972.

Bezvehnii, V. N., Rollov, E. V.: Subgroups of a free product of groups. Mod. Alg. **1,** 16–31 (1974) [Leningrad Gos. Ped. Inst.]

Bieri, R.: Gruppen mit Poincaré-Dualität. Comment. Math. Helv. **47,** 373–396 (1972).

Bieri, R.: Mayer-Vietoris sequences for HNN-groups and homological duality. Math. Z. **143,** 123–130 (1975).

Bieri, R.: Normal subgroups in duality groups and in groups of cohomological dimension 2. J. Pure Appl. Alg. **7,** 35–51 (1976).

Bieri, R.: Mayer-Vietoris sequences for HNN groups and homological duality. Math. Z. To appear.

Bieri, R., Eckmann, B.: Amalgamated free products of groups and homological duality. Comment. Math. Helv. **49,** 460–478 (1974).

Bieri, R., Eckmann, B.: Groups with homological duality generalizing Poincaré duality. Invent. Math. **20,** 103–124 (1973).

Bieri, R., Eckmann, B.: Finiteness properties of duality groups. Comment. Math. Helv. **49,** 74–83 (1974).

Biggs, N.: Cayley maps and symmetrical maps. Proc. Cambridge Philos. Soc. **72,** 381–386 (1972).

Binder, G. Ya.: The two-element bases of the symmetric group. Izv. Vyssh. Uchebn. Zaved. Matematika, no. 1 **(92),** 9–11 (1970).

Binz, E., Neukirch, J., Wenzel, G. H.: A subgroup theorem for free products of pro-finite groups. J. Algebra **19,** 104–105 (1971).

Birman, J. S.: Automorphisms of the fundamental group of a closed orientable 2-manifold. Proc. Amer. Math. Soc. **21,** 351–354 (1968).

Birman, J. S.: On braid groups. Comm. Pure Appl. Math. **22,** 41–72 (1969).

Birman, J. S.: Mapping class groups and their relationship to braid groups. Comm. Pure Appl.

Math. **22**, 213–238 (1969).

Birman, J. S.: Abelian quotients of the mapping class group of a 2-manifold. Bull. Amer. Math. Soc. **76**, 147–150 (1970).

Birman, J. S.: On Siegel's modular group. Math. Ann. **191**, 59–68 (1971).

Birman, J. S.: An inverse function theorem for free groups. Proc. Amer. Math. Soc. **41**, 634–638 (1974).

Birman, J. S.: Braids, links and mapping class groups. Ann. Math. Studies **82**, (1974).

Birman, J. S.: Mapping class groups and surfaces: a survey. Discontinuous Groups and Riemann Surfaces, Annals Studies **79**, 57–71 (1974).

Birman, J. S., Chillingsworth, D. R. J.: On the homeotopy group of a non-orientable surface. Proc. Cambridge Philos. Soc. **71**, 437–448 (1972).

Birman, J. S., Hilden, H. M.: On the mapping class groups of closed surfaces as covering spaces. Ann. of Math. Studies **66**, 81–115 (1971).

Blackburn, N.: Note on a theorem of Magnus. J. Austral. Math. Soc. **10**, 469–474 (1960).

Blackburn, N.: Conjugacy in nilpotent groups. Proc. Amer. Math. Soc. **16**, 143–148 (1965).

Blanc, C.: Une interprétation élémentaire des théorèmes fondamentaux de M. Nevanlinna. Comment. Math. Helv. **12**, 153–163 (1940).

Blanc, C.: Les réseaux Riemanniens. Comment. Math. Helv. **13**, 54–67 (1941).

Blanchfield, R. C.: Applications of free differential calculus to the theory of groups. Senior thesis, Princeton: Princeton University 1949.

Böge, S.: Definierende Relationen zwischen Erzeugenden der klassichen Gruppen. Abh. Math. Sem. Univ. Hamburg **30**, 165–178 (1967).

Bohnenblust, F.: The algebraic braid group. Ann. of Math. **48**, 127–136 (1947).

Boone, W. W.: Certain simple unsolvable problems in group theory, I, II, III, IV, V, VI. Nederl. Akad. Wetensch. Proc. Ser. A **57**, 231–237, 492–497 (1954), **58**, 252–256, 571–577 (1955), **60**, 22–27, 227–232 (1957).

Boone, W. W.: The word problem. Proc. Nat. Acad. Sci. U.S.A. **44**, 265–269 (1958).

Boone, W. W.: The word problem. Ann. of Math. **70**, 207–265 (1959).

Boone, W. W.: Partial results regarding word problems and recursively enumerable degrees of unsolvability. Bull. Amer. Math. Soc. **68**, 616–623 (1962).

Boone, W. W.: Word problems and recursively enumerable degrees of unsolvability. A sequel on finitely presented groups. Ann. of Math. **84**, 49–84 (1966).

Boone, W. W.: The theory of decision processes in group theory; a survey, Amer. Math. Soc., invited address; to appear in: Bull. Amer. Math. Soc.

Boone, W. W., Collins, D. J.: Embeddings into groups with only a few defining relations. J. Austral. Math. Soc. **18**, 1–7 (1974), pp. 37–74.

Boone, W. W., Haken, W., Poenaru, V.: On recursively unsolvable problems in topology and their classification. In: Contributions to Mathematical Logic (ed. K. Schütte). Amsterdam: North-Holland 1968.

Boone, W. W., Higman, G.: An algebraic characterization of the solvability of the word problem. J. Austral. Math. Soc. **18**, 41–53 (1974).

Boone, W. W., Rogers, H., Jr.: On a problem of J.H.C. Whitehead and a problem of Alonzo Church. Math. Scand. **19**, 185–192 (1966).

Boone, Pr, W. W., Higman, G.: An algebraic characterization of groups with soluble order problem. Studies in Logic **80**, 53–54 (1975).

Bordo, W., Rosenberger, G.: Eine Bemerkung zur Hecke-Gruppe $G(\lambda)$. Abh. Math. Sem. Univ. Hamburg **39**, 76–82 (1973).

Borisov, V. V.: Simple examples of groups with unsolvable word problem. Mat. Zametki **6**, 521–532 (1969).

Bovdi, A. A.: Dimension subgroups. Proc. Riga Sem. Alg. Latv. Gos. Univ., 5–7 (1969).

Boydron, Y.: Progressivité dans les produits libres. C. R. Acad. Sci. Paris Ser. A **273**, 799–780 (1971).

Boydron, Y.: Conjugaison des sous-groupes d'un groupe libre. Comptes Rendus Acad. Sci. Paris **276**, 1447–1448 (1975).

Boydron, Y.: Algorithmes dans les produits libres. Comptes Rendus Acad. Sci. Paris A **282**, 135–138 (1976).

Brahana, H. R.: Pairs of generators of the known simple groups whose orders are less than one million. Ann. of Math. **31**, 529–549 (1930).

Brahana, H. R.: On the groups generated by two operators of orders two and three whose product is of order eight. Amer. J. Math. **53**, 891–901 (1931).

Breiskorn, E.: Sur les groupes de tresses d'après V. I. Arnol'd. In: Sem. Bourbaki 1971–72 (Lecture Notes in Math., Vol. 317). Berlin-Heidelberg-New York: Springer 1973.

Breiskorn, E., Saito, K.: Artin-Gruppen und Coxeter-Gruppen. Invent. Math. **17**, 245–271 (1972).

Brenner, J. L.: Quelques groupes libres de matrices. C. R. Acad. Sci. Paris **241**, 1689–1691 (1955).

Brenner, J. L., MacLeod, R. A., Olesky, D. D.: Non-free groups generated by 2×2 matrices. Canad. J. Math. **27**, 237–245 (1975).

Brenner, J. L., Wiegold, J.: Two-generator groups, I. Michigan Math. J. **22**, 53–64 (1975).

Britton, J. L.: Solution of the word problem for certain types of groups, I, II. Proc. Glasgow Math. Assoc. **3**, 45–54 (1956), **3**, 68–90 (1957).

Britton, J. L.: The word problem for groups. Proc. London Math. Soc. **8**, 493–506 (1958).

Britton, J. L.: The word problem. Ann. of Math. **77**, 16–32 (1963).

Brown, K. S.: Euler characteristic of discrete groups and *G*-spaces. Invent. Math. **27**, 229–264 (1974).

Brown, R.: Groupoids and van Kampen's theorem. Proc. London Math. Soc. **17**, 385–401 (1967).

Brunner, A. M.: Transitivity systems of certain one-relator groups. In: Proc. Conf. Canberra 1973 (Lecture Notes in Math., Vol. 372, pp. 131–140). Berlin-Heidelberg-New York: Springer 1974.

Brunner, A. M.: The determination of Fibonacci groups. Bull. Austral. Math. Soc. **11**, 11–14 (1974).

Brunner, A. M.: A group with an infinite number of Nielsen inequivalent one-relator presentations. J. Algebra **42**, 81–84 (1976).

Buckley, J.: On the D-series of a finite group. Proc. Amer. Math. Soc. **18**, 185–186 (1967).

Bungaard, S., Nielsen, J.: On normal subgroups with finite index in F-groups. Mat. Tidsskr. B, 56–58 (1951).

Bungaard, S.: *See also* Nielsen, J.

Burde, G.: Zur Theorie der Zöpfe. Math. Ann. **151**, 101–107 (1963).

Burde, G.: *See* Zieschang, H.

Burns, R. G.: A note of free groups. Proc. Amer. Math. Soc. **23**, 14–17 (1969)

Burns, R. G.: On the intersection of finitely generated subgroups of a free group. Math. Z. **119**, 121–130 (1971).

Burns, R. G.: On the finitely generated subgroups of a free group. Trans. Amer. Math. Soc. **165**, 293–306 (1972).

Burns, R. G.: Finitely generated subgroups of HNN groups. Canad. J. Math. **25**, 1103–1112 (1973).

Burns, R. G.: On the rank of the intersection of subgroups of a Fuchsian group. In: Proc. Conf. Canberra 1973 (Lecture Notes in Math., Vol. 372, pp. 165–187). Berlin-Heidelberg-New York: Springer 1974.

Burns, R. G.: A proof of the Freiheitssatz and the Cohen-Lyndon theorem for one-relator groups. J. London Math. Soc. **7**, 508–514 (1974).

Burnside, W.: On an unsettled question in the theory of discontinuous groups. Quart. J. Math. **33**, 230–238 (1902).

Burnside, W.: The theory of groups of finite order. 2nd ed. 1911. New York: Dover 1955 [Reprint].

Camm, R.: Simple free products. J. London Math. Soc. **28**, 66–76 (1953).

Campbell, C. M.: *See* Robertson, E. F., Beetham, M. J.

Campbell, C. M., Robertson, E. F.: On matacyclic Fibonacci groups. Proc. Edinburgh Math. Soc. **19**, 253–256 (1974/75).

Campbell, C. M., Robertson, E. F.: A note on Fibonacci type groups. Can. Math. Bull. **18**, 173–175 (1975).

Campbell, C. M., Robertson, E. F.: Applications of the Todd-Coxeter algorithm to generalised Fibonacci groups. Proc. Roy. Soc. Edinburgh A **73**, 163–166 (1975).

Cannonito, F. B.: Hierarchies of computable groups and the word problem. J. Symbolic Logic **31**, 376–392 (1966).

Cannonito, F. B.: *See also* Boone, W. W.

Cayley, A.: On the theory of groups. Proc. London Math. Soc. **9,** 126–133 (1878).
Cayley, A.: The theory of groups: graphical representations. Amer. J. Math. **1,** 174–176 (1878).
Cayley, A.: On the theory of groups. Amer. J. Math. **2,** 139–157 (1889).
Cebotar, A. A.: Subgroups of groups with one defining relation that do not contain free subgroups of rank 2. Algebra i Logica **10,** 570–586 (1971).
Cebotar, A. A.: The center of a subgroup of a group with a single defining relation. Questions in the Theory of Groups and Semigroups. Tulsk Gas. Ped. Inst. Tula, 96–105 (1972).
Cebotar, A. A.: Those subgroups of groups with a single defining relation that have normal subgroups satisfying an identity. Sibirsk. Mat. Ž. **16,** 139–148 (1975).
Chandler, B.: The representation of a generalized free product in an associative ring. Comm. Pure Appl. Math. **21,** 271–288 (1968).
Chang, B.: The automorphism group of the free group with two generators. Michigan Math. J. **7,** 79–81 (1960).
Charnow, A.: A note on torsion free groups generated by a pair of matrices. Canad. Math. Bull. **17,** 747–748 (1975).
Chein, O.: IA automorphisms of free and free metabelian groups. Comm. Pure Appl. Math. **21,** 605–629 (1968).
Chein, O.: Subgroups of IA-automorphisms of a free group. Acta Math. **123,** 1–12 (1969).
Chein, O.: Induced automorphisms of free metabelian groups. Proc. Amer. Math. Soc. **31,** 1–9 (1972).
Chen, K. T., Fox, R. H., Lyndon, R. C.: Free differential calculus; IV. Ann. of Math. **63,** 294–397 (1958).
Chevalley, C., Herbrand, J.: Groupes topologiques, groupes fuchsiens, groupes libres. C. R. Acad. Sci. Paris **192,** 724–726 (1931).
Chillingsworth, D. R. J.: Winding numbers on surfaces, I, II, applications. Math. Ann. **196,** 218–249 (1972); **199,** 131–153 (1972).
Chillingsworth, D. R. J.: *See also* Birman, J. S.
Chipman, J. C.: Van Kampen's theorem for n-stage covers. Trans. Amer. Math. Soc. **192,** 357–401 (1967).
Chipman, J. C.: Subgroups of free products with amalgamated subgroups: a topological approach. Trans. Amer. Mach. Soc. **181,** 97–87 (1973).
Chiswell, I. M.: On groups acting on trees; Thesis. Ann Abor: Univ. Michigan 1973.
Chiswell, I. M.: The cohomological dimension of a 1-relator group. J. London Math. Soc. **11,** 381–382 (1975).
Chiswell, I. M.: Euler characteristics of groups. Math. Z. **147,** 1–11 (1976).
Chiswell, I. M.: Exact sequences associated with a graph of groups. J. Pure Appl. Alg. **8,** 63–74 (1976).
Chiswell, I. M.: Abstract length functions in groups. Math. Proc. Camb. Phil. Soc. **80,** 451–463 (1976).
Chiswell, I. M.: Abstract length functions in groups. Math. Proc. Camb. Phil. Soc. To appear.
Chiswell, I. M.: An example at an integer-valued length function. J. London Math. Soc. To appear.
Cohen, D. E.: Certain subgroups of free products. Matematika **7,** 117–124 (1960).
Cohen, D. E.: A topological proof in group theory. Proc. Cambridge Philos. Soc. **59,** 277–282 (1963).
Cohen, D. E.: Ends and free products of groups. Math. Z. **114,** 9–18 (1970).
Cohen, D. E.: Groups of cohomological dimension one (Lecture Notes in Math., Vol. 245). Berlin-Heidelberg-New York: Springer 1972.
Cohen, D. E.: Groups with free subgroups of finite index. In: Lecture Notes (in Math., Vol. 319, pp. 26–44). Berlin-Heidelberg-New York: Springer 1973.
Cohen, D. E.: Subgroups of HNN groups. J. Austral. Math. Soc. **17,** 394–405 (1974).
Cohen, D. E, Lyndon, R. C.: Free bases for normal subgroups of free groups. Trans. Amer. Math. Soc. **108,** 528–537 (1963).
Cohen, R.: Classes of automorphisms of free groups of infinite rank. Trans. Amer. Math. Soc. **177,** 99–120 (1973).
Cohn P. M.: Generalization of a theorem of Magnus. Proc. London Math. Soc. **2,** 297–310 (1952).
Cohn, P. M.: Universal algebra. New York-London; Harper and Row 1965.

Cohn, P. M.: On the structure of $\mathbb{GL}_2$ of a ring. Inst. Hautes Études Sci. Publ. Math. **30**, 5–53 (1966).
Cohn, P. M.: A presentation of SL for Euclidean imaginary number fields. Mathematika **15**, 156–163 (1968).
Coldewey, H.-D.: *See* Zieschang, H.
Collins, D. J.: A new non-Hopf group. Arch. Math. **19**, 581–583 (1968).
Collins, D. J.: On embedding groups and the conjugacy problem. J. London Math. Soc. **1**, 674–682 (1969).
Collins, D. J.: On recognising Hopf groups. Arch. Math. **20**, 235–240 (1969).
Collins, D. J.: Recursively enumerable degrees and the conjugacy problem. Acta Math. **122**, 115–160 (1969).
Collins, D. J.: Word and conjugacy problems in groups with only a few defining relations. Zeit. Math. Logik Grund. Math. **15**, 305–325 (1969).
Collins, D. J.: Free subgroups of small cancellation groups. Proc. London Math. Soc. **26**, 193–206 (1973).
Collins, D. J.: On a group embedding theorem of V. V. Borisov. Bull. London Math. Soc. To appear.
Collins, D. J.: *See also* Boone, W. W.
Comerford, L. P., Jr.: Real elements in small cancellation groups. Math. Ann. **208**, 279–293 (1974).
Comerford, L. P. Jr.: Powers and conjugacy in small cancellation groups. Arch. Math. **26**, 357–360 (1975).
Comerford, L. P. Jr. Truffault, B.: The conjugacy problem for free products of sixth-groups with cyclic amalgamation. Math. Z. **149**, 169–181 (1976).
Conway, J. H.: Advanced problem 5327. Amer. Math. Monthly **72**, 915 (1965).
Conway, J. H.: Solution to advanced problem 5327. Amer. Math. Monthly **74**, 91 (1967).
Cossey, J., Smythe, N.: HNN groups and groups with center. Knots, groups, and 3-manifolds. Ann. Math. Studies **84**, 101–118 (1975).
Coxeter, H. S. M.: Groups whose fundamental regions are simplexes. J. London Math. Soc. **6**, 132–136 (1931).
Coxeter, H. S. M.: Discrete groups generated by reflections. Ann. of Math. **35**, 588–621 (1934).
Coxeter, H. S. M.: The complete enumeration of finite groups of the form $R_i^2 = (R_iR_j)^{k_{ij}} = 1$. J. London Math. Soc. **10**, 21–25 (1935).
Coxeter, H. S. M.: The groups determined by the relation $S^l = T^m = (S^{-1}T^{-1}ST)^p = 1$. Duke Math. J. **2**, 61–73 (1936).
Coxeter, H. S. M.: An abstract definition for the alternating group in terms of two generators. J. London Math. Soc. **11**, 150–156 (1936).
Coxeter, H. S. M.: Abstract definition for the symmetry groups of the regular polytopes in terms of two generators. Part III: the rotation groups. Proc. Cambridge Philos. Soc. **33**, 315–324 (1937).
Coxeter, H. S. M.: The abstract groups $G^{m,n,p}$. Trans. Amer. Math. Soc. **45**, 73–150 (1939).
Coxeter, H. S. M.: A method for proving certain abstract groups to be infinite. Bull. Amer. Math. Soc. **46**, 246–251 (1940).
Coxeter, H. S. M.: The product of generators of a finite group generated by reflections. Duke Math. J. **18**, 765–782 (1951).
Coxeter, H. S. M.: Groups generated by unitary reflections of period two. Canad. J. Math. **9**, 243–272 (1957).
Coxeter, H. S. M.: On subgroups of the modular group. J. Math. Pures Appl. **37**, 317–319 (1958).
Coxeter, H. S. M.: Factor groups of the braid group. Proc. 4th Canad. Math. Cong, 95–122 (1959).
Coxeter, H. S. M.: The abstract group $G^{3,7,16}$. Proc. Edinburgh Math. Soc. **13**, 47–61 (1962); A correction; ib. 189.
Coxeter. H. S. M.: Cayley diagrams and regular complex polygons. Internat. Sympos. Comb. Math. Colo. State Univ. 1971, pp. 88–93. Amsterdam: North-Holland 1973.
Coxeter, H. S. M.: *See also* Todd, J. A.
Coxeter, H. S. M., Moser, W. O. J.: Generators and relations for discrete groups. Ergebnisse der Mathematik, Bd. 14, 3rd ed. Berlin-Heidelberg-New York: Springer 1972.
Craig, W.: Three uses of the Herbrand-Gentzen theorem in relating model theory to proof theory.

J. Symbolic Logic **22**, 269–285 (1957).
Crowe, D. W.: Some two-dimensional unitary groups generated by three reflections. Canad. J. Math. **13**, 418–426 (1961).
Crowell, R. H.: On the van Kampen theorem. Pacific J. Math. **9**, 43–50 (1959).
Crowell, R. H., Fox, R. H.: Introduction to knot theory. Ginn and Co. 1963.
Crowell, R. H., Smythe, N.: The subgroup theorem for amalgamated free products, HNN-constructions and colimits. In: Proc. Conf. Canberra 1973 (Lecture Notes in Math., Vol. 372, pp. 241–280). Berlin-Heidelberg-New York: Springer 1974.
Crowell, R. H., Smythe, N.: The Theory of Groupnets. To appear.
Curkin, V. A.: *See* Kargapolov, M. I.
Curran, P. M.: Cohomology of finitely presented groups. Pacific J. Math. **42**, 615–620 (1972).
Curtis, M. L.: *See* Andrews, J. J.
Dade, E. C.: Abelian groups of unimodular matrices. Illinois J. Math. **3**, 11–27 (1959).
Davis, M.: Computability and unsolvability, pp. 73–77. New York: McGraw Hill 1958.
Davis, M.: Hilbert's Tenth Problem is unsolvable. Amer. Math. Monthly **80**, 233–269 (1973).
De Groot, J.: Orthogonal isomorphic representations of free groups. Canad. J. Math. **8**, 256–262 (1956).
De Groot, J.: Die Gruppe der Abbildungsklassen. Acta Math. **69**, 135–206 (1938).
De Groot, J.: Über Abbildungen. Mat. Tidsskr. B, 25–48 (1939).
De Groot, J.: Über Abildungen geschlossener Flächen auf sich. Mat. Tidsskr. B, 146–151 (1950).
De Groot, J., Dekker, T.: Free subgroups of the orthogonal group. Composition Math. **12**, 134–136 (1954).
Dehn, M.: Über die Topologie des dreidimensionalen Raumes. Math. Ann. **69**, 137–168 (1910).
Dehn, M.: Über unendliche diskontinuerliche Gruppen. Math. Ann. **71**, 116–144 (1912).
Dehn, M.: Transformation der Kurve auf zweiseitigen Flächen. Math. Ann. **72**, 413–420 (1912).
Dekker, T. J.: On free groups of motions without fixed points. Nederl. Akad. Wetensch. Proc. Ser. A **61**, 348–353 (1958).
Dekker, T. J.: On free products of cyclic rotation groups. Canad. J. Math. **11**, 67–69 (1959).
Dekker, T. J.: On reflections in Euclidean spaces generating free products. Nieuw Arch. Wisk. **7**, 57–60 (1959).
Dekker, T. J.: *See* also De Groot, J.
Dey, I. M. S.: Schreier systems in free products. Proc. Glasgow Math. Assoc. **7**, 61–79 (1965).
Dixon, J. D.: Free subgroups of linear groups. In: Lecture Notes in Math., Vol. 319, pp. 45–56. Berlin-Heidelberg-New York: Springer 1973.
Djorup, F. M.: *See* Appel. K. I.
Doniyakhi, K. A.: Linear representation of the free product of cyclic groups. Leningrad. Gos. Univ. Učen. Zap. Ses. Mat. **10**, 158–165 (1940).
Douglas, J.: On finite groups with two independent generators. Proc. Nat. Acad. Sci. U.S.A. **37**, 604–610, 677–691, 749–760, 803–813 (1951).
Dubuque, P. E.: Sur les sous-groupes d'ordre fini dans un groupe infini. Mat. Sb. **10**, 147–150 (1942).
Dunwoody, M. J.: On relation groups. Math. Z. **81**, 180–186 (1963).
Dunwoody, M. J.: On T-systems of groups. J. Austral. Math. Soc. **3**, 172–179 (1963).
Dunwoody, M. J.: Some problems on free groups; Thesis. Austral. Nat. Univ. 1964.
Dunwoody, M. J.: The Magnus embedding. J. London Math. Soc. **44**, 115–117 (1969).
Dunwoody, M. J.: The ends of finitely generated groups. J. Algebra **12**, 339–344 (1969).
Dunwoody, M. J.: Nielsen transformations. In: Computational Problems in Abstract Algebra. Proc. Conf. Oxford 1967, pp. 45–46. London-New York: Pergamon 1970.
Dunwoody, M. J.: Relation modules. Bull. London Math. Soc. **4**, 151–155 (1972).
Dunwoody, M. J.: A group presentation associated with a 3-dimensional manifold. To appear.
Dunwoody, M. J., Pietrowski, A.: Presentations of the trefoil group. Canad. Math. Bull. **16**, 517–520 (1973).
Durnev, V. G.: Equations on free semigroups and groups. Math. Zametki **16**, 717–724 (1974).
Dyer, J. L.: On the residual finiteness of generalized free products. Trans. Amer. Math. Soc. **133**, 131–143 (1968).
Dyer, J. L.: On the isomorphism problem for polycyclic groups. Math. Z. **112**, 145–153 (1969).

Dyer, J. L.: A criterion for automorphisms of certain groups to be inner. J. Austral. Math. Soc. **21,** 179–184 (1976).

Dyer, J. L.: *See also* Landman-Dyer, J.

Dyer, J. L., Formanek, E.: The automorphism group of a free group is complete. J. London Math. Soc. **11,** 181–190 (1975).

Dyer, J. L., Formanek, E.: Complete automorpnism groups. Bull. Amer. Math. Soc. **81,** 435–437 (1975).

Dyer, J. L., Formanek, E.: Automorphism sequences of free nilpotent groups of class two. Math. Proc. Camb. Phil. Soc. **79,** 271–279 (1976).

Dyer, J. L., Scott, G. P.: Periodic automorphisms of free groups. Comm. Algebra **3,** 195–201 (1975).

Dyer, E., Vasquez, A. T.: Some small aspherical spaces. J. Austral. Math. Soc. **16,** 332–352 (1973).

Dyson, V. H.: The word problem and residually finite groups. Notices Amer. Math. Soc. **11,** 743 (1964).

Dyson, V. H.: A family of groups with nice word problems. J. Austral. Math. Soc. **17,** 414–425 (1974).

Dyson, V.: *See* Huber-Dyson, V.

Eckmann, B.: *See* Bieri, R.

Edmunds, C. C.: On the endomorphism problem for free groups. Comm. Algebra **3,** 7–20 (1975).

Edmunds, C. C.: Some properties of quadratic words in free groups. Proc. Amer. Math. Soc. **50,** 20–22 (1975).

Edmunds, C. C.: Products of commutators as products of squares. Canad. J. Math. **27,** 1329–1338 (1975).

Edmunds, C. C.: A short combinatorial proof of the Vaught conjecture. Canad. Bull. Math. **18,** 607–608 (1975).

Eilenberg, S., Ganea, T.: On the Lusternik-Schnirelmann category of abstract groups. Ann. of Math. **65,** 512–518 (1957).

Emerson, W.: Groups defined by permutations of a single word. Proc. Amer. Math. Soc. **21,** 386–390 (1969).

Epstein, D. B. A.: Finite presentations of groups and 3-manifolds. Quart. J. Math. **12,** 205–212 (1961).

Epstein, D. B. A.: Ends, topology of 3-manifolds and related topics. In: Proc. Univ. of Georgia Inst. 1961, pp. 110–117. Englewood Cliffs, Prentice-Hall 110–117 (1962).

Epstein, D. B. A.: A group with zero homology. Proc. Cambridge Philos. Soc. **64,** 99–601 (1968), addendum ib. 1237.

Epstein, D. B. A.: *See also* Zieschang, H.

Erdelyi, M.: Systems of equations over non-commutative groups. Acta Univ. Debrecen **2,** 145–149 (1955).

Evans, B.: A class of π_c groups closed under cyclic amalgamation. Bull. Amer. Math. Soc. **79,** 200–201 (1973).

Evans, B.: Cyclic amalgamations of residually finite groups. Pacific J. Math. **55,** 371–379 (1974).

Evans, B., Jaco, W.: Varieties of groups and three-manifolds. Topology **12,** 83–97 (1973).

Evans, R. J.: Free products of two real cyclic matrix groups. Glasgow Math. J. **15,** 121–128 (1974).

Federer, H., Jónsson, B.: Some properties of free groups. Trans. Amer. Math. Soc. **68,** 1–27 (1950).

Fenchel, W.: Estensioni di gruppi descontinui e transformazioni periodiche delle superficie. Rend. Accad. Naz. Lincei, Sc. fis.-mat. e nat., 326–329 (1948).

Fenchel, W.: Bemarkingen om endelige grupper af abbildungsklasser. Mat. Tidssk. B, 90–95 (1950).

Feuer, R. D.: Torsion-free subgroups of triangle groups. Proc. Amer. Math. Soc. **30,** 235–240 (1971).

Fiala, F.: Sur les polyèdres à faces triangulaires. Comment. Math. Helv. **19,** 83–90 (1946).

Fine, B.: The structure of $PSL_2(R)$; R, the ring of integers in a Euclidean quadratic imaginary number field. In: Discontinuous Groups and Riemann Surfaces, Ann. Math. Studies **79,** 145–170 (1974).

Fine, B.: The HNN and generalized free product structure of certain linear groups. Bull. Amer.

Math. Soc. **81**, 413–416 (1975).
Fine, B.: Fuchsian subgroups of the Picard group. Can. J. Math. **28**, 481–485 (1976).
Fine, B., Tretkoff, M.: The SQ-universality of certain arithmetically defined linear groups. J. London Math. Soc. **13**, 65–68 (1976).
Fischer, J.: The subgroups of a tree product of groups. Trans. Amer. Math. Soc. **210**, 27–50 (1975).
Fischer, J., Karrass, A., Solitar, D.: On one-relator groups having elements of finite order. Proc. Amer. Math. Soc. **33**, 297–301 (1972).
Ford, L. R.: Automorphic functions. 2nd ed. New York: Chelsea 1951.
Formanek, E.: *See* Bachmuth, S.
Formanek, E.: *See* Dyer, J. L.
Formanek, E.: Conjugate separability in polycyclic groups. J. Algebra **42**, 1–10 (1976).
Fouxe-Rabinovitch, D. I.: Beispiel einer diskreten Gruppe mit endlich vielen Erzeugenden und Relationen die kein vollständiges System der linearen Darstellungen zuläßt. Dokl. Akad. Nauk SSSR **29**, 549–550 (1940).
Fouxe-Rabinovitch, D. I: On a certain representation of a free group. Leningrad Gos. Univ. Uchen. Zap. Ser. Mat. **10**, 154–157 (1940).
Fouxe-Rabinovitch, D. I.: On the determinators of an operator of the free group. Mat. Sb. **7**, 197–208 (1940).
Fouxe-Rabinovitch, D. I.: Über die Nichteinfachheit einer lokal freien Gruppe. Mat. Sb. **7**, 327–328 (1940).
Fouxe-Rabinovitch, D. I.: Über die Automorphismengruppen der freien Produkte, I, II. Mat. Sb. **8**, 265–276 (1940); **9**, 183–220 (1941).
Fox, R. H.: On Fenchel's conjecture about F-groups. Mat. Tidsskr. B, 61–65 (1952).
Fox, R. H.: Free differential calculue I, II, III, V. Ann. of Math. **57**, 547–560 (1953); **59**, 196–210 (1954); **64**, 407–419 (1956); **71**, 408–422 (1960).
Fox, R. H.: *See also* Crowell, R. H., Chen, K. T.
Fox, R. H., Neuwirth, L.: The braid groups. Math. Scand. **10**, 119–126 (1962).
Frederick, K. N.: The Hopfian property for a class of fundamental groups. Comm. Pure Appl. Math. **16**, 1–8 (1963).
Fricke, R.: Über den arithmetischen Charakter der zu den Verzweigungen (2, 3, 7) und (2, 4, 7) gehörenden Dreiecksfunktionen. Math. Ann. **41**, 443–468 (1892).
Fricke, R., Klein, F.: Vorlesungen über die Theorie der automorphen Funktionen. Vols. I, II. Leipzig: Teubner 1897, 1901–1912.
Fridman, A. A.: On the relation between the word problem and the conjugacy problem in finitely presented groups, Trudy Moskov. Mat. Obsc. **9**, 329–356 (1960).
Fridman, A. A.: Degrees of unsolvability of the word problem for finitely presented groups, Moscow: Izdatelsvo Nauka 1967.
Fridman, A. A.: A solution of the conjugacy problem in a certain class of groups. Trudy Mat. Inst. Steklov 133 233–242 (1973).
Fried, M., Sacerdote, G. S.: Solving diophantine problems over all residue class fields of a number field and all finite fields. Ann. Math. **76**, 203–233 (1976).
Frucht, R.: Remarks on finite groups defined by generating relations. Canad. J. Math. **7**, 8–17 (1955).
Funcke, K.: Nicht frei äquivalente Darstellungen von Knotengruppen mit einer definierenden Relation. Math. Zeit. **141** 205–217 (1975).
Ganea, T.: *See* Eilenberg, S.
Garside, F. A.: The braid group and other groups. Quart. J. Math. **20**, 235–254 (1969).
Gassner, B. J.: On braid groups. Abh. Math. Sem. Univ. Hamburg **25**, 10–22 (1961).
Gerstenhaber, M.: On the algebraic structure of discontinuous groups. Proc. Amer. Math. Soc. **4**, 745–750 (1953).
Gerstenhaber, M., Rothaus, O. S.: The solution of sets of equations in groups. Proc. Nat. Acad. Sci. U.S.A. **48**, 1531–1533 (1962).
Gildenhuys, D.: On pro-*p* groups with a single defining relator. Invent. Math. **5**, 357–366 (1968).
Gildenhuys, D.: Generalizations of Lyndon's theorem on the cohomology of one-relator groups. Canad. J. Math. **28**, 473–480 (1976).
Gildenhuys, D.: The cohomology of groups acting on trees. J. Pure Appl. Alg. **6**, 265–274 (1975).

Gildenhuys, D.: One-relator groups that are residually of prime power order. J. Austral. Math. Soc. **19**, 388–409 (1975).

Gildenhuys, D.: Amalgams of Pro-p-groups with one defining relator. J. Alg. **42**, 11–25 (1976).

Gillette, R., Van Buskirk, J.: The word problem and consequences for the braid groups and mapping class groups of the 2-sphere. Trans. Amer. Math. Soc. **131**, 277–296 (1968).

Gladkii, A. V.: On groups with *k*-reducible bases. Dokl. Akad. Nauk SSSR **134**, 16–18 (1960).

Gladkii, A. V.: On simple Dyck words. Sibirsk Mat. Z. **2**, 36–45 (1961).

Goldberg, K.: Unimodular matrices of order 2 that commute. J. Washington Acad. Sci. **46**, 337–338 (1956).

Goldberg, K., Newman, M.: Pairs of matrices of order two which generate free groups. Illinois J. Math. **1**, 446–448 (1957).

Goldina, N. P.: Solution of some algorithmic problems for free and free nilpotent groups. Uspekhi Mat. Nauk **13**, 183–189 (1958).

Goldina, N. P.: *See also* Golovin, O. N.

Golod, E. S.: On nil-algebras and finitely approximable p-groups. Izv. Akad. Nauk SSSR Ser. Mat. **28**, 273–276 (1964).

Golod, E. S., Shafarevich, I. R.: On the class field tower. Izv. Akad. Nauk SSSR Ser. Mat. **28**, 261–272 (1964).

Golovin, O. N., Goldina, N. P.: Subgroups of free metabelian groups. Mat. Sb. **37**, 323–336 (1955).

Goryushkin, A. P.: Imbedding of countable groups in 2-generator groups. Mat. Zametki **16**, 231–235 (1974).

Gowdy, S.: On Greendlinger eighth-groups. Thesis. Temple Univ. 1971.

Gowdy, S. O.: On *r*-th roots in eighth-groups. Proc. Amer. Math. Soc. **51**, 253–259 (1975).

Greenberg, L.: Discrete groups of motions. Canad. J. Math. **12**, 414–425 (1960).

Greenberg, L.: Maximal Fuchsian groups. Bull. Amer. Math. Soc. **69**, 569–573 (1963).

Greenberg, L.: Note on normal subgroups of the modular group. Proc. Amer. Math. Soc. **17**, 1195–1198 (1966).

Greenberg, L.: Fundamental polygons for Fuchsian groups. J. Analyse Math. **18**, 99–105 (1967).

Greendlinger, M. D.: Dehn's algorithm for the word problem. Comm. Pure Appl. Math. **13**, 67–83 (1960).

Greendlinger, M. D.: On Dehn's algorithms for the conjugacy and word problems with applications. Comm. Pure Appl. Math. **13**, 641–677 (1960).

Greendlinger, M. D.: An analogue of a theorem of Magnus. Arch. Math. **12**, 94–96 (1961).

Greendlinger, M. D.: A class of groups all of whose elements have trivial centralizers. Math. Z. **78**, 91–96 (1962).

Greendlinger, M. D.: On Magnus's generalized word problem. Sibirsk. Mat. Zh. **5**, 955–957 (1964).

Greendlinger, M. D.: Solution by means of Dehn's generalized algorithm of the conjugacy problem for a class of groups which coincide with their anti-centers. Dokl. Akad. Nauk SSSR **158**, 1254–1256 (1964).

Greendlinger, M. D.: Solutions of the word problem for a class of groups by Dehn's algorithm and the conjugacy problem by a generalization of Dehn's algorithm. Dokl. Akad. Nauk SSSR **154**, 507–509 (1964).

Greendlinger, M. D.: Strengthening of two theorems for a class of groups. Sibirsk. Mat. Zh. **6**, 972–984 (1965).

Greendlinger, M. D.: On the word and conjugacy problems. Izv. Akad. Nauk SSSR Ser. Mat. **29**, 245–268 (1965).

Greendlinger, M. D.: The problem of conjugacy and coincidence with an anticenter in the theory of groups. Sibirsk. Mat. Z. **7**, 785–803 (1966).

Greendlinger, M. D.: Conjugacy of subgroups of free groups. Siber. Math. J. **11**, 1178–1180 (1970).

Greendlinger, M. D., Grindlinger, E. I. (editors): Questions in the Theory of Groups and Semigroups. Tulsk Gos. Ped. Inst. Tula 1972.

Gregorac, R. J.: On generalized free products of finite extensions of free groups. J. London Math. Soc. **41**, 662–666 (1966).

Gregorac, R. J.: A note on certain generalized free products. Proc. Amer. Math. Soc. **18**, 754–755 (1967).

Gregorac, R. J.: A note on finitely generated groups. Proc. Amer. Math. Soc. **18,** 756–758 (1967).
Gregorac, R. J.: *See* Allenby, R. B. J. T.
Griffith, P.: Extensions of free groups by torsion groups. Proc. Amer. Math. Soc. **24,** 677–679 (1970).
Griffiths, H. B.: A note on commutators in free products, I, II. Proc. Cambridge Philos. Soc. **50,** 178–188 (1954); **51,** 245–251 (1955).
Griffiths, H. B.: On the fundamental group of a surface, and a theorem of Schreier. Acta Math. **110,** 1–17 (1963).
Griffiths, H. B.: A covering-space approach to residual properties of groups. Michigan Math. J. **14,** 335–348 (1967).
Griffiths, H. B.: A covering-space approach to theorems of Greenberg in Fuchsian, Kleinian and other groups. Comm. Pure Appl. Math. **20,** 365–399 (1967).
Grossman, I., Magnus, W.: Groups and their graphs. New York: Random House 1964.
Grossman, E. K.: On the residual finiteness of certain mapping class groups. J. London Math. Soc. **9,** 160–164 (1974).
Grossman, E. K.: Representations of the automorphism groups of free groups. J. Alg. **30,** 388–399 (1974).
Grossman, E. K.: On certain permutation representations of mapping class groups. Math. Z. **146,** 105–112 (1976).
Grosswald, E.: On the structure of some subgroups of the modular group. Amer. J. Math. **72,** 809–834 (1950).
Grove, L. C.: *See* Benson, C. T.
Gruenberg, K. W.: Resolutions by relations. J. London Math. Soc. **35,** 481–494 (1960).
Gruenberg, K. W.: A new treatment of group extensions. Math. Z. **102,** 340–350 (1967).
Gruenberg, K. W.: Über die Relationenmoduln einer endlichen Gruppe. Math. Z. **118,** 30–33 (1970).
Gruenberg, K. W.: Cohomological topics in group theory. Lecture Notes in Math., Vol. 743. Berlin-Heidelberg-New York: Springer 1970.
Gruenberg, K. W.: Relation Modules of Finite Groups. CBMS Regional Conf. Series, 1976.
Gruenberg, K. W., Roggenkamp, K. W.: Decomposition of the augmentation ideal and of the relation modules of a finite group. Proc. London Math. Soc. **3,** 149–166 (1975).
Gruenberg, K. W.: *See also* Baumslag, G.
Grün, O.: Über eine Faktorgruppe freier Gruppen. J. Deutsch Math. **1,** 772–782 (1936).
Grünenfelder, L.: *See* Bachmann, F.
Grushko, I. A.: La résolution du problème d'identité dans les groupes à plusieurs relations d'un type spécial. Rec. Math. Moscow **3,** 543–550 (1938).
Grushko, I. A.: Über die Basen einem freien Produktes von Gruppen. Mat. Sb. **8,** 169–182 (1940).
Gupta, C. K., Gupta, N. D.: Power series and matrix representations of certain relatively free groups. In: Proc. Conf. Canberra 1973 (Lecture Notes in Math., Vol. 372, pp. 318–329). Berlin-Heidelberg-New York: Springer 1974.
Gupta, N. D.: *See* Gupta, C. K.
Gurevich, G. A.: On the conjugacy problem for groups with one defining relator. Dokl. Akad. Nauk. SSSR **207,** 18–20 (1972).
Gurevich, G. A.: On the conjugacy problem for groups with a single defining relation. Trudy Mat. Inst. Steklov **133,** 109–120 (1973).
Haken, H.: Zum Identitätsproblem bei Gruppen. Math. Z. **56,** 335–362 (1952).
Haken, W.: Connections between topological and group theoretical decision problems. In: Word Problems, pp. 427–441. Amsterdam: North-Holland 1973.
Haken, W.: *See also* Boone, W. W.
Hall, M., Jr.: Coset representations in free groups. Trans. Amer. Math. Soc. **67,** 421–432 (1949).
Hall, M., Jr.: Subgroups of finite index in free groups. Canad. J. Math. **1,** 187–190 (1949).
Hall, M., Jr.: A topology for free groups and related groups. Ann. of Math. **52,** 127–139 (1950).
Hall, M., Jr.: Subgroups of free products. Pacific J. Math. **3,** 115–120 (1953).
Hall, M., Jr.: The theory of groups. New York: Macmillan 1959.
Hall, M., Jr.: Generators and relations in groups—the Burnside problem. Lectures on Modern Mathematics, II, Wiley 1964, pp. 42–92.

Hall, M. Jr., Rado, T.: On Schreier systems in free groups. Trans. Amer. Math. Soc. **64**, 386–408 (1948).

Hall, P.: The splitting properties of relatively free groups. Proc. London Math. Soc. **4**, 343–356 (1954).

Hall, P.: Some word problems. J. London Math. Soc. **33**, 482–496 (1958).

Hall, P.: Nilpotent groups. Canad. Math. Cong. Univ. Alberta. Queen Mary College Math. Notes, 1970.

Hall, P.: Embedding a group in a join of given groups. J. Austral. Math. Soc. **17**, 434–495 (1974).

Harder, G.: A Gauss-Bonnet formula for discrete arithmetically defined groups. Ann. Sci. Ecole Norm. Sup. **4**, 409–455 (1971).

Harrison, N.: Real length functions in groups. Trans. Amer. Math. Soc. **174**, 77–106 (1972).

Harvey, W. J.: *See* Maclachlan, C.

Hempel, J.: Residual finiteness of surface groups. Proc. Amer. Math. Soc. **32**, 323 (1972).

Herbrand, J.: *See* Chevalley, C.

Higgins, P. J.: Presentations of groupoids, with applications to groups. Proc. Cambridge Philos. Soc. **60**, 7–20 (1964).

Higgins, P. J.: Grushko's theorem. J. Algebra **4**, 365–372 (1966).

Higgins, P. J.: Notes on categories and groupoids. London: Van Nostrand 1971.

Higgins, P. J., Lyndon, R. C.: Equivalence of elements under automorphisms of a free group. J. London Math. Soc. **8**, 254–258 (1974).

Higgins, P. J.: The fundamental groupoid of a graph of groups. J. London Math. Soc. **13**, 145–149 (1976).

Higman, G.: The units of group-rings. Proc. London Math. Soc. **46**, 231–248 (1940).

Higman, G.: A finitely generated infinite simple group. J. London Math. Soc. **26**, 61–64 (1951).

Higman, G.: Almost free groups. Proc. London Math. Soc. **1**, 284–290 (1951).

Higman, G.: A finitely related group with an isomorphic proper factor group. J. London Math. Soc. **26**, 59–61 (1951).

Higman, G.: Unrestricted free products and varieties of topological groups. J. London Math. Soc. **27**, 73–81 (1952).

Higman, G.: Subgroups of finitely presented groups. Proc. Royal Soc. London Ser. A **262**, 455–475 (1961).

Higman, G.: Finitely presented infinite simple groups. Notes on Pure Math. **8**, (1974). I. A. S. Austral. Nat. Univ.

Higman, G.: *See also* Boone, W. W.

Higman, G., Neumann, B. H., Neumann, H.: Embedding theorems for groups. J. London Math. Soc. **24**, 247–254 (1949).

Hilden, H.: *See* Birman, J. S.

Hirshon, R.: The intersection of the subgroups of finite index in some finitely presented groups. Proc. Amer. Math. Soc. **53**

Hmelevskii, Yu. I.: The solution of certain systems of equations in words. Dokl. Akad. Nauk SSSR **156**, 749–751 (1964).

Hmelevskii, Yu. I.: Word equations without coefficients. Dokl. Akad. Nauk SSSR **171**, 1047–1049 (1966).

Hmelevskii, Yu. I.: The solution of word equations with three unknowns. Dokl. Akad. Nauk SSSR **177**, 1023–1025 (1967).

Hmelevskii, Yu. I.: Systems of equations in a free group, I, II. Izv. **35**, 1237–1268 (1971); **36**, 110–179 (1972).

Hmelevskii, Yu. I.: Equations in free semigroups. Proc. Steklov Inst. Amer. Math. Soc. Transl. **107**, 272 (1976).

Hoare, A. H. M.: Group rings and lower central series. J. London Math. Soc. **1**, 37–40 (1969).

Hoare, A. H. M., Karrass, A., Solitar, D.: Subgroups of finite index of Fuchsian groups. Math. Z. **120**, 289–298 (1971).

Hoare, A. H. M., Karrass, A., Solitar, D.: Subgroups of infinite index in Fuchsian groups. Math. Z. **125**, 59–69 (1972).

Hoare, A. H. M., Karrass, A., Solitar, D.: Subgroups of NEC groups. Comm. Pure Appl. Math. **26**, 731–744 (1973).

Hoare, A. H. M.: On length functions and Nielsen methods in ree groups. J. London Math. Soc. **14**, 88–92.

Hoare, A. H. M.: *See also* Macheath, A. M.

Hopf, H.: Beiträge zur Klassifizierung der Flächenabbildungen. J. Reine Angew. Math. **165**, 225–236 (1931).

Hopf, H.: Fundamentalgruppe und zweite Bettische Gruppe. Comment. Math. Helv. **14**, 257–309 (1942).

Hopf, H.: Enden offener Räume und unendliche diskontinuierliche Gruppen. Comment. Math. Helv. **16**, 81–100 (1944).

Hopf, H.: Über die Bettischen Gruppen, die zu einer beliebigen Gruppe gehören. Comment. Math. Helv. **17**, 39–79 (1945).

Horowitz, R.: Characters of free groups represented in two-dimensional linear groups. Comm. Pure. Appl. Math. **25**, 635–649 (1972).

Horowitz, R.: Induced automorphisms on Fricke characters of free groups. Trans. Amer. Math. Soc. **208**, 41–50 (1975).

Houghton, C. H.: Ends of groups and the associated first cohomology groups. J. London Math. Soc. **6**, 81–92 (1972).

Houghton, C. H.: Ends of groups and baseless subgroups of wreath products. To appear.

Houghton, C. H., Segal, D.: Some sufficient conditions for groups to have one end. J. London Math. Soc. **10**, 89–96 (1975).

Howson, A. G.: On the intersection of finitely generated free groups. J. London Math. Soc. **29**, 428–434 (1954).

Hughes, I.: The second cohomology groups of one-relator groups. Comm. Pure Appl. Math. **19**, 299-308 (1966).

Hughes, I.: *See also* Bachmuth, S.

Huber-Dyson, V.: The word problem and residually finite groups. Notic Amer. Math. Soc. **11**, 743 (1964).

Huber-Dyson, V.: The undecidability of free groups with a length function. Univ. Calgary Math. Res. Paper **221**, 1–26 (1974).

Humphreys, J. F.: Two-generator conditions for polycyclic groups. J. London Math. Soc. **1**, 21–29 (1969).

Huppert, B.: Endliche Gruppen I. Die Grundlehren der math. Wissenschaften, Bd. 134. Berlin-Heidelberg-New York: Springer 1967.

Hurewicz, W.: Zu einer Arbeit von O. Schreier. Abh. Math. Sem. Univ. Hamburg **8**, 307–314 (1931).

Hurwitz, A.: Über Riemannsche Flächen mit gegebenen Verzweigungspunkten. Math. Ann. **39**, 1–61 (1891).

Hurwitz, R. D.: The conjugacy problem in certain product groups, Thesis, University of Illinois, 1974.

Hurwitz, R. D.: On the conjugacy problem in a free product with commuting subgroups. Math. Ann. **221**, 1–8 (1976).

Ihara, Y.: Algebraic curves mod p and arithmetic groups. Proc. Sympos. Pure Math. Amer. Math. Soc. **9**, 265–272 (1966).

Ihara, Y.: On discrete subgroups of the two by two projective linear groups over p-adic fields. J. Math. Soc. Japan **18**, 219–235 (1966).

Imrich, W.: On the Kurosh subgroup theorem. Seminar über Gruppen und Graphen. Univ. Graz 1975.

Ivanov, S. G.: The membership problem for a free product of groups with an amalgamated subgroup. Siber. Math. J. **16**, 1155–1171 (1975).

Ivanov, S. G.: Schreier systems in a free product of two groups with an amalgamated subgroup. Mat. Zap. Ural. Un-ta **9**, 13–33 (1975).

Iwasawa, K.: Einige Sätze über freie Gruppen. Proc. Imp. Acad. Tokyo **19**, 272–274 (1943).

Jaco, W.: Constructing 3-manifolds from group homomorphisms. Bull. Amer. Math. Soc. **74**, 936–940 (1968).

Jaco, W.: Heegaard splittings and splitting homomorphisms. Trans. Amer. Math. Soc. **144**, 365–379 (1969).

Jaco, W.: Finitely presented subgroups of three-manifold groups. Invent. Math. **13**, 335–346 (1971).

Jaco, W.: Geometric realizations for free quotients. J. Austral. Math. Soc. **11**, 411–418 (1972).

Jaco, W.: *See also* Evans, B.

Jennings, S. A.: The structure of the group ring of a p-group over a modular field. Trans. Amer. Math. Soc. **50**, 175–185 (1941).

Jennings, S. A.: The group ring of a class of infinite nilpotent groups. Canad. J. Math. **7**, 169–187 (1955).

Johnson, D. L.: A note on the Fibonacci groups. Israel J. Math. **17**, 277–282 (1974).

Johnson, D. L.: Extensions of Fibonacci groups. Bull. London Math. Soc. **7**, 101–104 (1974).

Johnson, D. L.: Some infinite Fibonacci groups. Proc. Edinburgh Math. Soc. **19**, 311–314 (1974/75).

Johnson, D. L.: Presentations of Groups. London Math. Soc. Lecture Note Ser. **66**, Cambridge, 1976.

Johnson, D. L., Mawdesley, H.: Some groups of Fibonacci type. J. Austral. Math. Soc. **20**, 199–204 (1975).

Johnson, D. L., Wamsley, J. W.: Minimal relations for certain finite p-groups. Israel J. Math. **8**, 349–356 (1970).

Johnson, D. L., Wamsley, J. M., Wright, D.: The Fibonacci groups. Proc. London Math. Soc. **20**, 577–592 (1974).

Jones, E. C.: Advanced Problem 5636. Amer. Math. Monthly **72**, 1124 (1969).

Jones, J. M. T.: Direct products and the Hopf property. J. Austral. Math. Soc. **17**, 174–196 (1974).

Jónnson, B.: *See* Federer, H.

Justin, J.: Propriétés combinatoires de certains semi-groupes. C. R. Acad. Sci. Paris Ser A **269**, 1113–1115 (1969).

Justin, J.: Groupes et semigroupes à croissance linéaire. C. R. Acad. Sci. Paris Ser. A **273**, 212–213 (1971).

Justin, J.: Characterization of the repetitive commutative semigroups. J. Algebra. To appear.

Kalme, C.: A note on the connectivity of components of Kleinian groups. Trans. Amer. Math. Soc. **137**, 301–307 (1969).

Kalashnikov, V., Kurosh, A.: Free products of groups with amalgamated central subgroup. Dokl. Akad. Nauk SSSR **6**, 285–286 (1935).

Kaplansky, I.: A note on groups without isomorphic subgroups. Bull. Amer. Math. Soc. **51**, 529–530 (1945).

Kargapolov, M. I.: Finitely generated linear groups. Algebra i Logika **6**, 17–20 (1967).

Kargopolov, M. I.: Finite approximability of supersolvable groups with respect to conjugacy. Alg. i Logika **6**, 63–68 (1967).

Kargapolov, M. I., Merzlyaakov, Yu. I., Remeslennikov, V. N.: On a method of group adjunction. Perm. Gos. Univ. Ucen. Zap. **17**, 9–11 (1960).

Kargapolov, M. I., Remeslennikov, V. N.: The conjugacy problem for free solvable groups. Algebra i Logika **5**, 15–25 (1966).

Kargapolov, M. I., Remeslennikov, V. N., Romanovskii, N. S., Romankov, V. A., Curkin, V. A.: Algorithmic questions of o-powered groups. Algebra i Logika **8**, 643–659 (1969).

Karrass, A.: *See* Baumslag, G., Fischer, J., Hoare, A. H. M., Magnus, W.

Karrass, A., Magnus, W., Solitar, D.: Elements of finite order in groups with a single defining relation. Comm. Pure Appl. Math. **13**, 57–66 (1960).

Karrass, A., Pietrowski, A., Solitar, D.: Finite and infinite cyclic extensions of free groups. J. Austral. Math. Soc. **16**, 458–466 (1972).

Karrass, A., Pietrowski, A., Solitar, D.: An improved subgroup theorem for HNN groups with some applications. Canad. J. Math. **26**, 214–224 (1974).

Karrass, A., Pietrowski, A., Solitar, D.: Finitely generated groups with a free subgroup of finite index. J. Austral. Math. Soc. To appear.

Karrass, A., Solitar, D.: Note of a theorem of Schreier. Proc. Amer. Math. Soc. **66**, 696–697 (1957).

Karrass, A., Solitar, D.: Subgroup theorems in the theory of groups given by defining relations. Comm. Pure Appl. Math. **11**, 547–571 (1958).

Karrass, A., Solitar, D.: On free products. Proc. Amer. Math. Soc. **9**, 217–221 (1958).

Karrass, A., Solitar, D.: On the failure of the Howson property for a group with a single defining relation. Math. Z. **108**, 235–236 (1969).

Karrass, A., Solitar, D.: On finitely generated subgroups of a free group. Proc. Amer. Math. Soc. **22**, 209–213 (1969).

Karrass, A., Solitar, D.: On finitely generated subgroups of a free product. Math. Z. **108**, 285–287 (1969).

Karrass, A., Solitar, D.: On groups with one defining relation having an abelian normal subgroup. Proc. Amer. Math. Soc. **23**, 5–10 (1969).

Karrass, A., Solitar, D.: The subgroups of a free product of two groups with an amalgamated subgroup. Trans. Amer. Math. Soc. **150**, 227–255 (1970).

Karrass, A., Solitar, D.: Subgroups of HNN groups and groups with one defining relation. Canad. J. Math. **23**, 627–643 (1971).

Karrass, A., Solitar, D.: The free product of two groups with a malnormal amalgamated subgroup. Canad. J. Math. **23**, 933–959 (1971).

Karrass, A., Solitar, D.: On the presentation of Kleinian function groups. To appear.

Karrass, A., Solitar, D.: On a theorem of Cohen and Lyndon about free bases for normal subgroups. Canad. J. Math. **24**, 1086–1091 (1972).

Karrass, A., Solitar, D.: On finitely generated subgroups which are of finite index in generalized free products. Proc. Amer. Math. Soc. **37**, 22–28 (1973).

Kashincev, E. V.: Generalization of a result of Greendlinger. Ivanov. Gos. Ped. Inst. Uchen. Zap. **61**, 152–155 (1969).

Katz, R., Magnus, W.: Residual properties of free groups. Comm. Pure Appl. Math. **22**, 1–13 (1964).

Keen, L.: Canonical polygons for finitely generated Fuchsian groups. Acta Math. **115**, 1–16 (1966).

Keller, O.-H.: Eine Darstellung der Komposition endlicher Gruppen durch Streckenkomplexe. Math. Ann. **128**, 177–199 (1954).

Keller, R. Diplomarbert, Bochum (1973).

Kesten, H.: Symmetric random walks on groups. Trans. Amer. Math. Soc. **92**, 336–354 (1959).

Kirkinskii, A. S., Remeslennikov, V. N.: The isomorphism problem for solvable groups. Math. Zametki **18**, 437–439 (1975).

Klassen, V. P.: The occurrence problem for a certain class of groups. Algebra i Logika **9**, 306–312 (1970).

Klassen, V. P.: On the occurrence and conjugation problems for certain group extensions. Questions in the Theory of Groups and Semigroups, 87–95. Tulsk Gos. Ped. Inst. Tula 1972.

Klein, F.: Neue Beiträge zur Riemannischen Funktionentheorie. Math. Ann. **21**, 141–218 (1883).

Klein, F.: *See* Fricke, R.

Klein, F., Fricke, R.: Vorlesungen über die Theorie der Elliptischen Modulfunktionen, I, II. Leipzig, 1890–1892.

Knapp, A. W.: Doubly generated Fuchsian groups. Michigan Math. J. **15**, 289–304 (1968).

Kneser, M.: Erzeugende und Relationen verallgemeinerter Einheitengruppen. J. Reine Angew. Math. **214**, 345–349 (1964).

Kopitov, V. M.: The solvability of the occurrence problem in finitely generated solvable matrix groups over an algebraic number field. Algebra i Logika **7**, 53–63 (1968).

Kostrikin, A. I.: On presenting groups by generators and defining relations. Izv. Akad. Nauk SSSR Ser. Mat. **28**, 1119–1122 (1965).

Kostrikin, A. I.: Algebraische Zahlentheorie. Ber. Tagung. Math. Forschung. Oberwolfach. Mannheim: Bibliog. Inst. 1969.

Knopp, M. I., Lehner, J., Newman, M.: Subgroups of F-groups. Math. Ann. **160**, 312–318 (1965).

Kra, I.: Automorphic forms and Kleinian groups. New York: Benjamin 1972.

Krause, H. U.: Gruppenstruktur und Gruppenbild, Thesis, Zürich: ETH Zürich 1953.

Kravitz, S.: On the geometry of Teichmüller spaces and the structure of their modular group. Ann. Acad. Sci. Fenn. Ser. A VI **278**, (1959).

Król, M.: On free generators of the commutator subgroup of a free group. Bull. Acad. Polon. Sci. Sér. Sci. Math. Astronom. Phys. **9**, 279–282 (1961).

Kubota, R.: The subgroup theorem. Arch. Math. **16**, 1–5 (1965).

Kuhn, H. W.: Subgroup theorems for groups presented by generators and relations. Ann. of

Math. **56,** 22–46 (1952).
Kuo Lo, T.-N.: On groups of finite cohomological dimension. J. Algebra **24,** 460–464 (1973).
Kurosh, A. G.: Die Untergruppen der freien Produkte von beliebigen Gruppen. Math. Ann. **109,** 647–660 (1934).
Kurosh, A. G.: Zum Zerlegungsproblem der Theorie der freien Produkte. Rec. Math. Moscow **2,** 995–1001 (1937).
Kurosh, A. G.: The theory of groups, I, II, 2nd ed. (transl. and ed. K. A. Hirsch). New York: Chelsea 1960.
Kurosh, A. G., *See also* Kalashnikov, V.
Kuznetsov, A. V.: Algorithms as operations in algebraic systems, Izv. Akad. Nauk SSSR Ser. Mat. (1958).
Labute, J. P.: On the descending central series of groups with a single defining relation. J. Algebra **14,** 16–23 (1970).
Landman-Dyer, J.: On the isomorphism problem for polycyclic groups. Math. Z. **112,** 145–153 (1969).
Laudenbach, F.: Topologie de la dimension trois. Homotopie et isotopie. Astérisque **12,** Soc. Math. France, 1974.
Lazard, M.: Détermination et généralisation des groupes de dimension des groupes libres. C. R. Acad. Sci. Paris **236,** 1222–1224 (1953).
Lazard, M.: Sur les groupes nilpotents et les anneaux de Lie. Ann. École Norm. Sup. **71,** 101–190 (1953).
Lazard, M.: *See also* Bass, H.
Leech, J. W.: Coset enumeration on digital computors. Proc. Cambridge Philos. Soc. **59,** 257–267 (1963).
Leech, J. W.: Generators for certain normal subgroups of (2, 3, 7). Proc. Cambridge Philos. Soc. **61,** 321–332 (1965).
Leech, J. W.: Note on the abstract group (2, 3, 7; 9). Proc. Cambridge Philos. Soc. **62,** 7–10 (1966).
Leech, J. W.: Coset enumeration. In: Proc. Conf. Oxford 1967 pp. 21–35. Oxford; Pergamon 1970.
Lehner, J.: Representations of a class of infinite groups. Michigan Math. J. **7,** 233–236 (1960).
Lehner, J.: On the generation of discontinuous groups. Pacific J. Math. **13,** 169–170 (1963).
Lehner, J.: Discontinuous groups and automorphic functions. Math. Surveys **8.** Amer. Math. Soc., (1964).
Lehner, J.: A short course in automorphic functions. Winston-Holt 1966.
Lehner, J.: Lectures on modular forms. Nat. Bureau Standards Appl. Math. Ser. **61,** 1969.
Lehner, J.: *See also* Knopp, M. I.
Lehner, J., Newman, M.: Real two-dimensional representations of the modular group and related groups. Amer. J. Math. **87,** 945–954 (1965).
Lehner, J., Newman, M.: Real two-dimensional representations of the free product of two finite cyclic groups. Proc. Cambridge Philos. Soc. **62,** 135–141 (1966).
Lentin, A.: Contribution à une théorie des équations dans les monoïdes libres. Doctorat d'Etat, Paris 1969.
Lentin, A.: Equations dans les monoïdes libres. Math. Sci. Humaines **31,** 5–16 (1970).
Lentin, A.: Équations dans les monoïdes libres. Paris: Gauthier-Villars 1972.
Levi, F. W.: Über die Untergruppen der freien Gruppen, I, II. Math. Z. **32,** 315–318 (1930); **37,** 90–97 (1933).
Levi, F. W.: The commutator group of a free product. J. Indian Math. Soc. **4,** 136–144 (1940).
Levi, F. W.: On the number of generators of a free product, and a lemma of Alexander Kurosch. J. Indian Math. Soc. **5,** 149–155 (1941).
Levi, F. W.: *See also* Baer, R.
Levin, F.: Solutions of equations over groups. Bull. Amer. Math. Soc. **68,** 603–604 (1962).
Levin, F.: One variable equations over groups. Arch. Math. **15,** 179–188 (1964).
Levin, F.: Factor groups of the modular group. J. London Math. Soc. **43,** 195–203 (1968).
Levinson, H.: On the genera of graphs of group presentations, I, II. Ann. New York Acad. Sci. **175,** 277–284 (1970); J. Combinatorial Theory **12,** 205–225 (1972).
Levinson, H., Maskit, B.: Special embeddings of Cayley diagrams. J. Comb. Theory B **18,** 12–17

(1975).
Levinson, H.: *See also* Rapaport, E. S.
Lewin, J.: A finitely presented group whose group of automorphisms is infinitely generated. J. London Math. Soc. **42**, 610–613 (1967).
Lewin, J.: On the intersection of augmentation ideals. J. Algebra **16**, 519–522 (1970).
Lewin, J., Lewin, T.: On center by abelian by one-relator groups. Comm. Pure Appl. Math. **26**, 767–774 (1973).
Lewin, J., Lewin, T.: The group algebra of a torsion-free one-relator group can be embedded in a field. Bull. Amer. Math. Soc. **81**, 947–949 (1975).
Lewin, T. (= Taylor, T.): *See* Baumslag, G., Lewin, J.
Lickorish, W. B. R.: Homeomorphisms of non-orientable 2-manifolds. Proc. Cambridge Philos. Soc. **59**, 307–317 (1963).
Lickorish, W. B. R.: A finite set of generators for the homeotopy group of a 2-manifold. Proc. Cambridge Philos. Soc. **60**, 769–778 (1964); Corrigendum **62**, 679–681.
Liebeck, H.: A test for commutators. Glasgow Math. J. **17**, 31–36 (1976).
Lipschutz, M.: *See* Lipschutz, S.
Lipschutz, S.: Elements in S-groups with trivial centralizers. Comm. Pure Appl. Math. **13**, 679–683 (1964).
Lipschutz, S.: On a finite matrix representation of the braid group. Arch. Math. **12**, 7–12 (1961).
Lipschutz, S.: On powers of elements in S-groups. Proc. Amer. Math. Soc. **13**, 181–186 (1962).
Lipschutz, S.: On square roots in eighth-groups. Comm. Pure Appl. Math. **15**, 39–43 (1962).
Lipschutz, S.: Note on a paper by Shepperd on the braid group. Proc. Amer. Math. Soc. **14**, 225–227 (1963).
Lipschutz, S.: An extension of Greendlinger's results on the word problem. Proc. Amer. Math. Soc. **15**, 37–43 (1964).
Lipschutz, S.: Powers in eighth-groups. Proc. Amer. Math. Soc. **16**, 1105–1106 (1965).
Lipschutz, S.: Generalization of Dehn's result on the conjugacy problem. Proc. Amer. Math. Soc. **17**, 759–762 (1966).
Lipschutz, S.: On powers in generalized free products of groups. Arch. Math. **19**, 575–576 (1968).
Lipschutz, S.: On the conjugacy problem and Greendlinger's eighth-groups. Proc. Amer. Math. Soc. **23**, 101–106 (1969).
Lipschutz, S.: On Greendlinger groups. Comm. Pure Appl. Math. **23**, 743–747 (1970).
Lipschutz, S.: On conjugate powers in eight-groups. Bull. Amer. Math. Soc. **77**, 1050–1051 (1971).
Lipschutz, S.: Note on independent equation problems in groups. Arch. Math. **22**, 113–116 (1971).
Lipschutz, S.: On conjugacy in Greendlinger eighth-groups. Arch. Math. **23**, 121–124 (1972).
Lipschutz, S.: On powers, conjugacy classes and small-cancellation groups. In: Lecture Notes in Math., Vol. 319, pp. 126–132. Berlin-Heidelberg-New York: Springer 1973.
Lipschutz, S.: Identity theorems in small-cancellation groups. Comm. Pure Appl. Math. **26**, 775–780 (1973).
Lipschutz, S.: On the word problem and T-fourth groups. In: Word Problems, pp. 443–452. Amsterdam: North-Holland 1973.
Lipschutz, S.: The conjugacy problem and cyclic amalgamations. Bull. Amer. Math. Soc. **81**, 114–116 (1973).
Lipschutz, S., Lipschutz, M.: A note on root decision problems in groups. Canad. J. Math. **25**, 702–705 (1975).
Lipschutz, S., Miller, C. F. III: Groups with certain solvable and unsolvable decision problems. Comm. Pure Appl. Math. **24**, 7–15 (1971).
Litvinieva, Z. K.: The conjugacy problem for finitely presented groups. Dal'nevostočn Mat. Sb. **1**, 54–71 (1970).
Lloyd, E. K.: Riemann surface transformation groups. J. Combinatorial Theory **13**, 17–27 (1972).
Lorents, A. A.: Solution of systems of equations in one unknown in free groups. Dokl. Akad. Nauk SSSR **148**, 1253–1256 (1963).
Lorents, A. A.: Coefficient-free equations in free groups. Dokl. Akad. Nauk SSSR **160**, 538–540 (1965).
Lorents, A. A.: Representations of sets of solutions of systems of equations with one unknown in a free group. Dokl. Akad. Nauk SSSR **178**, 290–292 (1968).

Losey, G.: On dimension subgroups. Trans. Amer. Math. Soc. **97**, 474–486 (1960).
Losey, G.: On the structure of $Q_2(G)$ for finitely generated groups. Canad. J. Math. **25**, 353–359 (1973).
Lyndon, R. C.: Cohomology theory of groups with a single defining relation. Ann. of Math. **52**, 650–665 (1950).
Lyndon, R. C.: On the Fouxe-Rabinovich series for free groups. Port. Math. **12**, 115–118 (1953).
Lyndon, R. C.: The equation $a^2b^2 = c^2$ in free groups. Michigan Math. J. **6**, 155–164 (1959).
Lyndon, R. C.: Equations in free groups. Trans. Amer. Math. Soc. **96**, 445–457 (1960).
Lyndon, R. C.: Groups with parametric exponents. Trans. Amer. Math. Soc. **96**, 518–533 (1960).
Lyndon, R. C.: Dependence and independence in free groups. J. Reine Angew. Math. **210**, 148–173 (1962).
Lyndon, R. C.: Length functions in groups. Math. Scand. **12**, 209–234 (1963).
Lyndon, R. C.: Grushko's theorem. Proc. Amer. Math. Soc. **16**, 822–826 (1965).
Lyndon, R. C.: Dependence in groups. Colloq. Math. **14**, 275–283 (1966).
Lyndon, R. C.: Equations in free metabelian groups. Proc. Amer. Math. Soc. **17**, 728–730 (1966).
Lyndon, R. C.: On Dehn's algorithm. Math. Ann. **166**, 208–228 (1966).
Lyndon, R. C.: A maximum principle for graphs. J. Combinatorial Theory **3**, 34–37 (1967).
Lyndon, R. C.: On the Freiheitssatz. J. London Math. Soc. **5**, 95–101 (1972).
Lyndon, R. C.: Two notes on Rankin's book on the modular group. J. Austral. Math. Soc. **16**, 454–457 (1973).
Lyndon, R. C.: On products of powers in groups. Comm. Pure Appl. Math. **26**, 781–784 (1973).
Lyndon, R. C.: Geometric methods in the theory of abstract infinite groups. Permutations: actes du colloque, Paris V, 1972, pp. 9–14. Paris: Gauthier-Villars 1974.
Lyndon, R. C.: On non-Euclidean crystallographic groups. In: Proc. Conf. Canberra 1973 (Lecture Notes in Math., Vol. 372, pp. 437–442). Berlin-Heidelberg-New York: Springer 1974.
Lyndon, R. C.: On the combinatorial Riemann-Hurwitz formula. Convegni sui gruppi infiniti, Rome 1973. New York and London: Academic Press 1976 435–439.
Lyndon, R. C.: *See also* Boone, W. W., Chen, K. T., Cohen, D. E., Higgins, P. J.
Lyndon, R. C., McDonough, T., Newman, M.: On products of powers in groups. Proc. Amer. Math. Soc. **40**, 419–420 (1973).
Lyndon, R. C., Newman, M.: Commutators as products of squares. Proc. Amer. Math. Soc. **39**, 267–272 (1973).
Lyndon, R. C., Schützenberger, M. P.: The equation $a^M = b^Nc^P$ in a free group. Michigan Math. J. **9**, 289–298 (1962).
Lyndon, R. C., Ullman, J. L.: Groups of elliptic linear fractional transformations. Proc. Amer. Math. Soc. **18**, 1119–1124 (1967).
Lyndon, R. C., Ullman, J. L.: Pairs of real 2-by-2 matrices that generate free products. Michigan Math. J. **15**, 161–166 (1968).
Lyndon, R. C., Ullman, J. L.: Groups generated by two parabolic linear fractional transformations. Canad. J. Math. **21**, 1388–1403 (1969).
Macbeath, A. M.: Fuchsian groups. Dundee: Queen's College 1961.
Macbeath, A. M.: On a theorem by J. Nielsen. Quart. J. Math. **13**, 235–236 (1962).
Macbeath, A. M.: Packings, free products and residually finite groups. Proc. Cambridge Philos. Soc. **59**, 555–558 (1963).
Macbeath, A. M.: On a theorem of Hurwitz. Glasgow Math. J. **5**, 90–96 (1961).
Macbeath, A. M.: Geometrical realizations of isomorphisms between plane groups. Bull. Amer. Math. Soc. **71**, 629–630 (1965).
Macbeath, A. M.: The classification of non-Euclidean plane crystallographic groups. Canad. J. Math. **6**, 1192–1205 (1967).
Macbeath, A. M.: Generators of the linear fractional groups. Symposium on Number Theory, pp. 14–32. Houston: Amer. Math. Soc. 1967.
Macbeath, A. M.: Action of automorphisms of a compact Riemann surface on the first homology group. Bull. London Math. Soc. **5**, 103–108 (1973).
Macbeath, A. M., Hoare, A. H. M.: Groups of hyperbolic crystallography. Math. Proc. Camb. Phil. Soc. **79**, 235–249 (1976).
Macbeath, A. M., Singerman, D.: Spaces of subgroups and Teichmüller space. Proc. London

Math. Soc. **31**, 211–256 (1975).
MacDonald, B. R.: Automorphisms of GL(S, R). Trans. Amer. Math. Soc. **215**, 145–159 (1976).
MacDonald, I. D.: On a class of finitely presented groups. Canad. J. Math. **14**, 602–613 (1962).
MacDonald, I. D.: On cyclic commutator subgroups. J. London Math. Soc. **38**, 419–422 (1963).
MacHenry, T.: A remark concerning commutator subgroups of free groups, Comm. Pure Appl. Math. **26**, 785–786 (1973).
Macintyre, A.: Omitting quantifier free types in generic structures, J. Symbolic Logic **37**, 512–520 (1972).
Macintyre, A.: On algebraically closed groups, Ann. of Math. **96**, 53–97 (1972).
Maclachlan, C., Harvey, W. J.: On the mapping-class groups and Teichmüller spaces. Proc. London Math. Soc. **30**, 495–512 (1975).
Maclachlin, C.: *See* Harvey, W. J.
MacLane, S.: A proof of the subgroup theorem for free products. Mahematika **5**, 13–19 (1958).
MacLane, S.: Homology. Die Grundlehren der math. Wissenschaften, Bd. 114, 3rd print. corr. Berlin-Heidelberg-New York: Springer 1975.
MacLeod, R. A.: *See* Brenner, J. L.
Magnus, W.: Über diskontinuierliche Gruppen mit einer definierenden Relation (Der Freiheitssatz). J. Reine Angew. Math. **163**, 141–165 (1930).
Magnus, W.: Untersuchungen über einige unendliche diskontinuierliche Gruppen. Math. Ann. **105**, 52–74 (1931).
Magnus, W.: Das Identitätsproblem für Gruppen mit einer definierenden Relation. Math. Ann. **106**, 295–307 (1932).
Magnus, W.: Über Automorphismen von Fundamentalgruppen berandeter Flächen. Math. Ann. **109**, 617–646 (1934).
Magnus, W.: Über *n*-dimensionale Gittertransformationen. Acta Math. **64**, 353–367 (1934).
Magnus, W.: Beziehungen zwischen Gruppen und Idealen in einem speziellen Ring. Math. Ann. **111**, 259–280 (1935).
Magnus, W.: Über Beziehungen zwischen höheren Kommutatoren. J. Reine Angew. Math. **177**, 105–115 (1937).
Magnus, W.: Über freie Faktorgruppen und freie Untergruppen gegebener Gruppen. Monatsh. Math. **47**, 307–313 (1939).
Magnus, W.: On a theorem of Marshall Hall. Ann. of Math. **40**, 764–768 (1939).
Magnus, W.: Residually finite groups. Bull. Amer. Math. Soc. **75**, 305–316 (1969).
Magnus, W.: Braids and Riemann surfaces. Comm. Pure Appl. Math. **25**, 151–161 (1972).
Magnus, W.: Rational representations of Fuchsian groups and non-parabolic subgroups of the modular group. Nachr. Akad. Wiss. Göttingen Math.-Phys. Kl. II, 179–189 (1973).
Magnus, W.: Noneuclidean Tesselations and their Groups, New York and London: Academic Press 1974.
Magnus, W.: Braid groups: a survey. In: Proc. Conf. Canberra 1973 (Lecture Notes in Math., Vol. 372, pp. 494–498). Berlin-Heidelberg-New York: Springer 1974.
Magnus, W.: Two generator subgroups of PSL(2, *C*). Nachr. Akad. Wiss. Göttingen Math.-Phys. Kl. II, **7**, 81–94 (1975).
Magnus, W., Karrass, A., Solitar, D.: Combinatorial group theory. New York: Wiley 1966.
Magnus, W., Peluso, A.: On knot groups. Comm. Pure Appl. Math. **20**, 749–770 (1967).
Magnus, W.: *See also* Grossman, I., Karrass, A., Katz, R.
Magimovski, V. L.: Directly decomposable groups with one defining relation. Sibirsk. Mat. Zh. **8**, 1370–1384 (1967).
Makanin, G. S.: The conjugacy problem in the braid group. Dokl. Akad. Nauk SSSR **182**, 495–496 (1968).
Makanin, G. S.: On systems of equations in free groups. Sibirsk. Mat. Zh. **13**, 587–595 (1972).
Malcev, A. I.: On isomorphic matrix representations of infinite groups. Mat. Sb. **8**, 405–422 (1940).
Malcev, A. I.: On homomorphisms onto finite groups. Uchen. Zap. Karel. Ped. Inst. Ser. Fiz.-Mat. Nauk **18**, 49–60 (1958).
Malcev, A. I.: The undecidability of the elementary theory of finite groups. Dokl. Akad. Nauk SSSR **138**, 771–774 (1961).
Malcev, A. I.: On the equation $zxyx^{-1}y^{-1}z^{-1} = aba^{-1}b^{-1}$ in a free group. Algebra i Logika **1**,

45–50 (1962).
Mangler, W.: Die Klassen topologischer Abbildungen einer geschlossenen Fläche auf sich. Math. Z. **44**, 541–554 (1939).
Marden, A.: On finitely generated Fuchsian groups. Comment. Math. Helv. **42**, 81–85 (1967).
Marden, A.: Schottky groups and circles. In: Contributions to Analysis. Academic Press, 1974, 273–278.
Markov, A.: Über die freie Äquivalenz der geschlossenen Zöpfe. Mat. Sb. **43**, 73–78 (1936).
Markov, A.: Foundations of the algebraic theory of braids. Trudy Mat. Inst. Steklov **16**, 55 (1945).
Markov, A. A.: On certain insoluble problems concerning matrices. Dokl. Akad. Nauk SSSR **57**, 539–542 (1947).
Markov, A. A.: Zum Problem der Darstellbarkeit von Matrizen. Z. Math. Logik Grundlagen Math. **4**, 157–168 (1958).
Markov, A. A.: The insolubility of the problem of homeomorphy. Dokl. Akad. Nauk SSSR **121**, 218–220 (1958).
Markov, A. A.: Unsolvability of certain problems in topology. Dokl. Akad. Nauk SSSR **123**, 978–980 (1958).
Markov, A. A.: Insolubility of the problem of homeomorphy. In: Proc. Internat. Cong. Cambridge 1958, pp. 300–306. Cambridge: Cambridge Univ. Press 1960, 300–306.
Maschke, H.: The representation of finite groups, especially of the rotation groups of the regular bodies in three- and four-dimensional space, by Cayley's color diagrams. Amer. J. Math. **18**, 156–194 (1896).
Maskit, B.: *See* Levinson, H.
Maskit, B.: A theorem of planar covering surfaces with applications to 3-manifolds. Ann. of Math. **81**, 361–365 (1965).
Maskit, B.: A characterization of Schottky groups. J. Analyse Math. **19**, 227–230 (1967).
Maskit, B.: On Klein's combination theorem I, II, III. Trans. Amer. Math. Soc. **120**, 499–509 (1965); **131**, 32–39 (1968); Ann. of Math. Studies **66**, 297–316 (1971).
Maskit, B.: On Poincaré's theorem for fundamental polygons. Advances Math. **7**, 219–230 (1971).
Massey, W. S.: Algebraic topology: an introduction. New York: Harcourt, Brace, and World 1967.
Mathieu, Y., Vincent, B.: A propos des groupes de noeuds qui sont desproduits libres amalgamés non triviaux. C. R. Acad. Paris **682**, A1045–1047 (1975).
Matiyasevich, Yu. V.: Enumerable sets are Diophantine. Dokl. Akad. Nauk SSSR **191**, 279–282 (1970). English translation: Soviet Math. Dokl. **11**, 354–357 (1970).
Matiyasevich, Yu. V.: Diophantine representation of enumerable predicates, Izv. Akad. Nauk SSSR Ser. Mat. **35**, 3–30 (1971).
Matsumoto, M.: Générateurs et relations des groupes de Weyl généralisés. C. R. Acad. Sci. Paris Sér. A **258**, 3419–3422 (1964).
Mayoh, B. H.: Groups and semigroups with solvable word problems. Proc. Amer. Math. Soc. **18**, 1038–1039 (1967).
Mawdesley, H.: *See* Johnson, D. L.
McCool, J.: Elements of finite order in free product sixth-groups. Glasgow Math. J. **9**, 128–145 (1969).
McCool, J.: The order problem and the power problem for free product sixth-groups. Glasgow Math. J. **10**, 1–9 (1969).
McCool, J.: Embedding theorems for countable groups. Canad. J. Math. **22**, 827–835 (1970).
McCool, J.: The power problem for groups with one defining relator. Proc. Amer. Math. Soc. **28**, 427–430 (1971).
McCool, J.: A presentation for the automorphism group of a free group of finite rank. J. London Math. Soc. **8**, 259–266 (1974).
McCool, J.: On Nielsen's presentation of the automorphism group of a free group. J. London Math. Soc. **10**, 265–170 (1975).
McCool, J.: Some finitely presented subgroups of the automorphism group of a free group. J. Algebra **35**, 205–213 (1975).
McCool, J., Pietrowski, A.: On free products with amalgamation of two infinite cyclic groups. J. Algebra **18**, 377–383 (1971).

McCool, J., Pietrowski, A.: On recognizing certain one relator presentations. Proc. Amer. Math. Soc. **36**, 31–33 (1972).

McCool, J., Schupp, P. E.: On one relator groups and HNN extensions. J. Austral. Math. Soc. **16**, 249–256 (1973).

McDonough, T.: *See* Lyndon, R. C.

McKenzie, R., Thompson, R. J.: An elementary construction of unsolvable word problems in group theory. In: Word Problems, pp. 457–478. Amsterdam: North-Holland 1973.

Mendelsohn, N. S.: An algorithmic solution for a word problem in group theory. Canad. J. Math. **16**, 509–516 (1964); correction, **17**, 505 (1965).

Mendelsohn, N. S.: *See also* Ree, R.

Mennicke, J. L.: Einige endliche Gruppen mit drei Erzeugenden und drei Relationen. Arch. Math. **10**, 409–418 (1959).

Mennicke, J. L.: A note on regular coverings of closed orientable surfaces. Proc. Glasgow Math. Assoc. **5**, 49–66 (1961).

Mennicke, J. L.: Finite factor groups of the unimodular group. Ann. of Math. **81**, 316–337 (1965).

Mennicke, J. L.: Eine Bemerkung über Fuchssche Gruppen. Invent. Math. **2**, 301–305 (1967); corrigendum, **6**, 106 (1968).

Mennicke, J. L.: On Ihara's modular group. Invent. Math. **4**, 202–228 (1967).

Mennicke, J. L.: *See also* Behr, H.

Merzlyaakov, J. U.: *See* Kargapolov, M. I.

Meskin, S.: On some groups with a single defining relation. Math. Ann. **184**, 193–196 (1969).

Meskin, S.: Nonresidually finite one-relator groups. Trans. Amer. Math. Soc. **164**, 105–114 (1972).

Meskin, S.: One relator groups with center. J. Austral. Math. Soc. **16**, 319–323 (1973).

Meskin, S.: Periodic automorphisms of the two-generator free group. In: Proc. Conf. Canberra 1973 (Lecture Notes in Math., Vol. 372, pp. 494–498). Berlin-Heidelberg-New York: Springer 1974.

Meskin, S.: A finitely generated residually finite group with an unsolvable word problem. Proc. Amer. Math. Soc. **43**, 8–10 (1974).

Meskin, S.: The isomorphism problem for a class of one-relator groups. Math. Ann. **217**, 53–57 (1975).

Meskin, S., Pietrowski, A., Steinberg, A.: One-relator groups with center. J. Austral. Math. Soc. **16**, 319–323 (1973).

Metzler, W.: Über den Homotopietyp zweidimensionaler CW-Komplexe und Elementartransformationen bei Darstellungen von Gruppen durch Erzeugende und definierende Relationen. Preprint.

Mikhailova, K. A.: The occurrence problem for direct products of groups. Dokl. Akad. Nauk SSSR **119**, 1103–1105 (1958).

Mikhailova, K. A.: The occurrence problem for free products of groups. Dokl. Akad. Nauk SSSR **127**, 746–748 (1959).

Mikhailova, K. A.: The occurrence problem for direct products of groups. Mat. Sb. **70**, 241–251 (1966).

Mikhailova, K. A.: The occurence problem for free products of groups. Mat. Sb. **75**, 199–210 (1968).

Mikalev, A. V.: *See* Zaleskii, A. E.

Miller, C. F. III: On Britton's theorem A. Proc. Amer. Math. Soc. **19**, 1151–1154 (1968).

Miller, C. F. III: On group-theoretic decision problems and their classification. Ann. of Math. Studies **68**. Princeton: Princeton University Press 1971.

Miller, C. F. III: *See also* Lipschutz, S.

Miller, C. F. III, Schupp, P. E.: Embeddings into Hopfian groups. J. Algebra **17**, 171–176 (1971).

Miller, C. F. III, Schupp, P. E.: The geometry of HNN extensions. Comm. Pure Appl. Math. **26**, 787–802 (1973).

Miller, G. A.: On the groups generated by two operators. Bull. Amer. Math. Soc. **7**, 424–426 (1900).

Miller, G. A.: On the groups generated by two operators of orders two and three respectively whose product is of order six. Quart. J. Math. **33**, 76–79 (1901).

Miller, G. A.: Groups defined by the orders of two generators and the order of their product.

Amer. J. Math. **24,** 96–100 (1902).
Miller, G. A.: The groups generated by two operators which have a common square. Arch. Math. Phys. **9,** 6–7 (1908).
Miller, G. A.: Finite groups which may be defined by two operators satisfying two conditions. Amer. J. Math. **31,** 167–182 (1909).
Miller, G. A.: Groups generated by two operators of order three whose product is of order four. Bull. Amer. Math. Soc. **26,** 361–369 (1920).
Millington, M. H.: Subgroups of the classical modular group. J. London Math. Soc. **1,** 351–357 (1969).
Milnor, J.: Advanced problem 3603. Amer. Math. Monthly **75,** 685–686 (1968).
Milnor, J.: A note on curvature and fundamental groups. J. Differential Geometry **2,** 1–7 (1968).
Milnor, J.: Growth of finitely generated solvable groups. J. Differential Geometry **2,** 447–449 (1968).
Mital, J. N., Passi, I. B. S.: Annihilators of relation modules. J. Austral. Math. Soc. **16,** 228–233 (1973).
Mochizuki, H. Y.: *See* Bachmuth, S.
Moldavanskii, D. I.: Certain subgroups of groups with one defining relation. Sibirsk. Mat. Z. **8,** 1370–1384 (1967).
Moldavanskii, D. I.: The intersection of finitely generated subgroups. Sibirsk. Mat. Z. **9,** 1422–1426 (1968).
Moldavanskii, D. I.: Conjugacy of subgroups of a free group. Algebra i Logika **8,** 691–694 (1969).
Moldavanskii, D. I.: A certain theorem of Magnus. Ivanov. Gos. Ped. Inst. Uchen. Zap. **44,** 26–28 (1969).
Moldavanskii, D. I.: Nielsen's method for a free product of groups. Ivanov. Gos. Ped. Inst. Uchen. Zap. **61,** 170–182 (1969).
Moran, S.: Dimension subgroups modulo n. Proc. Cambridge Philos. Soc. **68,** 579–582 (1970).
Moser, W. C. J.: *See* Coxeter, H. S. M.
Mostowski, A. W.: On automorphisms of relatively free groups. Fund. Math. **50,** 403–411 (1961/62).
Mostowski, A. W.: On the decidability of some problems in special classes of groups. Fund. Math. **59,** 123–135 (1966).
Mostowski, A. W.: Decision problems in group theory. Tech. Report **19,** Univ. Iowa, 1969.
Murasugi, K.: The center of a group with a single defining relation. Math. Ann. **155,** 246–251 (1964).
Murasugi, K.: The center of the group of a link. Proc. Amer. Math. Soc. **16,** 1052–1057 (1965), errata, **18,** 1142 (1967).
Mycielski, J.: *See* Balcerzyk, S.
Nagao, H.: On $GL(2, K[x])$. J. Inst. Polytech. Osaka City Univ. Ser. A **10,** 117–121 (1959).
Nagata, M.: On automorphism group of $k[x, y]$. Lectures on Math. Kyoto **5,** (1972).
Neukirch, J.: *See* Binz, E.
Neumann, B. H.: Die Automorphismengruppe der freien Gruppen. Math. Ann. **107,** 367–386 (1932).
Neumann, B. H.: Some remarks on infinite groups. J. London Math. Soc. **12,** 120–127 (1937).
Neumann, B. H.: On the number of generators of a free product. J. London Math. Soc. **18,** 12–20 (1943).
Neumann, B. H.: Adjunction of elements to groups. J. London Math. Soc. **18,** 4–11 (1943).
Neumann, B. H.: On a special class of infinite groups. Nieuw Arch. Wisk. **23,** 117–127 (1950).
Neumann, B. H.: A two-generator group isomorphic to a proper factor group. J. London Math. Soc. **25,** 247–248 (1950).
Neumann, B. H.: A note on algebraically closed groups. J. London Math. Soc. **27,** 227–242 (1952).
Neumann, B. H.: On a problem of Hopf. J. London Math. Soc. **28,** 351–353 (1953).
Neumann, B. H.: An essay on free products of groups with amalgamations. Philos. Trans. Roy. Soc. London Ser. A **246,** 503–554 (1954).
Neumann, B. H.: On a conjecture of Hanna Neumann. Proc. Glasgow Math. Assoc. **3,** 13–17 (1956).
Neumann, B. H.: On some finite groups with trivial multiplicator. Publ. Math. Debrecen **4,** 190–

194 (1956).
Neumann, B. H.: On characteristic subgroups of free groups. Math. Z. **94**, 143–151 (1966).
Neumann, B. H.: The isomorphism problem for algebraically closed groups. In: Word Problems, pp. 553–562. Amsterdam: North-Holland 1973.
Neumann, B. H.: *See also* Higman, G.
Neumann, B. H., Neumann, H.: A remark on generalised free products. J. London Math. Soc. **25**, 202–204 (1950).
Neumann, B. H., Neumann, H.: Zwei Klassen charakteristischer Untergruppen und ihrer Faktorgruppen. Math. Nachr. **4**, 106–125 (1951).
Neumann, B. H., Neumann, H.: Embedding theorems for groups. J. London Math. Soc. **34**, 465–479 (1959).
Neumann, H.: Generalised free products with amalgamated subgroups, I, II. Amer. J. Math. **70**, 590–625 (1948); **71**, 491–540 (1949).
Neumann, H.: Generalised free sums of cyclical groups. Amer. J. Math. **72**, 671–685 (1950).
Neumann, H.: On the intersection of finitely generated free groups. Publ. Math. Debrecen **4**, 36–39 (1956); addendum, **5**, 128 (1957).
Neumann, H.: Varieties of Groups. Ergebnisse der Mathematik, Bd. 37. Berlin-Heidelberg-New York: Springer 1967.
Neumann, H.: *See also* Higman, G., Neumann, B. H.
Neumann, P. M.: The SQ-universality of some finitely presented groups. J. Austral. Math. Soc. **16**, 1–6 (1973).
Neumann, P. M., Newman, M. F.: On Schreier varieties of groups. Math. Z. **98**, 196–199 (1967).
Neumann, P. M., Wiegold, J.: Schreier varieties of groups. Math. Z. **85**, 392–400 (1964).
Neuwirth, L. P.: An alternative proof of a theorem of Iwasawa on free groups. Proc. Cambridge Philos. Soc. **57**, 895–896 (1961).
Neuwirth, L. P.: Knot groups. Ann. of Math. Studies **56**, (1965).
Neuwirth, L. P.: An algorithm for the construction of 3-manifolds from 2-complexes. Proc. Cambridge Philos. Soc. **64**, 603–613 (1968).
Neuwirth, L. P.: Some algebra for 3-manifolds. In: Topol. of Manifolds (Proc. Inst. Univ. Georgia 1969, pp. 179–184). Chicago: Markhan 1970.
Neuwirth, L. P.: The status of some problems related to knot groups. In: Topology Conference (Lecture Notes in Math., Vol. 375, pp. 209–230). Berlin-Heidelberg-New York: Springer 1974.
Newman, B. B.: Some results on one-relator groups. Bull. Amer. Math. Soc. **74**, 568–571 (1968).
Newman, B. B.: The soluble subgroups of a one-relator group with torsion. J. Austral. Math. Soc. **16**, 278–285 (1973).
Newman, M.: Some free products of cyclic groups. Michigan Math. J. **9**, 369–373 (1962).
Newman, M.: Free subgroups and normal subgroups of the modular group. Illinois J. Math. **8**, 262–265 (1964).
Newman, M.: Classification of normal subgroups of the modular group. Trans. Amer. Math. Soc. **126**, 267–277 (1967).
Newman, M.: Pairs of matrices generating discrete free groups and free products. Michigan Math. J. **15**, 155–160 (1968).
Newman, M.: *See also* Knopp, M. I., Lehner, J., Lyndon, R. C.
Newman, M. F.: *See* Neumann, P. M.
Nielsen, J.: Die Isomorphismen der allgemeinen unendlichen Gruppe mit zwei Erzeugenden. Math. Ann. **78**, 385–397 (1918).
Nielsen, J.: Über die Isomorphismen unendlicher Gruppen ohne Relation. Math. Ann. **79**, 269–272 (1919).
Nielsen, J.: Om Regning med ikke kommutative Faktoren og dens Anvendelse i Gruppeteorien. Mat. Tidsskr. B, 77–94 (1921).
Nielsen, J.: Die isomorphismengruppe der freien Gruppen. Math. Ann. **91**, 169–209 (1924).
Nielsen, J.: Die Gruppe der dreidimensionalen Gittertransformationen. Danske Vid. Selsk. Mat.-Fys. Medd. **12**, 1–29 (1924).
Nielsen, J.: Über topologische Abbildungen geschlossener Flächen. Abh. Math. Sem. Univ. Hamburg **3**, 246–260 (1924).
Nielsen, J.: Untersuchungen zur Topologie der geschlossenen zweiseitigen Flächen, I, II, III.

Acta Math. **50,** 189–358 (1927); **53,** 1–76 (1929); **58,** 87–167 (1931).
Nielsen, J.: Über Gruppen linearer Transformationen. Mitt. Math. Gesellsch. Hamburg **8,** 82–104 (1940).
Nielsen, J.: Abbildungsklassen endlicher Ordnung. Acta Math. **75,** 23–115 (1942).
Nielsen, J.: Surface transformation classes of algebraically finite type. Danske Vid. Selsk. Math.-Fys. Medd. **21,** 1–89 (1944).
Nielsen, J.: The commutator group of the free product of cyclic groups. Mat. Tidsskr. B, 49–56 (1948).
Nielsen, J.: Nogle grundlaeggende begreber vedrorende diskontinuerte grupper af lineaere substitutioner i en kompleks variabel. 11th Scand. Math. Cong. Trondheim 1946, pp. 61–70.
Nielsen, J.: A basis for subgroups of free groups. Math. Scand. **3,** 31–43 (1955).
Nielsen, J.: *See also* Bungaard, S.
Nielsen, J., Bundgaard, S.: Forenklede Bevizer for nogle Satningen i Flacktopologien. Mat. Tidssk. B, 1–16 (1946).
Nivat, M.: Sur le noyau d'un homomorphisme du monoïde libre dans un groupe libre. Sem. Schützenberger-Lentin-Nivat 69/70, Paris 1970.
Novikov, P. S.: On algorithmic unsolvability of the problem of identity. Dokl. Akad. Nauk SSSR **85,** 709–712 (1952).
Novikov, P. S.: Unsolvability of the conjugacy problem in the theory of groups. Izv. Akad. Nauk SSSR Ser. Mat. **18,** 485–524 (1954).
Novikov, P. S.: On the algorithmic unsolvability of the word problem in group theory. Trudy Mat. Inst. Steklov **44,** 143 (1955).
Novikov, P. S.: The unsolvability of the problem of the equivalence of words in a group and several other problems in algebra. Czechoslovak Math. J. **6,** 450–454 (1956).
Novikov, P. S.: Über einige algorithmische Probleme der Gruppentheorie. Jber. Deutsch. Math. Verein. **61,** 88–92 (1958).
Novikov, P. S., Adyan, S. I.: Commutative subgroups and the conjugacy problem in free periodic groups of odd exponent. Izv. Akad. Nauk SSSR Ser. Mat. **32,** 1176–1190 (1968).
Novikov, P. S., Adyan, S. I.: Defining relations and the word problem for free periodic groups of odd exponent. Izv. Akad. Nauk SSSR Ser. Mat. **32,** 971–979 (1968).
Ojanguren, M.: Algebraischer Beweis zweier Formeln von H. Hopf aus der Homologietheorie der Gruppen. Math. Z. **94,** 391–395 (1966).
Ojanguren, M.: Sur les présentations libres des groupes finis. C. R. Acad. Sci. Paris Sér. A-B **264,** A60–61 (1967).
Ojanguren, M.: Freie Präsentierungen endlicher Gruppen und zugehörige Darstellungen. Math. Z. **106,** 293–311 (1968).
Olesky, D. D.: *See* Brenner, J. L.
Olshanskii, A.Yu.: The characteristic subgroups of free groups. Izv. Akad. Nauk SSSR Ser. Mat. **29,** 179–180 (1974).
Ordman, E. T.: Subgroups of amalgamated free products. Bull. Amer. Math. Soc. **76,** 358–360 (1970).
Ordman, E. T.: On subgroups of amalgamated free products. Proc. Cambridge Philos. Soc. **69,** 13–23 (1971).
Osborne, R. P.: On the 4-dimensional Poincaré conjecture for manifolds with 2-dimensional spines. Canad. Math. Bull. **17,** 549–552 (1974).
Osborne, R. P., Stevens, R. S.: Group presentations corresponding to spines of 3-manifolds, I, II, III, Iv. To appear.
Oxley, P.: Ends of groups and a related construction, Thesis. Queen Mary College, 1971.
Papakyriakopoulos, C. D.: On solid tori. Proc. London Math. Soc. **32,** 281–299 (1957).
Papakyriakopoulos, C. D.: On Dehn's lemma and the asphericity of knots. Ann. of Math. **66,** 1–26 (1957).
Parmenter, M. M., Passi, I. B. S., Sehgal, S. K.: Polynomial ideals in group rings. Canad. J. Math. To appear.
Passi, I. B. S.: Polynomial maps on groups. J. Algebra **9,** 121–151 (1968).
Passi, I. B. S.: Dimension subgroups. J. Algebra **9,** 152–182 (1968).
Passi, I. B. S.: Polynomial functors. Proc. Cambridge Philos. Soc. **66,** 505–512 (1969).

Passi, I. B. S., Sehgal, S. K.: Lie dimension groups. Comm. Algebra **3**, 59–73 (1975).
Passi, I. B. S., Sharma, S.: The third dimension subgroup mod n. J. London Math. Soc. **9**, 176–182 (1975).
Patterson, S. J.: On the cohomology of Fuchsian groups. Glasgow Math. J. **16**, 123–140 (1975).
Peczynski, N.: Eine Kennzeichnung der Relationen der Fundamentalgruppe einer nicht-orientierbaren geschlossenen Fläche, Diplomarbeit, Bochum; Ruhr-Univ. 1972.
Peczynski, N., Rosenberger, G., Zieschang, H.: Von Untergruppen der Triangel-Gruppen. Invent. Math. to appear.
Peczynski, N., Rosenberger, G., Zieschang, H.: Uber Erzeugende ebener diskontinuierlicher Gruppen. Abstract. In: Proc. Conf. Canberra 1973 (Lecture Notes in Math., Vol. 372, pp. 562–564). Berlin-Heidelberg-New York: Springer 1974.
Peczynski, N., Rosenberger, G., Zieschang, H.: Uber Erzeugende ebener diskontinuierlicher Gruppen. Inventiones Math. **29**, 161–180 (1975).
Peiffer, R.: Über Identitäten zwischen Relationen. Math. Ann. **121**, 67–99 (1949).
Peluso, A.: A residual property of free groups. Comm. Pure. Appl. Math. **19**, 435–437 (1967).
Peluso, A.: *See also* Magnus, W.
Petresco, J.: Sur les commutateurs. Math. Z. **61**, 348–356 (1954).
Petresco, J.: Sur les groupes libres. Bull. Sci. Math. **80**, 6–32 (1956).
Petresco, J.: Sur le théorème de Kuroš dans les produits libres. Ann. Sci. École Norm. Sup. **75**, 107–123 (1958).
Petresco, J.: Algorithmes de décision et de construction dans les groupes libres. Math. Z. **79**, 32–43 (1962).
Petresco, J.: Systèmes minimaux de relations fondamentales dans les groupes de rang fini. Sem. Dubreil-Pisot, Paris 1955/56.
Petresco, J.: Prégroupes de mots et problème des mots. Sem. Dubreil-Dubreil-Jacotin-Lesieur-Pisot, Paris, 1967/68.
Pietrowski, A.: The isomorphism problem for one-relator groups with non-trivial centre. Math. Z. **136**, 95–106 (1974).
Pietrowski, A.: *See also* Dunwoody, M. J., Karrass, A., McCool, J.
Piollet, D.: Sur les systèmes d'équations strictement quadratiques dans un monoïde libre. C. R. Acad. Sci. Paris Ser. A **273**, 967–970 (1971).
Piollet, D.: Sur les équations quadratiques dans un groupe libre. C. R. Acad. Sci. Paris Sér. A **274**, 1697–1699 (1972).
Piollet, D.: Equations quadratiques dans le groupe libre. J. Algebra **33**, 395–404 (1975).
Poénaru, V.: Groupes Discrets. Lecture Notes in Math., Vol. 421. Berlin-Heidelberg-New York: Springer 1974.
Poénaru, V.: *See* Boone, W. W.
Poincaré, H.: Théorie des groupes fuchsiens. Acta Math. **1**, 1–62 (1882).
Poincaré, H.: Mémoire sur les groupes kleinéens. Acta Math. **3**, 49–92 (1883).
Prener, R.: *See* Anshel, M.
Pressburger, N.: Über die Vollständigkeit eines gewissen Systems der Arithmetik ganzer Zahlen, in welchem die addition als einzige Operation hervortritt. Comptes Rendus 1er Congr. Math. Pays Slaves, 92–101 (1929).
Pride, S.: Certain subgroups of one-relator groups. Math. Z. **146**, 1–6 (1976).
Pride, S. J.: Residual properties of free groups. I, II, III. Pacific J. Math. **43**, 725–733 (1972); Bull. Austral. Math. Soc. 7, 113–120 (1972); Math. Z. **132**, 245–248 (1973).
Pride, S. J.: On the Nielsen equivalence of pairs of generators for certain HNN-groups. In: Proc. Conf. Canberra 1973 (Lecture Notes in Math., Vol. 372, pp. 580–588). Berlin-Heidelberg-New York: Springer 1974.
Pride, S. J.: On the generation of one-relator groups. Trans. Amer. Math. Soc. **210**, 331–364 (1975).
Prisco, R.: On free products, conjugating factors, and Hopfian groups, Thesis. Adelphi Univ. 1967.
Purzitsky, N.: Two-generator discrete free products. Math. Z. **126**, 209–223 (1972).
Purzitsky, N.: Canonical generators of Fuchsian groups. Illinois J. Math. **18**, 484–490 (1974).
Purzitsky, N.: Real two-generator representation of two-generator free groups. Math. Z. **127**, 95–104 (1972).
Purzitsky, N.: All two-generator Fuchsian groups. Math. Z. **147**, 87–92 (1976).

Purzitsky, N., Rosenberger, G.: Two generator Fuchsian groups of genus one. Math. Z. **128,** 245–251 (1972); correction, ibid. **132,** 261–262 (1973).
Quillen, D. G.: On the associated graded ring of a group ring. J. Algebra **10,** 411–418 (1968).
Rabin, M. O.: Recursive unsolvability of group theoretic problems. Ann. of Math. **67,** 172–174 (1958).
Rademacher, H.: Über die Erzeugenden von Kongruenzuntergruppen der Modulgruppe. Abh. Math. Sem. Univ. Hamburg **7,** 134–148 (1929).
Rado, T.: *See* Hall,M., Jr.
Rankin, R. A.: The modular group and its subgroups. Bombay: Ramanujan Inst. 1969.
Rapaport, E. S.: On free groups and their automorphisms. Acta Math. **99,** 139–163 (1958).
Rapaport, E. S.: Note on Nielsen transformations. Proc. Amer. Math. Soc. **10,** 228–235 (1959).
Rapaport, E. S.: Cayley color groups and Hamilton lines, Scripta Math. **24,** 51–58 (1959).
Rapaport, E. S.: On the commutator subgroup of a knot group. Ann. of Math. **71,** 157–162 (1960).
Rapaport, E. S.: On the defining relations of a free product. Pacific J. Math. **14,** 1389–1393 (1964).
Rapaport, E. S.: Groups of order 1. Proc. Amer. Math. Soc. **15,** 828–833 (1964).
Rapaport, E. S.: Remarks on groups of order 1. Amer. Math. Monthly **75,** 714–720 (1968).
Rapaport, E. S.: Groups of order 1: some properties of presentations. Acta Math. **121,** 127–150 (1968).
Rapaport, E. S.: Finitely presented groups: the deficiency. J. Algebra **24,** 531–543 (1973).
Rapaport, E. S., Levinson, H. W.: Planarity of Cayley diagrams. Proc. Colloq. Kalamazoo 1972.
Rapaport, E. S.: *See* Strasser, E. R.
Ree, R.: Commutator groups of free products of torsion free abelian groups. Ann. of Math. **66,** 380–394 (1957).
Ree, R.: On certain pairs of matrices which do not generate a free group. Canad. Math. Bull. **4,** 49–51 (1961).
Ree, R., Mendelsohn, N. S.: Free subgroups of groups with a single defining relation. Arch. Math. **19,** 577–580 (1968).
Reidemeister, K.: Knoten und Gruppen. Abh. Math. Sem. Univ. Hamburg **5,** 8–23 (1926).
Reidemeister, K.: Über endliche diskrete Gruppen. Abh. Math. Sem. Univ. Hamburg **5,** 33–39 (1927).
Reidemeister, K.: Über Identitäten von Relationen. Abh. Math. Sem. Univ. Hamburg **16,** 114–118 (1949).
Reidemeister, K.: Einführung in die kombinatorische Topologie. New York: Chelsea 1950.
Reidemeister, K.: Complexes and homotopy chains. Bull. Amer. Math. Soc. **56,** 297–307 (1950).
Reidemeister, K., Brandis, A.: Über freie Erzeugendensysteme der Wegegruppen eines zusammenhängenden Graphen. Sammelband zu Ehren des 250. Geburtstages Eulers, pp. 284–292. Berlin; Akademie-Verlag 1959.
Reiner, I.: Automorphisms of the modular group. Trans. Amer. Math. Soc. **80,** 35–50 (1955).
Reiner, I.: Subgroups of the unimodular group. Proc. Amer. Math. Soc. **12,** 173–174 (1961).
Remeslennikov, V. N.: Conjugacy in polycyclic groups. Algebra i Logika **8,** 404–411 (1969).
Remeslennikov, V. N.: Finite approximability of groups with respect to conjugacy. Sibirsk. Mat. Zh. **12,** 1085–1099 (1971).
Remeslennikov, V. N.: *See also* Kargapolov, M. I.
Remeslennikov, V. N.: *See* Kirkinskii, A. S.
Remeslennikov, V. N., Sokolov, V. G.: Some properties of a Magnus embedding. Algebra i Logika **9,** 566–578 (1970).
Remmers, J. H.: A geometric approach to some algorithmic problems for semigroups, Thesis. Univ. Michigan 1971.
Rhemtulla, A.: A problem of bounded expressibility in free products. Proc. Cambridge Philos. Soc. **64,** 573–584 (1968).
Ribes, L.: Cohomological characterization of amalgamated products of groups. J. Pure Appl. Alg. **4,** 309–317 (1974).
Riley, R.: Parabolic representations of knot groups. Proc. London Math. Soc. **24,** 217–242 (1972).
Riley, R.: Hecke invariants of knot groups. Glasgow Math. J. **15,** 17–26 (1974).
Rips, I. A.: On the fourth integer dimension subgroup. Israel J. Math. **12,** 342–346 (1972).
Robertson, E. F.: *See* Campbell, C. M.

Robinson, D. J. S.: Residual properties of some classes of infinite soluble groups. Proc. London Math. Soc. **18,** 495–520 (1968).

Robinson, D. J. S.: Finiteness conditions and generalized soluble groups. Berlin-Heidelberg-New York: Springer 1972.

Robinson, G. De B.: On the fundamental region of a group, and the family of configurations which arise therefrom. J. London Math. Soc. **6,** 70–75 (1931).

Roggenkamp, K. W.: *See* Gruenberg, K. W.

Roggenkamp, K. W.: Relation modules of finite groups and related topics. Alg. i Log. **12,** 351–359; 365 (1973).

Rollov, E. V.: *See* Bezvehnii, V. N.

Romanovskii, N. S.: *See* Kargapolov, M. I.

Romanovski, N. S.: A freedom theorem for groups with one defining relation in the varieties of nilpotent and solvable groups of given class. Mat. Sb. **89,** 93–99 (1970).

Romanovski, N. S.: On some algorithmic problems for solvable groups. Alg. i Log. **13,** 26–34

Romankov, V. A.: *See* Kargapolov, M. I.

Room, T. G.: The generation by two operators of the symplectic group over GF(2). J. Austral. Math. Soc. **1,** 38–46 (1959/60).

Rosenberger, G.: Automorphismen und Erzeugende für Gruppen mit einer definierenden Relation. Math. Z. **129,** 259–267 (1972).

Rosenberger, G.: Fuchssche Gruppen, die freies Produkt zweier zyklischer Gruppen sind, und die Gleichungen $x^2 + y^2 + z^2 = xyz$. Math Ann. **199,** 213–227 (1972).

Rosenberger, G.: Eine Bemerkung zu den Triangel-Gruppen. Preprint.

Rosenberger, G.: Das eingeschränkte Isomorphieproblem für Fuchssche Gruppen. Preprint.

Rosenberger, G.: Das eingeschränkte Isomorphieproblem für Fuchssche Gruppen von Geschlecht $g \geqslant 1$. Preprint.

Rosenberger, G.: Von diskreten Gruppen, die von drei Elementen der Ordnung zwei erzeugt werden. Preprint.

Rosenberger, G.: Über Triangel-Gruppen. Math. Zeit. **132,** 239–244 (1973).

Rosenberger, G.: Zum Rang- und Isomorphieproblem für freie Produkte mit Amalgam, Habilitationschrift. Hamburg 1974.

Rosenberger, G.: Zum Isomorphieproblem für Gruppen mit einer definierenden Relation. III. J. Math. **20,** 614–621 (1976).

Rosenberger, G.: *See also* Bordo, W., Peczynski, N.

Rosenberger, G.: On the isomorphism problem for one-relator groups. Arch. Math. To appear.

Rosenberger, G.: Anwendung der Nielsenschen Kürzungsmethode in Gruppen mit einer definierenden Relation. To appear.

Rosenberger, G.: Produkte von Potenzen und Kommutatoren in freien Gruppen. To appear.

Rosset, S.: A property of groups of nonexponential growth. Proc. Amer. Math. Soc. **54,** 24–26 (1976).

Rothaus, O. S.: *See* Gerstenhaber, M.

Rothaus, O. S.: On the non-triviality of some group extensions given by generators and relations. Bull. Amer. Math. Soc. **82,** 284–286 (1976).

Rotman, J. J.: Covering complexes with applications to algebra. Rocky Mountain J. Math. **3,** 641–674 (1973).

Rotman, J. J.: The Theory of Groups: An Introduction. 2nd ed. Boston: Allyn and Bacon 1973.

Ryshkov, S. S.: On maximal finite groups of integer $(n \times n)$ matrices. Dokl. Akad. Nauk SSSR **204,** 561–564 (1972).

Sacerdote, G. S.: Some unsolvable decision problems in group theory. Proc. Amer. Math. Soc. **36,** 231–238 (1972).

Sacerdote, G. S.: Elementary properties of free groups. Trans. Amer. Math. Soc. **178,** 127–138 (1972).

Sacerdote, G. S.: *SQ*-universal 1-relator groups. In: Lecture Notes in Math., Vol. 319, p. 168). Berlin-Heidelberg-New York: Springer 1973.

Sacerdote, G. S.: On a problem of Boone. Math. Scand. **31,** 111–117 (1973).

Sacerdote, G. S.: Almost all free products of groups have the same positive theory. J. Algebra **27,** 475–485 (1974).

Sacerdote, G. S.: All theorem-A groups are HNN groups, submitted to Canad. J. Math.
Sacerdote, G. S.: A characterization of the subgroups of finitely presented groups, to appear in Bull. Amer. Math. Soc.
Sacerdote, G. S.: Subgroups of finitely presented groups, submitted to J. London Math. Soc.
Sacerdote, G. S.: Some logical problems concerning free and free product groups. Rocky Mountain J. Math. **6**, 401–408 (1976).
Sacerdote, G. S.: *See* Fried, M.
Sacerdote, G. S., Schupp, P. E.: *SQ*-universality of HNN and 1-relator groups. J. London Math. Soc. **7**, 733–740 (1974).
Sacerdote, G. S.: On the groups of Britton's theorem A. Can. J. Math. **28**, 635–639 (1976).
Shafarevich, I. R.: *See* Golod, E. S.
Sag. T. W., Wamsley, J. W.: Minimal presentations for groups of order 2^n, $n \leqslant 6$. J. Austral. Math. Soc. **15**, 461–469 (1973).
Sag. T. W., Wamsley, J. W.: On computing the minimal number of defining relations for finite groups. Math. Comp. **27**, 361–362 (1973).
Sah, C.-H.: Groups related to compact Riemann surfaces. Acta Math. **123**, 13–42 (1969).
Saito, K.: *See* Breiskorn, E.
Sanatani, S.: On planar group diagrams. Math. Ann. **172**, 203–208 (1967).
Sandling, R.: The dimension subgroup problem. J. Algebra **21**, 216–231 (1972).
Sandling, R.: Dimension subgroups over arbitrary coefficient rings. J. Algebra **21**, 250–265 (1972).
Sandling, R.: Subgroups dual to dimension subgroups. Proc. Cambridge Philos. Soc. **71**, 33–38 (1972).
Sandling, R.: Modular augmentation ideals. Proc. Cambridge Philos. Soc. **71**, 25–32 (1972).
Sanov, I. N.: A property of a representation of a free group. Dokl. Akad. Nauk SSSR **57**, 657–659 (1947).
Sansone, G.: I sottogruppi del gruppo di Picard e due teoremi sui finiti analoghi al teorema Dyck. Rend. Circ. Mat. Palermo **47**, 273–333 (1923).
Shchepin, G. G.: On the occurence problem for a nilpotent product of finitely presented groups Dokl. Akad. Nauk SSSR **160**, 294–297 (1965).
Shchepin, G. G.: On the occurence problem in finitely defined groups. Sibirsk. Mat. Z. **9**, 443–448 (1968).
Scott, P.: Normal subgroups of 3-manifold groups. J. London Math. Soc. **13**, 5–12 (1976).
Schenkman, E.: The equation $a^nb^n = c^n$ in a free group. Ann. of Math. **70**, 562–564 (1959).
Schenkman, E.: Some two generator groups with two relations. Arch. Math. **18**, 362–363 (1967).
Schiek, H.: Bemerkung über eine Relation in freien Gruppen. Math. Ann. **126**, 375–376 (1953).
Schiek, H.: Gruppen mit Relationen $X^3 = 1$, $(XY)^3 = 1$. Arch. Math. **6**, 341–347 (1955).
Schiek, H.: Gruppen mit Relationen $(abc)^2 = e$. Math. Nachr. **13**, 247–256 (1955).
Schiek, H.: Ähnlichkeitsanalyse von Gruppenrelationen. Acta Math. **96**, 157–252 (1956).
Schiek, H.: Adjunktionsproblem und inkompressible Relationen, I, II. Math. Ann. **146**, 314–320 (1962); **141**, 163–170 (1965).
Schiek, H.: Das Adjunktionsproblem der Gruppentheorie. Math. Ann. **147**, 158–165 (1962).
Schiek, H.: Equations over groups. In: Word Problems, pp. 563–568. Amsterdam: North Holland 1973.
Schmidt, O. J.: Abstract theory of groups. 2nd ed. San Francisco-London: Freeman 1966.
Schreier, O.: Über die Gruppen $A^aB^b = 1$. Abh. Math. Sem. Univ. Hamburg **3**, 167–169 (1924).
Schreier, O.: Die Untergruppen der freien Gruppen. Abh. Math. Sem. Univ. Hamburg **5**, 161–183 (1927).
Schubert, H.: Die eindeutige Zerlegbarkeit eines Knotens in Primknoten. S.-B. Heidelberger Akad. Wiss. Math.-Natur. Kl. 57–104 (1949).
Schupp, P. E.: On Dehn's algorithm and the conjugacy problem. Math. Ann. **178**, 119–130 (1968).
Schupp, P. E.: On the substitution problem for free groups. Proc. Amer. Math. Soc. **23**, 421–423 (1969).
Schupp, P. E.: A note on recursively enumerable predicates in groups. Fund. Math. **65**, 61–63 (1969).
Schupp, P. E.: On the conjugacy problem for certain quotient groups of free products. Math. Ann. **186**, 123–129 (1970).

Schupp, P. E.: On Greendlinger's Lemma. Comm. Pure Appl. Math. **23,** 233–240 (1970).
Schupp, P. E.: Small cancellation theory over free products with amalgamation. Math. Ann. **193,** 255–264 (1971).
Schupp, P. E.: A survey of small cancellation theory. In: Word Problems, pp. 569–589. Amsterdam: North-Holland 1973.
Schupp, P. E.: A survey of SQ-universality. In: A Conference on Group Theory (Lecture Notes in Math., Vol. 319, pp. 183–188). Berlin-Heidelberg-New York: Springer 1973.
Schupp, P. E.: Some reflections on HNN extensions. In: Proc. Conf. Canberra 1973 (Lecture Notes in Math., Vol. 372, pp. 611–632). Berlin-Heidelberg-New York: Springer 1974.
Schupp, P. E.: A strengthened Freiheitssatz. Math. Ann. **221,** 73–80 (1976).
Schupp, P. E.: Embeddings into simple groups. J. London Math. Soc. **13,** 90–94 (1976).
Schupp, P. E.: *See also* McCool, J., Miller, C. F. III, Sacerdote, G. S.
Schur, I.: Über die Darstellungen der endlichen Gruppen durch gebrochene lineare Substitutionen. J. Reine Angew. Math. **127,** 20–50 (1904).
Schützenberger, M. P.: Sur l'équation $a^{2+n} = b^{2+m}c^{2+p}$ dans un groupe libre. C. R. Acad. Sci. Paris **248,** 2435–2436 (1959).
Schützenberger, M. P.: *See also* Lyndon, R. C.
Scott, G. P.: Finitely generated 3-manifold groups are finitely presented. J. London Math. Soc. **6,** 437–440 (1973).
Scott, G. P.: An embedding theorem for groups with a free subgroup of finite index. Bull. London Math. Soc. **6,** 304–306 (1974).
Scott, P.: *See* Dyer, J. L.
Scott, W. R.: Algebraically closed groups. Proc. Amer. Math. Soc. **2,** 118–121 (1951).
Searby, D. G., Wamsley, J. W.: Minimal presentations for certain metabelian groups. Proc. Amer. Math. Soc. **32,** 342–348 (1972).
Segal, D.: *See* Houghton, C. H.
Segal, I. E.: The non-existence of a relation which is valid for all finite groups. Bol. Soc. Mat. São Paulo **2,** 3–5 (1947).
Sehgal, S. K.: *See* Parmenter, M. M., Passi, I. B. S.
Seifert, H.: Konstruktion dreidimensionaler Mannigfaltigkeiten. Jber. Deutsch. Math. Ver. **38,** 248–260 (1929).
Seifert, H.: Bemerkungen zur stetigen Abbildung von Flächen. Abh. Math. Sem. Univ. Hamburg **12,** 29–37 (1938).
Seksenbaev, K.: On the theory of polycyclic groups. Algebra i Logika **4,** 79–83 (1965).
Selberg, A.: On discontinuous groups in higher-dimensional symmetric spaces, pp. 147–164. Colloq. Function Theory, Bombay, 1960.
Serre, J.-P.: Sur la dimension cohomologique des groupes profinis. Topology **3,** 413–420 (1965).
Serre, J.-P.: Cohomologie des groupes discrets. C. R. Acad. Sci. Paris Sér. A-B **268,** 268–271 (1969).
Serre, J.-P.: Cohomologie des groupes discrets. Ann. of Math. **70,** 77–169 (1971).
Serre, J.-P.: Arbres, amalgames et $\mathbb{SL}_2$. Notes Collège de France 1968/69, ed. avec H. Bass; Springer Lecture Notes, To appear.
Serre, J.-P.: Amalgames et points fixes. In: Proc. Conf. Canberra 1973 (Lecture Notes in Math., Vol. 372, pp. 633–640). Berlin-Heidelberg-New York: Springer, 1974.
Serre, J.-P.: Problems. In: Proc. Conf. Canberra 1973 (Lecture Notes in Math., Vol. 372, pp. 734–735). Berlin-Heidelberg-New York: Springer 1974.
Serre, J.-P.: *See also* Bass. H.
Seymour, J. E.: Conjugate powers and unique roots in certain small cancellation groups, Thesis. University of Illinois 1974.
Shapiro, J., Sonn, J.: Free factor groups of one-relator groups. Duke Math. J. **41,** 83–88 (1974).
Sharma, S.: *See* Passi, I. B. S.
Shenitzer, A.: Decomposition of a group with a single defining relation into a free product. Proc. Amer. Math. Soc. **6,** 273–279 (1955).
Shepperd, J. A. H.: Braids which can be plaited with their threads tied together at each end. Proc. Royal Soc. Ser. A **265,** 229–244 (1961/62).
Siegel, C. L.: Bemerkung zu einem Satze von Jakob Nielsen. Mat. Tidsskr. B, 66–70 (1950).

Siegel, C. L.: Über einige Ungleichungen bei Bewegungsgruppen in der nichteuklidischen Ebene. Math. Ann. **133,** 127–138 (1957).

Sieradski, A.: J. Combinatorial isomorphisms and combinatorial homotopy equivalences. J. Pure Appl. Alg. **7,** 59–95 (1976).

Simmons, H.: The word problem for absolute presentations. J. London Math. Soc. **6,** 275–280 (1973).

Singerman, D.: Subgroups of Fuchsian groups and finite permutation groups. Bull. London Math. Soc. **2,** 319–323 (1970).

Singerman, D.: Finitely maximal Fuchsian groups. J. London Math. Soc. **6,** 29–38 (1972).

Singerman, D.: On the structure of non-Euclidean crystallographic groups. Proc. Cambridge Philos. Soc. **76,** 233–240 (1974).

Singerman, D.: Symmetries of Riemann surfaces with large automorphism groups. Math. Ann. **210,** 17–32 (1974).

Singerman, D.: Automorphisms of maps, permutation groups and Riemann surfaces. Bull. London Math. Soc. **8,** 65–68 (1976).

Singerman, D.: *See also* Macbeath, A. M.

Sinkov, A.: The groups determined by the relations $S^l = T^m = (S^{-1}T^{-1}ST)^p = 1$. Duke Math. J. **2,** 74–83 (1936).

Sinkov, A.: On the group-defining relations (2, 3, 7; p). Ann. of Math. **38,** 577–584 (1937).

Sinkov, A.: Necessary and sufficient conditions for generating certain simple groups by two operators of periods two and three. Amer. J. Math. **59,** 67–76 (1937).

Sinkov, A.: On generating the simple group $\mathbb{LF}(2, 7^n)$ by two operators of periods two and three. Bull. Amer. Math. Soc. **44,** 449–455 (1938).

Sinkov, A.: A note on a paper by J. A. Todd. Bull. Amer. Math. Soc. **45,** 762–765 (1939).

Sinkov, A.: The number of abstract definitions of $\mathbb{LF}(2, p)$ as a quotient group of (2, 3, n). J. Algebra **12,** 525–532 (1969).

Smythe, N.: *See* Crowell, R. H., Cossey, J.

Smythe, N.: A generalization of Grushko's theorem to the mapping cylinder group. Abstract, Notices Amer. Math. Soc. **23,** A–419 (1976).

Sokolov, V. G.: *See* Remeslennikov, V. N.

Soldatova, V. V.: On groups with δ-basis, for $\delta < 1/4$, and one additional condition. Sibirsk. Mat. Zh. **7,** 627–637 (1966).

Soldatova, V. V.: On a class of finitely presented groups. Dokl. Akad. Nauk SSSR **172,** 1276–1277 (1967).

Soldatova, V. V.: Solution of the word problem for a certain class of groups. Ivanov. Gos. Ped. Inst. Uchen. Zap. **44,** 17–25 (1969).

Soldatova, V. V.: The centralizer of an arbitrary element. Ivanov. Gos. Ped. Inst. Uchen. **61,** 209–224 (1969).

Solitar, D.: *See* Fischer, J., Hoare, A. H. M., Karrass, A., Magnus, W.

Solomon, L.: The solution of equations in groups. Arch. Math. **20,** 241–247 (1969).

Sonn, J.: *See* Shapiro, J.

Specht, W.: Freie Untergruppen der binären unimodularen Gruppe. Math. Z. **72,** 319–331 (1959/60).

Specker, E.: Die erste Cohomologiegruppe von Überlagerungen und Homotopie-Eigenschaften dreidimensionaler Mannigfaltigkeiten. Comment. Math. Helv. **23,** 303–333 (1949).

Specker, E.: Endenverbände von Räumen und Gruppen. Math. Ann. **122,** 167–174 (1950).

Speiser, A.: Theorie der Gruppen von endlicher Ordnung. Basel: Birkhäuser 1956.

Stallings, J. R.: On the recursiveness of sets of presentations of 3-manifold groups. Fund. Math. **51,** 191–194 (1962/63).

Stallings, J. R.: A finitely presented group whose 3-dimensional integral homology is not finitely generated. Amer. J. Math. **85,** 541–543 (1963).

Stallings, J. R.: A topological proof of Grushko's theorem on free products. Math. Z. **90,** 1–8 (1965).

Stallings, J. R.: Centerless groups—an algebraic formulation of Gottlieb's theorem. Topology **4,** 129–134 (1965).

Stallings, J. R.: A remark about the description of free products of groups. Proc. Cambridge

Philos. Soc. **62**, 129–134 (1966).
Stallings, J. R.: Groups of dimension 1 are locally free. Bull. Amer. Math. Soc. **74**, 361–364 (1968).
Stallings, J. R.: On torsion-free groups with infinitely many ends. Ann. of Math. **88**, 312–334 (1968).
Stallings, J. R.: Groups of cohomological dimension one. Proc. Sympos. Pure Math. Amer. Math. Soc. **17**, 124–128 (1970).
Stallings, J. R.: Group theory and three-dimensional manifolds. Yale Monographs **4**, (1971).
Stallings, J. R.: Characterization of tree products of finitely many groups. To appear.
Stallings, J. R.: Quotients of the powers of the augmentation ideal in a group ring. Knots, Groups, and 3-Manifolds, ed. L. P. Neuwirth. Ann. Math. Studies **84**, 101–118 (1975).
Stammbach, U.: Anwendungen der Homologietheorie der Gruppen auf Zentralreihen und auf Invarianten von Präsentierungen. Math. Z. **94**, 157–177 (1966).
Stammbach, U.: Ein neuer Beweis eines Satzes von Magnus. Proc. Cambridge Philos. Soc. **63**, 929–930 (1967).
Stammbach, U.: Über freie Untergruppen gegebener Gruppen. Comment. Math. Helv. **43**, 132–136 (1968).
Stebe, P. F.: Residual finiteness of a class of knot groups. Comm, Pure Appl. Math. **21**, 563–583 (1968).
Stebe, P. F.: On free products of isomorphic free groups with a single finitely generated amalgamated subgroup. J. Algebra **11**, 359–362 (1969).
Stebe, P. F.: A residual property of certain groups. Proc. Amer. Math. Soc. **26**, 37–42. (1970).
Stebe, P. F.: Conjugacy separability of certain free products with amalgamation. Trans. Amer. Math. Soc. **156**, 119–129 (1971).
Stebe, P. F.: Conjugacy separability of the groups of hose knots. Trans. Amer. Math. Soc. **159**, 79–90 (1971).
Stebe, P. F.: Conjugacy separability of certain Fuchsian groups. Trans. Amer. Math. Soc. **163**, 173–188 (1972).
Stebe, P. F.: Conjugacy separability of groups of integer matrices. Proc. Amer. Math. Soc. **32**, 1–7 (1972).
Stebe, P. F.: *See also* Anshel, M.
Steinberg, A.: On free nilpotent quotient groups. Math. Z. **85**, 185–196 (1964).
Steinberg, A.: On equations in free groups. Michigan Math. J. **18**, 87–95 (1971).
Steinberg, A.: *See also* Baumslag, G., Meskin, S.
Steinberg, R.: Générateurs, relations et revêtements de groupes algébriques. Colloq. Bruxelles 1962. Louvain-Paris 1963.
Steinberg, R.: Generators for simple groups. Canad. J. Math. **14**, 277–283 (1962).
Stender, P. V.: On the application of the sieve method to the solvability of the word problem for relations. Mat. Sb. **32**, 97–108 (1953).
Stender, P. V.: On primitive elements in a free group of rank 2. Izv. Vyssh. Uchebn. Zaved. Matematica, 101–106 (1962).
Stevens, R. S.: Classification of 3-manifolds with certain spines. Thesis. Colorado State Univ. 1974.
Stevens, R. S.: *See also* Osborn, R. P.
Stork, D. F.: Structure and applications of Schreier coset graphs. Comm. Pure Appl. Math. **24**, 797–805 (1971).
Strasser, E. R. (= Rapaport, E. S.): Knot-like groups. Knots, Groups, and 3-Manifolds. Ann. Math. Studies **88**, 119–133 (1975).
Strasser, E. R. (= Rapaport, E. S.), Levinson, H. W.: Planarity of Cayley diagrams: planar presentations. Proc. Conf. Boca Raton 1975. Utilitas Math., Winnipeg 1975, pp. 567–593.
Strebel, R.: *See* Baumslag, G.
Sunday, J. G.: Presentations of the groups $\mathbb{SL}(2, m)$ and $\mathbb{PSL}(2, n)$. Canad. J. Math. **24**, 1129–1131 (1972).
Suprunenko, D. A.: On the order of an element of a group of integral matrices. Dokl. Akad. Nauk BSSR **7**, 221–223 (1963).
Svark, A. A.: A volume invariant of coverings. Dokl. Akad. Nauk SSSR **105**, 32–34 (1955).
Swan, R. G.: Periodic resolutions for finite groups. Ann. of Math. **72**, 267–291 (1960).
Swan, R. G.: Minimal resolutions for finite groups. Topology **4**, 193–208 (1965).

Swan, R. G.: Generators and relations for certain special linear groups. Bull. Amer. Math. Soc. **74**, 576–581 (1968).
Swan R. G.: Groups of cohomological dimension one. J. Algebra **12**, 585–610 (1969).
Swan, R. G.: Generators and relations for certain special linear groups. Advances Math. **6**, 1–77 (1971).
Swierczkowski, S.: On a free group of rotations of Euclidean space. Nederl. Akad. Wetensen. Proc. Ser. A **61**, 376–378 (1958).
Tang, C. Y.: *See* Allenby, R. B. J. T.
Takahasi, M.: Bemerkungen über den Untergruppensatz in freien produkten. Proc. Imp. Acad. Tokyo **20**, 589–594 (1944).
Takahasi, M.: On partitions of free products of groups. Osaka Math. J. **1**, 49–51 (1949).
Takahasi, M.: Note on locally free groups. J. Inst. Polytech. Osaka City Univ. Ser. A. Math. **1**, 65–70 (1950).
Takahasi, M.: Note on chain conditions in free groups. Osaka Math. J. **3**, 221–225 (1951).
Takahasi, M.: Note on word subgroups in free products of groups. J. Inst. Polytech. Osaka City Univ. Ser. A. Math. **2**, 13–18 (1951).
Takahasi, M.: Primitive locally free groups. J. Inst. Polytech. Osaka City Univ. Ser. A. **5**, 81–85 (1954).
Tartakovskii, V. A.: On the problem of equivalence for certain types of groups. Dokl. Akad. Nauk SSSR **58**, 1909–1910 (1947).
Tartakovskii, V. A.: On the process of extinction. Dokl. Akad. Nauk SSSR **58**, 1605–1608 (1947).
Tartakovskii, V. A.: The sieve method in group theory. Mat. Sb. **25**, 3–50 (1949).
Tartakovskii, V. A.: Application of the sieve method to the solution of the word problem for certain types of groups. Math. Sb. **25**, 251–274 (1949).
Tartakovskii, V. A.: Solution of the word problem for groups with a k-reduced basis for $k > 6$. Izv. Akad. Nauk SSSR Ser Math. **13**, 483–494 (1949).
Tartakovskii, V. A.: On primitive composition. Mat. Sb. **30**, 39–52 (1952).
Taussky, O.: Matrices of rational integers. Bull. Amer. Math. Soc. **66**, 327–345 (1960).
Taussky, O., Todd, J.: Commuting bilinear transformations and matrices. J. Washington Acad. Sci. **46**, 373–375 (1956).
Taylor, T.: *See* Baumslag, G.
Thompson, R. J.: A finitely presented infinite simple group. Unpublished.
Thompson, R. J.: *See* McKenzie, R.
Threlfall, W.: Gruppenbilder. Abh. Sächs. Akad. Wiss. Leipzig Math.-Natur. Kl. **41**, 1–54 (1932).
Tietze, H.: Über die topologischen Invarianten mehrdimensionaler Mannigfaltigkeiten. Monatsh. Math. Phys. **19**, 1–118 (1908).
Tits, J.: Groupes et géométries de Coxeter. Inst. Hautes Etudes Sci. Publ. Math. (1961).
Tits, J.: Le problème des mots dans les groupes de Coxeter. In: Sympos. Math. Rome 1967/68, pp. 175–185. London: Academic Press 1969.
Tits, J.: Sur le groupe des automorphismes d'un arbre. Essays on Topology. Mém. dédiées à G. de Rham. Springer, 1970, 188–211.
Tits, J.: Free subgroups in linear groups. J. Algebra **20**, 250–270 (1972).
Tits, J.: Buildings of spherical type and finite BN-pairs. Appendix 3: Generators and relations (Lecture Notes in Math., Vol. 386). Berlin-Heidelberg-New York: Springer 1974.
Todd, J.: *See* Taussky, O.
Todd, J. A., Coxeter, H. S. M.: A practical method for enumerating cosets of a finite abstract group. Proc. Edinburgh Math. Soc. **5**, 25–34 (1936).
Toh, K. H.: Problems concerning residual finiteness in nilpotent grous. Mimeographed. Univ. of Malaya.
Topping, I. M.: Free generators and the free differential calculus, Thesis. State Univ. New York, Stony Brook, 1973.
Tretkoff, M.: *See* Fine, B.
Tretkoff, M.: A topological proof of the residual finiteness of certain amalgamated free products. Comm. Pure Appl. Math. **26**, 855–859 (1973).
Tretkoff, M.: Covering space proofs in combinatorial group theory. Comm. Algebra **3**, 429–457 (1975).

Tretkoff, C.: Nonparabolic subgroups of the modular group. Glasgow Math. J. **16,** 90–102 (1975).
Trott, S.: A pair of generators for the unimodular group. Canad. Math. Bull. **3,** 245–252 (1962).
Trotter, H.: An algorithm for the Todd-Coxeter method of coset enumeration. Canad. Math. Bull. **7,** 357–368 (1964).
Truffault, B.: Sur le problème des mots pour les groupes de Greendlinger. C. R. Acad. Sci. Paris Sér. A-B **267,** 1–3 (1968).
Truffault, B.: Note sur un théorème de Lipschutz. Arch. Math. **25,** 1–2 (1974).
Truffault, B.: Centralisateurs des éléments d'ordre fini dans les groupes de Greendlinger. Math. Z. **136,** 7–11 (1974).
Truffault, B.: Centralisateurs des éléments dans les groupes de Greendlinger. C. R. Acad. Sci. Paris Sér. A **279,** 317–319 (1974).
Truffault, B.: *See* Comerford, L. P., Jr.
Tukia, P.: On discrete groups of the unit disk and their automorphisms. Ann. Acad. Sci. Fennicae A. I. **504,** 1–45 (1972).
Ullman, J. L.: *See* Lyndon, R. C.
Valiev, M. K.: A theorem of G. Higman. Algebra i Logika **9,** 9–22 (1968).
Valiev, M. K.: Examples of universal finitely presented groups. Dokl. Akad. Nauk SSSR **211,** 265–268 (1973).
van der Waerden, B. L.: Free products of groups. Amer. J. Math. **70,** 527–528 (1948).
van Est, W. T.: Finite groups with generators A, B, C in the relation $A^a = B^b = C^c = ABC = 1$. Nieuw Arch. Wisk. **1,** 16–26 (1953).
van Kampen, E. R.: On the connection between the fundamental groups of some related spaces. Amer. J. Math. **55,** 261–267 (1933).
van Kampen, E. R.: On some lemmas in the theory of groups. Amer. J. Math. **55,** 268–273 (1933).
van Vleck, E. B.: On the combination of non-loxodromic substitutions. Trans. Amer. Math. Soc. **20,** 299–312 (1912).
Vasquez, A. T.: *See* Dyer, E.
Verdier, J.-L.: Caractéristique d'Euler-Poincaré. Bull. Soc. Math. France **101,** 441–445 (1973).
Vogt, E.: *See* Zieschang, H.
Volvachev, R. T.: On the order of an element of a matrix group. Vesci Akad. Nauk BSSR Ser. Fiz.-Mat. Nauk, 11–16 (1965).
Wagner, D. H.: On free products of groups. Trans. Amer. Math. Soc. **84,** 352–378 (1957).
Waldhausen, F.: Gruppen mit Zentrum und 3-dimensionale Mannigfaltigkeiten. Topology **6,** 505–517 (1967).
Waldhausen, F.: On irreducible 3-manifolds which are sufficiently large. Ann. of Math. **87,** 56–88 (1968).
Waldhausen, F.: The word problem in fundamental groups of sufficiently large irreducible 3-manifolds. Ann. of Math. **88,** 272–280 (1968).
Waldhausen, F.: Algebraic K-theory of generalized free products. Preprint.
Waldinger, H. On the subgroups of the Picard group. Proc. Amer. Math. Soc. **16,** 1373–1378 (1965).
Wall, C. T. C.: Rational Euler characteristics. Proc. Cambridge Philos. Soc. **57,** 182–184 (1961).
Wall, C. T. C.: Finiteness conditions for CW complexes, II. Proc. Roy. Soc. Ser. A **295,** 129–139 (1966).
Wamsley, J. W.: The multiplicator of finite nilpotent groups. Bull. Austral. Math. Soc. **3,** 1–8 (1970).
Wamsley, J. W.: A class of three-generator, three-relation, finite groups. Canad. J. Math. **22,** 36–40 (1970).
Wamsley, J. W.: The deficiency of metacyclic groups. Proc. Amer. Math. Soc. **24,** 724–726 (1970).
Wamsley, J. W.: Minimal presentations for certain group extensions. Israel J. Math. **9,** 459–463 (1971).
Wamsley, J. W.: The deficiency and the multiplicator of finite nilpotent groups. J. Austral. Math. Soc. **13,** 124–128 (1972).
Wamsley, J. W.: A class of two generator two relation finite groups. J. Austral. Math. Soc. **14,** 38–40 (1972).
Wamsley, J. W.: On a class of groups of prime-power order. Israel J. Math. **11,** 297–298 (1972).

Wamsley, J. W.: Minimal presentations for finite groups. Bull. London Math. Soc. **5**, 129–144 (1973).
Wamsley, J. W.: On certain pairs of matrices which generate free groups. Bull. London Math. Soc. **5**, 109–110 (1973).
Wamsley, J. W.: A class of finite groups with deficiency zero. Proc. Edinburgh Math. Soc. **19**, 25–29 (1974).
Wamsley, J. W.: Some finite groups with zero deficiency. J. Austral. Math. Soc. **18**, 73–75 (1974).
Wamsley, J. W.: Some groups with trivial Schur multiplicator. J. Austral. Math. Soc. To appear.
Wamsley, J. W.: The deficiency of wreth products of groups. J. Algebra. **27**, 48–56 (1973).
Wamsley, J. W.: Presentations of class two p-groups. Trans. Amer. Math. Soc. To appear.
Wamsley, J. W.: On a class of finite groups. J. Austral. Math. Soc. **19**, 290–291 (1975).
Wamsley, J. W.: *See also* Johnson, D. L., Sag, L. W., Searby, D. G.
Wehrfritz, B. A. F.: 2-generator conditions in linear groups. Arch. Math. **22**, 237–240 (1971).
Wehrfritz, B. A. F.: Infinite linear groups. An account of the group-theoretic properties of infinite groups of matrices. Ergebnisse der Math., Bd. 76. Berlin-Heidelberg-New York: Springer 1973.
Wehrfritz, B. A. F.: Conjugacy separating representations of free groups. Proc. Amer. Math. Soc. **40**, 52–56 (1973).
Wehrfritz, B. A. F.: Two examples of soluble groups that are not conjugacy separable. J. London Math. Soc. **7**, 312–316 (1974).
Weinbaum, C. M.: Visualizing the word problem, with an application to sixth groups. Pacific J. Math. **16**, 557–578 (1966).
Weinbaum, C. M.: Partitioning a primitive word into a generating set. Math. Ann. **181**, 157–162 (1969).
Weinbaum, C. M.: On relators and diagrams for groups with one defining relation. Illinois J. Math. **16**, 308–322 (1972).
Weinbaum, C. M.: The word and conjugacy problem for the knot group of any tame prime alternating knot. Proc. Amer. Math. Soc. **22**, 22–26 (1971).
Weir, A. J.: The Reidemeister-Schreier and Kuros subgroup theorems. Mathematika **3**, 47–55 (1956).
Wenzel, G. H.: *See* Binz, E.
White, A. T.: Graphs, Groups and Surfaces. Math. Stud. **8**, Amsterdam: North-Holland 1973.
Whitehead, J. H. C.: On certain sets of elements in a free group. Proc. London Math. Soc. **41**, 48–56 (1936).
Whitehead, J. H. C.: On equivalent sets of elements in a free group. Ann. of Math. **37**, 782–800 (1936).
Wicks, M. J.: Commutators in free products. J. London Math. Soc. **37**, 433–444 (1962).
Wicks, M. J.: The equation $x^2y^2 = g$ over free products. Proc. Cong. Singapore Nat. Acad. Sci., 238–248 (1971).
Wicks, M. J.: A general solution of binary homogeneous equations over free groups. Pacific J. Math. **41**, 543–561 (1972).
Wicks, M. J.: The arithmetic of a group. Bull. Singapore Math. Soc., 25–40 (1973).
Wicks, M. J.: A relation in free products. Proc. Conf. Canberra 1973. Springer Lecture Notes 372 (1974) 709–716.
Wicks, M. J.: The symmetries of classes of elements in a free group of rank two. Math. Ann. **212**, 21–44 (1974).
Wicks, M. J.: Presentations of some classical groups. Bull. Austral. Math. Soc. **13**, 1–12 (1975).
Wiegold, J.: Some remarks on generalised products of groups with amalgamations. Math. Z. **75**, 57–78 (1961).
Wiegold, J.: *See also* Neumann, P. M., Zrenner, J. L.
Wilkens, D. L.: On non-archimedean length in groups. Mathematika **23**, 57–61 (1976).
Wilkens, D. L.: On non-archimedean length in groups. Preprint.
Wilkie, H. C.: On non-Euclidean crystallographic groups. Math. Z. **91**, 87–102 (1966).
Williams, J. S.: Nielsen equivalence of presentations of some solvable groups. Math. Z. **137**, 351–362 (1964).
Williams, J. S.: Free presentations and relation modules of finite groups. J. Pure Appl. Algebra **3**, 203–217 (1973).

Witt, E.: Treue Darstellung Liescher Ringe. J. Reine Angew. Math. **177**, 152–160 (1937).

Wolf, J. A.: Growth of finitely generated solvable groups and curvature of Riemannian manifolds. J. Differential Geometry **2**, 421–446 (1968).

Wright, D.: *See* Johnson, D. L.

Wright, D.: The amalgamated free product structure of $Gl_2(K[X_1, \ldots, X_n])$. Bull. Amer. Math. Soc. **82**, 724–726 (1976).

Wussing, H.: Die Genesis des Abstrakten Gruppenbegriff. Berlin: VEB Deutcher Verlag Wiss. 1969.

Zaleskii, A. E., Mikhalev, A.V.: Group rings. Itogi Nauki i Teknii **2**, 5–119 (1973) [J. Sov. Math. 4, 1–78 (1975)]

Zassenhaus, H.: Ein Verfahren, jeder endlichen p-Gruppe einen Lie-Ring mit der Charakteristik p zuzuordnen. Abh. Math. Sem Univ. Hamburg **13**, 200–207 (1940).

Zassenhaus, H.: A presentation of the groups PSL(2, p) with three defining relations. Canad. J. Math. **21**, 310–311 (1969).

Ziegler, M.: Gruppen mit vorgeschreibenem Wortproblem. Math. Ann. **219**, 43–51 (1976).

Zieschang, H.: Über Worte $S_1^{a_1} S_2^{a_2} \cdots S_p^{a_p}$ in einer freien Gruppen mit p freien Erzeugenden. Math. Ann. **147**, 143–153 (1962).

Zieschang, H.: Über einfache Kurven auf Vollbrezeln. Abh. Math. Sem. Univ. Hamburg **25**, 231–250 (1962).

Zieschang, H.: On the classification of simple systems of paths on a surface of genus 2. Dokl. Akad. Nauk SSSR **152**, 841–844 (1963).

Zieschang, H.: On a problem of Neuwirth concerning knot groups. Dokl. Akad. Nauk SSSR **153**, 1017–1019 (1963).

Zieschang, H.: Über einfache Kurvensysteme auf einer Vollbrezel vom Geschlecht 2. Abh. Math. Sem. Univ. Hamburg **26**, 237–247 (1964).

Zieschang, H.: Alternierende Produkte in freien Gruppen, I, II. Abh. Math. Sem. Univ. Hamburg **27**, 13–31 (1964); **28**, 219–233 (1965).

Zieschang, H.: Automorphisms of planar groups. Dokl. Akad. Nauk SSSR **155**, 57–60 (1964).

Zieschang, H.: On simple systems of curves on handlebodies. Mat. Sb. **66**, 230–239 (1965).

Zieschang, H.: Über Automorphismen ebener diskontinuierlicher Gruppen. Math. Ann. **166**, 148–167 (1966).

Zieschang, H.: Discrete groups of motions of the plane and planar group diagrams. Uspekhi Mat. Nauk **21**, 195–212 (1966).

Zieschang, H.: Algorithmen für einfache Kurven auf Flächen, I, II. Math. Scand. **17**, 17–40 (1965); **25**, 49–58 (1969).

Zieschang, H.: A theorem of Nielsen, some of its applications and generalizations. In: Proc. 4th Allunion Conf. Topology, Tashkent, 1963; pp. 184–201. (1967).

Zieschang, H.: Über die Nielsensche Kürzungsmethode in freien Produkten mit Amalgam. Invent. Math. **10**, 4–37 (1970).

Zieschang, H.: On extensions of fundamental groups of surfaces and related groups. Bull. Amer. Math. Soc. **77**, 1116–1119 (1971); addendum, **80**, 366–367 (1974).

Zieschang, H.: Lifting and projecting homeomorphisms. Arch. Math. **24**, 416–421 (1973).

Zieschang, H.: Homology groups of surfaces. Math. Ann. **206**, 1–21 (1973).

Zieschang, H.: Addendum to: "On extensions of fundamental groups of surfaces and related groups." Bull. Amer. Math. Soc. **80**, 366–367 (1974).

Zieschang, H.: Generators of the free product with amalgamation of two infinite cyclic groups. Math. Ann. To appear.

Zieschang, H.: *See also* Peczynski, N.

Zieschang, H., Burde, G.: Neuwirthsche Knoten und Flächenabbildungen. Abh. Math. Sem. Univ. Hamburg **31**, 239–246 (1967).

Zieschang, H., Epstein, D. B. A.: Curves on 2-manifolds: a counterexample. Acta Math. **115**, 109–110 (1966).

Zieschang, H., Vogt, E., Coldewey, H.-D.: Flächen und ebene diskontinuierliche Gruppen. Berlin-Heidelberg-New York: Springer 1970.

Russian Names in Cyrillic

There is no universal agreement on how Russian names should be transliterated. For readers desire to consult Russian sources, we here list the names of cited Russian authors in the origina

Adyan, S. I. Адян С. И.
Aselderov, Z. M. Асельдеров, З. М.
Bezverkhnii, V. N Безверхний, Б. Н.
Borisov, V V. Борисов, В. В.
Bovdi, A. A. Бовди, А. А.
Chebotar A. A. Чеботарь, А. А.
Curkin, V. A. Цуркин, В. А.
Doniyakhi, K. A. Донияхи, Х. А.
Dubuque, P. E. Дюбюк, П. Е.
Durnev, V. G. Дурнев, В. Г.
Fridman, A. A. Фридман, А. А.
Fouxe-Rabinovitch, D. I. Фукс-Рабинович, Д. И.
Gladkii, A. B. Гладкий, А. В.
Goldina N. P. Гольдина, Н. П.
Golod, E. S. Голод, Е. С.
Golovin O. N. Головин, О. Н.
Greendlinger, M. D. Гриндлингер, М. Д.
Grushko, I. A. Грушко, И. А.
Gurevich, G. A. Гуревич, Г. А.
Hmelevskii, Yu. I. Хмелевский, Ю. И.
Kalashnikov, V. A. Калашников, В. А.
Kargapolov, M. I. Каргаполов, М. И.
Kashinchev, E. V. Кашинчев, Е. В.
Klassen, V. P. Классен, В. П.
Kopitov, V. M. Копитов, В. М.
Kostrikin, A. I. Кострикин, А. И.
Kurosh, A. G. Курош, А. Г.
Kuznetsov, A. V. Кузнецов, А. В.
Lorents, A. A. Лоренц, А. А.
Magimovskii, V. L. Магимовский, В. Л.
Makanin, G. S. Маканин, Г. С.
Malcev, A. I. Мальцев, А. И
Markov, A. A. Марков, А. А.
Matiyasevich, Yu. V. Матиясевич, Ю. В
Merzlyakov, Yu. I. Мерзляков, Ю. И.
Mikhailova, K. A. Михайлова, К. А.
Moldavanskii, D. I. Молдаванский, Д. I
Novikov, P. S. Новиков, П. С.
Olshanskii, A. Yu. Ольшанский, А. Ю.
Remeslennikov, V. N. Ремесленников, В
Romankov, V. A. Романков, В. А.
Romanovskii, N. S. Романовский, Н. С.
Shafarevich, I R. Шафареич, И. Р.
Sanov, I. N. Санов, И. Н.
Shchepin, G. G. Щепин, Г. Г.
Seksenbaev, K. Сексенбаев, К.
Sokolov, V. G. Соколов, В. Г.
Soldatova, V. V. Солдатова, В. В.
Stender, P. V. Стендер, П. В.
Suprunenko, D. A. Супруненко, Д. А.
Svark, A. A. Сварк, А. А.
Tartakovskii, V. A. Тартаковский, В. А
Valiev, M. K. Валиев, М. К.
Volvachev, R. T Волвачев, Р. Т.

Index of Names*

*Includes Chapters I-V, but not Bibliography.

Subject Index

Printing: Weihert-Druck GmbH, Darmstadt
Binding: Buchbinderei Schäffer, Grünstadt

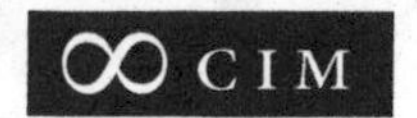

M. Aigner Combinatorial Theory ISBN 978-3-540-61787-7
A. L. Besse Einstein Manifolds ISBN 978-3-540-74120-6
N. P. Bhatia, G. P. Szegő Stability Theory of Dynamical Systems ISBN 978-3-540-42748-3
J. W. S. Cassels An Introduction to the Geometry of Numbers ISBN 978-3-540-61788-4
R. Courant, F. John Introduction to Calculus and Analysis I ISBN 978-3-540-65058-4
R. Courant, F. John Introduction to Calculus and Analysis II/1 ISBN 978-3-540-66569-4
R. Courant, F. John Introduction to Calculus and Analysis II/2 ISBN 978-3-540-66570-0
P. Dembowski Finite Geometries ISBN 978-3-540-61786-0
A. Dold Lectures on Algebraic Topology ISBN 978-3-540-58660-9
J. L. Doob Classical Potential Theory and Its Probabilistic Counterpart ISBN 978-3-540-41206-9
R. S. Ellis Entropy, Large Deviations, and Statistical Mechanics ISBN 978-3-540-29059-9
H. Federer Geometric Measure Theory ISBN 978-3-540-60656-7
S. Flügge Practical Quantum Mechanics ISBN 978-3-540-65035-5
L. D. Faddeev, L. A. Takhtajan Hamiltonian Methods in the Theory of Solitons ISBN 978-3-540-69843-2
I. I. Gikhman, A. V. Skorokhod The Theory of Stochastic Processes I ISBN 978-3-540-20284-4
I. I. Gikhman, A. V. Skorokhod The Theory of Stochastic Processes II ISBN 978-3-540-20285-1
I. I. Gikhman, A. V. Skorokhod The Theory of Stochastic Processes III ISBN 978-3-540-49940-4
D. Gilbarg, N. S. Trudinger Elliptic Partial Differential Equations of Second Order ISBN 978-3-540-41160-4
H. Grauert, R. Remmert Theory of Stein Spaces ISBN 978-3-540-00373-1
H. Hasse Number Theory ISBN 978-3-540-42749-0
F. Hirzebruch Topological Methods in Algebraic Geometry ISBN 978-3-540-58663-0
L. Hörmander The Analysis of Linear Partial Differential Operators I – Distribution Theory and Fourier Analysis ISBN 978-3-540-00662-6
L. Hörmander The Analysis of Linear Partial Differential Operators II – Differential Operators with Constant Coefficients ISBN 978-3-540-22516-4
L. Hörmander The Analysis of Linear Partial Differential Operators III – Pseudo-Differential Operators ISBN 978-3-540-49937-4
L. Hörmander The Analysis of Linear Partial Differential Operators IV – Fourier Integral Operators ISBN 978-3-642-00117-8
K. Itô, H. P. McKean, Jr. Diffusion Processes and Their Sample Paths ISBN 978-3-540-60629-1
T. Kato Perturbation Theory for Linear Operators ISBN 978-3-540-58661-6
S. Kobayashi Transformation Groups in Differential Geometry ISBN 978-3-540-58659-3
K. Kodaira Complex Manifolds and Deformation of Complex Structures ISBN 978-3-540-22614-7
Th. M. Liggett Interacting Particle Systems ISBN 978-3-540-22617-8
J. Lindenstrauss, L. Tzafriri Classical Banach Spaces I and II ISBN 978-3-540-60628-4
R. C. Lyndon, P. E Schupp Combinatorial Group Theory ISBN 978-3-540-41158-1
S. Mac Lane Homology ISBN 978-3-540-58662-3
C. B. Morrey Jr. Multiple Integrals in the Calculus of Variations ISBN 978-3-540-69915-6
D. Mumford Algebraic Geometry I – Complex Projective Varieties ISBN 978-3-540-58657-9
O. T. O'Meara Introduction to Quadratic Forms ISBN 978-3-540-66564-9
G. Pólya, G. Szegő Problems and Theorems in Analysis I – Series. Integral Calculus. Theory of Functions ISBN 978-3-540-63640-3
G. Pólya, G. Szegő Problems and Theorems in Analysis II – Theory of Functions. Zeros. Polynomials. Determinants. Number Theory. Geometry ISBN 978-3-540-63686-1
W. Rudin Function Theory in the Unit Ball of $\mathbb{C}^n$ ISBN 978-3-540-68272-1
S. Sakai C*-Algebras and W*-Algebras ISBN 978-3-540-63633-5
C. L. Siegel, J. K. Moser Lectures on Celestial Mechanics ISBN 978-3-540-58656-2
T. A. Springer Jordan Algebras and Algebraic Groups ISBN 978-3-540-63632-8
D. W. Stroock, S. R. S. Varadhan Multidimensional Diffusion Processes ISBN 978-3-540-28998-2
R. R. Switzer Algebraic Topology: Homology and Homotopy ISBN 978-3-540-42750-6
A. Weil Basic Number Theory ISBN 978-3-540-58655-5
A. Weil Elliptic Functions According to Eisenstein and Kronecker ISBN 978-3-540-65036-2
K. Yosida Functional Analysis ISBN 978-3-540-58654-8
O. Zariski Algebraic Surfaces ISBN 978-3-540-58658-6